MCP HAHNEMANN UNIVERSITY
HAHNEMANN LIBRARY

D1649225

THE WILLS EYE HOSPITAL ATLAS OF CLINICAL OPHTHALMOLOGY

SECOND EDITION

THE WILLS EYE HOSPITAL ATLAS OF CLINICAL OPHTHALMOLOGY

SECOND EDITION

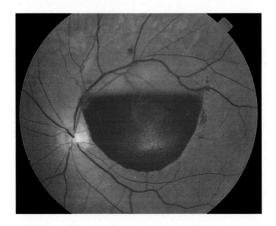

Valsalva induced boat-shaped sub-hyaloid hemorrhage overlying the macula of a 23-year-old lifeguard, sustained while struggling to launch his lifeboat into a rough Jersey shore surf.

Edited by

WILLIAM TASMAN, M.D.

Professor and Chairman
Department of Ophthalmology
Jefferson Medical College
Thomas Jefferson University
Ophthalmologist-in-Chief
Wills Eye Hospital
Philadelphia, Pennsylvania

EDWARD A. JAEGER, M.D.

Professor of Ophthalmology
Jefferson Medical College
Thomas Jefferson University
Attending Surgeon
Wills Eye Hospital
Philadelphia, Pennsylvania

Associate Editors

James J. Augsburger
Jonathan B. Belmont
William E. Benson
Gary C. Brown
Joseph H. Calhoun
Elisabeth J. Cohen

Helen V. Danesh-Meyer
David H. Fischer
Joseph C. Flanagan
Peter R. Laibson
Robert A. Mazzoli
Christopher J. Rapuano
Carl D. Regillo

Peter J. Savino
Bruce M. Schnall
Carol L. Shields
Jerry A. Shields
S. Gregory Smith
George L. Spaeth

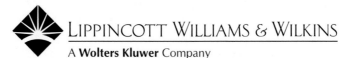

LIPPINCOTT WILLIAMS & WILKINS
A **Wolters Kluwer** Company
Philadelphia • Baltimore • New York • London
Buenos Aires • Hong Kong • Sydney • Tokyo

Acquisitions Editor: Jonathan Pine
Developmental Editor: Kerry Barrett
Production Editor: Janice Stangel/Penny Bice
Manufacturing Manager: Colin Warnock
Cover Designer: Mark Lerner
Compositor: Maryland Composition

© 2001 by Lippincott Williams & Wilkins
530 Walnut Street
Philadelphia, PA 19106 USA
LWW.com

All rights reserved. This book is protected by copyright. No part of this book may be reproduced in any form or by any means, including photocopying, or utilized by any information storage and retrieval system without written permission for the copyright owner, except for brief quotations embodied in critical articles and reviews. Materials appearing in this book prepared by individuals as part of their official duties as U.S. government employees are not covered by the above-mentioned copyright.

Printed in China

Library of Congress Cataloging-in-Publication Data

The Wills Eye Hospital atlas of clinical ophthalmology / edited by William Tasman, Edward A. Jaeger; associate editors, James J. Augsburger . . . [et al.].—2nd ed.
    p.; cm.
  Includes bibliographical references and index.
  ISBN 0-7817-2774-X
    1. Eye—Diseases—Atlases. 2. Ophthalmology—Atlases. I. Title: Atlas of clinical ophthalmology. II. Tasman, William, 1929–III. Jaeger, Edward A. IV. Wills Eye Hospital (Philadelphia, Pa.)
[DNLM: 1. Eye Diseases—Atlases. WW 17 W741 2001]
  RE71.W55 2001
  617.7'1—dc21

                                                                    2001020374

Care has been taken to confirm the accuracy of the information presented and to describe generally accepted practices. However, the authors, editors, and publisher are not responsible for errors or omissions or for any consequences from application of the information in this book and make no warranty, expressed or implied, with respect to the currency, completeness, or accuracy of the contents of the publication. Application of this information in a particular situation remains the professional responsibility of the practitioner.

The authors, editors, and publisher have exerted every effort to ensure that drug selection and dosage set forth in this text are in accordance with current recommendations and practice at the time of publication. However, in view of ongoing research, changes in government regulations, and the constant flow of information relating to drug therapy and drug reactions, the reader is urged to check the package insert for each drug for any change in indications and dosage and for added warnings and precautions. This is particularly important when the recommended agent is a new or infrequently employed drug.

Some drugs and medical devices presented in this publication have Food and Drug Administration (FDA) clearance for limited use in restricted research settings. It is the responsibility of the health care provider to ascertain the FDA status of each drug or device planned for use in their clinical practice.

10 9 8 7 6 5 4 3 2 1

To the past and present members of
the Wills Eye Hospital Attending, Resident, and Fellow staffs
whose dedication to patient care, teaching, and sharing of knowledge
has been the hallmark of Wills since 1832.

CONTENTS

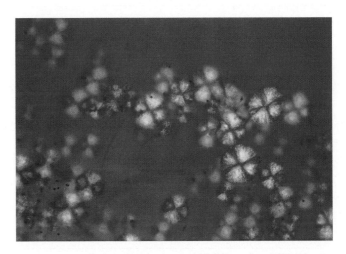

Asteroid Hyalosis: Asteroid bodies in the vitreous show a characteristic Maltese cross pattern of vivid birefringence during polarization microscopy. Millipore filter preparation, hematoxylin—eosin with crossed polarizers, ×250. (Courtesy Ralph C. Eagle, Jr., M.D., Philadelphia, Pennsylvania)

CONTRIBUTORS

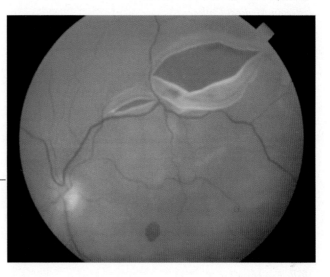

Two retinal tears in the superior arcade and a macular hole secondary to trauma in a mentally challenged 17-year-old with head-banging tendencies.

EDITORS

James J. Augsburger, M.D.
Professor and Chairman
Department of Ophthalmology
University of Cincinnati College of Medicine
Cincinnati, Ohio
Ophthalmologist-in-Chief
The University Hospital
Cincinnati, Ohio
Chapter 7

Jonathan B. Belmont, M.D.
Associate Surgeon
Retina Department
Co-Director
Uveitis Service, Retina Department
Wills Eye Hospital
Philadelphia, Pennsylvania
Chapter 8

William E. Benson, M.D.
Professor of Ophthalmology
Jefferson Medical College
Thomas Jefferson University
Director
Retina Service
Wills Eye Hospital
Philadelphia, Pennsylvania
Chapter 4

Gary C. Brown, M.D.
Professor of Ophthalmology
Jefferson Medical College
Thomas Jefferson University
Director
Retina Vascular Unit
Wills Eye Hospital
Philadelphia, Pennsylvania
Chapter 5

Joseph H. Calhoun, M.D.
Chief
Pediatric Ophthalmology
Wills Eye Hospital
Philadelphia, Pennsylvania
Chapter 11

Elisabeth J. Cohen, M.D.
Professor of Ophthalmology
Jefferson Medical College
Thomas Jefferson University
Director
Cornea Service
Wills Eye Hospital
Philadelphia, Pennsylvania
Chapter 1

Helen V. Danesh-Meyer, F.R.A.C.O.
Discipline of Ophthalmology
University of Auckland
Auckland, New Zealand
Chapter 9

David H. Fischer, M.D.
Associate Professor of Ophthalmology
Jefferson Medical College
Thomas Jefferson University
Associate Ophthalmologist
Hospital of the University of Pennsylvania
Associate Surgeon
Director of Uveitis
Retina Service
Wills Eye Hospital
Philadelphia, Pennsylvania
Chapter 8

Joseph C. Flanagan, M.D.
Professor of Ophthalmology
Jefferson Medical College
Thomas Jefferson University
Director
Oculoplastic Service
Wills Eye Hospital
Philadelphia, Pennsylvania
Chapter 10

Peter R. Laibson, M.D.
Professor of Ophthalmology
Jefferson Medical College
Thomas Jefferson University
Co-Director
Cornea Department
Wills Eye Hospital
Philadelphia, Pennsylvania
Chapter 1

Robert A. Mazzoli, M.D., F.A.C.S.
Clinical Assistant Professor
Surgery (Ophthalmology)
Uniformed Services University of the Health Sciences
Chairman
Ophthalmology
Director
Ophthalmic Plastic, Reconstructive, and Orbital Surgery
Madigan Army Medical Center
Tacoma, Washington
Chapter 10

Christopher J. Rapuano, M.D.
Associate Professor of Ophthalmology
Jefferson Medical College
Thomas Jefferson University
Co-Director
Refractive Surgery
Cornea Service
Wills Eye Hospital
Philadelphia, Pennsylvania
Chapter 1

Carl D. Regillo, M.D.
Associate Professor of Ophthalmology
Jefferson Medical College
Thomas Jefferson University
Associate Surgeon
Wills Eye Hospital
Philadelphia, Pennsylvania
Chapter 4

Peter J. Savino, M.D.
Professor of Ophthalmology
Jefferson Medical College
Thomas Jefferson University
Director
Neuro-Ophthalmology Service
Wills Eye Hospital
Philadelphia, Pennsylvania
Chapter 9

Bruce M. Schnall, M.D.
Associate Surgeon
Pediatric Ophthalmology
Wills Eye Hospital
Philadelphia, Pennsylvania
Chapter 11

Carol L. Shields, M.D.
Associate Professor of Ophthalmology
Jefferson Medical College
Thomas Jefferson University
Attending Surgeon
Ocular Oncology
Wills Eye Hospital
Philadelphia, Pennsylvania
Chapter 6

Jerry A. Shields, M.D.
Professor of Ophthalmology
Jefferson Medical College
Thomas Jefferson University
Director
Oncology Service
Wills Eye Hospital
Philadelphia, Pennsylvania
Chapter 6

S. Gregory Smith, M.D.
Attending Surgeon
Cataract and Primary Eye Care Services
Wills Eye Hospital
Philadelphia, Pennsylvania
Chapter 2

George L. Spaeth, M.D.
Louis J. Esposito Glaucoma Research Professor
Jefferson Medical College
Director
Glaucoma Service
Wills Eye Hospital
Philadelphia, Pennsylvania
Chapter 3

CONTRIBUTORS

Neal H. Atebara, M.D.
Assistant Clinical Professor
Department of Surgery
University of Hawaii School of Medicine
Retina Center of Hawaii
Staff Surgeon, Ophthalmology
Queen's Medical Center
Honolulu, Hawaii

Augusto Azuara-Blanco, M.D., Ph.D.
Consultant Ophthalmic Surgeon
Aberdeen Royal Infirmary
Aberdeen, United Kingdom
Chapter 3

Edward H. Bedrossian, Jr., M.D., F.A.C.S.
Assistant Professor
Department of Ophthalmology
Jefferson Medical College
Thomas Jefferson University
Attending Surgeon
Oculoplastic Surgery Department
Wills Eye Hospital
Philadelphia, Pennsylvania
Chapter 10

Ralph C. Eagle, Jr., M.D.
Director
Department of Pathology
The Noel T. and Sara L. Simmonds Professor
of Ophthalmic Pathology
Wills Eye Hospital
Professor of Ophthalmology and Pathology
Jefferson Medical College
Thomas Jefferson University
Philadelphia, Pennsylvania
Chapter 2

Jeffrey D. Henderer, M.D.
Assistant Professor of Ophthalmology
Jefferson Medical College
Thomas Jefferson University
Assistant Surgeon
Wills Eye Hospital
Philadelphia, Pennsylvania
Chapter 3

Edward A. Jaeger, M.D.
Professor of Ophthalmology
Jefferson Medical College
Thomas Jefferson University
Attending Surgeon
Wills Eye Hospital
Philadelphia, Pennsylvania
Chapter 2

L. Jay Katz, M.D.
Professor of Ophthalmology
Jefferson Medical College
Thomas Jefferson University
Attending Surgeon
Wills Eye Hospital
Philadelphia, Pennsylvania
Chapter 3

Marlene R. Moster, M.D.
Professor of Ophthalmology
Jefferson Medical College
Thomas Jefferson University
Attending Surgeon
Glaucoma Service
Wills Eye Hospital
Philadelphia, Pennsylvania
Chapter 3

Jonathan S. Myers, M.D.
Instructor of Ophthalmology
Jefferson Medical College
Thomas Jefferson University
Assistant Surgeon
Wills Eye Hospital
Philadelphia, Pennsylvania
Chapter 3

Robert B. Penne, M.D.
Instructor
Ophthalmology
Jefferson Medical College
Thomas Jefferson University
Associate Surgeon
Oculoplastic Department
Wills Eye Hospital
Philadelphia, Pennsylvania
Chapter 10

Douglas J. Rhee, M.D.
Assistant Professor
Department of Ophthalmology
Jefferson Medical College
Thomas Jefferson University
Assistant Surgeon
Wills Eye Hospital
Philadelphia, Pennsylvania
Chapter 3

Mary A. Stefanyszyn, M.D.
Clinical Instructor of Ophthalmology
Jefferson Medical College
Thomas Jefferson University
Associate in Surgery
Wills Eye Hospital
Philadelphia, Pennsylvania
Chapter 10

William Tasman, M.D.
Professor and Chairman
Department of Ophthalmology
Jefferson Medical College
Thomas Jefferson University
Ophthalmologist-in-Chief
Wills Eye Hospital
Philadelphia, Pennsylvania
Chapters 2 and 5

Annette K. Terebuh, M.D.
Private Practice
Bellefontaine, Ohio
Chapter 3

Richard P. Wilson, M.D.
Professor of Ophthalmology
Jefferson Medical College
Thomas Jefferson University
Attending Surgeon
Glaucoma
Wills Eye Hospital
Philadelphia, Pennsylvania
Chapter 3

PREFACE

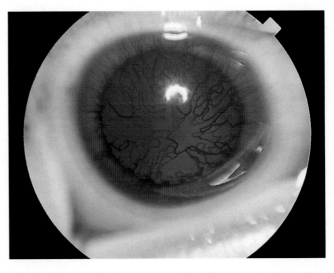

Persistent tunica vasculosis in a premature infant with retinopathy of prematurity.

As this second edition goes to press, Wills is moving to its fourth home during its 168-year history. Thus, it is an exciting time and perhaps fitting that this second edition is being published as this transition is being made. In the first edition, we pointed out how many artists have focused on the eye as almost a theme in many of their paintings. Eye disorders, as a matter of fact, can be traced to artists such as Monet who developed cataracts. During the development of these cataracts, his portrayal, for example, of the Japanese footbridge at his home in Giverny, changed considerably.

What has not changed, however, is the importance of visual illustrations of eye diseases. Since our first edition, it has now become quite common to store these images on computer disks, which facilitates storage and organization of the material. As these changes take place, Wills medical staff continues to contribute to the literature and to the collection of photographs in our archives. The second edition of this *Atlas* contains 11 chapters and over 1400 illustrations, which cover ocular conditions from the front of the eye to the back. As before, we have developed a CD-ROM version of the Atlas complete with animation and voice over, which has been expanded from the first edition.

We hope that readers will find this second effort a helpful resource.

ACKNOWLEDGMENTS

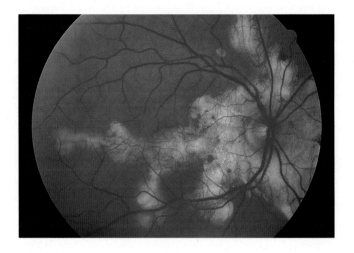

Serpiginous choroiditis in a 49-year-old male who was visually symptomatic for 15 months. Vision in the right eye was 20/200. (Photograph courtesy of Jay Klancnik, M.D. and Mary Jude Cox, M.D.).

The editors would like to gratefully acknowledge all the individuals who contributed to the initial development of this textbook and to those who participated in this second edition. This includes members of the Wills Eye Hospital staff as well as members of our private office staffs. Without their assistance in manuscript preparation, slide discovery, and information gathering, the textbook would not have been produced in such a timely fashion.

Daniel P. Montzka, M.D., a wizard on the computer, provided invaluable assistance in the initial editing of the printed manuscript and continues to be extremely instrumental in revising the companion CD-ROM. Ralph C. Eagle, Jr., M.D., provided many of the histopathology slides, descriptions, and clinical-pathologic correlations. He has added considerable material to the CD-ROM version of the second edition. We are also grateful to Neal Atebara, M.D., for providing illustrations throughout the text and coordinating the optics section in the CD-ROM.

We would especially like to thank Robert E. Curtin II, Jack Scully, and Roger Barone of the Wills Eye Hospital Audio Visual Department for their dedicated efforts in coordinating the illustrations as well as assisting in preparation of the CD-ROM.

Finally, we would like to express our appreciation to the staff of Lippincott, Williams & Wilkins for their invaluable assistance in the development of this textbook. Developmental Editor Kerry Barrett provided expert editorial assistance and was always readily available. Without her pleasant and persistent attention to detail and her editorial expertise, the end product would have been much more difficult to attain. J. Stuart Freeman, Jr., the irrepressible retiring Senior Editor at Lippincott, originally suggested the idea of compiling the extensive and varied Wills Eye Hospital Clinical experience in the form of an atlas. Present Senior Executive Editor, Jonathan Pine, has continued Stuart's tradition and has been very supportive. We greatly appreciated the encouragement and direction of these individuals and we hope this second edition continues to justify their confidence.

External Diseases

Elisabeth J. Cohen
Christopher J. Rapuano
Peter R. Laibson

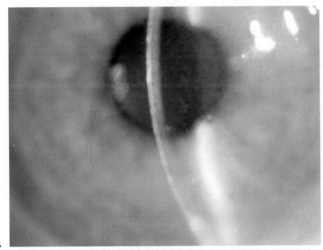

A

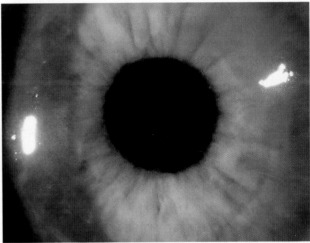

B

Recurrent lattice corneal dystrophy in a corneal transplant before (A) and after (B) excimer laser phototherapeutic keratectomy.

ANATOMY OF THE CORNEA

BLEPHARITIS
Infectious Blepharitis
Stye, Hordeolum, and Chalazion
Seborrheic Blepharitis
Atopic Blepharitis
Contact Dermatitis
Molluscum Contagiosum
Blepharitis Caused by Lice Infestation

CONJUNCTIVITIS
Viral Conjunctivitis
Allergic Conjunctivitis
Bacterial Conjunctivitis
Chronic Follicular Conjunctivitis

HERPES SIMPLEX KERATITIS
Acute Dendritic Herpes Simplex Keratitis
Other Manifestations of Ocular Herpes Simplex Virus Infection
Trophic Epithelial Defects
Stromal Keratitis
Associated Uveitis
Corneal Scarring

HERPES ZOSTER OPHTHALMICUS
Dermatologic Involvement
Ocular Involvement

CORNEAL ULCERS
Sterile Infiltrates
Bacterial Ulcers
Fungal Keratitis
Acanthamoeba Keratitis

EPISCLERITIS AND SCLERITIS
Episcleritis
Anterior Scleritis

NONINFECTIOUS CORNEAL DISEASE
Dry Eye Syndrome
Filamentary Keratopathy
Exposure or Neurotrophic Keratopathy
Ocular Rosacea
Stevens-Johnson Syndrome
Ocular Cicatricial Pemphigoid
Vitamin A Deficiency
Mucopolysaccharidoses
Sphingolipidoses
Cystinosis
Wilson's Disease
Adrenochrome Deposits
Floppy Eyelid Syndrome
Superior Limbic Keratoconjunctivitis
Thygeson's Superficial Punctate Keratopathy
Terrien's Marginal Degeneration
Mooren's Ulcer
Rheumatoid Melt
Megalocornea
Microcornea
Sclerocornea
Kerectasia

DEVELOPMENTAL ANGLE ANOMALIES
Posterior Embryotoxon
Axenfeld's Anomaly and Syndrome
Rieger's Anomaly and Syndrome
Peters' Anomaly

TRAUMA
Corneal Abrasion
Corneal Laceration
Corneal Foreign Body
Corneal Rust Ring
Chemical Burn
Hyphema
Birth Trauma

EPITHELIAL CORNEAL DYSTROPHIES
Cogan's Microcytic Dystrophy
Map-Dot Fingerprint Dystrophy
Meesmann's Dystrophy
Corneal Dystrophies of Bowman's Layer

STROMAL DYSTROPHIES
Granular Dystrophy
Lattice Corneal Dystrophy
Gelatinous Drop-like Dystrophy
Macular Corneal Dystrophy
Crystalline Dystrophy of Schnyder
Central Cloudy Dystrophy of François

ENDOTHELIAL DYSTROPHIES
Cornea Guttata
Fuchs' Dystrophy
Posterior Polymorphous Dystrophy
Congenital Hereditary Endothelial Dystrophy

DEGENERATIONS
Keratoconus
Arcus Senilis
Lipid Degeneration
Pterygium
Pinguecula
White Limbal Girdle of Vogt
Spheroidal Degeneration
Coats' Ring
Salzmann's Degeneration
Band Keratopathy

COMPLICATIONS OF CORNEAL SURGERY
Whorl Keratopathy After Penetrating Keratoplasty
Subepithelial Corneal Infiltrates in Corneal
    Graft Rejection
Endothelial Graft Rejection of Corneal Transplants

COMPLICATIONS OF REFRACTIVE SURGERY
Infection in Radial Keratotomy
Perforation of the Cornea in Radial Keratotomy
Corneal Haze in Excimer Laser Photorefractive Keratectomy Surgery
LASIK Complications
LASIK Button-hole
LASIK Free Cap
LASIK Flap Dislocation
LASIK Infection
LASIK Diffuse Lamellar Keratitis
LASIK Epithelial Ingrowth
LASIK Flap Striae
LASIK Iron Line
LASIK Interface Debris

TUMORS
Limbal Dermoid
Pyogenic Granuloma
Conjunctival Intraepithelial Neoplasia
Malignant Melanoma of the Conjunctiva and Cornea
Lymphomatous Infiltration

ANATOMY OF THE CORNEA

The precorneal tear film is generally considered as the most anterior aspect of the cornea and is about 7 μm thick. It is firmly adsorbed onto the anterior layer of the corneal epithelium by mucoproteins of the mucoid tear film layer attached to the microvilli of the superficial epithelial cells.

Beneath the precorneal tear film, the corneal *epithelium* is 50 μm thick and is composed of five to eight layers of epithelial cells (Fig. 1.1). The inner layer consists of basal epithelial cells that are responsible for producing the epithelial basement membrane, which maintains adherence of the epithelium to Bowman's layer. Above the basal epithelial layer are several rows of wing cells that are somewhat flattened. Progressively flatter and thinner layers of epithelial cells progress to the outer surface layer, which contains the microvilli. The epithelium constitutes about 10% of the corneal thickness.

Beneath the epithelium is *Bowman's layer*, which is the most anterior layer of the corneal stroma. It is a uniform collagen layer firmly anchored at the limbus. Bowman's layer does not swell as the stroma does, because Bowman's layer is composed of firmly compacted collagen fibrils.

The *stroma*, which makes up 90% of the cornea, has three components: collagen fibers, or lamella, surrounded by a ground substance and interspersed with occasional stromal keratocytes. The regular arrangement of the collagen fibrils and its relation to the mucopolysaccharide ground substance provides corneal clarity.

Beneath the stroma is *Descemet's membrane*, an acellular, strong, elastic membrane that is the basement membrane of the corneal endothelium and is produced by a secretion of the corneal endothelium. It grows throughout life and becomes slightly thicker with advanced age. It is usually 3 μm thick at birth and can grow to 30 to 40 μm in old age. In certain diseases, such as endothelial and Fuchs' dystrophies,

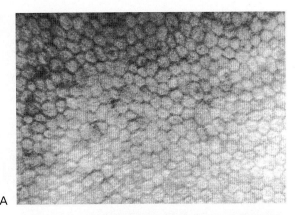

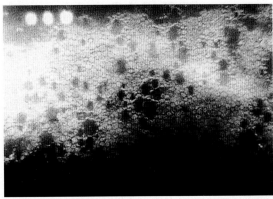

FIGURE 1.2. A: Specular microscopy of normal corneal endothelium. The endothelial cell count was approximately 3,200 cells/mm². **B:** Endothelial specular microscopy revealed endothelial dystrophy with areas of endothelial cell drop-out. Between the areas of endothelial drop-out, the endothelial cell count was relatively normal. This patient did not have stromal or epithelial edema.

Descemet's membrane is even thicker, and the nonbanded posterior portion can be extremely thick compared with the normal membrane.

The *endothelium* is a single layer of cells responsible for corneal stromal hydration. The endothelial cells seldom divide, and with aging, inflammation, trauma, or endothelial dystrophy, the endothelial cell count diminishes. The cell count may be 5,000 to 6,000 mm² at birth but 1,000 or less later in life (Fig. 1.2A,B). As the endothelial cells die out and disappear, the adjacent endothelial cells thin and spread out to take their place, diminishing the endothelial cell count.

BLEPHARITIS

Infectious Blepharitis

Blepharitis is a common condition of the eyelids causing chronic ocular irritation and foreign body sensation. It is associated with thickening of the eyelids, telangiectatic vessels along the lid margins, and plugging of the meibomian glands

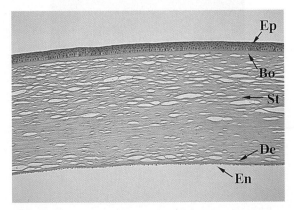

FIGURE 1.1. The anatomy of the cornea. (Ep, epithelium; Bo, Bowman's layer; St, stroma; De, Descemet's membrane; En, endothelium.)

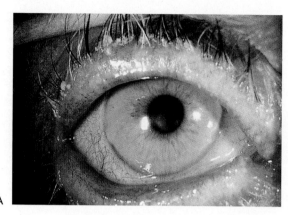
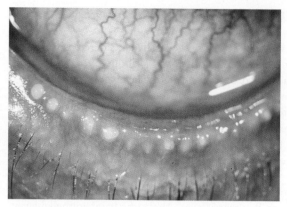

FIGURE 1.3. A: Blepharitis is associated with crusting of the eyelashes, thickening of the eyelids, telangiectatic vessels along the lid margins, and plugging of the meibomian glands. **B:** The meibomian glands become plugged in posterior blepharitis with or without rosacea.

(Fig. 1.3A,B). There is usually crusting along the eyelashes and sometimes misdirection and loss of eyelashes. *Staphylococcus* bacteria are the most common offending organisms. In many patients, blepharitis is associated with rosacea, manifested by telangiectatic vessels on the facial skin, and with rhinophyma in more advanced cases (Fig. 1.4).

Good lid hygiene with mechanical scrubbing of the lid margins, warm compresses, and antibiotic ointment at bedtime using bacitracin or erythromycin is the standard treatment for blepharitis. Patients whose condition is unresponsive, those who have rosacea, or those who have corneal complications such as margin infiltrates benefit from the use of systemic tetracycline (250 mg, orally four times each day for 1 week, then twice daily) or doxycycline (100 mg, orally twice daily for 1 week, then once daily). Systemic erythromycin is an alternative to systemic doxycycline for patients who are unable to tolerate doxycycline and for children who cannot take doxycycline because it stains developing teeth.

Stye, Hordeolum, and Chalazion

Patients with blepharitis are prone to hordeola, styes, and chalazia, which are inflammations of the eyelid glands. A stye, or external hordeolum, is an abscess of a gland of Zeis at the lid margin (Fig. 1.5A). An internal hordeolum is an infection within the meibomian gland deeper in the tarsus (Fig. 1.5B). Both are acute, painful lid nodules, tender to the touch, which produce lid swelling and redness and which may point as the abscess localizes. Chalazia are subacute, nontender nodules associated with granuloma formation in response to meibomian gland lipid extravasated within the tarsus (Fig. 1.5C).

Hordeola typically respond to warm compresses within several days. Occasionally, incision and drainage are necessary. Chalazia usually respond to 15-minute warm compresses four

times each day for 2 weeks, but they may require steroid injection or surgical excision. The underlying lid disease in both cases should be treated with warm compresses and antibiotic ointment. Recurrent chalazia can be prevented in many cases by systemic tetracycline. Recurrent chalazia removed surgically should be sent for pathologic analysis. Sebaceous cell carcinoma can masquerade as recurrent chalazia.

Seborrheic Blepharitis

Seborrheic blepharitis refers to crusting of the eyelids associated with seborrheic dermatitis of the eyebrows and scalp

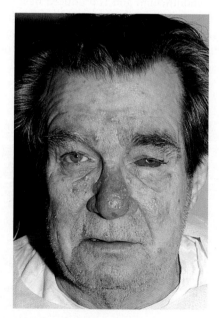

FIGURE 1.4. Blepharitis may be associated with rosacea that is manifested by telangiectatic vessels on the skin and, as in the advanced case shown here, with rhinophyma.

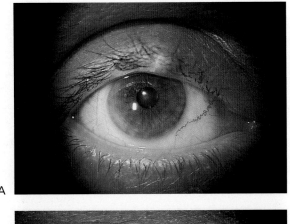

A

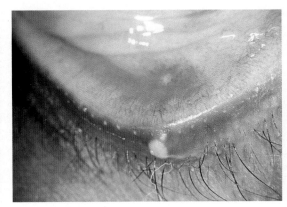

B

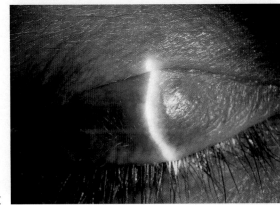

C

FIGURE 1.5. A: Stye of the upper eyelid. **B:** Hordeolum pointing on the inner aspect of the lid and at the meibomian gland opening at the lid margin. **C:** A chalazion is a nontender nodule of the lid consisting of a granulomatous reaction to meibomian lipid.

without meibomian gland inflammation or staphylococcal infection. Crusting of the lashes can occur without inflammation of the lid margin posterior to the lashes (Fig. 1.6).

Treatment consists of warm compresses, lid scrubs, and shampoo for the treatment of seborrhea.

Atopic Blepharitis

Atopic blepharitis occurs in patients who have atopic dermatitis involving the eyelids. In atopic blepharitis, lichenification of the eyelids often is complicated by cracking of the eyelids nasally and temporally (Fig. 1.7).

Lubrication of the eyelids with ophthalmic ointments may be sufficient in mild cases, but patients often require application of steroid ophthalmic ointment to the eyelids once or twice daily to control symptoms. They must be closely monitored for complications of steroids, including intraocular pressure elevation, because the steroids are absorbed into the eye. Topical antihistamines and mast cell stabilizers have variable efficacy. In severe cases, topical cyclosporine can be effective in decreasing or eliminating the need for topical corticosteroids. Optimization of systemic treatment of atopy is indicated and may reduce or eliminate the need for application of steroids to the eyelids. Atopic patients are prone to colonization with staphylococci and

streptococci, and they may benefit from the application of bacitracin or erythromycin ointment at bedtime.

Contact Dermatitis

Contact dermatitis is a type IV delayed hypersensitivity reaction to topical ophthalmic medication. A periocular

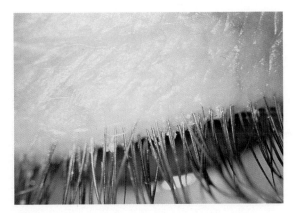

FIGURE 1.6. Seborrheic blepharitis is associated with crusting of the eyelids without meibomian gland inflammation and with seborrheic dermatitis of the eyebrows and scalp.

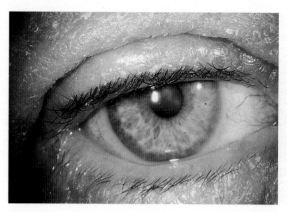

FIGURE 1.7. In atopic blepharitis, there is an eczematoid reaction of the eyelids.

eczematoid reaction develops after several days or longer of exposure to the offending medication (Fig. 1.8). Neomycin and atropine are common causes, but any ophthalmic medication can be involved.

Discontinuing the topical medication is sufficient treatment in most cases. In severe cases, topical steroid ointment can be used to speed recovery. Patients should be informed that they are allergic to the medication causing the reaction. If the patient is on multiple medications, the physician may discontinue them all or only the most likely one, depending on the severity of the reaction.

Molluscum Contagiosum

Molluscum contagiosum is a DNA pox virus infection that causes single or multiple umbilicated lid lesions that may cause a toxic follicular conjunctivitis (Fig. 1.9A,B). In immunocompromised hosts, such as patients with acquired immunodeficiency syndrome, lesions may be greater in number, but they are not associated with conjunctivitis.

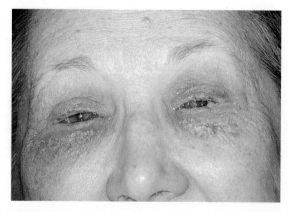

FIGURE 1.8. Contact dermatitis is a delayed hypersensitivity reaction to topical ophthalmic medication causing a periocular eczematoid reaction.

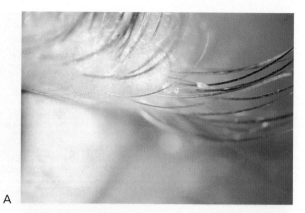

A

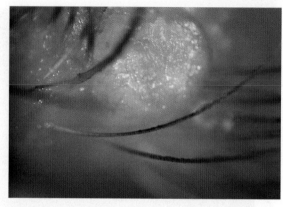

B

FIGURE 1.9. A: Molluscum contagiosum is associated with single or multiple umbilicated lid lesions. **B:** At higher magnification, the depressed center of these lesions is more apparent.

Treatment requires excision of the lesions in most cases. Observation of the lesions may be sufficient for patients without conjunctivitis.

Blepharitis Caused by Lice Infestation

Infestation of the eyelids by pubic lice (*Phthiriasis pubis,* crabs) is a cause of chronic blepharoconjunctivitis. It is a sexually transmitted disease.

Patients with lice infestation experience irritation of the eyelids and mild crusting. Slit lamp examination reveals globular nits (i.e., eggs) attached to the eyelash shaft. Fully developed adult lice are seen among the eyelashes, often partially embedded in the skin (Fig. 1.10). Movement of the lice's appendages can be seen. Characteristically, blood-tinged debris is present along the base of the lashes.

The lice and eggs should be removed mechanically, using fine forceps if feasible. Trimming the lashes is another treatment option. Any petroleum-based jelly applied to the eyelids three times daily for 10 days smothers the lice. Bacitracin or erythromycin ointment can be used for this purpose. An application of physostigmine (Eserine) ointment paralyzes the adult lice but does not affect the nits; therefore a second application may be necessary in 7 days.

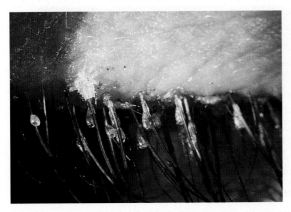

FIGURE 1.10. Eyelid infestation with *Phthiriasis pubis*. An adult crab louse can be seen at the lash line with numerous nits (i.e., eggs) attached firmly to the eyelash shafts.

The accompanying pupillary miosis produced by physostigmine ointment is uncomfortable, and this treatment is rarely used anymore. Nonocular, moist, hair-bearing areas should be treated with Kwell shampoo. Clothes and bedding should be thoroughly washed.

CONJUNCTIVITIS

Viral Conjunctivitis

Acute follicular conjunctivitis is most commonly caused by adenoviral infection and is referred to as epidemic keratoconjunctivitis (EKC). EKC is often associated with an upper respiratory tract infection and preauricular adenopathy. It spreads from one eye to the other, and the eye infected second is less involved. Less common causes of acute follicular conjunctivitis include herpes simplex infection and acute hemorrhagic conjunctivitis.

The onset of adenoviral conjunctivitis is sudden, with diffuse lid swelling and conjunctival redness. The eyes are uncomfortable, produce tears, and have a foreign body sensation. Follicles appear as elevations in the inferior palpebral conjunctiva, with vessels coming from the periphery (Fig. 1.11A). There may be subconjunctival and lid hemorrhages, a discharge, and pseudomembranes in severe cases (Fig. 1.11B, C). Corneal involvement follows a typical pattern, with intraepithelial microcysts developing during the first few days, followed by fluorescein-staining epithelial hyperplasia. Subepithelial infiltrates (Fig. 1.11D) appear during the second week as the ocular injection and infection are resolving. The subepithelial infiltrates gradually get smaller and resolve in most cases over several months.

Viral conjunctivitis is highly contagious, and precautions, including hand washing and disinfection of exposed surfaces, are necessary for the patient and physician to avoid spreading the disease by hand-eye-hand contamination. There is no specific treatment for viral conjunctivitis. Most cases are treated supportively with cool compresses and lubricating drops. In severe cases associated with acute incapacitating discomfort, pseudomembranes, corneal erosions, or significantly reduced vision as a result of subepithelial infiltrates, topical corticosteroids are used, although they may prolong the course of the disease.

Allergic Conjunctivitis

A history of atopy and papillary reaction of the superior tarsus seen when the upper eyelid is everted are common to a variety of forms of allergic conjunctivitis. Itching is the major symptom of ocular allergy. Seasonal (i.e., hay fever) and perennial allergic conjunctivitis are usually associated with rhinitis. The conjunctival injection is mild to moderate.

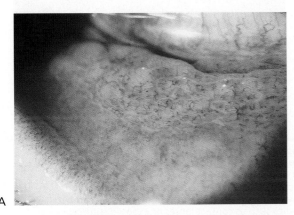

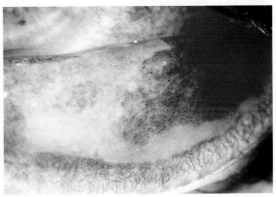

A   B

FIGURE 1.11. A: Viral conjunctivitis is associated with an acute follicular reaction. In follicles, vessels course on the surface from the periphery of the lesions toward the center rather than emerging in the center, as is the case in papillae. **B:** Acute adenoviral conjunctivitis with subconjunctival hemorrhage and pseudomembrane formation. *(continued)*

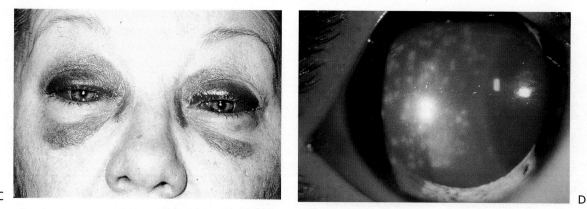

FIGURE 1.11. *Continued.* **C:** In severe adenoviral conjunctivitis, the patient may have lid ecchymoses in addition to subconjunctival hemorrhages. **D:** During the second week, subepithelial infiltrates develop in patients with epidemic keratoconjunctivitis. In most cases, the infiltrates gradually resolve over many months.

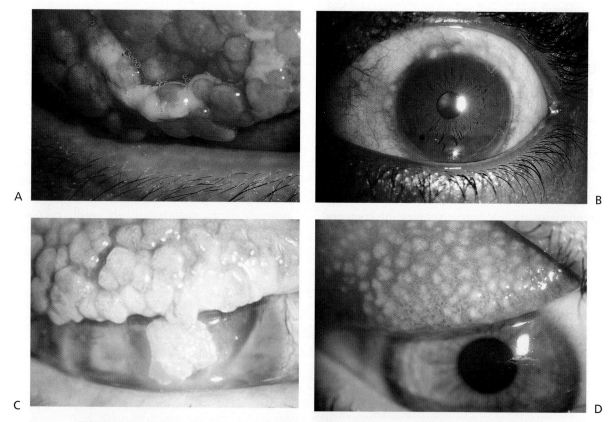

FIGURE 1.12. **A:** Vernal keratoconjunctivitis is associated with giant papillae or cobblestones of the superior tarsus and with a ropy, adherent, mucous discharge. **B:** Trantas dots are infiltrates at the limbus that are composed predominantly of eosinophils. **C:** In severe vernal keratoconjunctivitis, superficial sterile shield ulcers require topical steroid treatment. **D:** Giant papillary conjunctivitis is characterized by papillae of the superior tarsus, which are thought to be caused by an allergic reaction to the coating on foreign bodies such as contact lenses or exposed sutures.

Velvety papillae are maximal along the superior border of the superior tarsus.

In *vernal keratoconjunctivitis*, giant papillae or cobblestones cover the entire superior tarsus, and there is often a ropy, adherent mucous discharge (Fig. 1.12A). Some patients have limbal follicles or Horner-Trantas dots, which are composed of eosinophils (Fig. 1.12B). In severe forms of vernal keratoconjunctivitis, shield ulcers of the cornea develop, usually superiorly (Fig. 1.12C).

Giant papillary conjunctivitis appears similar to a mild form of vernal conjunctivitis (Fig. 1.12D). It is seen in patients with contact lenses, exposed sutures, or ocular prostheses.

Atopic keratoconjunctivitis is associated with atopic blepharitis and papillary conjunctivitis. In severe cases, it can be complicated by corneal neovascularization and scarring and by anterior cortical cataracts (Fig. 1.13).

Treatment varies according to the type of allergic conjunctivitis. Avoidance of the allergen, when possible, and systemic control of allergies are helpful. Cool compresses and topical lubrication may suffice in mild cases. Topical antihistamines (e.g., levocabastine) and nonsteroidal anti-inflammatory agents (e.g., ketorolac) are useful in treating acute seasonal conjunctivitis. Topical mast cell stabilizers (e.g., lodoxamide, cromolyn, etc.) are indicated for vernal conjunctivitis and are useful in treating chronic allergic conditions, including giant papillary and atopic conjunctivitis. Daily or frequent lens replacement and improved lens cleaning, after a period of discontinuing lens wear in more severe cases, are also important in the treatment of lens-related giant papillary conjunctivitis. Topical corticosteroids are necessary for the treatment of shield ulcers and severe flare-ups of vernal and atopic conjunctivitis, but they should be avoided if possible in other types of ocular allergies.

Bacterial Conjunctivitis

Bacterial conjunctivitis is characterized by conjunctival injection, papillary reaction, and purulent or mucopurulent discharge (Fig. 1.14). It is caused by a wide variety of microorganisms and may be acute, hyperacute, or chronic.

The patient with *acute conjunctivitis* notices a sudden onset of redness of the eye that is accompanied by a discharge and sticking together of the eyelids in the morning. Tearing and irritation may be experienced, but significant pain is rare. The condition is usually unilateral but may be bilateral. There is injection of the epibulbar and palpebral conjunctiva, and a papillary reaction is found in the inferior palpebral conjunctiva. The discharge may vary from frank pus to a scant mucopurulent excretion. The lashes are frequently crusted. The most common bacteria associated with acute conjunctivitis are *Staphylococcus*, *Streptococcus*, and *Haemophilus influenzae*.

Hyperacute conjunctivitis is usually bilateral and is characterized by the sudden onset of conjunctival redness and chemosis, lid swelling, and copious purulent discharge (Fig. 1.15 A, B). Pain, tenderness to touch, and preauricular lymphadenopathy are common. The most common pathogens causing hyperacute conjunctivitis are gonococcus and meningococcus, but other organisms, such as *Staphylococcus aureus* and *Streptococcus*, may produce this picture. In untreated gonococcal infection, corneal involvement occurs frequently. In gonococcal conjunctivitis, corneal ulcers typically begin at the superior limbus (Fig. 1.16A). Corneal ulcers rapidly progress if inadequately treated, and they may perforate within 1 to 2 days (Fig. 1.16B). Hyperacute conjunctivitis may be associated with pseudomembrane formation and subsequent conjunctival scarring or symblepharon.

Chronic conjunctivitis is a condition with low-grade symptoms and findings that can be annoyingly persistent. The symptoms are nonspecific and include foreign body sensation, intermittent redness, and mild mattering of the lids. Clinical signs may be minimal, with mild conjunctival

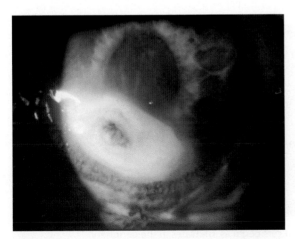

FIGURE 1.13. In severe atopic keratoconjunctivitis, corneal scarring, neovascularization, and melting can develop.

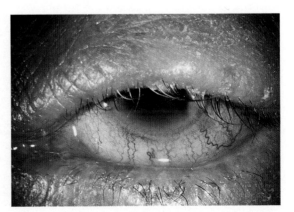

FIGURE 1.14. Acute bacterial conjunctivitis with mild lid swelling, conjunctival injection, and discharge along the lid margin.

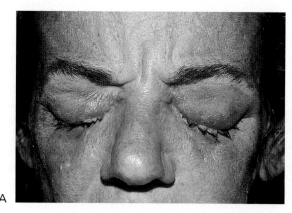
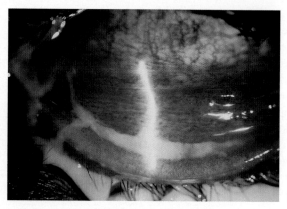

A   B

FIGURE 1.15. A: Hyperacute gonococcal conjunctivitis, with copious mucopurulent discharge and lid swelling. **B:** Hyperacute conjunctivitis caused by meningococcal infection with mucopurulent discharge.

injection and discharge. Blepharitis, styes, and chalazia often accompany chronic conjunctivitis.

Acute bacterial conjunctivitis is treated with broad-spectrum antibiotic drops, such as trimethoprim-polymyxin (Polytrim), the fluoroquinolones (i.e., Ocuflox, Ciloxan), or an aminoglycoside (e.g., Tobrex, gentamicin). Supplementary ointments, such as bacitracin or erythromycin at bedtime, may be helpful, and ointments are more effective in children. Neomycin with polymyxin B and sodium sulfacetamide preparations have been used for many years, but allergic reactions to these agents are common. In routine cases, cultures are not obtained because most cases are self-limited or respond to treatment. When unusual circumstances, persistent disease, or corneal involvement is present, culture and sensitivity studies are indicated. Underlying dacryocystitis can cause refractory mucopurulent conjunctivitis requiring systemic antibiotics.

In hyperacute conjunctivitis, smears and cultures are necessary, particularly if gonococcal or meningococcal infection is suspected (Fig. 1.17). The treatment of gonococcal conjunctivitis is a single injection of ceftriaxone (1 g) if the cornea is not involved or admission for a 5-day course of intravenous ceftriaxone if the cornea is involved. Topical therapy is ineffective, but bacitracin or ciprofloxacin can be used to supplement systemic therapy. Patients should also be treated with systemic tetracycline for *Chlamydia* infection and evaluated for other sexually transmitted diseases, including syphilis and human immunodeficiency virus infection.

Chronic Follicular Conjunctivitis

Chronic follicular conjunctivitis can be caused by *Chlamydia* infection, trachoma in endemic regions of the world, and drug reactions to epinephrine, antivirals, and a variety of ophthalmic medications.

Follicles occur more frequently in the inferior fornix than in the superior tarsus (Fig. 1.18A,B). In *Chlamydia* infection, peripheral subepithelial infiltrates may be present (Fig. 1.19A), and if the diagnosis is delayed, superior pannus can develop (Fig. 1.19B). Corneal neovascularization is less com-

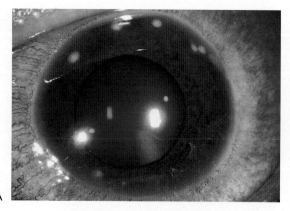
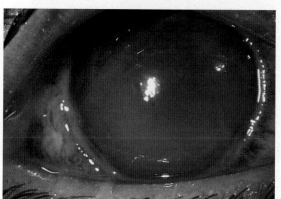

A   B

FIGURE 1.16. A: In gonococcal conjunctivitis, corneal ulcers begin as infiltrates in the periphery, usually superiorly. **B:** The rapidly progressing corneal ulcers caused by gonococcal infection can thin and perforate within several days.

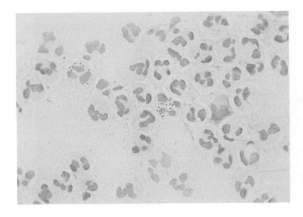

FIGURE 1.17. Gram stain of a conjunctival smear from a patient with gonococcal conjunctivitis. Figure 1.15A reveals many polymorphonuclear cells and intracellular gram-negative diplococci.

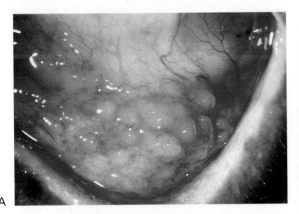
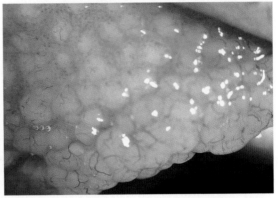

A

B

FIGURE 1.18. A: In chronic follicular conjunctivitis, follicles occur most frequently in the inferior palpebral conjunctiva. **B:** Occasionally, a follicular reaction develops on the superior tarsus in patients with chronic follicular conjunctivitis caused by *Chlamydia* infection.

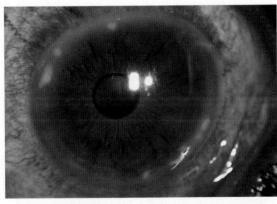
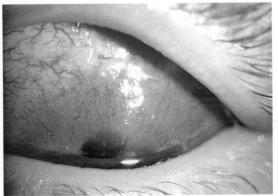

A

B

FIGURE 1.19. A: In cases of *Chlamydia* infection, peripheral subepithelial infiltrates develop several weeks after initial infection. **B:** Occasionally, severe chlamydial conjunctivitis causes corneal pannus formation.

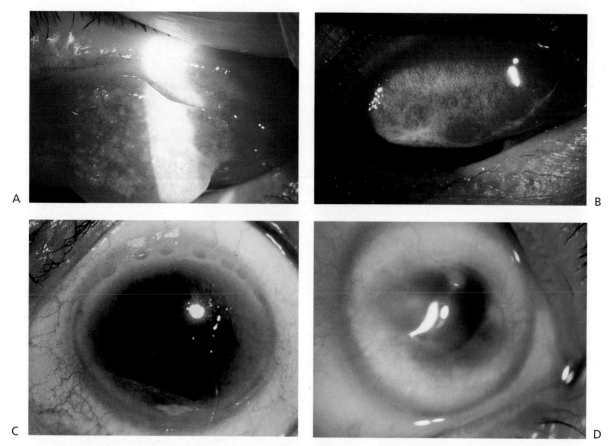

FIGURE 1.20. A: In trachoma, a mixed papillary follicular reaction of the superior tarsus is followed by conjunctival scarring. **B:** Linear conjunctival scars parallel to the lid margin due to trachoma are called Arlt's lines. **C:** Herbert's pits are depressed limbal scars. (Courtesy of the Wills collection.) **D:** Trachoma can result in corneal scarring and neovascularization.

mon than in trachoma. In the infected newborn as opposed to the adult, there is more purulent discharge, and follicles are absent.

In trachoma, there is a mixed follicular papillary reaction, predominantly of the superior tarsus, followed by conjunctival scarring, dry eyes, and trichiasis due to cicatricial entropion (Fig. 1.20A–D). Limbal inflammation is followed by the formation of depressed scars called Herbert's pits.

Chlamydia infection is diagnosed by immunofluorescence tests, tissue cultures of corneal scrapings, or both. Polymerase chain reaction testing is available. *Chlamydia* conjunctivitis in adults is treated with systemic doxycycline or tetracycline for 3 weeks. Erythromycin (250 mg four times daily) can be used as an alternative systemic medication if the patient is allergic to doxycycline or tetracycline or is less than age 8. A single dose of 1 g azithromycin is also effective. In newborns, inclusion conjunctivitis requires systemic erythromycin treatment of the infant and the parents. Trachoma is treated with topical or systemic tetracycline or erythromycin or systemic azithromycin. Eradication of the disease is difficult in endemic areas with poor hygiene be-

cause of reinfection, but periodic systemic azithromycin has the potential to eradicate this leading cause of preventable blindness affecting over 100 million people in the Middle East, Africa, and Southeast Asia.

HERPES SIMPLEX KERATITIS

Acute Dendritic Herpes Simplex Keratitis

Acute dendritic herpes simplex keratitis is characterized by the sudden onset of superficial corneal ulceration in the form of a dendrite after invasion of the epithelium by the herpes simplex virus (HSV). A dendrite is a branching epithelial ulceration with swollen, raised edges and terminal bulbs caused by active infection of the corneal epithelium with HSV type I (Fig. 1.21A). Primary infections with HSV are usually inapparent, and the virus becomes latent in the trigeminal ganglion. The precipitating factors leading to virus reactivation include fever, ultraviolet exposure, trauma, and stress. The use of topical or systemic corticosteroids is associated with the worsening of dendritic keratitis.

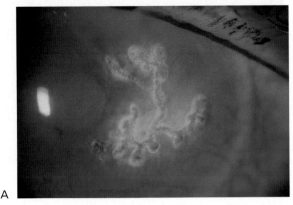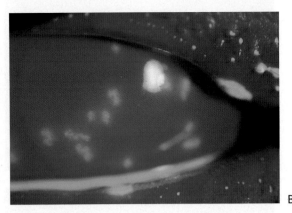

FIGURE 1.21. **A:** The hallmark of herpes simplex keratitis is the dendrite, a branching, epithelial ulceration with swollen, raised edges and terminal bulbs. **B:** In primary herpes simplex virus infections, multiple small dendrites may develop.

Patients notice pain, tearing, foreign body sensation, redness, and sensitivity to light. These symptoms may be mistaken for acute conjunctivitis, and it is important to keep HSV keratitis in the differential diagnosis of a red eye and acute follicular conjunctivitis. Fluorescein staining reveals the typical tree-branching appearance. Occasionally, multiple, small dendrites may be present (Fig. 1.21B). Ghost dendrites, which may follow dendrites, are dendritiform opacities in the superficial stroma (Fig. 1.22A). Dendrites recurring after penetrating keratoplasties for severe corneal scarring as a result of HSV begin in the periphery and may extend into the graft (Fig. 1.22B).

Acute HSV dendritic keratitis is treated with topical antiviral medication using trifluridine drops eight times each day or vidarabine ointment five times each day for 10 to 14 days. Topical steroids are contraindicated.

Other Manifestations of Ocular Herpes Simplex Virus Infection

Other manifestations of ocular HSV infections include lid blisters, follicular conjunctivitis, conjunctival dendrites, and geographic ulcers. The grouped vesicular lid eruption is extensive in primary infection (Fig. 1.23A). Healing occurs without scarring. Lid margin HSV ulcers (Fig. 1.23B) can be associated with infection of the adjacent corneal and conjunctival epithelium (Fig. 1.23C). Follicular conjunctivitis frequently accompanies primary HSV infection, but it can also be a manifestation of recurrent infection. Dendrites can involve the corneal and conjunctival epithelium. Geographic ulcers are large dendrites with similar epithelial borders but larger central epithelial defects (Fig. 1.24A). Rose bengal vividly stains the virus-infected epithelium

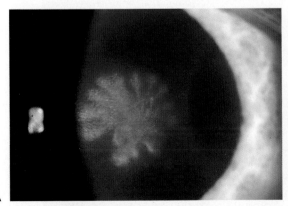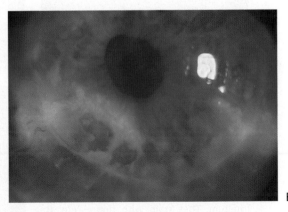

FIGURE 1.22. **A:** Ghost dendrites sometimes develop after herpes simplex dendrites. The ghost dendrites are superficial corneal opacities with the same shape as the original dendrite. They usually fade gradually without additional therapy but may leave superficial scarring. **B:** When dendrites develop after corneal transplantation for herpes simplex keratitis, they usually develop in the periphery and then extend onto the donor cornea.

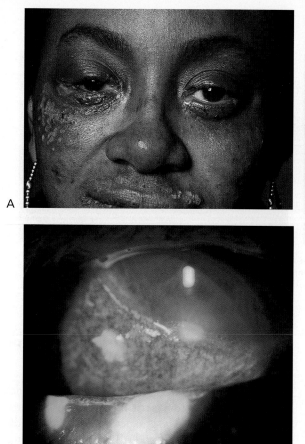

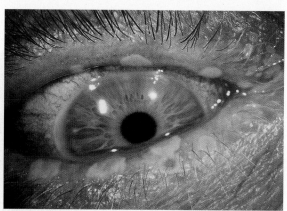

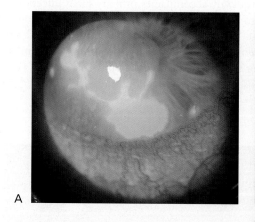

FIGURE 1.23. A: In overt primary herpes simplex virus infection, there is a vesicular lid rash that usually does not scar. **B:** Recurrent herpes simplex disease may produce more limited ulcerative blepharitis. **C:** When the lid margin is involved, there may be infection of the adjacent conjunctiva and cornea.

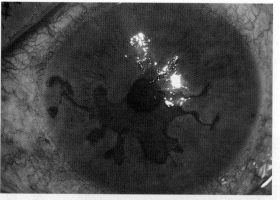

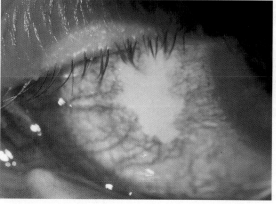

FIGURE 1.24. A: Geographic ulcers are large, dendritic infections of the corneal epithelium. They stain with fluorescein. **B:** Geographic ulcers and dendrites stain with rose bengal, with the greatest staining occurring along the edge of the ulcer where there is active viral infection. **C:** Herpes simplex virus infections can also cause conjunctival geographic ulcers.

along the border of geographic ulcers (Fig. 1.24B). HSV is also a cause of geographic conjunctival ulcers (Fig. 1.24C).

HSV blepharitis does not require treatment if the lesions are away from the lid margin. If the lid margin is involved, topical antivirals should be used in the eye prophylactically five times each day for 7 days. Follicular conjunctivitis in a patient with a history of recurrent HSV keratitis in the involved eye should also be treated with topical antivirals five times each day. Geographic ulcers are treated with topical trifluridine eight times each day. Prolonged use of antivirals results in toxicity manifested initially by superficial punctate keratitis in a whorl pattern. Treatment is discontinuation of the toxic antiviral medication and the use of preservative-free lubricating drops. Systemic acyclovir alone is effective in the treatment of dendritic keratitis but is not indicated unless standard topical antiviral therapy is unsuccessful. Systemic acyclovir is used in adults with overt primary infections, although this is not an approved use of the drug.

Trophic Epithelial Defects

Noninfectious trophic epithelial defects occur in patients with a history of recurrent HSV keratitis. The trophic defects are epithelial erosions with smooth, rolled edges (Fig. 1.25A). They are presumed to be associated with decreased corneal sensitivity caused by recurrent HSV keratitis. They

may be complicated by corneal melting and perforation (Fig. 1.25B) and with microbial superinfection (Fig. 1.25C).

Trophic defects are treated with lubrication, antibiotic ointment, discontinuation of toxic antivirals, and sometimes with patching. A partial temporary tarsorrhaphy is very helpful in promoting epithelial healing when lubrication is insufficient. Progressive melting and small perforations are managed with tissue adhesive and a bandage lens, but an emergency patch graft or penetrating keratoplasty may be necessary for larger perforations.

Stromal Keratitis

Nonnecrotizing Stromal Keratitis

HSV stromal keratitis is divided into nonnecrotizing and necrotizing diseases. Nonnecrotizing HSV stromal keratitis appears as localized corneal edema (Fig. 1.26A,B). Disciform keratitis is a common form of nonnecrotizing HSV stromal keratitis associated with a round area of full-thickness corneal edema that is often accompanied by localized granulomatous keratic precipitates.

The HEDS study showed that topical corticosteroids accompanied by antiviral prophylaxis are safe and effective treatment for nonnecrotizing HSV stromal keratitis, shortening the time until resolution. Topical steroids are often begun with prednisolone (1%, four times daily) and pro-

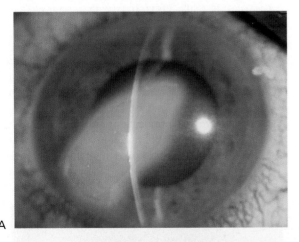

A

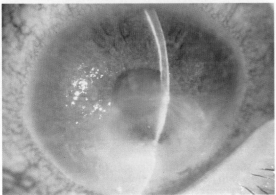

B

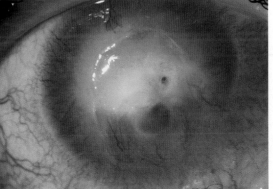

C

FIGURE 1.25. A: Persistent trophic epithelial defects have rounded borders. **B:** Trophic defects can be complicated by corneal thinning, melting, and perforation, **(C)** and by microbial superinfection. Cultures grew *Staphylococcus aureus* in this case.

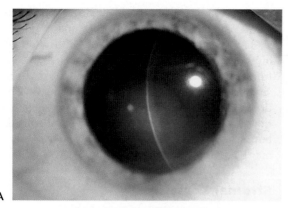
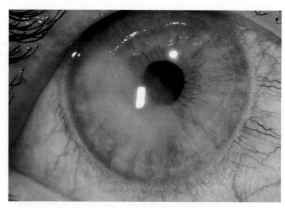

A   B

FIGURE 1.26. A: Disciform keratitis is a form of nonnecrotizing herpes simplex virus (HSV) stromal keratitis associated with a round area of full-thickness corneal edema and localized granulomatous keratic precipitates. **B:** Nonnecrotizing HSV stromal keratitis is associated with localized corneal edema, which may not have a disciform shape.

phylactic topical antivirals three or four times daily. It is necessary to taper topical steroids slowly, often using 0.125% prednisolone from four times daily to once weekly.

The HEDS treatment studies showed that systemic acyclovir is not effective in the treatment of stromal HSV keratitis. The HEDS prevention studies showed that systemic acyclovir 400 mg po bid is effective in significantly reducing recurrences and is most beneficial in patients with a history of stromal keratitis, as they are prone to recurrent stromal keratitis, which results in scarring and loss of vision.

Necrotizing Stromal Keratitis

Necrotizing HSV stromal keratitis, in the past called viral interstitial keratitis, has areas of white stromal infiltrates in addition to corneal edema (Fig. 1.27A,B). Corneal neovascularization is also frequently present. When patients with recurrent HSV keratitis develop staining infiltrates, it is important to rule out microbial superinfection with bacteria or unusual organisms by performing smears and cultures.

Necrotizing HSV keratitis is treated like nonnecrotizing stromal keratitis, with topical steroids and prophylactic antivirals as previously discussed. Necrotizing stromal keratitis is uncommon, and there were not enough patients in the HEDS study to determine whether systemic acyclovir has a role in its treatment.

Uveitis

Acute granulomatous uveitis or iridocyclitis is another manifestation of ocular HSV disease. Herpetic stromal keratitis may or may not be active at the time of the uveitis.

The onset of HSV anterior uveitis is acute, with pain, redness, and sensitivity to lights. Granulomatous keratic precipitates and anterior chamber flare and cells are seen. Uveitis can result in localized iris atrophy and an irregular, sometimes dilated pupil (Fig. 1.28A,B). Herpetic uveitis is often associated with increased intraocular pressure, which may be an indicator of active viral replication in the anterior chamber.

Treatment of herpetic uveitis includes topical cortico-

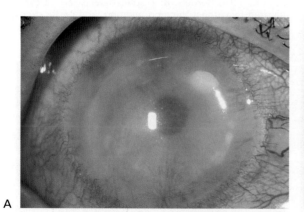
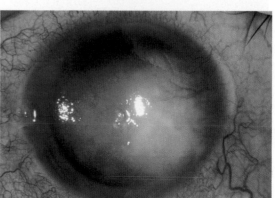

A   B

FIGURE 1.27. A,B: Necrotizing herpes simplex virus stromal keratitis is characterized by white stromal infiltrates in addition to corneal edema, usually with neovascularization.

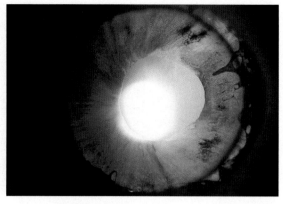
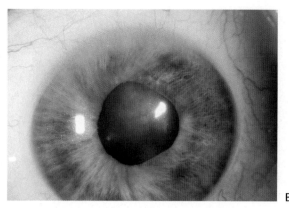

A

B

FIGURE 1.28. A: Herpes simplex virus (HSV) uveitis can result in localized iris atrophy that is best seen in retroillumination. **B:** The same patient, seen in broad illumination, has an irregular pupil secondary to HSV uveitis.

steroids, prophylactic topical antivirals, cycloplegia, and topical and systemic glaucoma medications such as β blockers or carbonic anhydrase inhibitors as needed to control intraocular pressure. Miotics and Xalatan are avoided. The optic nerve and visual fields should be followed closely.

The HEDS study of acyclovir treatment for herpetic iridocyclitis was terminated because of a lack of enrollment, but a probable benefit of treatment was observed among patients treated with acyclovir 400 mg five times a day for 10 weeks compared to placebo.

Corneal Scarring

HSV keratitis can lead to extensive corneal scarring. It is second only to trauma as the most common cause of unilateral corneal blindness in the United States.

Corneal scarring is manifested by localized opacification, usually with variable thinning and surface irregularity, resulting in reduced vision (Fig. 1.29). Corneal scarring may be severe enough to require corneal transplantation for visual rehabilitation.

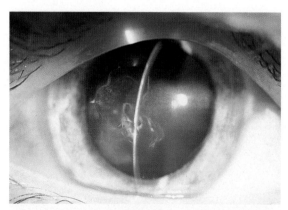

FIGURE 1.29. Recurrent herpes simplex virus keratitis can result in corneal scarring and reduced vision, necessitating a corneal transplant in some cases.

HERPES ZOSTER OPHTHALMICUS
Dermatologic Involvement

The hallmark of herpes zoster ophthalmicus is a vesicular skin eruption resulting in scarring in the distribution of one of the branches of the trigeminal nerve. Of the three divisions of cranial nerve V, the first or ophthalmic division is the most commonly affected. Zoster can sometimes occur without a rash, but the diagnosis is much more difficult.

The organism responsible for herpes zoster is the herpes varicella virus, which also causes chickenpox. After the primary chickenpox infection, the varicella virus persists in a latent state in the trigeminal ganglion or sensory ganglion of the spinal cord. Acute zoster infection may develop later in life after a reactivation of the virus. The patient notices progressive discomfort or neuralgic pain on the affected side in the scalp, forehead, temple area, and behind the eye. The pain may precede the rash by a day or two and initially puzzle the clinician. The rash is vesicular and results in scarring. Skin involvement strictly obeys the midline (Fig. 1.30). The three main branches of the ophthalmic division are the supraorbital, lacrimal, and nasociliary. One or more branches may be involved. Because the globe is innervated by the nasociliary branch, the likelihood of ocular involvement increases to 75% if this branch is affected. This branch also supplies the skin on the bridge and tip of the nose. If this area is not affected, only approximately one third of the eyes become involved.

The patient often develops conjunctival injection and discharge even without intraocular involvement. If the rash involves the eyelid, cicatricial contraction may result in corneal exposure and/or trichiasis.

Patients with acute herpes zoster ophthalmicus are treated with acyclovir (800 mg, five times daily) for 7 to 10 days. Alternative treatment includes famciclovir (500 mg tid) or valacyclovir (1,000 mg tid), but the latter is not used

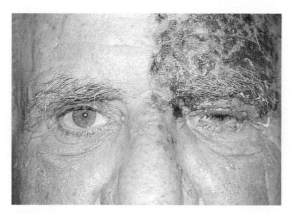

FIGURE 1.30. The hallmark of herpes zoster is a vesicular skin eruption of the first division of the fifth cranial nerve that strictly obeys the midline and results in scarring.

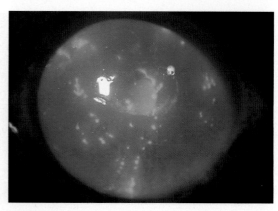

FIGURE 1.31. Early in the course of the disease, patients with herpes zoster ophthalmicus have conjunctivitis and punctate keratitis, which may have a dendritic appearance mimicking herpes simplex virus keratitis.

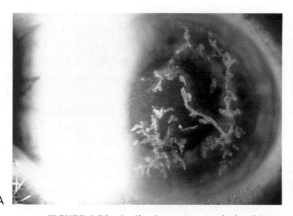

A

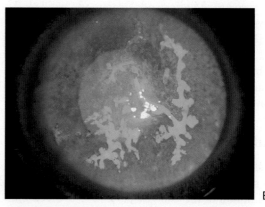

B

FIGURE 1.32. A: Classic zoster pseudodendrites are elevated mucous plaques with tapered ends, which have a delayed onset. **B:** They stain with fluorescein, but are not ulcerated.

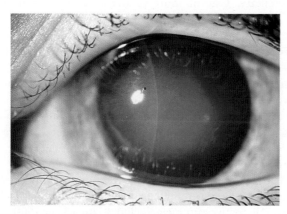

FIGURE 1.33. Disciform keratitis secondary to herpes zoster appears similar to disciform keratitis secondary to herpes simplex.

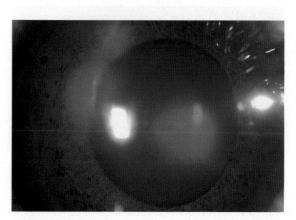

FIGURE 1.34. In nummular keratitis, the subepithelial infiltrates are larger and more variable in size than those in adenoviral conjunctivitis.

in immunocompromised hosts. Use of systemic corticosteroids to prevent postherpetic neuralgia is controversial, and they are much less frequently used than in the past. Topical antibiotics and cold compresses are helpful for conjunctivitis. A dermatologist may be consulted for additional topical treatment of the vesicular lesions.

Ocular Involvement

Acute Lesions

Acutely, patients with herpes zoster ophthalmicus have conjunctivitis and punctate keratitis when the eye is involved. Acute epithelial involvement with punctate keratitis may have a dendriform appearance, mimicking HSV dendritic keratitis (Fig. 1.31). The typical appearance of the rash aids greatly in the diagnosis of herpes zoster, but its appearance may be delayed.

Treatment of conjunctivitis and punctate keratitis is nonspecific, with cool compresses and topical lubrication with or without prophylactic topical antibiotics. Topical antivirals are not effective or indicated. Acyclovir is effective against herpes zoster but is not available as a topical ophthalmic medication in the United States.

Zoster Epithelial Keratitis

Classic zoster pseudodendrites occur later in the course of the disease, after the rash has healed. Zoster pseudodendrites are mucous plaques that are elevated, stain with fluorescein, and have tapered ends (Fig. 1.32A,B). They differ from herpes simplex dendrites, which are epithelial ulcerations with a depressed center and terminal bulbs.

Zoster dendrites are treated with lubrication, using frequent preservative-free drops and ointment. Topical antivirals are contraindicated because they are ineffective and toxic. Topical steroids can be used as needed to treat zoster keratouveitis, which is frequently also present.

Zoster Stromal Keratitis

Herpes zoster is associated with various forms of stromal keratitis occurring several weeks or more after the acute infection. Zoster can be associated with disciform keratitis that is similar in appearance to herpes simplex disciform keratitis (Fig. 1.33). This condition can follow chickenpox or zoster. Nummular keratitis with scattered subepithelial infiltrates larger and more variable in size than those seen in adenoviral conjunctivitis can develop (Fig. 1.34). Interstitial keratitis with localized corneal edema and deep corneal neovascularization and lipid infiltrates can also occur (Fig. 1.35 A, B).

Stromal keratitis is treated with topical corticosteroids. Mild inflammation may be responsive to low-dose topical steroids. Steroids must be tapered over many months or years. Some patients require long-term, low-dose steroids such as 0.125% prednisolone once each week to prevent flare-ups. Topical antivirals are not used.

Neurotrophic Keratitis

Neurotrophic keratitis with or without corneal melting is a late manifestation of herpes zoster and is related to permanently decreased corneal sensation. Trophic epithelial defects are erosions with smooth borders that are frequently located inferocentrally (Fig. 1.36). Corneal sensation is decreased or absent. Persistent epithelial defects can be complicated by corneal melting, resulting in impending or frank perforation (Fig. 1.37) or by microbial superinfection.

Trophic epithelial defects can be prevented by using preservative-free lubricating drops and ointment in patients with ocular surface irregularities after zoster infection. Trophic defects are treated with bland antibiotic ointments usually without pressure patching. Temporary or permanent lateral tarsorrhaphy can facilitate healing and prevent recurrent surface breakdown. Corneal melts are treated similarly to trophic defects to promote epithelial healing. A tis-

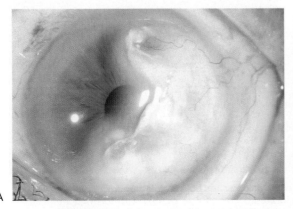
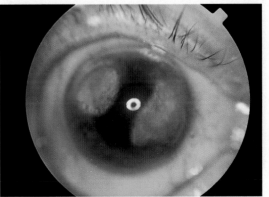

FIGURE 1.35. **A:** Interstitial keratitis in herpes zoster patients is associated with localized corneal edema, deep corneal neovascularization, and frequently, lipid keratopathy. **B:** Lipid keratopathy secondary to herpes zoster ophthalmicus. (Courtesy of E. Jaeger, M.D.)

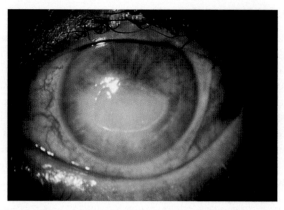

FIGURE 1.36. Neurotrophic keratitis in herpes zoster patients is associated with inferocentral corneal erosions with smooth borders.

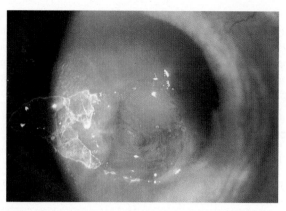

FIGURE 1.37. Persistent neurotrophic epithelial defects can be complicated by corneal melting.

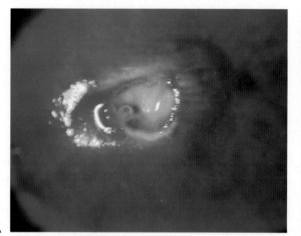

A

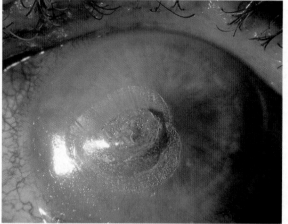

B

FIGURE 1.38. Small perforation secondary to herpes zoster ophthalmicus before **(A)** and after **(B)** application of tissue adhesive and a bandage contact lens.

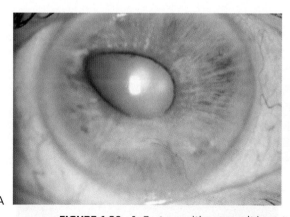

A

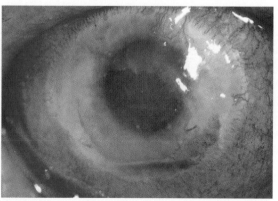

B

FIGURE 1.39. **A:** Zoster uveitis can result in sector iris atrophy and an irregular pupil. This patient also has an inferior corneal scar following a perforated bacterial ulcer treated with fortified antibiotics and tissue adhesive. **B:** Zoster uveitis may be severe and associated with hyphemas. This patient also has a neurotrophic epithelial defect.

sue adhesive covered by a bandage lens is used for impending and small perforations (Fig. 1.38A, B). Larger perforations require patch grafts. Topical steroids promote melting in patients with persistent epithelial defects. They should be avoided in patients not already on them and tapered gradually in patients using them.

Zoster Uveitis

Uveitis may accompany keratitis or occur independently. Zoster uveitis is usually associated with granulomatous keratic precipitates and frequently causes increased intraocular pressure. Zoster uveitis can result in sector iris atrophy and an irregular pupil (Fig. 1.39A) more frequently than herpes simplex uveitis. In severe cases, zoster uveitis can be associated with a hyphema (Fig. 1.39B).

Treatment of zoster uveitis consists of cycloplegia and topical steroids on a gradually tapering regimen without topical antivirals. Increased intraocular pressure is treated as needed with aqueous suppressants without miotic agents or Xalatan.

Zoster Episcleritis and Scleritis

Zoster can be associated with episcleritis and scleritis. The clinical features of pain, localized redness, tenderness and swelling of the conjunctiva, episclera, and sclera are similar to those seen in nonzoster cases. Unlike other causes of episcleritis and scleritis, nodular episcleritis can evolve into nodular scleritis in zoster (Fig. 1.40A). Scleritis may be accompanied by localized stromal keratitis (Fig. 1.40B).

Episcleritis is responsive to topical steroids, but scleritis requires systemic nonsteroidal antiinflammatory agents and steroids if the nonsteroidal antiinflammatories are ineffective. Sclerokeratitis is treated with topical steroids for the cornea and systemic medication to control the scleritis.

CORNEAL ULCERS

Sterile Infiltrates

Staphylococcal hypersensitivity keratitis is manifested by sterile marginal infiltrates. Sterile infiltrates are also seen in patients who wear contact lenses.

Staphylococcal marginal infiltrates are usually located superiorly or inferiorly, near where the lid margin rests against the cornea. The infiltrates are frequently concentric to the limbus and have an intervening clear space (Fig. 1.41). The epithelial defect, if present, is usually smaller than the infiltrate. Conjunctival injection is usually localized to the area of the infiltrate. The anterior chamber is quiet.

Sterile infiltrates in contact lens wearers are small (<1 mm), peripheral, often multiple, and nonstaining (Fig. 1.42). They are not associated with pain, corneal edema, or anterior chamber inflammation.

Staphylococcal hypersensitivity infiltrates are responsive to treatment with weak topical steroids. In addition, treatment of the underlying lid disease with warm compresses, antibiotic ointment, and often with systemic tetracycline is indicated to prevent recurrent episodes.

Sterile infiltrates in contact lens wearers are treated by discontinuing use of the lenses. Low-dose antibiotics are frequently prescribed. The cause of the infiltrate may be hypoxia or a reaction to solutions used for disinfection. After the infiltrate resolves, the fit of the lens should be checked, a hydrogen peroxide system of disinfection should be used, and lens use should be limited to daily wear. If the infiltrate is possibly infected, it should be treated as a bacterial ulcer. Steroids are generally to be avoided in lens-related sterile in-

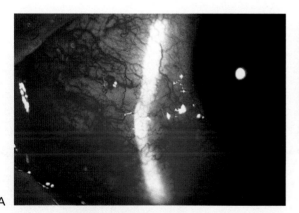
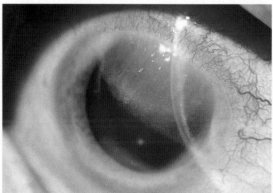

A   B

FIGURE 1.40. A: Nodular scleritis is characterized by a localized area of scleral and episcleral swelling associated with marked pain. The condition requires systemic treatment with nonsteroidal antiinflammatory agents. Nodular episcleritis has a similar appearance but is responsive to topical steroids. **B:** In herpes zoster, there can be scleral keratitis with localized scleral inflammation and adjacent corneal edema.

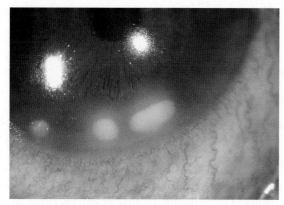

FIGURE 1.41. Staphylococcal hypersensitivity keratitis is characterized by infiltrates located in the periphery, concentric to the limbus, with an intervening clear space between the infiltrate and the limbus.

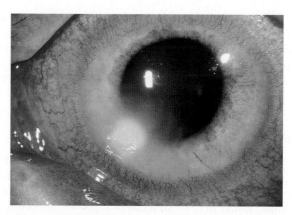

FIGURE 1.43. Infected corneal ulcers are characterized by corneal infiltrates associated with overlying epithelial defects and an anterior chamber reaction. This ulcer caused by *Staphylococcus aureus* extends toward the center of the cornea and is associated with surrounding corneal edema.

filtrates because the problem resolves with lens discontinuation, and the physician does not want to mistreat an early, undiagnosed infected ulcer.

Bacterial Ulcers

Corneal ulcers caused by bacteria present as acutely painful infiltrates associated with overlying epithelial defects and an anterior chamber reaction. Frequently, corneal edema surrounds the infiltrate. There may or may not be a mucopurulent discharge, but its presence points to an infectious cause. The most frequent causative organisms are *Staphylococcus, Pseudomonas, Streptococcus,* and *Moraxella,* but a wide variety of bacteria may be cultured.

S. aureus corneal ulcers have a more central or radial component than staphylococcal marginal infiltrates (Fig. 1.43). They are associated with more inflammation, including diffuse injection, surrounding corneal edema, and an anterior chamber reaction.

Pseudomonas is the most common cause of ulcers in persons wearing cosmetic soft contact lenses. Ulcers may be se-

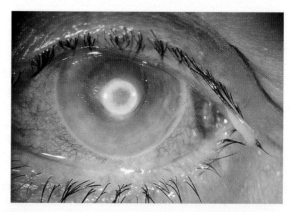

FIGURE 1.44. Severe *Pseudomonas* ulcers typically are associated with adherent mucopurulent discharge and can have a ring appearance caused by dense infiltration and edema at the periphery of the ulcer and central corneal thinning.

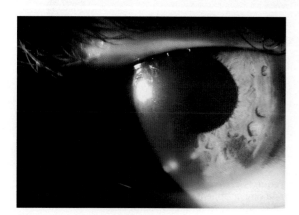

FIGURE 1.42. Sterile infiltrates in contact lens wearers are small, peripheral, often multiple, and nonstaining.

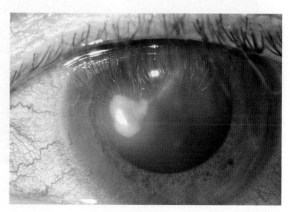

FIGURE 1.45. Small *Pseudomonas* infections may lack the appearance of typical, severe *Pseudomonas* ulcers. This patient has a radial extension resembling radial keratoneuritis.

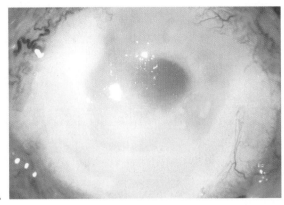

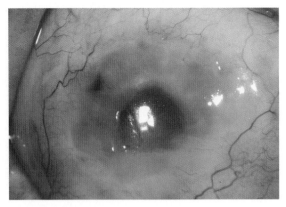

A   B

FIGURE 1.46. A: *Pseudomonas* corneal ulcers that extend to the limbus and onto the sclera are more serious than those that are limited to the cornea. These ulcers require long-term systemic therapy. **B:** A follow-up photograph of the same patient shows a resolved *Pseudomonas* corneal ulcer with scleral extension after prolonged systemic ciprofloxacin treatment.

vere, with marked corneal inflammation, edema, and an adherent mucopurulent discharge (Fig. 1.44). Early *Pseudomonas* infections may not have the characteristic features of more advanced cases (Fig. 1.45). When pseudomonal infection extends onto the sclera, the prognosis for saving the eye is improved by treatment with oral ciprofloxacin (Fig. 1.46A,B).

Streptococcal infections can cause severe suppurative keratitis, especially in eyes with preexisting ocular surface disease (Fig. 1.47). Less commonly, streptococcal infections have a crystalline appearance without inflammation (Fig. 1.48). Although gram-negative infections usually are more serious than gram-positive infections, severe streptococcal infections can be as serious as *Pseudomonas* ulcers. Crystalline keratopathy caused by *Streptococcus* occurs in patients on topical corticosteroids, usually after penetrating keratoplasty.

Moraxella is a relatively common cause of ulcers in eyes with preexisting surface disease and in debilitated patients. The organism tends to grow slowly, the ulcer tends to re-

spond slowly to treatment, and perforations are more common than with other organisms (Fig. 1.49A,B).

The standard treatment of corneal ulcers includes immediate, intensive treatment every 15 to 30 minutes with broad-spectrum fortified antibiotics (i.e., tobramycin or gentamicin 15 mg/mL and cefazolin 50 mg/mL or vancomycin 12 to 25 mg/mL) or one of the fluoroquinolones, ciprofloxacin or ofloxacin. Corneal smears and cultures usually are not performed for small ulcers, but are indicated in large ulcers (>1 to 2 mm), ulcers not responding to initial treatment, and when an unusual organism is suspected by the history or appearance. Many prefer fortified antibiotics for severe ulcers requiring hospitalization and fluoroquinolones for less serious infections treated on an outpatient basis. Antibiotics are modified on the basis of culture results and gradually tapered as the infection responds. Systemic therapy is indicated only for perforated ulcers, those with scleral extension, and gonococcal infections.

Nocardia and atypical mycobacteria are uncommon

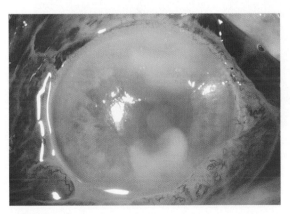

FIGURE 1.47. Streptococcal infection can be associated with severe suppuration.

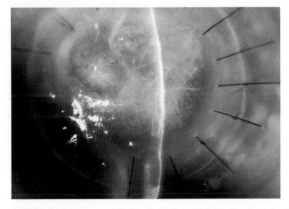

FIGURE 1.48. Streptococcal infection can be associated with crystalline keratopathy without significant inflammation, usually in patients who are on a regimen of topical steroids after corneal transplantation.

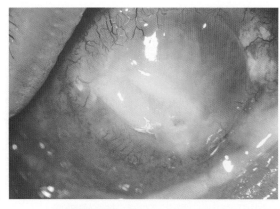
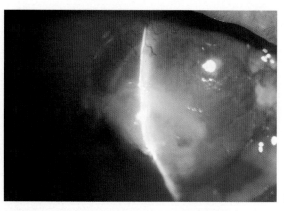

A
B

FIGURE 1.49. A: *Moraxella* ulcers are associated with dense, full thickness corneal infiltrates. **B:** In this case, the cornea perforated, and the anterior chamber is flat. Blood tinged infiltrate and radial folds towards the ulcer are signs associated with perforation.

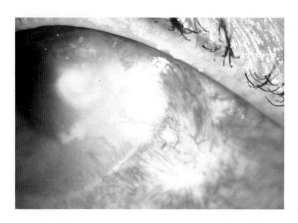

FIGURE 1.50. *Nocardia* infection developed in this patient after a partial-thickness laceration at the time of a farm-related injury. (From Donnenfeld ED, Cohen EJ, Barza M, Baum J. Treatment of *Nocardia* keratitis with topical trimethoprim-sulfamethoxazole. *Am J Ophthalmol* 1985;99:602, with permission.)

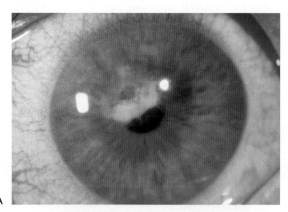
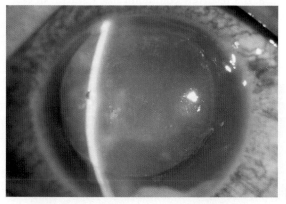

A
B

FIGURE 1.51. A: This recalcitrant corneal ulcer was diagnosed by corneal biopsy and cultures to be caused by atypical mycobacteria. **B:** This severe atypical mycobacteria infection occurred following laser in situ keratomileusis.

causes of indolent corneal ulcers (Figs. 1.50, 1.51 A,B). Both are acid-fast organisms present in the soil. Both infections can develop weeks after injury with vegetable-contaminated matter. Atypical mycobacterial infections have been associated with inadequate sterilization of surgical instruments. Both infections are slowly progressive, often recalcitrant to medical treatment. Diagnosis is aided by the addition of acid-fast stains to the standard Gram and Giemsa stains. On the Gram stain, the organisms can be confused with gram-positive rods and thought to be diphtheroids. Lowenstein-Jensen culture media are used to isolate atypical mycobacteria. Both types of infections are treated with fortified amikacin drops. Topical and/or oral clarithromycin is also used in atypical mycobacteria infections.

Fungal Keratitis

Fungal corneal ulcers are caused by a wide variety of filamentous organisms after trauma with vegetable-contaminated matter and by *Candida* in eyes with preexisting ocular surface disease.

Fusarium and *Aspergillus* are the most commonly isolated filamentous organisms. Ulcers typically have a feathery border and satellite lesions, and the infiltrate extends beyond the epithelial defect (Fig. 1.52A,B). The physician cannot count on this typical appearance. Giemsa-stained smears and cultures on appropriate media are necessary to make the

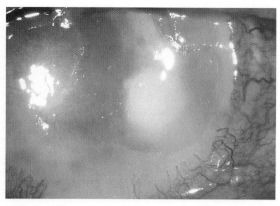

FIGURE 1.53. Corneal ulcer in a patient with pseudophakic bullous keratopathy was determined by cultures to be caused by *Candida albicans* infection.

diagnosis (Fig. 1.52C). *Candida* ulcers look similar to bacterial ulcers and are usually not suspected on the basis of the history or clinical appearance (Fig. 1.53).

Fungal ulcers are less responsive to medical therapy than bacterial ulcers. The drug of choice for filamentous infections is natamycin, but drug penetration and efficacy are limited. Amphotericin (0.15%) is the drug of choice for *Candida*. Oral fluconazole is also used in fungal infections. Topical steroids enhance fungal infections and therefore are contraindicated. Penetrating keratoplasty is indicated for in-

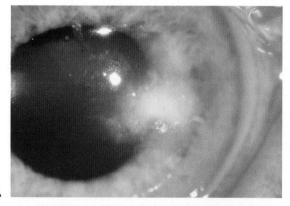

A

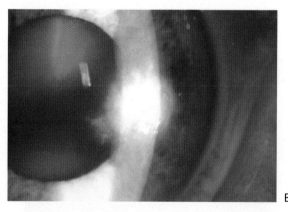

B

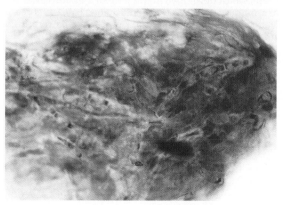

C

FIGURE 1.52. A: This corneal ulcer in a patient using extended wear aphakic soft contact lenses was caused by a filamentous fungal organism, *Fusarium.* **B:** The ulcer has a typical feathery border. **C:** Giemsa-stained corneal smears obtained from the patient in Figure 1.51 revealed septate, filamentous organisms.

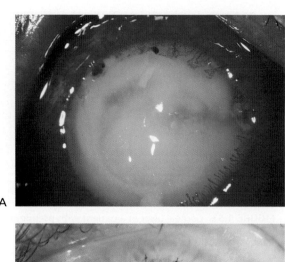

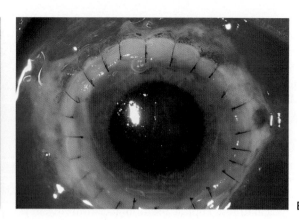

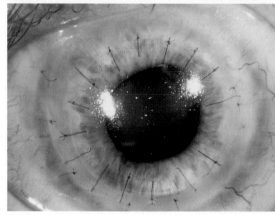

FIGURE 1.54. A: Corneal ulcer caused by *Fusarium* was unresponsive to intensive, appropriate medical treatment. **B:** The patient underwent a large, penetrating keratoplasty (PK) to save the eye. This graft failed as expected. **C:** Subsequently, a smaller PK was performed successfully for visual rehabilitation in a similar patient with fungal keratitis.

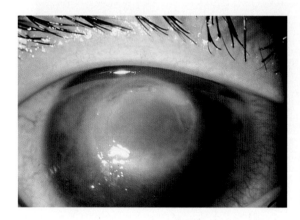

FIGURE 1.55. The hallmark of *Acanthamoeba* keratitis is a ring infiltrate, which developed in this patient 2 months after the onset of symptoms. (From Cohen EJ, Buchanan HW, Laughrea GS, et al. Diagnosis and management of *Acanthamoeba* keratitis. *Am J Ophthalmol* 1985;100:390, with permission.)

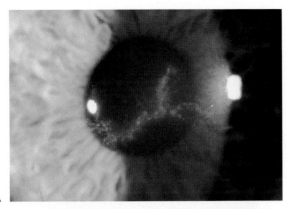 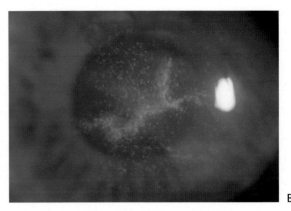

FIGURE 1.56. A: An early manifestation of *Acanthamoeba* keratitis is a dendritiform epithelial lesion. **B:** The lesion stains with fluorescein.

fection that progresses despite maximal appropriate medical therapy (Fig. 1.54A–C).

Acanthamoeba Keratitis

Acanthamoeba keratitis is an uncommon parasitic infection associated with the use of contact lenses, inadequate lens disinfection, and exposure to contaminated water such as swimming pools. It is frequently misdiagnosed as HSV keratitis, but unlike HSV keratitis, *Acanthamoeba* keratitis is associated with pain that is often out of proportion to the slit lamp findings.

The hallmark of advanced *Acanthamoeba* keratitis is a ring infiltrate (Fig. 1.55). Earlier signs of *Acanthamoeba* infection include dendritiform epithelial lesions (Figs. 1.56A,B and 1.57), radial keratoneuritis, and nonspecific stromal keratitis. Advanced disease can be associated with corneal necrosis and thinning (Fig. 1.58A) and complicated by bacterial superinfection (Fig. 1.58B).

Early diagnosis is critical for increasing the success of medical treatment. The organisms can be identified on Giemsa-stained smears (Fig. 1.59) or with calcifluor white stains when epithelial disease is present. Cultures are done on nonnutrient agar with an *Escherichia coli* overlay or buffered charcoal-yeast extract agar.

The medications used for treatment include topical propamidine, neomycin, clotrimazole, Baquacil, and chlorohexidine. Progressive infection may require penetrating keratoplasty, but there is a definite risk of recalcitrant,

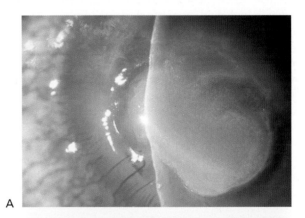

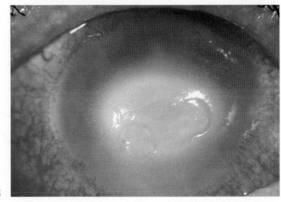

FIGURE 1.58. A: Advanced *Acanthamoeba* keratitis can be complicated by corneal thinning and necrosis. **B:** *Acanthamoeba* keratitis can also be complicated by bacterial superinfection, in this case by *Streptococcus* organisms.

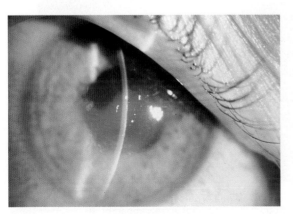

FIGURE 1.57. This large, geographic, dendritiform lesion of the corneal epithelium is caused by *Acanthamoeba* infection.

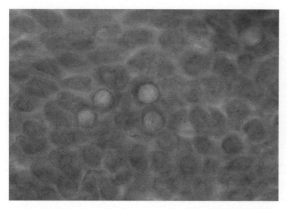

FIGURE 1.59. If there is epithelial infection caused by *Acanthamoeba*, the diagnosis can be made by Giemsa-stained smears that reveal the characteristic cysts.

recurrent infection after surgery. Since the use of Baquacil, medical treatment is much more successful than previously.

EPISCLERITIS AND SCLERITIS

Episcleritis

Inflammation of the episclera is typically a recurrent, but self-limited condition of young adults. It is usually not associated with underlying systemic abnormalities.

Episcleritis can be simple and flat (Fig. 1.60A) or nodular (Fig. 1.60B), may affect one sector or be diffuse, and may involve one or both eyes. Nodules are pink and can be moved slightly over the underlying sclera with a cotton-tipped applicator. The cornea is typically unaffected, and patients notice mild-to-moderate ocular redness and pain.

A systemic workup is usually not indicated for episcleritis. It usually resolves without treatment. More severe cases can be treated with topical steroids and systemic non-steroidal antiinflammatory agents such as aspirin or ibuprofen.

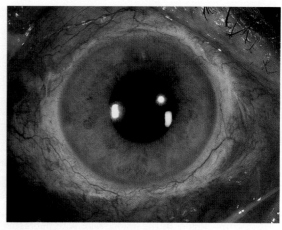

FIGURE 1.61. Anterior scleritis. The sectorial, diffuse area of scleral inflammation was moderately painful and did not blanch in response to instillation of a 2.5% solution of phenylepinephrine.

Anterior Scleritis

Anterior scleritis involves inflammation of the sclera, overlying conjunctiva, and episclera. Half of the patients with scleritis have an identifiable underlying systemic illness associated with the scleritis.

Anterior scleritis is divided into diffuse (i.e., flat, widespread inflammation; Fig. 1.61), nodular (i.e., localized, immovable, tender nodules; Fig. 1.62), and necrotizing forms (i.e., associated with thinning of the sclera). Necrotizing scleritis can occur with inflammation, which is quite painful and often associated with a systemic inflammatory disease such as Wegener's granulomatosis (Fig. 1.63), or can occur without inflammation, a form that is relatively painless and occurs primarily in patients with severe rheumatoid arthritis (Fig. 1.64). Sometimes, scleritis can be infectious and associated with corneal ulceration (Fig. 1.65). There can be extreme thinning of the sclera, even to the point of perforation.

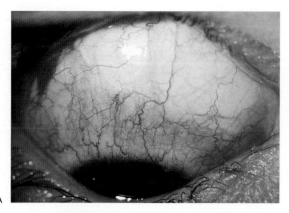
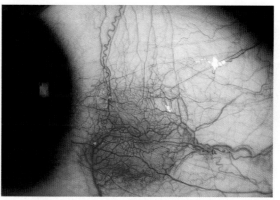

A   B

FIGURE 1.60. A: Diffuse episcleritis in the superior perilimbal area. The conjunctival redness blanched with 2.5% phenylepinephrine, leaving the darker, radial episcleral vessels apparent. **B:** Nodular episcleritis. A slightly mobile, moderately tender, elevated nodule is evident, typically with overlying conjunctival injection.

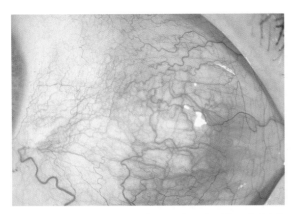

FIGURE 1.62. Nodular scleritis is associated with painful, localized swelling and elevation of the episclera and sclera.

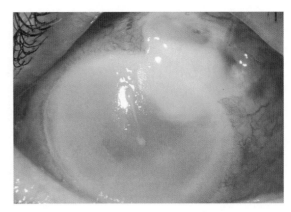

FIGURE 1.65. Scleral infections can be caused by an extension of corneal infection into the sclera. This case, caused by streptococcal infection, occurred several days after cataract surgery and resulted in loss of the eye.

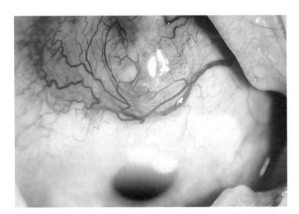

FIGURE 1.63. In necrotizing scleritis, there is localized episcleral and scleral inflammation with scleral necrosis and thinning. In this case, the scleritis is associated with peripheral keratitis.

A systemic workup typically includes a physical examination and determinations of a complete blood count, erythrocyte sedimentation rate, urinalysis, fluorescent treponemal antibody (FTA-ABS) test for syphilis, rheumatoid factor, antinuclear antibody test (ANA), antineutrophil cytoplasmic antibody test (ANCA), and purified protein derivative test (PPD). Scleritis can be treated with systemic nonsteroidal antiinflammatory agents. More severe scleritis, especially necrotizing scleritis, requires systemic steroids and sometimes requires cytotoxic agents. Topical steroids are ineffective. Subconjunctival steroid injections are usually contraindicated, but recent reports suggest they may be effective and not a risk factor for perforation. Rarely, surgery is necessary to preserve the globe.

NONINFECTIOUS CORNEAL DISEASE

Dry Eye Syndrome

Dry eye syndrome is a condition in which the tear film does not adequately coat the conjunctiva and cornea. It may result from a decreased quantity of otherwise normal tears or an abnormal quality of the tear film causing increased evaporation.

The primary symptoms include ocular burning and foreign body sensation. The symptoms are usually exacerbated by prolonged use of the eyes and by environmental factors such as wind, heat, smoke, and low humidity. Paradoxically, patients may complain of excess tearing if the eye becomes so irritated that reflex tearing mechanisms are activated. A decreased tear lake and a decreased tear film breakup time are common. Other signs include punctate fluorescein or rose bengal staining of the cornea and conjunctiva, typically inferiorly or in the interpalpebral zone (Fig. 1.66A). Excess mucus, filaments, or both may be seen. A Schirmer's test performed with the patient's eye anesthetized, typically reveals reduced baseline tear secretion (<5 mm).

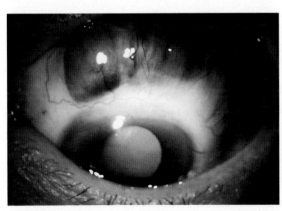

FIGURE 1.64. Scleromalacia perforans is a noninflammatory form of necrotizing scleritis characterized by scleral thinning, usually occurring in patients with advanced rheumatoid arthritis.

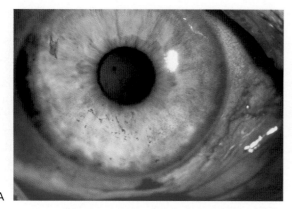
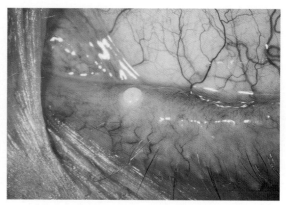

FIGURE 1.66. A: Dry eye syndrome is revealed by rose bengal staining of the interpalpebral cornea and conjunctiva. **B:** Silicone plug is present in the inferior punctum.

The numerous underlying causes that should be considered include systemic medications, such as antihistamines and oral contraceptives; collagen vascular diseases, such as Sjögren's syndrome and rheumatoid arthritis; ocular cicatricial pemphigoid; Stevens-Johnson syndrome; and vitamin A deficiency. A stepwise approach to treatment is appropriate, beginning with regular artificial tear drops several times a day for mildly dry eyes. For moderate dry eye syndrome, preservative-free tears are used up to every 1 to 2 hours during the day, with artificial tear ointment use at night. In severe cases, more viscous drops, more frequent applications of ointment, and temporary or permanent punctal occlusion by plugs or cautery are used (Fig. 1.66B). Lateral tarsorrhaphy may be required if less aggressive therapy fails.

Filamentary Keratopathy

Filaments are strands of epithelial cells and mucus attached to the surface of the cornea at the end of the strand (Fig. 1.67). Filaments are typically caused by corneal surface disease, most commonly dry eye syndrome. Other causes include superior limbic keratoconjunctivitis, recurrent erosions, bullous keratopathy, and patching. Patients have a red eye and complain of moderate-to-severe pain and foreign body sensation. The filaments stain with fluorescein and the unattached end moves with blinking.

Filaments may be removed with fine forceps or a cotton-tipped applicator after topical anesthesia. The underlying condition should be appropriately treated. Lubrication with preservative-free artificial tear drops and treatment with topical acetylcysteine (10%) usually works well. Punctal occlusion is indicated when filaments are secondary to severe dry eyes, and temporary punctal occlusion may be helpful in superior limbic keratitis. Occasionally, a bandage soft contact lens may be tried for filamentary keratitis in the absence of dry eyes.

Exposure or Neurotrophic Keratopathy

Exposure keratopathy results from inadequate eyelid closure that causes corneal drying. It often occurs in conjunction with neurotrophic keratopathy, which is corneal surface dis-

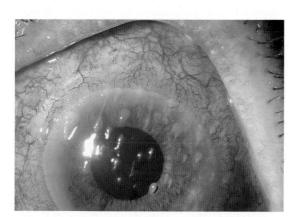

FIGURE 1.67. In filamentary keratopathy, strands of epithelial cells intertwined with mucous debris are attached to the cornea. The filaments stain with fluorescein.

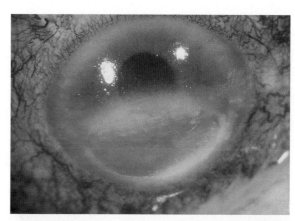

FIGURE 1.68. Exposure keratopathy can be complicated by an inferior corneal epithelial defect, in this case due to a Bell's palsy in a diabetic patient who also had decreased corneal sensation.

ease secondary to decreased corneal sensation. Patients with exposure keratopathy typically complain of mild-to-moderate pain and foreign body sensation, but patients with neurotrophic keratopathy have few symptoms. Superficial punctate fluorescein staining is found in the area of the palpebral fissure and in the lower one third of the cornea. The conjunctiva is often injected and may also stain with fluorescein or rose bengal. More advanced cases can have corneal infiltration, ulceration, or perforation (Fig. 1.68).

The underlying cause of the exposure (e.g., eyelid deformity, proptosis from thyroid disease) or neurotrophic keratopathy (e.g., acoustic neuroma) should be evaluated and treated. Mild conditions can be managed with artificial tear drops and ointments, and more advanced conditions may require eyelid taping at bedtime, patching, tarsorrhaphy, or conjunctival flap surgery.

Ocular Rosacea

Rosacea is a chronic, inflammatory condition that mainly affects the skin of the face. Patients develop mild-to-severe erythema along with telangiectasias and papules of the cheeks, nose, and forehead (Fig. 1.69A). Similar features can develop on the eyelid margins (Fig. 1.69B), affecting the meibomian gland secretions and creating ocular redness, burning, and a foreign body sensation. In more advanced cases, peripheral corneal neovascularization, infiltration, and even ulceration and perforation can occur. Rhinophyma can develop in severely affected patients, especially males.

Warm compresses, eyelid hygiene, and topical antibiotic ointment applied to the eyelid margins are the mainstays of treatment. Oral tetracycline, doxycycline, minocycline, or erythromycin can be extremely helpful in quieting the inflammation of the eyelid margins and meibomian glands. In patients requiring long-term treatment with oral medications, the initial dose is often tapered.

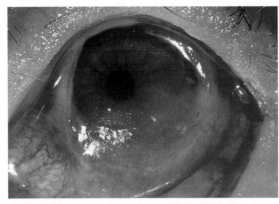

FIGURE 1.70. One month after the acute onset of Stevens-Johnson syndrome, there is still active conjunctival and corneal inflammation and already significant symblepharon formation.

Stevens-Johnson Syndrome

Stevens-Johnson syndrome (i.e., erythema multiform major) is a severe hypersensitivity reaction affecting the skin and mucous membranes. Precipitating factors include drugs such as penicillin, sulfa, and antiseizure medications and infections such as HSV infection or mycoplasma pneumonia.

The acute phase, which can last 6 or more weeks, is characterized by bullous eruptions of the skin (i.e., target lesions) and mucosal ulceration. Ocular manifestations include an acute pseudomembranous conjunctivitis, persistent corneal epithelial defects, and symblepharon formation (Fig. 1.70). The mortality rate can be as high as 20% to 33%. Chronic ocular findings include symblepharon, dry eye syndrome, trichiasis, corneal vascularization, scarring, erosions, and ulceration.

During the acute phase, topical steroids, antibiotics, and lubricants are used. Systemic steroids are controversial. Long-term treatment with lubrication and correction of eyelid abnormalities such as trichiasis are typically required.

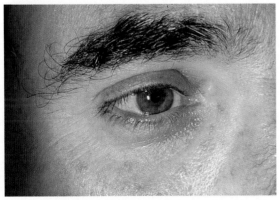 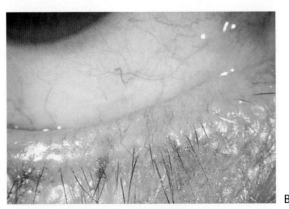

FIGURE 1.69. A: The skin changes of acne rosacea include telangiectasias, erythema, and papules of the cheeks, nose, and forehead. (Courtesy of Guy F. Webster, M.D., Ph.D., Philadelphia, PA.) **B:** Eyelid margin telangiectasias are typically seen in ocular rosacea.

Keratoprosthesis surgery can be considered for end-stage disease in patients with good optic nerve and retinal function.

Ocular Cicatricial Pemphigoid

Ocular cicatricial pemphigoid is a chronic vesiculobullous disease of mucous membranes and skin that typically has a gradual onset. Its underlying cause is most likely autoimmune, although it has also been associated with certain topical medications.

Patients with ocular cicatricial pemphigoid usually are older than 60 years of age, and more women than men are affected. It is usually bilateral, with a pattern of remissions and exacerbations. The hallmarks of ocular cicatricial pemphigoid are conjunctival symblepharon and inferior forniceal foreshortening (Fig. 1.71A). The condition often produces progressive conjunctival scarring, dry eye syndrome, trichiasis, entropion, and corneal neovascularization, scarring, and ulceration (Fig. 1.71B,C).

A diagnostic conjunctival biopsy for immunofluorescent studies can be performed. Treatment includes intensive lubrication and prevention of secondary problems from glaucoma and eyelid abnormalities. Immunosuppressant therapy with dapsone, cyclophosphamide, or methotrexate is indicated for progressive disease. The clinical course and response to treatment vary greatly.

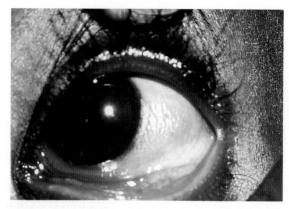

FIGURE 1.72. In vitamin A deficiency, the conjunctiva is extremely dry and lacks its normal luster. Notice the absence of a normal tear lake. (Courtesy of D.E. Silverstone, M.D., New Haven, CT.)

Vitamin A Deficiency

Vitamin A deficiency, also called xerophthalmia, is seen in extremely malnourished patients or those with defective vitamin A absorption or metabolism, as after gastrointestinal surgery. A slit lamp examination reveals bilateral conjunctival and corneal dryness (Fig. 1.72). Triangular gray-white spots (i.e., Bitot's spots) can be seen on the perilimbal conjunctiva in the palpebral fissure.

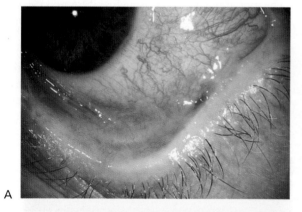

A

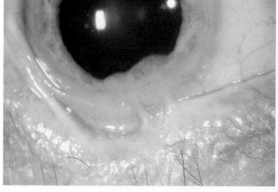

B

C

FIGURE 1.71. A: The hallmark of ocular cicatricial pemphigoid (OCP) is inferior forniceal foreshortening. **B:** Severe symblepharon formation can create adhesions between the eyelid and cornea. **C:** In end stage OCP there is obliteration of the fornices and keratinization of the ocular surface.

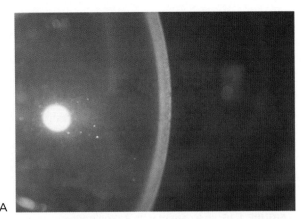
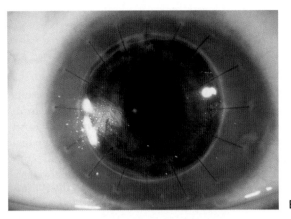

A   B

FIGURE 1.73. A: In Maroteaux-Lamy syndrome, clouding involves the entire cornea and is full thickness. This clouding usually develops after birth. **B:** Successful corneal transplantation may improve vision, but visual recovery may be limited by associated conditions such as optic atrophy, which was present preoperatively in this case due to meningeal involvement that became much worse when the patient developed hydrocephalus.

The underlying cause should be evaluated and treated. Systemic vitamin A replacement therapy is often necessary. Intensive lubrication with preservative-free artificial tears and ointments is required for the surface disease.

Mucopolysaccharidoses

The mucopolysaccharidoses are a family of inherited disorders of carbohydrate metabolism allowing mucopolysaccharides to accumulate in tissue. These conditions are autosomal recessive, except for Hunter's syndrome, which is an X-linked recessive condition.

Most of these disorders cause corneal clouding, retinopathy, and optic nerve disease. Sanfilippo's syndrome and Hunter's syndrome typically do not cause cloudy corneas. Corneal clouding usually involves full thickness cornea and is usually not present at birth (Fig. 1.73A). If the corneal clouding is severe, penetrating keratoplasty is recommended (Fig.1.73B). Genetic counseling is indicated.

Sphingolipidoses

Sphingolipidoses are a family of inherited lipid storage disorders. All are autosomal recessive except for Fabry's disease, which is an X-linked recessive condition. These disorders generally affect the retina. Fabry's disease can also cause renal failure. Patients with Fabry's disease and carriers demonstrate cornea verticillata, golden brown, whorl-like lines at the base of the corneal epithelium (Fig. 1.74). Milder corneal changes can occur from medications such as chloroquine, hydroxychloroquine, indomethacin, and amiodarone. Patients with Fabry's disease can also develop conjunctival and retinal vascular abnormalities.

Because visual acuity is not affected by cornea verticillata,

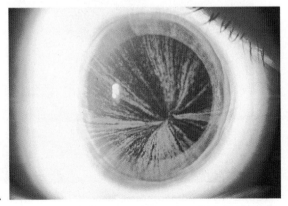
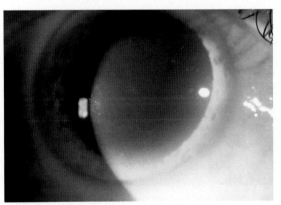

A   B

FIGURE 1.74. A: Cornea verticillata, characterized by brownish, whorl-like patterns in the epithelium, is seen in patients who have or are carriers of Fabry's disease (i.e., sphingolipidosis). **B:** Cornea verticillata can also be seen in patients using systemic medications such as chloroquine, hydroxychloroquine, indomethacin, and amiodarone (as in this case).

no treatment is needed. Genetic counseling is recommended.

Cystinosis

Cystinosis is an autosomal recessive metabolic defect resulting in cystine crystal deposition in tissue. The infantile form is fatal without kidney transplantation. The adult form demonstrates anterior segment crystals but not kidney disease. All patients demonstrate cystine crystals in the conjunctiva, cornea, and iris (Fig. 1.75). Severe forms also have lenticular and retinal crystals. The crystals typically do not affect visual acuity, but patients may be photophobic.

In severe cases, penetrating keratoplasty can be considered. Genetic counseling should be provided.

Wilson's Disease

Wilson's disease is an autosomal recessive degeneration of liver and kidney function that can cause neurologic damage. The primary ophthalmic finding is a Kayser-Fleischer's ring, a brownish green band of copper deposition in the deep peripheral cornea (Fig. 1.76). It typically is 1 to 3 mm wide and is deep in the peripheral cornea at the level of Descemet's membrane. It occurs first superiorly and then inferiorly and is detected earliest by gonioscopy.

The ocular findings do not require treatment. Referral to an internist and neurologist for a complete workup and treatment can be life saving.

Adrenochrome Deposits

Adrenochrome deposits are melanin-like pigment accumulations of oxidized epinephrine. They can be found imbedded in the conjunctiva, typically interiorly (Fig. 1.77). Patients usually have a history of topical epinephrine use for glaucoma.

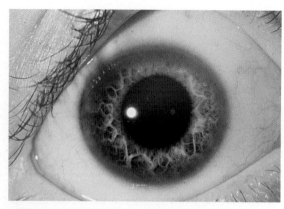

FIGURE 1.76. In a patient with Wilson's disease, a dense Kayser-Fleischer's ring, which is a brownish green band of copper deposition, is seen in the deep peripheral cornea.

Floppy Eyelid Syndrome

Floppy eyelid syndrome typically develops in obese patients with extremely lax eyelids, which can evert spontaneously or with minimal manipulation. Classically, the eyelids evert and rub on the pillow or sheets while the patient is sleeping.

Patients complain of ocular irritation, redness, and foreign body sensation. They have extremely lax, rubbery, redundant upper eyelids that evert with minimal force. There is a fine, diffuse papillary reaction of the upper tarsal conjunctiva (Fig. 1.78). The cornea may reveal superficial punctate staining, peripheral neovascularization, or a frank epithelial defect.

A protective plastic shield over the eyes at night can prevent the eyelids from rubbing on external surfaces. Taping the eyelids closed at night can also prevent spontaneous eversion. Occasionally, a surgical eyelid tightening procedure is required.

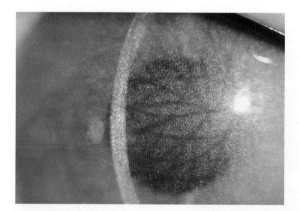

FIGURE 1.75. In cystinosis, cystine crystals are apparent throughout the full thickness of the cornea. Depending on the severity of the disease, crystals can also be seen in the conjunctiva, iris, lens, and retina.

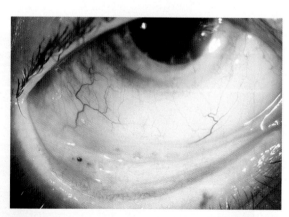

FIGURE 1.77. Adrenochrome deposits are brownish black, melanin-like pigment accumulations that are often evident in the inferior conjunctiva in patients on long-term regimens of epinephrine drops.

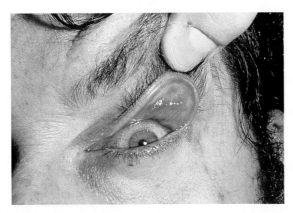

FIGURE 1.78. Floppy eyelid syndrome. The patient has an extremely lax upper eyelid that everts easily on examination and often everts spontaneously during sleep or with minimal manipulation during eye examination.

Superior Limbic Keratoconjunctivitis

Superior limbic keratoconjunctivitis is a bilateral, inflammatory condition of the conjunctiva and cornea of unknown cause that is characterized by remissions and exacerbations. Patients complain of mild to severe ocular dryness, irritation, and foreign body sensation. External examination reveals a superior sectorial conjunctivitis. Slit lamp examination demonstrates a thickened, inflamed superior bulbar conjunctiva with punctate fluorescein or rose bengal staining (Fig. 1.79). There is a fine, velvety, papillary response of the upper palpebral conjunctiva, and there is often punctate staining of the superior peripheral cornea. Filaments can be seen superiorly.

Because many of these patients have associated thyroid dysfunction, thyroid function tests should be obtained. Treatment of superior limbic keratoconjunctivitis involves a stepwise approach that includes lubrication, punctal occlu-sion by silicone plugs, ½% silver nitrate solution applications, local thermal cautery, and local conjunctival resection.

Thygeson's Superficial Punctate Keratopathy

Thygeson's superficial punctate keratopathy is a bilateral inflammatory condition of the cornea. Its cause is unknown, and it undergoes remissions and exacerbations. Symptoms include mild-to-moderate light sensitivity and foreign body sensation, with or without mildly decreased vision. Slit lamp examination reveals a noninflamed conjunctiva. The cornea demonstrates small, punctate, white, slightly elevated, snowflake-shaped epithelial and subepithelial opacities that usually have mild superficial staining (Fig. 1.80).

In mild cases, artificial tear drops may significantly improve the symptoms. Most patients require a tapering dose of mild topical steroids to control the symptoms, and occasionally, a bandage soft contact lens is used.

Terrien's Marginal Degeneration

Terrien's marginal degeneration is a slowly progressive, unilateral or bilateral, essentially noninflammatory, peripheral corneal thinning disorder seen more commonly in men.

The patients' eyes are white, typically with no history of inflammation or an epithelial defect. Vision may be decreased from irregular astigmatism. Slit lamp examination reveals a mildly to severely thinned peripheral cornea, which usually begins superiorly and can spread nasally and temporally. There are commonly lipid deposits at the leading edge of the vascularized, thinned cornea (Fig. 1.81).

The primary problem is decreased vision from irregular astigmatism, which can usually be successfully treated with a rigid gas-permeable contact lens. Rarely, the thinning is so

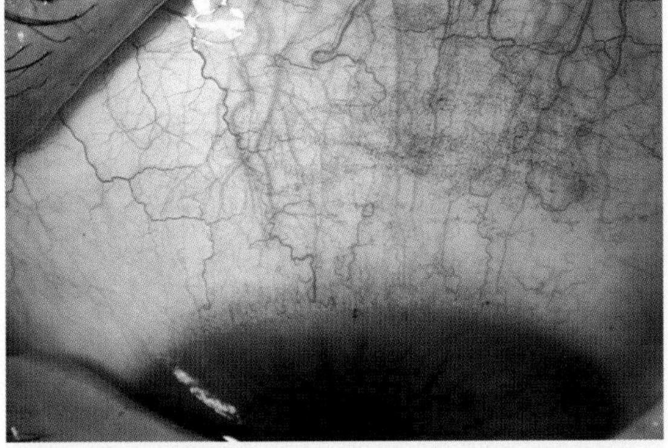

FIGURE 1.79. In superior limbic keratoconjunctivitis, there is superior, radial, conjunctival injection and fine staining with rose bengal.

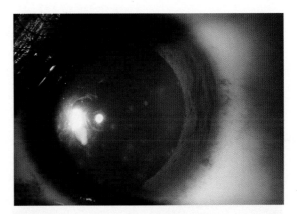

FIGURE 1.80. In Thygeson's superficial punctate keratopathy, small, white, slightly elevated, snowflake epithelial or subepithelial opacities are evident. These opacities usually stain with fluorescein.

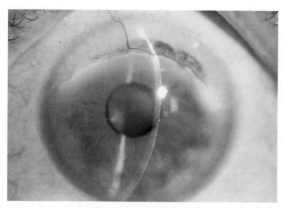

FIGURE 1.81. Superior, mildly vascularized corneal thinning with lipid at the leading edge is characteristic of Terrien's marginal degeneration.

severe that perforation with mild trauma is possible. In such cases, a lamellar corneoscleral graft may be required for tectonic purposes.

Mooren's Ulcer

Mooren's ulcer is a unilateral or bilateral, chronic, progressive, painful thinning and ulceration of the peripheral cornea. The underlying cause is unknown.

Mooren's ulcers typically begin in the nasal or temporal periphery or both areas. The ulceration can progress rapidly circumferentially and centrally, with an undermined leading edge (Fig. 1.82). It may progress more slowly toward the sclera. The ulceration may go down to Descemet's membrane and may lead to perforation. Older patients tend to have a more benign form that involves only one eye and responds well to treatment. Younger patients, many of whom are of African descent, tend to have a more aggressive form of the disease that involves both eyes and is minimally responsive to treatment.

The workup, which is similar to that for scleritis, attempts to identify an underlying cause. Ocular treatment, depending on the severity, includes topical lubricants, topical antibiotics, topical and systemic steroids, and other immunosuppressive agents, such as cyclophosphamide or methotrexate. Surgical options include conjunctival resection, cryotherapy, conjunctival flap, cyanoacrylate glue, and lamellar or penetrating keratoplasty.

Rheumatoid Melt

Unilateral or bilateral peripheral corneal ulceration can develop in patients with collagen vascular diseases. Slit lamp examination reveals a peripheral or occasionally a central corneal epithelial defect and ulceration. There may be mild-to-moderate associated inflammation (Fig. 1.83). If the epithelial defect does not heal, the ulceration can become larger and deeper and even progress to perforation.

The underlying collagen vascular disorder should be treated. The goal of ocular treatment is to decrease inflammation and heal the epithelial defect. Healing is typically accomplished using topical lubricants or antibiotics, and occasionally using systemic steroids and other immunosuppressive agents. Punctal occlusion and temporary or permanent lateral tarsorrhaphy can work well to heal the epithelium. Tissue adhesive or corneal surgery may be needed if other treatments fail.

Megalocornea

Megalocornea is considered to be nonprogressive corneal enlargement (>13 mm horizontally), not the result of congenital glaucoma. It is usually bilateral. Because it is an X-linked recessive disorder, it is found mostly in males.

The enlarged cornea is clear and has a normal thickness (Fig. 1.84). The enlarged corneal ring stretches the zonular fibers and predisposes the eye to develop a subluxed lens, glaucoma, or both. Routine follow-up examinations are re-

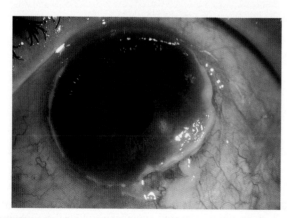

FIGURE 1.82. A severe, painful, peripheral corneal ulcerative process with an undermined leading edge and peripheral neovascularization is typical of a Mooren's ulcer. The underlying cause is unknown.

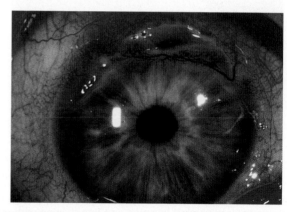

FIGURE 1.83. A peripheral corneal ulceration to the level of Descemet's membrane superiorly is found in this patient with rheumatoid arthritis and is known as a rheumatoid melt.

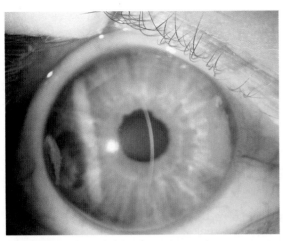

FIGURE 1.84. Megalocornea is a clear cornea with a horizontal diameter greater than 13 mm that is not the result of congenital glaucoma. The enlarged corneal ring predisposes the eye to develop a subluxed lens or glaucoma.

quired, especially monitoring for lens and glaucoma problems.

Microcornea

Microcornea exists when the horizontal corneal diameter is less than 10 to 11 mm. It can be unilateral or bilateral, autosomal dominant or recessive, and found in males and females.

The microcornea can be clear or cloudy (Fig. 1.85). These corneas are associated with hyperopia, because the corneas are often flat. The anterior chamber angles are crowded, predisposing the patient to angle closure glaucoma, but microcornea is also associated with open angle glaucoma. Routine follow-up examination is required, especially to monitor for glaucoma.

Sclerocornea

Sclerocornea involves nonprogressive scleralization of the peripheral or entire cornea. It is usually bilateral and occurs

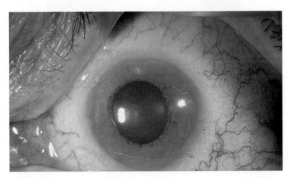

FIGURE 1.85. Microcornea is a small cornea that measures less than 10 to 11 mm horizontally. This patient's cornea was 9 mm in diameter.

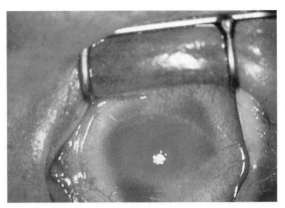

FIGURE 1.86. Sclerocornea is associated with greater corneal opacification peripherally than centrally.

in males and females. The scleral tissue masks only the limbus in mild cases and the entire cornea in severe cases (Fig. 1.86). The cornea is typically flat, with approximately the same curvature as the sclera.

Glasses or contact lenses can be used if the central cornea is clear to correct hyperopia associated with central corneal flattening. A corneal transplant can be attempted if the visual axis is involved. The prognosis for graft survival is worse than for Peters' anomaly, but has improved with the use of topical cyclosporine postoperatively.

Kerectasia

Kerectasia is a rare, severe ectasia of the cornea. It is probably not a developmental abnormality but is instead a result of an intrauterine corneal infection with corneal ulceration and often perforation. Fortunately, most cases are unilateral. The cornea is opaque and severely ectatic, bulging through the eyelid fissure and extending anterior to the eyelid margins (Fig. 1.87). Anterior segment reconstruction can be attempted, but the prognosis is extremely poor.

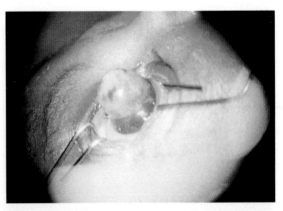

FIGURE 1.87. Kerectasia. This severe, anterior staphyloma was probably caused by an intrauterine corneal infection with ulceration and possible perforation.

DEVELOPMENTAL ANGLE ANOMALIES

Posterior Embryotoxon

Posterior embryotoxon is a prominent, slightly anteriorly displaced Schwalbe's ring. It is a variant of normal and does not have significant sequelae. A white, slightly irregular line just anterior to the limbus on the posterior cornea is seen on slit lamp examination (Fig. 1.88). It may be present in only a portion (several clock hours) of the cornea. No treatment is required.

Axenfeld's Anomaly and Syndrome

Axenfeld's anomaly is posterior embryotoxon with adherent iris stands (Fig. 1.89). Axenfeld's syndrome is Axenfeld's anomaly and glaucoma, which occurs in one half of the patients with Axenfeld's anomaly. Both conditions are autosomal dominant.

Peripheral iris processes are connected to a prominent, anteriorly displaced Schwalbe's ring (Fig. 1.90). If these are excessive, the angle is compromised, and glaucoma develops. Corneal edema may occur, probably caused by a decrease in the endothelial cells that migrate down the iris processes.

Routine follow-up examinations are needed, especially to monitor for corneal edema and glaucoma.

Rieger's Anomaly and Syndrome

Rieger's anomaly is the Axenfeld's anomaly plus iris stromal atrophy. One half of these eyes develop glaucoma. Rieger's syndrome is the Rieger's anomaly plus skeletal, dental, and other abnormalities. Both conditions are autosomal dominant.

Hypoplastic areas of iris stroma accompany the iris strands to the anteriorly displaced Schwalbe's ring (Fig. 1.91A). There may be associated peripheral anterior synechiae, corectopia, and pseudopolycoria (Fig. 1.91B).

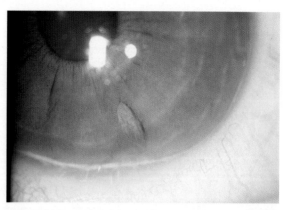

FIGURE 1.89. The anteriorly displaced Schwalbe's ring (i.e., posterior embryotoxon) with iris strands is prominent in this patient with Axenfeld's anomaly. An adjacent iris crypt is shown.

Typically, the pupil appears to be pulled toward the area of peripheral anterior synechiae, with iris stromal atrophy, which can progress to stretch holes, occurring 180 degrees away. Corneal edema can occur.

Routine follow-up examinations are needed, especially to monitor for glaucoma, cataract, and corneal edema.

Peters' Anomaly

Peters' anomaly is a spectrum of disorders that all include a central corneal scar with defects of the posterior cornea. One half of these eyes have glaucoma. Peters' anomaly is typically sporadic but can be inherited.

Along with the central corneal scar and abnormalities of the endothelium, Descemet's membrane, and posterior stroma, there may be iris adhesions to the posterior cornea (Fig. 1.92A,B). Occasionally, a cataract develops that may also be adherent to the posterior cornea.

Management options, which depend on severity, include observation, sector iridectomy, and penetrating keratoplasty with or without cataract and glaucoma surgery.

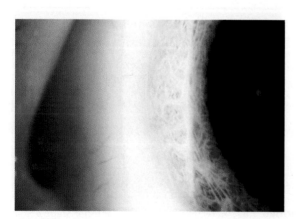

FIGURE 1.88. Posterior embryotoxon. A prominent, anteriorly displaced Schwalbe's ring occurs in many normal eyes.

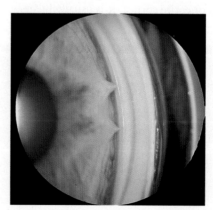

FIGURE 1.90. A gonioscopic view reveals iris strands adherent to the Schwalbe's ring in the eye of a patient with Axenfeld's anomaly. The intraocular pressure was normal in this patient.

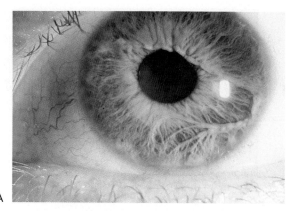

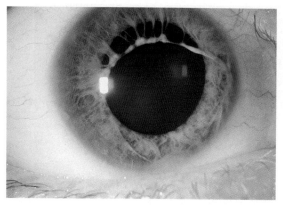

FIGURE 1.91. A: Rieger's anomaly. Iris strands extending to an anteriorly displaced Schwalbe's ring are associated with a large area of iris hypoplasia. **B:** The same patient's other eye revealed more severe iridocorneal adhesions and areas of iris atrophy.

TRAUMA

Corneal Abrasion

A corneal abrasion is the absence of an area of corneal epithelium that is usually caused by trauma. The patient complains of mild-to-severe ocular pain, foreign body sensation, tearing, and photophobia. Slit lamp examination reveals an area of fluorescein staining of the cornea (Fig. 1.93). A corneal abrasion can be associated with eyelid swelling, conjunctival injection, a mild anterior chamber reaction, and mild miosis. Corneal stromal edema may be seen with severe or with longstanding abrasions.

Treatment of routine traumatic corneal abrasions includes cycloplegia and frequent antibiotic ointment, and occasional pressure patching with a bandage soft contact lens. Corneal abrasions in contact lens wearers or those with a higher risk of infection, such as abrasions from vegetable matter or false fingernails, are treated with cycloplegia, antibiotic ointment, and no pressure patching, as pressure patching may encourage bacterial infection, particularly *Pseudomonas* infection. Patients are followed closely until the abrasion heals. If a corneal infiltrate develops, corneal smears and cultures and more aggressive antibiotic therapy are necessary.

Corneal Laceration

Trauma to the eye can cause a partial-thickness or full-thickness defect in the cornea (Fig. 1.94).

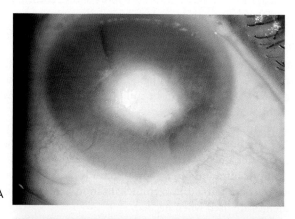

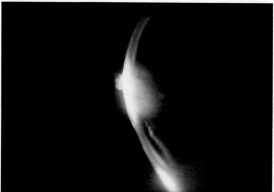

FIGURE 1.92. A: Peters' anomaly. A dense central corneal scar and iris abnormalities are found in the patient's eye. **B:** The slit lamp view of the same eye reveals iris adhesions to the posterior cornea.

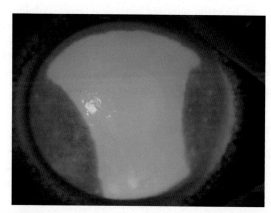

FIGURE 1.93. A large, traumatic corneal abrasion stains brightly with the cobalt blue light after topical fluorescein instillation.

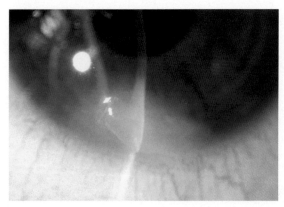

FIGURE 1.94. This eye demonstrates a peripheral corneal laceration with a formed anterior chamber. However, because it was Seidel-positive with poorly opposed wound edges, it was emergently surgically repaired.

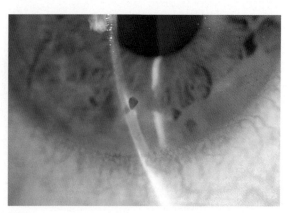

FIGURE 1.95. Corneal foreign body. The end of a thorn is apparent deep in the corneal stroma. Because it did not perforate Descemet's membrane, this eye was not Seidel-positive.

A Seidel test is used to help determine whether a laceration involves the partial or full thickness of the cornea. The area in question is painted with fluorescein dye and examined at the slit lamp with the cobalt blue light to determine if aqueous is leaking out, causing fluorescence or a lightening of the yellow-green dye. Trauma severe enough to cause a corneal laceration may also lead to iris prolapse, scleral laceration, cataract formation, and hyphema.

Corneal lacerations can be treated with observation or surgical repair, depending on the size and depth of the laceration and on associated ocular damage. Generally, large partial-thickness and most full-thickness corneal lacerations are surgically repaired. Patients with full-thickness corneal lacerations are treated with several days of systemic antibiotics to prevent endophthalmitis.

Corneal Foreign Body

A corneal foreign body can result from minor or more severe corneal trauma. Patients complain of ocular redness, pain, light sensitivity, and a foreign body sensation. A foreign body is detected by slit lamp examination.

Surface foreign bodies, such as a seed cover or an insect wing, can be easily removed with fine forceps while using the slit lamp. Deeper foreign bodies also may be removable using the slit lamp. However, very deep and full-thickness foreign bodies are best removed in the operating room (Fig. 1.95). Antibiotics and follow-up evaluations are important to prevent corneal and intraocular infection.

Corneal Rust Ring

Metal corneal foreign bodies can rapidly deposit rust in the underlying and surrounding corneal tissue. A reddish brown, circular opacity in the anterior stroma has an overlying epithelial defect (Fig. 1.96).

The metal foreign body should be removed first. Occasionally, the rust ring can be removed in one piece with a foreign body spud or 23-gauge needle. More often, the rust ring should be removed with a small hand-held rust ring drill. The corneal abrasion is then treated and followed to ensure healing.

Chemical Burn

Chemical burns may be caused by acids or alkali. Injuries from either can be mild or severe. Alkali tends to penetrate the cornea more rapidly and cause more severe corneal and intraocular damage than acid.

The clinical manifestations of chemical burns vary from mild conjunctivitis to superficial punctate keratopathy to epithelial erosions, which can lead to corneal opacities and corneal perforation, depending on the severity of the injury (Fig. 1.97). There also can be mild to extensive damage of the conjunctiva and eyelids.

No matter how severe the burn, immediate treatment includes copious irrigation and removal of any particulate matter. After a neutral pH has been reached, topical antibiotics, lubricants, and often topical steroids are used to prevent infection and aid in reepithelialization. Antiglaucoma medicines are used when needed.

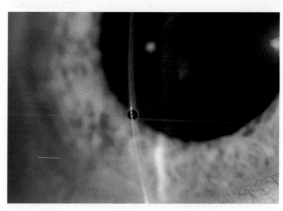

FIGURE 1.96. Corneal rust ring. A small, reddish brown, circular opacity remained in the cornea after the removal of an iron foreign body.

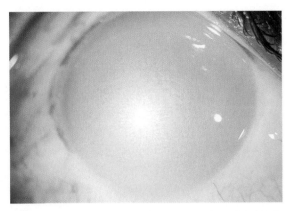

FIGURE 1.97. Alkali burn. Significant corneal, conjunctival, and scleral damage occurred after a severe alkali injury. Notice the opacified cornea and the conjunctival and scleral blanching, indicating severe damage to the surrounding blood vessels.

Topical steroids should be discontinued after 7 to 10 days because they can promote corneal melting and perforation. Close follow-up is required until reepithelialization has occurred. Long term corneal defects (weeks to months) have been treated with oral tetracycline, fibronectin, nerve growth factor and autologous serum, among others, in experimental designs.

Hyphema

A hyphema is defined as blood in the anterior chamber, most commonly from blunt or penetrating trauma or intraocular surgery.

A microhyphema is composed of red blood cells suspended in the aqueous fluid, and a frank hyphema is the layering of blood or a clot in the anterior chamber. There can be associated conjunctival, corneal, iris, and scleral damage (Fig. 1.98A). A longstanding hyphema, especially in an eye with compromised corneal endothelium or elevated intraocular pressure, may cause blood staining of the cornea. Blood staining clears from the periphery of the cornea but can take months (Fig. 1.98B).

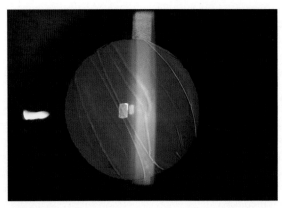

FIGURE 1.99. Oblique breaks in Descemet's membrane are evident using retroillumination. The trauma was caused by forceps used during delivery.

Postoperative hyphemas tend to resolve without rebleeding. Traumatic hyphemas from blunt trauma are treated with bed rest, atropine drops, oral antifibrinolytic agents such as aminocaproic acid, and occasionally with topical steroids to prevent rebleeding. The intraocular pressure should be monitored and treated if elevated. Patients with hyphema who are sickle disease positive or trait positive are at greater risk for the development of complications and should be monitored carefully. Hyphema patients are at risk for developing angle recession glaucoma in the future.

Birth Trauma

A mechanical forceps injury to the cornea during delivery can cause a break in Descemet's membrane, leading to corneal edema. It is usually unilateral. Corneal stromal edema is evident within days of a forceps-assisted birth. Descemet's membrane breaks are typically vertical or oblique (Fig. 1.99). The corneal edema generally clears over weeks to months but may recur many years later.

Cycloplegic and hypertonic agents can be used for symptomatic relief. After the edema clears, the eyes often reveal

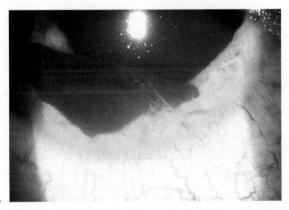

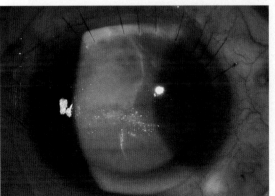

A   B

FIGURE 1.98. A: In hyphema, a blood clot is in the anterior chamber after a corneal laceration with damage to the iris. **B:** Central, red-brown corneal blood staining is clearing from the periphery months after a complete hyphema.

myopic astigmatism, which can cause amblyopia if not appropriately treated.

EPITHELIAL CORNEAL DYSTROPHIES

Cogan's Microcytic Dystrophy

Cogan's microcytic dystrophy is an anterior corneal dystrophy affecting the epithelium and epithelial basement membrane. It is part of the spectrum of dystrophies known as epithelial basement membrane corneal dystrophies. This dystrophy may be inherited, although it can also occur spontaneously.

The intraepithelial cysts range in size from barely discernible pinpoint spots to larger, oval, and irregularly shaped cysts, all within the corneal epithelium (Fig. 1.100). The cysts consist of cytoplasmic and nuclear debris and may be found in all layers of the corneal epithelium. They are usually centrally located, unilateral or bilateral, and do not incite corneal vascularization or associated stromal haze (Fig. 1.101). They are recognized as part of a dystrophic process involving the basement membrane of the corneal epithelium. When the cysts are numerous, large, and present in the visual axis, they may cause blurred vision from irregular astigmatism. Patients who have these cysts are more prone to recurrent corneal erosions if their corneas are damaged, and they may also suffer spontaneous corneal erosions. The cysts are accompanied by map-like or fingerprint lines that are fine, linear changes surrounding the cysts.

When the cysts are few and small, they cause no symptoms. When they are larger and accompanied by maps and fingerprints in the visual axis, blurred vision occurs. Lubricating drops, such as artificial tears, during the day and ointment at bedtime may make the slightly symptomatic (from erosions) patient comfortable. If the cysts are more numerous, if they affect vision, or if there are recurrent erosions, mechanical debridement of the epithelium, cysts, and the underlying basement membrane is important. If the

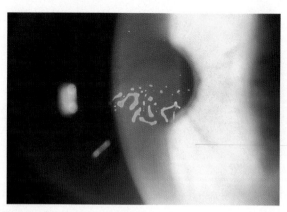

FIGURE 1.101. A close-up view of an area of Cogan's microcysts shows a pinpoint microcyst, a slightly larger intraepithelial milky white microcyst, and several large geographic figures that are also microcysts. In this patient, this condition caused a slightly elevated epithelium and irregular astigmatism with blurred vision, because the visual axis was involved.

basement membrane is left, the cysts may recur. If mechanical debridement is not helpful and the patient suffers from recurrent erosions, anterior stromal reinforcement (puncture) is sometimes performed. Excimer laser phototherapeutic keratectomy just into Bowman's membrane, approximately 5 to 8 μm deep, has been successful.

Map-Dot Fingerprint Dystrophy

The map-dot fingerprint dystrophy is an anterior, epithelial basement membrane dystrophy that includes Cogan's microcysts (i.e., the dots), map-like changes produced by areas of basement membrane present within the epithelium, and fingerprints, which are parallel rows of basement membrane within the epithelium (Figs. 1.102 and 1.103).

The dots, or Cogan's microcysts, are intraepithelial, milky cysts that occur at the edge of grayish, fine map lines.

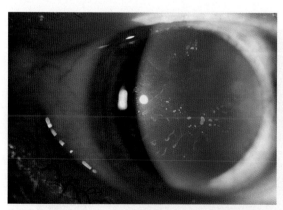

FIGURE 1.100. Cogan's microcystic dystrophy is composed of intraepithelial microcysts appearing as tiny, milky white dots. The microcysts appear against a background of map-like changes.

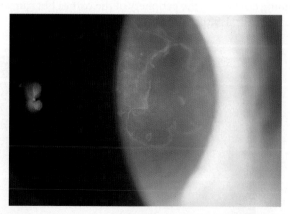

FIGURE 1.102. A close-up view of the map-like changes that represent the pattern of the basement membrane within the corneal epithelium. This condition may slightly elevate the corneal epithelium and, when in the visual axis, cause irregular astigmatism and blurred vision.

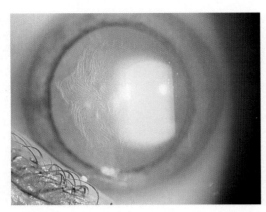

FIGURE 1.103. Part of the map-dot fingerprint changes can be seen in retroillumination against the dilated pupil. Parallel rows of thickened basement membrane in a map-like pattern give it a fingerprint-like appearance.

Usually, maps occur without the microcysts. The microcysts represent desquamating epithelial cells that are entrapped beneath the abnormal basement membrane sheets within the epithelium, preventing these cells, which later form cysts, from sloughing. The parallel thickening of basement membrane in adjacent rows forms the fingerprint lines.

With minimal map-dot fingerprint changes in the visual axis, lubricating drops and a bland ointment at bedtime are all that is required. In many cases, patients with mild map-dot fingerprint alterations of the superficial cornea need no treatment. When the changes are in the visual axis and obscure vision, mechanical debridement is the treatment choice. If there are recurrent corneal erosions associated with this disease, anterior stromal reinforcement (puncture) is sometimes helpful to enhance adhesion of the epithelium to prevent the erosions. For the most part, patients with map-dot fingerprint dystrophy can be observed. Lubricating ointments may be all that is required for minor symptoms. In more severe cases, excimer laser physiotherapeutic keratectomy or anterior stromal puncture is used. This is a self-limited disease that occurs in patients between 20 and 60 years of age, and it is seldom symptomatic in patients older than 60 years of age.

Meesmann's Dystrophy

Also called juvenile epithelial corneal dystrophy, Meesmann's dystrophy is a disorder of the corneal epithelium that is inherited in an autosomal dominant pattern. Multiple, fine, pinpoint or small cysts are seen in the corneal epithelium. Pathologic analysis reveals a fibrogranular, "peculiar" substance that stains for mucopolysaccharide within the epithelial cells.

The epithelial cysts are numerous, occurring almost from limbus to limbus, and do not affect the stroma (Fig. 1.104). The cysts are seen early in life, are usually stationary, and cause minor interference with visual acuity. Patients may

develop recurrent corneal erosions, for which mechanical debridement is sometimes helpful. The cysts recur with regeneration of the epithelium. Lubricating drops or ointment is usually all that is needed for this very mild dystrophy. Lamellar corneal transplantation and superficial keratectomy are unnecessary. The use of soft contact lenses has been helpful in some cases but is usually not required.

Corneal Dystrophies of Bowman's Layer

Reis in 1917 and Bucklers in 1949 described a dystrophy that was dominantly inherited and usually appeared in the first decade of life. Painful corneal erosions and moderately to significantly reduced vision were the main symptoms. Unfortunately, histopathology was not included in their reports. This dystrophy consisted of geographic opacities in the region of Bowman's layer and superficial stroma. Recurrent corneal erosions were common and occurred with significant pain in the first and second decades of life. Eventually, scarring ensued with corneal anesthesia, which led to marked decrease in vision. Reis-Bucklers' corneal dystrophy is now considered by many authors to be the same as a superficial variant of granular dystrophy. It is still confused with the honeycomb dystrophy of Thiel and Benhke.

There are two schools of thought concerning these changes. First, those who tend to lump them all together and call them variants of the same dystrophy (Reis-Bucklers'), and those who separate them. These dystrophies involving Bowman's layer generally have similar symptoms and are treated alike. Light and electron microscopy have helped in differentiating these dystrophies of Bowman's layer. The clinical course and light and electron microscopic findings have recently been reviewed by Kuchle and colleagues. They feel the dystrophies involving Bowman's layer should be divided into two groups: first, corneal dystrophy of Bowman's layer type I (CDB-I), which is the "true" Reis-

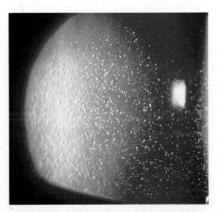

FIGURE 1.104. Meesmann's corneal dystrophy, which is best viewed in retroillumination against the dilated pupil, produces multiple, pinpoint cysts within the corneal epithelium. These cysts usually do not cause significant visual loss and do not stain with any diagnostic dyes.

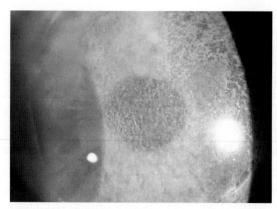

FIGURE 1.105. CDB-I or "true" Reis-Bucklers' corneal dystrophy. This also has been called superficial variant of granular dystrophy because of the rod-like granules noted in the superficial cornea in the region of Bowman's layer and superficial stroma.

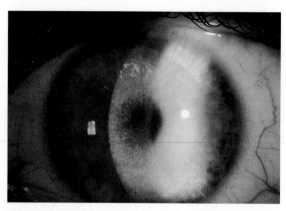

FIGURE 1.107. Following excimer laser phototherapeutic keratectomy, this patient had a recurrence of CDB-I "true" Reis-Bucklers' corneal dystrophy or superficial variant of granular dystrophy. Repeat excimer laser phototherapeutic keratectomy can be done as the pathology is superficial and the laser does not ablate into the deeper cornea. Eventually, a lamellar corneal transplant and possibly a penetrating corneal transplant may be necessary in a few patients.

Bucklers' dystrophy and also has been called the superficial variant of granular dystrophy; and corneal dystrophy of Bowman's layer type II (CDB-II), or the honeycomb dystrophy, which was originally described by Thiel and Benhke.

CDB-I is characterized by an autosomal dominant inheritance pattern with frequent recurrent corneal erosions starting early in life, leading to marked visual loss (Figs. 1.105, 1.106, and 1.107). The corneal dystrophy of Bowman's layer type II (CDB-II) (honeycomb-shaped or Thiel-Benhke's dystrophy), has a similar inheritance pattern and similar symptoms, but visual loss starts a little later in life and may not be as severe (Figs. 1.108 and 1.109).

The light microscopy findings in CDB-I consist of granular deposits in the region of Bowman's layer compared to CDB-II, where there was a fibrocellular, avascular, undulating layer giving the appearance of saw-tooth configuration between the epithelium and the stroma and replacing, for the most part, Bowman's layer. This did not

stain very well with Mason's trichrome in CDB-II but was markedly positive in CDB-I or the true Reis-Bucklers' dystrophy (superficial variant of granular dystrophy).

Electron microscopy differentiated these two entities involving Bowman's layer quite well. In CDB-I, there were rod-shaped granules present in the region of this pathology replacing Bowman's layer similar to the rod-shaped bodies in classical granular corneal dystrophy. In CDB-II, the subepithelial presence of an atypical peculiar collagen substance or "curly" filaments characterizes this dystrophy. This is now considered to be the honeycomb-shaped dystrophy of Thiel-Benhke.

In the early stages of both CDB-I and CDB-II, treatment consists of lubricating drops, patching, occasional bandage soft contact lenses, and antibiotic ointment to prevent infection. In the first decade of life when these dystrophies first occur, visual acuity is usually good between the episodes of

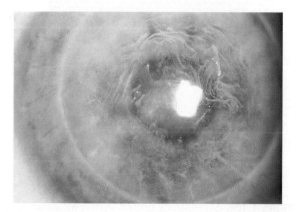

FIGURE 1.106. Recurrence of CDB-I after a corneal transplant. Notice the marked irregularity of the light reflex and the wavy pathology in the region of Bowman's layer. This patient required phototherapeutic keratectomy for visual recovery.

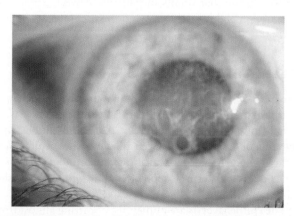

FIGURE 1.108. CDB-II or Thiel-Benhke's corneal dystrophy. In this dystrophy, also described as honeycomb-shaped, there are "curly" filaments in the superficial cornea in the region of Bowman's layer rather than the rod-like granules typical of CDB-I.

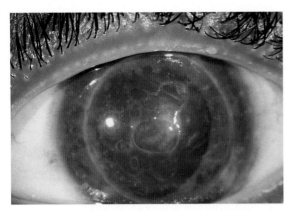

FIGURE 1.109. Recurrence of CDB-II in a patient who had a corneal transplant for severe dystrophic changes involving the superficial as well as the midcornea. This patient was first thought to have Reis-Bucklers' dystrophy but light and electron microscopy eventually revealed that curly filaments were present in the region of Bowman's layer and this represents CDB-II or Thiel-Benhke's honeycomb dystrophy. The treatment as in CDB-I is excimer laser phototherapeutic keratectomy and then when sufficient stroma is involved, either lamellar or penetrating corneal transplantation.

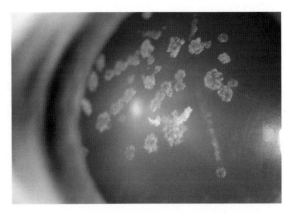

FIGURE 1.110. In granular dystrophy, hyaline deposits are sharply demarcated in the stroma and are surrounded by clear cornea.

corneal erosions. In the second and third decades, as scarring occurs, vision becomes more blurred and surgical treatment is necessary. Superficial kerectomy has been done to remove the scarring in the region of Bowman's layer. Usually a very superficial portion of the stroma is removed along with Bowman's layer and epithelium. It is generally easy to find a superficial stromal lamella where the pathology is minimal or has not occurred, allowing for a fairly smooth dissection. Now, excimer laser phototherapeutic keratectomy is the treatment of choice for this superficial corneal disease. There is recurrence of pathology after excimer laser phototherapeutic kerectomy, but considerably better vision is achieved for 1 to 4 years with this treatment and the necessity for corneal transplantation is delayed (Fig. 1.107).

Eventually, the disease recurs despite the dissections and excimer laser treatments, and either a lamellar or penetrating keratoplasty is required (Fig. 1.109). Recurrence of disease in the corneal transplant is common for both CDB-I and CDB-II, but the visual acuity is usually better as the superficial cornea may be clearer despite recurrence of disease in the graft. It is better to do a lamellar corneal transplant first because if the disease does recur in the graft, a repeat lamellar or penetrating keratoplasty may be necessary. These corneal dystrophies involving Bowman's layer usually do not cause recurrent erosion or pain after the third or fourth decades of life, although visual loss may be considerable.

STROMAL DYSTROPHIES

Granular Dystrophy

Granular dystrophy is a dominantly inherited, fairly common, and recognizable corneal dystrophy that has varied

manifestations and pathologic features. Treatment is seldom necessary in the first few decades of life as symptoms occur later as the dystrophy progresses.

As with most dominantly inherited corneal dystrophies, the pathology is central rather than peripheral and does not cause inflammation or vascularization of the cornea. Characteristic of this dystrophy are clear areas between the hyaline deposits in the stroma, which allows for good vision late into the course of the disease (Figs. 1.110 and 1.111). In some families, however, the clear stroma in the middle of the pathologic areas is compromised, causing decreased vision (Fig. 1.112). Recurrent corneal erosions can occur later in the course of the disease, but much of the visual loss is caused by the stromal hyaline deposits.

A new variation of granular dystrophy, called *Avellino dystrophy*, has been recognized. It has amyloid deposits in addition to the hyaline stromal deposits. Several families with this unusual combination have been traced back to Avellino, Italy, for which this granular dystrophy variation was named. Symptoms are similar to those of granular dystrophy, but the corneal changes are somewhat different (Fig. 1.113). Some of the stromal opacities are more irregular and elongated. Avellino dystrophy also is dominantly inherited.

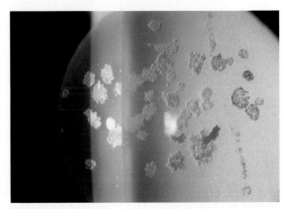

FIGURE 1.111. Retroillumination reveals the clarity of the stroma between deposits of hyaline in a case of granular corneal dystrophy.

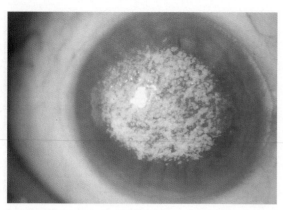

FIGURE 1.112. Granular dystrophy with confluent opacities can lead to superficial corneal erosions and blurred vision. Notice the irregular light reflex. In this case, there is no clear space between the hyaline deposits, and vision is significantly blurred. Penetrating keratoplasty is indicated.

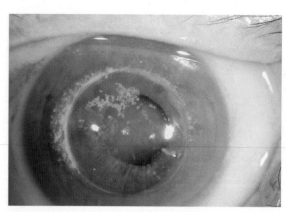

FIGURE 1.114. Recurrent granular dystrophy in a corneal transplant. This patient's original corneal transplant was done about 15 years before this photograph was taken. Notice the remaining granular dystrophy beyond the edge of the graft. Superficial granular deposits in the stroma have recurred. The patient still had good vision at the time of this photograph; regrafting was not indicated for another 10 years.

In the first few decades of life, no treatment is needed because vision is good and erosions usually do not occur. In some families, confluent pathology in the central cornea is found during the fourth decade and beyond. Depending on the extent of the central opacity and the response to visual correction with contact lenses and other means, penetrating corneal transplantation may be the treatment of choice. Excimer laser phototherapeutic keratectomy and lamellar keratoplasty usually are not options because of the depth of the defect in the middle and deeper stroma. Recurrence of hyaline and amyloid degeneration in the new transplant tissue is common (Fig. 1.114). The prognosis for corneal transplantation in granular dystrophy is generally excellent, with well over 90% of the corneas remaining clear for at least several years. Eventually, granular deposits may form in the superficial stroma and cause recurrent opacification and possible recurrent erosion.

The genetics of granular, lattice, and macular dystrophy have revealed that they all involve a mutation at the BIGH-3 gene.

Lattice Corneal Dystrophy

Amyloid deposits in the cornea characterize this dominantly inherited stromal dystrophy. Recurrent erosions may occur in the fourth decade and beyond, which lead to decreased corneal sensation, scar formation, and significantly decreased vision.

Lattice corneal dystrophy is a bilateral corneal dystrophy with linear deposits of hyaline in the stroma. Patients with this dystrophy must be differentiated from patients with prominent corneal nerves and blood vessels in the cornea, both linear findings that can be confused with lattice dystrophy. The epithelium and sub-Bowman's stroma are generally spared until the fourth decade of life (Fig. 1.115) or

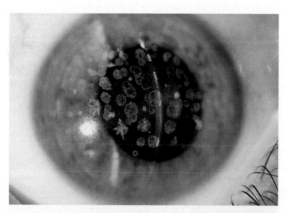

FIGURE 1.113. In granular corneal dystrophy, granular-appearing amyloid and hyaline degenerative changes were found in the stroma. This is the Avellino variation of granular dystrophy seen in families whose origin can be traced to the small hill town of Avellino, Italy.

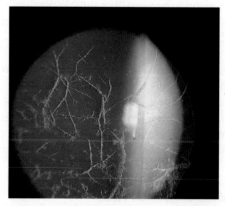

FIGURE 1.115. Retroillumination of lattice corneal dystrophy. Notice the typical thick, linear pattern of amyloid degeneration in the stroma. The relatively good light reflex indicates excellent vision, and the surrounding stroma is clear in this early case of amyloid deposits in the stroma.

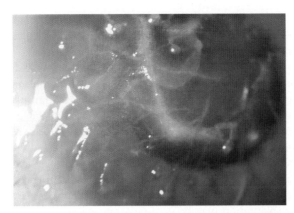

FIGURE 1.116. Recurrent erosion in lattice dystrophy shows marked filamentary keratitis and thick lattice changes. These erosions were painful and led to significant corneal scarring and the need for a corneal transplant.

later, when superficial erosions and filamentary keratitis occur (Fig. 1.116). These erosions may mimic the appearance of dendritic keratitis from HSV infection. The cornea becomes anesthetic, and Bowman's membrane and superficial stroma are replaced by scar tissue. These erosions are painful, and the marked irregular astigmatism and confluent scar formation causes decreased vision. As the corneal nerves are destroyed, the cornea becomes much less sensitive.

Symptoms can vary in any family and between families, with later generations developing problems earlier in life. With the continued erosions and laying down of more scar tissue with each erosive episode, it may take several years to a decade or more before vision is decreased enough to warrant surgical treatment.

At first, with only stromal lattice changes, no treatment is necessary. As the superficial pannus builds up, the irregular astigmatism that occurs can be treated with a soft or rigid gas-permeable contact lens. When this is insufficient, the superficial cornea may be peeled by superficial keratectomy or phototherapeutic keratectomy with excimer laser. Eventually, these means fail because repeated keratectomy becomes too deep to provide good vision. A penetrating corneal transplant is then required. These grafts are visually successful early, but amyloid deposits recur in the new graft tissue. These deposits are first seen in the periphery where sutures were placed and are later seen in the central stroma of the donor button (Fig. 1.117). Repeat corneal transplantation is also successful, but amyloid deposits develop in subsequent grafts. Lamellar corneal transplants are an alternative to penetrating grafts if the dissection bed can be extremely smooth. Automated microtomes are being developed which will do this.

Gelatinous Drop-like Dystrophy

Gelatinous drop-like dystrophy is another dystrophy that is caused by localized amyloid deposits. In this case, the deposits are superficial and cause visual loss early. It is a recessive disease that is usually seen in the first and second decades of life, causing severe loss of vision. There are no systemic findings associated with this amyloid dystrophy. The cornea develops multiple, confluent, epithelial and subepithelial, gelatinous, mulberry-like deposits that obscure vision (Fig. 1.118). Histopathologic analysis reveals mounds of amyloid between the corneal epithelium and Bowman's membrane and deeper deposits of amyloid in the stroma, similar to lattice dystrophy.

Superficial keratectomy is preferred over lamellar corneal transplantation or penetrating keratoplasty because the amyloid deposits and visual loss recur after each keratectomy.

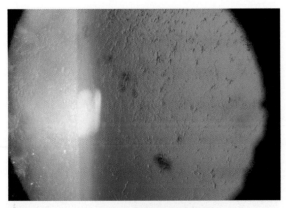

FIGURE 1.117. Recurrent lattice dystrophy is seen as fine deposits using retroillumination in the patient in Figure 1.116, who received a corneal transplant. About 4 years later, superficial deposits were detected in the cornea. These recurrences start along the suture tracks in the donor button and then can be seen, in some cases, in the superficial stroma.

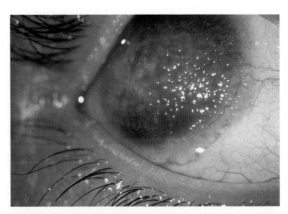

FIGURE 1.118. Gelatinous drop-like dystrophy. The mulberry appearance of superficial corneal deposits is easily recognized by the marked broken-light reflex from the corneal surface. The appearance of localized, superficial amyloid deposits characterizes this condition, for which superficial keratectomy is preferred over lamellar corneal transplants or penetrating grafts. The disease is often recurrent.

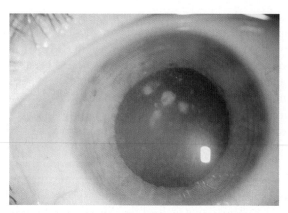

FIGURE 1.119. The diffuse corneal haze with highlighted white deposits typifies macular corneal dystrophy. The dystrophy is present from limbus to limbus and in all layers of the cornea, but visual acuity is not disturbed early in the course of the disease. Penetrating keratoplasty is indicated in the later course of this recessive corneal dystrophy.

Macular Corneal Dystrophy

Macular corneal dystrophy is the only major autosomal recessive stromal dystrophy. It results from the abnormal synthesis of keratin sulfate proteoglycan, occurs early in life, and causes visual loss in the first or second decade of life. Two types of this dystrophy have been described, one with systemic involvement and one without.

With accumulation of glycosaminoglycans within stromal keratocytes, the endothelium, and the stroma, there is a diffuse limbus-to-limbus haze in all layers of the stroma (Fig.1.119) accompanied by corneal thinning. Central, focal, white deposits are seen in the stroma against a background of variable stromal haze. These deposits become more diffuse, as does the background haze, leading to further visual loss (Fig. 1.120). Erosions do not occur, and vision may not be decreased as the corneal surface remains

smooth at first. With further deposits of glycosaminoglycan and a buildup of focal, white deposits, corneal opacification increases and corneal transplantation is needed.

Depending on the corneal background haze and focal, white deposits, penetrating corneal transplantation may be required for better vision. Generally, corneal transplantation may take place between 10 and 35 years of age, unlike treatment for the other stromal dystrophies. Disease recurs in the new graft, but the hazy opacity appears less often and later than does the recurrence of dystrophic changes in granular and lattice dystrophy grafts. Because all corneal layers are affected with recurrences, repeat penetrating corneal transplantation may be necessary, but is less likely and occurs later than in granular or lattice dystrophies.

Crystalline Dystrophy of Schnyder

The crystalline dystrophy of Schnyder is an autosomal dominant dystrophy that is less often seen than granular, lattice, and macular stromal dystrophies. It is largely inherited from people of Scandinavian background. An early sign of this stromal dystrophy is the characteristic crystals appearing in irregular, central, ring-like deposits in the first few years after birth.

The needle-shaped crystals are first faintly seen in a central, ring-like configuration. During the first four or five decades of life, these stromal crystals do not interfere with the epithelial surface, and vision is usually good (Fig. 1.121). Arcus senilis is usually prominent but does not always accompany the crystals. Significantly elevated triglycerides and serum cholesterol may be found in some affected individuals and family members. Some affected individuals may also demonstrate genu valgum, xanthelasma, and cardiovascular problems.

With age, more cholesterol crystals are deposited in the stroma, along with triglycerides and cholesterol esters. The cornea becomes more diffusely opacified, and the entire

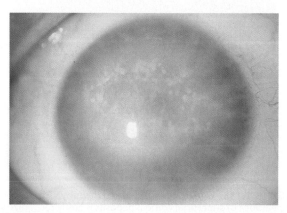

FIGURE 1.120. More severe involvement of macular corneal dystrophy than that seen in Figure 1.119, with a central corneal diffuse haze and decreased vision. Even though the light reflex is sharp, vision is decreased (20/70). Penetrating keratoplasty is indicated.

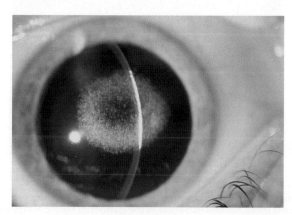

FIGURE 1.121. Although the opacity looks dense, this 28-year-old patient with Schnyder's crystalline dystrophy has 20/20 vision. The periphery of the cornea is clear, and the deposits are located in the superficial one third of the stroma.

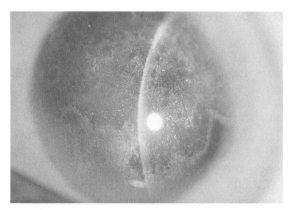

FIGURE 1.122. Later in the course of Schnyder's crystalline dystrophy, the deposits become diffuse, and no portion of the cornea is spared. When vision is significantly reduced by diffuse deposits and irregular astigmatism, penetrating keratoplasty is indicated.

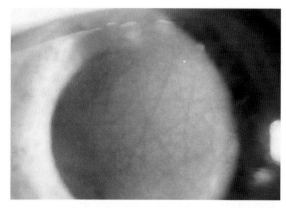

FIGURE 1.124. Central cloudy dystrophy of François should not be confused with posterior crocodile shagreen, shown here. In this normal, mild, corneal degeneration, there is no decompensation of the cornea and no corneal or epithelial edema. Both conditions are benign, and they can be differentiated by the linear pattern of haze in the deep cornea in posterior crocodile shagreen.

stroma, from limbus to limbus, is involved. The cornea takes on a more opaque whitish appearance and vision diminishes (Fig. 1.122). Corneal transplantation is generally required after age 45 years.

No treatment is required during the first decades of life because vision is usually excellent. Later, with further deposits of crystals and lipid permeating the corneal stroma, corneal transplantation is required. The transplants stay clear for many years, but cholesterol crystals, triglycerides, and cholesterol esters eventually enter the new graft and cause a haze 10 to 20 years after transplantation. Repeat corneal transplantation may be necessary and is also successful.

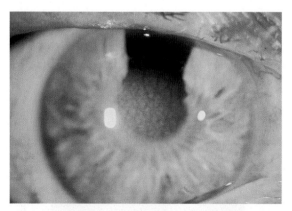

FIGURE 1.123. Central cloudy dystrophy of François produces a cloudy appearance of the stroma adjacent to Descemet's membrane. The light reflex is sharp, and these changes were noticed before the patient had an intracapsular cataract operation with sector iridectomy. This condition can be confused with Fuchs' dystrophy, but in the Fuchs' form, the stroma and the epithelium are edematous. In this case, there is no corneal thickening, and the epithelium is clear. These forms must be differentiated, because cataract surgery does not lead to corneal decompensation for central cloudy dystrophy of François as it may in Fuchs' dystrophy.

Central Cloudy Dystrophy of François

This dystrophy may be confused with posterior mosaic crocodile shagreen. Both involve the deep stroma and have somewhat similar appearances. Both are innocuous and do not interfere with vision.

Central cloudy dystrophy of François is a dominantly inherited dystrophy in some families. It mainly involves the axial cornea and occurs deep in the stroma. There are grayish, small, uniform patches with clearer areas outlining the patchy cloudy areas (Fig. 1.123).

Vision is not affected because the changes do not involve the endothelium and because the cornea is not prone to the onset of late edema after cataract surgery or even without surgery. The disease does not follow the course of Fuchs' dystrophy, with which it has been confused. The deep patchy changes of posterior crocodile shagreen, with grayish, polygonal patches of various sizes surrounded by clear lines, can be differentiated from the dystrophy of François by its crocodile-like skin pattern (Fig. 1.124).

Observation alone is indicated, because the pathologic changes of this dystrophy do not progress and do not lead to corneal clouding, edema, or vision-threatening opacity.

ENDOTHELIAL DYSTROPHIES

Cornea Guttata

Also called endothelial dystrophy, cornea guttata are mushroom-shaped excrescences or bumps on Descemet's membrane concomitant with decreased cell numbers and flattening of the endothelial cell layer. Usually, thickening of Descemet's membrane is evident and progresses, with the endothelial cells diminishing and the guttae increasing. Cornea guttata are seen more frequently with aging. They have been described in normal populations, affecting 5% to 70%, with higher numbers for older populations. Most patients with cornea guttata do not progress to Fuchs' dystrophy.

The classic appearance is that of beaten silver pattern, which is seen with a broad slit beam by specular microscopy. The slit lamp changes are more central and seldom reach the corneal periphery (Fig. 1.125). Many patients who undergo cataract surgery have endothelial dystrophy. They do not develop Fuchs' dystrophy postoperatively but are subject to more postoperative corneal edema as their endothelial cell counts are diminished. These corneas usually clear postoperatively unless endothelial guttata are numerous and the endothelial cell count is significantly diminished before surgery.

Most persons with endothelial guttata do not progress to or develop stromal and epithelial edema. The name "Fuchs" is applied to the dystrophy when corneal stromal and epithelial edema occur, and the determination is based on severe endothelial dystrophy.

Observation is indicated for endothelial guttata. Because over 90% of the patients with this condition do not develop corneal edema (i.e., Fuchs' dystrophy), they should be told about the benign nature of their corneal disorder. If cataract surgery is contemplated, the patient should be told of the slight increase in postoperative problems (e.g., corneal edema) with this surgery. Phacoemulsification and extracapsular cataract extraction can lead to postoperative corneal edema if guttata are present. The edema usually clears in a few weeks after the surgery. Corneal transplantation is not required for endothelial dystrophy. Patients who have marked endothelial dystrophy and require cataract surgery but have normal corneal thickness (no edema) should not undergo a corneal transplant but should instead have only cataract surgery and posterior chamber lens implantation.

Fuchs' Dystrophy

Stromal corneal swelling with evidence of epithelial corneal edema in the presence of endothelial guttata is called Fuchs' corneal dystrophy, also known as late hereditary endothelial dystrophy. Fuchs never saw cornea guttata because the slit lamp biomicroscope had not been invented, but his name remains attached to this disease because he was the first to describe it.

About 10% of cases of Fuchs' dystrophy are inherited. It is thought to be an autosomal dominant trait in some families. Fuchs' dystrophy occurs more commonly in women than men. The earliest diagnosis of Fuchs' dystrophy can be made in a patient with cornea guttata who develops stromal swelling as measured by pachymetry or where stromal swelling is noted at the slit lamp. Early epithelial edema may be seen as bedewing and may be present only on awakening because of corneal decompensation overnight, when there is no evaporation from the corneal surface because the eyelids are closed. Later in the course of the disease, when there is more confluent endothelial involvement and less endothelial cell function, epithelial and stromal edema occur continually, and vision is blurred all day. The corneal edema can develop into macroedema from the bedewing, and marked corneal irregularity can further blur vision (Fig. 1.126). The edematous epithelial cells eventually may lead to bullous keratopathy, which is usually not painful, unlike the bullous keratopathy accompanying cataract surgery (Fig. 1.127).

In the early phases of epithelial edema, hypertonic eye drops (usually sodium chloride) during the day and hypertonic ointment at bedtime may help deturgess the cornea and smooth the epithelial surface to provide better vision. Lowering the intraocular pressure with a β-blocking agent can also decrease the stromal and epithelial edema. A bandage soft contact lens for daily wear can smooth the corneal

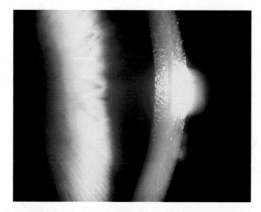

FIGURE 1.125. Endothelial dystrophy. Notice the beaten copper or silver appearance of the endothelium, which indicates cornea guttata changes in the corneal endothelium. The cornea was of normal thickness, and there was no epithelial edema. This condition is best seen by specular microscopy. No more than 10% of the patients with endothelial dystrophy eventually develop Fuchs' dystrophy.

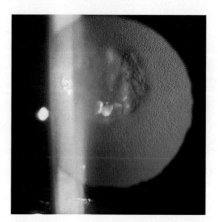

FIGURE 1.126. Fuchs' dystrophy is seen in retroillumination as a marked irregularity of the cornea surrounded by endothelial dystrophy. The cornea was thickened to approximately 0.7 mm, but the localized corneal edema allowed vision around this corneal opacity.

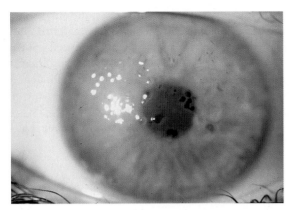

FIGURE 1.127. Notice the epithelial macroedema, and bullous changes. The patient's vision was significantly reduced because of epithelial edema, and a penetrating keratoplasty was indicated.

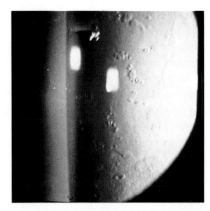

FIGURE 1.129. Grouped small vesicles in a patient with polymorphous dystrophy are seen using retroillumination. The endothelial changes are minimal, and this patient has normal corneal thickness and normal vision.

surface and provide better vision, but this is a temporizing treatment. A hair dryer held at arm's length with the warm air blown onto the cornea may more rapidly deturgess the cornea and improve vision after awakening. This also is a temporary expedient. Penetrating corneal transplantation is the only treatment when the corneal edema cannot be helped by other means and is usually successful, with better than 90% of the transplants providing clear corneas. The disease does not recur in the graft because the donor endothelium in the new graft remains intact.

Posterior Polymorphous Dystrophy

Widely variable clinical manifestations characterize this autosomal dominant dystrophy. Most patients do not require transplantation, and the disease is usually not found until later in life, when unusual single or groups of vesicles are seen on routine examination. Specular microscopy of these areas reveals the disease most clearly (Fig. 1.128).

Clinical Features. Few cases are recognized in the first decades of life, because most patients have good vision until later. The endothelial changes are usually first seen on a routine examination, when individual (Fig. 1.129) or grouped (Fig. 1.130) endothelial vesicles are seen with the broad slit lamp beam; the vesicles are surrounded by normal-appearing endothelium. This condition is better visualized by retroillumination against the red reflex of a dilated pupil. In most cases, stromal edema and epithelial edema do not occur, but when the endothelium is compromised sufficiently, corneal stromal and epithelial edema may be seen.

About 25% of patients may develop peripheral anterior synechiae, as seen by gonioscopy. Patients with extensive peripheral anterior synechiae may develop glaucoma, which can be difficult to treat. In these cases, differentiation between the iridocorneal endothelial (ICE) syndrome must be made. Posterior polymorphous dystrophy is bilateral and dominantly inherited, but ICE syndrome is not inherited and is unilateral. All patients with ICE syndrome develop

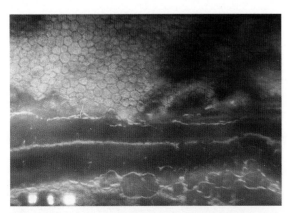

FIGURE 1.128. Specular microscopy of posterior polymorphous dystrophy. Posterior polymorphous dystrophy produces areas of normal endothelium surrounded by large areas of markedly abnormal endothelium with linear drop-out of endothelial cells and large cystic areas of endothelial cell absence.

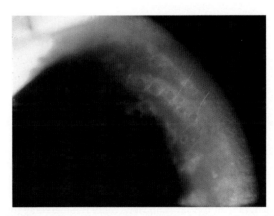

FIGURE 1.130. Notice the linear vesicles in this patient with posterior polymorphous dystrophy. There was slight corneal edema over these areas of vesicles, but because most of the endothelium was healthy, the patient had relatively good vision.

glaucoma, although this is not the case with posterior polymorphous dystrophy.

Most patients with posterior polymorphous dystrophy only require observation because the few single or grouped endothelial vesicles do not cause corneal edema. If corneal stromal and epithelial edema occur, it is treated like the edema caused by Fuchs' dystrophy. For the few patients who develop severe edema from posterior polymorphous dystrophic changes, penetrating corneal transplantation is the treatment of choice. Keratoplasty for this dystrophy is highly successful if glaucoma is not present or can be controlled. The corneal transplants stay clear in more than 90% of cases, and host endothelium does not replace donor endothelium.

Congenital Hereditary Endothelial Dystrophy

Congenital hereditary endothelial dystrophy may be inherited as an autosomal dominant or recessive trait. The endothelium may be severely compromised early, leading to marked corneal edema and visual loss during the first few years of life.

This disease, which may appear at birth in some cases, must be differentiated from congenital glaucoma. In congenital hereditary endothelial dystrophy, the intraocular pressure is normal, and the cornea is not enlarged but is thickened. In other forms of this dystrophy, the cornea may be clear at birth, but decompensation occurs during the first decade, as the endothelial cells die out. The endothelial cells seen at keratoplasty are remarkably atrophic or missing and the stroma may be three times the normal corneal thickness (Fig. 1.131). No reason for endothelial cell death is known, but the nonbanded posterior part of Descemet's membrane, which usually develops after the fifth month of pregnancy, is abnormal.

Penetrating corneal transplantation is the only treatment when vision is significantly reduced from stromal and epithelial edema. Keratoplasty success is reduced compared with the results for Fuchs' dystrophy and posterior polymorphous dystrophy because of the marked difference between the host and donor corneal stroma and because of the lack of host endothelial cell viability. However, the operation still provides a chance for visual improvement. The success rate varies but is about 75%.

DEGENERATIONS

Keratoconus

Keratoconus is a mostly bilateral, occasionally hereditary (10%), paracentral corneal ectasia. This noninflammatory condition is a common disorder. The incidence has been estimated to be between 4 and 100 per 10,000 members of the general population. This disease occurs in both sexes equally. The marked variation in symptoms, from severe blurred vision to no visual loss despite computerized topographic evidence of keratoconus corneal changes, makes incidence reporting difficult.

Keratoconus can be associated with Down syndrome (Fig. 1.132), atopic disease, and vernal catarrh; in all cases, eye rubbing is common. It also occurs with retinitis pigmentosa, certain retinal degeneration, aniridia, and Marfan's syndrome. The earliest manifestation of keratoconus is the frequent need to change the prescription for glasses, even before there is slit lamp evidence of the disease. At this point, there is usually inferior corneal steepening, which is seen earliest with inferior keratometry or with computerized corneal topography. As the disease progresses, certain clinical signs appear, such as apical protrusion and slight thinning of the apex seen by using the slit lamp. Vogt's striae, which are folds in Descemet's membrane that disappear in response to pressure, are also a diagnostic sign (Fig. 1.133). A Fleischer's ring may be visible all around the

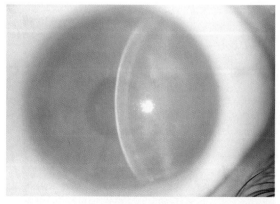

FIGURE 1.131. In this slit lamp view, there is a markedly thickened cornea and diffuse corneal edema from limbus to limbus. This typifies congenital hereditary endothelial dystrophy, which occurred in this patient within the first few years of life and required corneal transplantation.

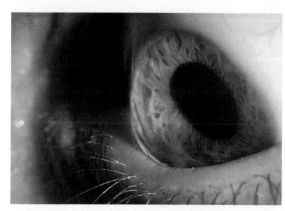

FIGURE 1.132. Keratoconus in a patient with Down syndrome is revealed by a positive Munson's sign and marked central and paracentral ectasia of the cornea.

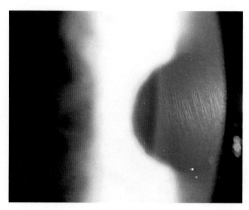

FIGURE 1.133. Vogt's striae occur centrally in a patient with keratoconus. By applying digital pressure on the eye while looking through the slit lamp, these striae in the deep cornea, mostly Descemet's membrane, disappear, which is characteristic of keratoconus.

cone or at the base of the cone. This is an iron line that is deposited because of corneal surface irregularity. With more protrusion, apical scarring forms, which can make contact lens use more difficult. Further protrusion stretches Descemet's membrane and can cause it to rupture. Aqueous then flows into the stroma, leading to marked swelling and further loss of vision. This condition is called a corneal hydrops (Fig. 1.134).

Keratoconus in its early stages is managed with glasses or soft contact lenses. As the cornea irregularity becomes more pronounced, rigid gas-permeable contact lenses are needed to restore visual acuity. Approximately 90% of patients with keratoconus are managed without the need for corneal surgery. Epikeratophakic lamellar procedures had been indicated, particularly for patients with Down syndrome. Because epikeratophakic tissue is no longer commercially available, this procedure is seldom done. Lamellar keratoplasty with new microkeratomes or facilitated lamellar dissection with air or fluid is being done.

Penetrating corneal transplants are indicated when patients no longer achieve good vision with rigid gas-permeable contact lenses or are unable to wear their contact lenses. Fortunately, penetrating keratoplasty is successful in 97% of these cases, providing 20/40 vision or better. Some form of graft rejection is encountered in about one third of these corneal transplants; fewer than 2% must be repeated because of irreversible rejection.

Pellucid marginal degeneration is a variation of keratoconus in which there is marked corneal steepening and anterior protrusion of the inferior cornea near the 6-o'clock limbus. It is considerably rarer than keratoconus. Unlike keratoconus, in which the corneal steepening appears in the paracentral cornea, this ectasia occurs close to the limbus but not directly at the limbus. The central cornea remains normal until later in the disease course, and visual acuity is good. A fine inferior pannus can occur, and the cornea can protrude significantly, making contact lens wear difficult or impossible (Fig. 1.135).

A fairly steep change from normal-appearing cornea centrally to extreme thinning and anterior bowing forward near the limbus is typically seen in cases of pellucid degeneration. As with keratoconus, the early stages of pellucid degeneration are usually managed with glasses, and later with rigid gas-permeable contact lenses. As long as a rigid gas-permeable contact lens can be worn, vision is usually acceptable, because the central cornea does not usually develop scarring.

Arcus Senilis

This degenerative corneal change is typified by peripheral corneal lipid deposits in an arc or complete circle and is en-

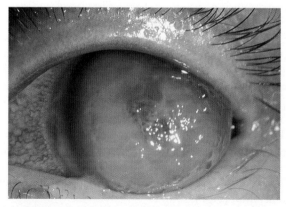

FIGURE 1.134. Hydrops in a patient with Down syndrome who has keratoconus. Abrupt ruptures in Descemet's membrane in severe keratoconus in response to eye rubbing may cause the aqueous to quickly expand into the stroma and cause marked swelling of the cornea, as much as five or six times the normal corneal thickness in some cases. This patient slowly improved over time, and the cornea returned to its previous configuration, although it was a little flatter and with more scarring. In most cases, hydrops resolves without surgery.

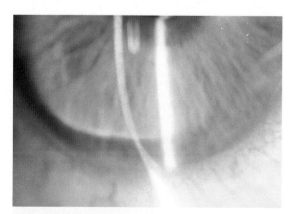

FIGURE 1.135. Pellucid degeneration is seen as marked steepening of the inferior cornea adjacent to but not directly at the limbus. This is a forme fruste of keratoconus with marked inferior steepening. Vision may be good until late in the course of the degeneration, because the central cornea is not ectatic. As the inferior cornea steepens, rigid gas-permeable contact lenses become more uncomfortable to wear, and the patient requires corneal transplantation.

countered with aging and certain systemic diseases of abnormal lipid metabolism.

Arcus senilis usually occurs as an aging process. It begins inferiorly and superiorly and later, but less commonly, it may encircle the cornea. It is not accompanied by peripheral corneal vascularization and is typified by a clear interval between the limbus and the lipid deposits. The lipid deposits have a more clearly defined peripheral border and a more diffuse central border (Fig. 1.136). The lipid is most concentrated in the deeper cornea near Descemet's membrane but occurs in more advanced cases in all layers of the stroma. Diseases characterized by abnormal lipid deposits include hyperlipoproteinemia I and III and corneal dystrophies such as Schnyder's crystalline dystrophy.

Observation alone is indicated, because the peripheral lipid deposits in arcus senilis and in circular senilis do not interfere with vision and do not cause peripheral thinning or degenerative changes.

Lipid Degeneration

The appearance of a whitish or yellowish, arc-like configuration in front of an area of corneal opacification with blood vessels signifies the abnormal deposition of lipid in the cornea stroma.

This secondary lipid degeneration occurs when blood vessels grow into the stroma and are associated with old stromal inflammation or infection. After the stromal inflammation heals, many vessels collapse and disappear or remain empty of blood; these are called ghost vessels. When blood persists in these blood vessels, there may be a very slow leakage of lipids from the vessel capillary wall, which deposits lipid material at the leading edge of the vascularized stroma in an arc shape (Fig. 1.137). If the lipid is peripheral, no visual consequences occur, but central lipid degeneration may cause visual loss. The lipid is deposited in all layers of the stroma.

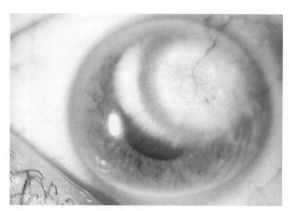

FIGURE 1.137. Lipid degeneration. In this cornea, which was previously inflamed, there is an arc of yellowish deposit in front of the corneal scar opacity with feeding vessels. When blood persists in these blood vessels, there may be a very slow leakage of lipids from the capillary walls, which deposit lipid material at the leading edge of the vascularized stroma. This is lipid degeneration. As long as vision is not affected, observation alone is indicated. Closing off the vessels may slow down or stop the deposition of lipid, but in most cases, this is unnecessary.

Obstructing the flow of blood in the stromal vessels can halt further deposition of lipid temporarily. Usually, the vessels open again after being closed. These vessels can be closed by several methods, including partial removal or cutting, cautery, laser, and chemical means. Generally, peripheral secondary lipid deposits can be observed when they do not affect the visual axis. They seldom spread centrally, and vision remains good. When these deposits occur in significant amounts in the central cornea, penetrating corneal transplantation may be necessary for improved visual acuity.

Pterygium

A pterygium is a triangular-shaped fibrovascular, degenerative tissue growing onto the cornea. It usually begins nasally but can start temporally and grow onto normal corneal tissue. Exposure to ultraviolet light is considered to be the major cause of pterygium growth, although the precise mechanism or trigger events are unknown. Pterygia are far more common in people living within 20 degrees of the equator than in the far northern or southern regions away from the equator.

Pterygia may start out as a pinguecula in the nasal or temporal conjunctiva. The stimulus to cross the limbus and grow onto the cornea is not understood. A sheath of vessels is carried onto the cornea behind a leading edge of elastotic degeneration (Fig. 1.138).

Capillaries in the head of the pterygium may grow further onto the cornea and lead to more opacification. Areas where red blood cells are seen to accumulate at the leading edge and where they are not confined by capillary walls indicate activity of the pterygium and further progression onto the cornea. When the pterygium stops growing, an iron line, known as Stocker's line, may occur in front of it

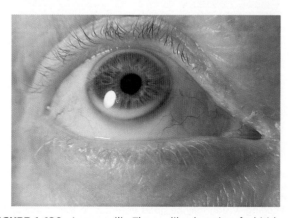

FIGURE 1.136. Arcus senilis. The arc-like deposits of whitish yellow lipid are detected interiorly and superiorly, almost circumventing the limbus and leaving the lucid area that typifies arcus senilis formation.

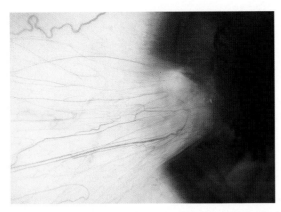

FIGURE 1.138. Early pterygium with vessels and the opacified pterygium head advancing onto the cornea. Observation alone is indicated when the pterygium enters the cornea. In many cases, it does not advance farther. Pterygia that are not advancing, do not affect vision, and are not cosmetic problems require observation alone.

in clear cornea. The pterygium may advance onto the cornea and then become dormant, never threatening vision, or it may proceed across the cornea and compromise the visual axis causing significantly blurred vision.

Observation alone is indicated for early pterygia that are not cosmetically disfiguring, do not threaten the visual axis, and are not growing further onto the cornea. If pterygia removal is necessary, there are several means of removing the pterygia, but the most important consideration is preventing their recurrence, which is usually worse than the primary pterygia (Fig. 1.139). Methods to remove the pterygia that have the lowest recurrence rates are under investigation. Removing the pterygium and replacing it with a conjunctival transplant from the upper bulbar conjunctiva of the same eye is effective, with only a 5% to 10% recurrence rate. Removing the pterygium and applying beta radiation with a

strontium 90 applicator has about a 20% recurrence rate. The bare sclera technique alone, without covering the pterygium bed, is no longer done. The latest means of preventing recurrence is with the use of mitomycin C, but the dose and complication rate are still being investigated.

Pinguecula

The asymptomatic appearance of yellowish lipid deposits in the conjunctiva of the nasal interpalpebral region characterizes a pinguecula. When a pinguecula advances onto the cornea, it is then called a pterygium, but a pterygium does not necessarily have to start with a pinguecula.

Pinguecula formation occurs in many older people and is considered a degenerative process. A yellowish deposit may occur in the conjunctiva nasally, near the limbus, and sometimes temporally (Fig. 1.140). These deposits are elastotic degeneration of the substantia propria and may represent abnormal elastic fibers. Exposure to ultraviolet light, drying, and dust can cause pinguecula formation. Occasionally, a pinguecula can become inflamed and form pingueculitis, an inflamed and vascularized lesion.

Pingueculitis is treated with a short course of topical steroids. Almost all noninflamed pinguecula can be observed without the need for surgery. If they enlarge and become a cosmetic problem, local excision easily removes the pathology. Pinguecula recurrences are slow and uncommon.

White Limbal Girdle of Vogt

The common type II limbal girdle of Vogt is an opacity occurring more often at the nasal limbus than the temporal limbus. It is a limbal degeneration directly related to aging that is found in almost everyone older than 80 years of age. Seen in 55% of patients 40 to 60 years of age, this can be considered a normal finding, although it may look like the

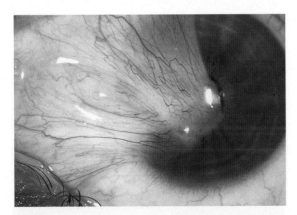

FIGURE 1.139. A recurrent pterygium has grown into the previous bed and has advanced into the visual axis. Removal of this pterygium with conjunctival transplantation is necessary. A diamond burr can be used to smooth the central cornea to allow better vision. Occasionally, lamellar corneal transplantation is needed if the visual axis is compromised.

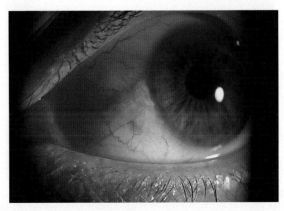

FIGURE 1.140. The pinguecula is an area of elastotic degeneration appearing in the conjunctiva at the limbus but not on the cornea. Most pingueculae remain in place and do not cross the limbus to the cornea. Almost all patients older than 80 years of age have some pinguecula formation.

beginning of band keratopathy. There are subepithelial deposits of hyaline degeneration and elastosis similar to pinguecula. These are seen in an arc-like configuration peripheral to where Bowman's membrane ends (Fig. 1.141). The very thin, small, finger-like extensions found centrally do not progress.

Because there are no symptoms and the degeneration does not progress, no treatment is necessary. It should not be confused with band keratopathy.

Spheroidal Degeneration

Spheroidal degeneration has had various names. It has been called climatic droplet keratopathy, Labrador keratopathy, keratinoid degeneration, and chronic actinic keratopathy. It is a nonhereditary degeneration that is usually related to climatic conditions but referred to as spheroidal degeneration because of the spherical appearance of the yellowish droplets.

The yellowish droplets typify this form of degeneration. They may start in the conjunctiva, at the limbus, or in the cornea. Clusters of fine to coarse yellowish droplets or larger, oval deposits are seen beneath the epithelium. They may be associated with corneal opacities and sometimes with blood vessels. They may take on a band-shaped appearance in more advanced cases (Fig. 1.142), but usually only the exposed area of the interpalpebral fissure is involved.

There are several forms. One form is associated with previous corneal disease and trauma, and another is a degenerative aging change that is usually seen nasally and later temporally. It occurs in different geographic regions and with increasing frequency with age. The degeneration is more prevalent in the northern regions (hence, the name Labrador keratopathy). The cause is unknown, but it is as-

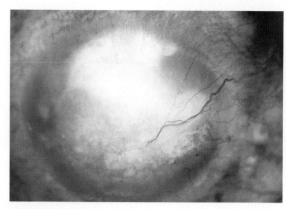

FIGURE 1.142. Spheroidal degeneration. Notice the golden yellow appearance of the degenerative area in a patient with chronic corneal disease.

sociated with corneal drying and exposure to the sun, wind, sand, ice, and ultraviolet light. The droplets are proteinaceous material in the anterior stroma and Bowman's layer, and they are extracellular.

In most cases, the lesions are asymptomatic and need only to be observed. Where there is central corneal pathology, superficial keratectomy permanently cures the condition. Most of the time, the pathology is located nasally and temporally, and observation alone is indicated.

Coats' Ring

Coats' ring is an oval deposit of iron that is a small remnant of a previous corneal injury, as from a foreign body. Coats' ring is usually located in the region of Bowman's layer and consists of discrete white dots, located for the most part in the inferior cornea where the trauma has occurred. The white dots consist of iron deposits and are probably remnants of the previous injury.

Observation alone is indicated, because the ring does not extend superficially or deep into the cornea. It is an interesting and unusual finding (Fig. 1.143).

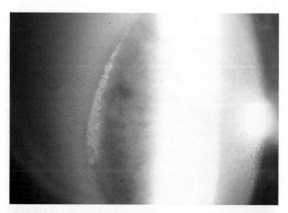

FIGURE 1.141. The limbal girdle of Vogt consists of fine radial white lines at the temporal or nasal limbus and represents elastotic and hyaline changes. Most patients older than 60 years of age have some form of limbal girdle, and almost all patients who are very elderly have some limbal girdle of Vogt. This is a normal finding, and it does not grow farther onto the cornea as does band keratopathy.

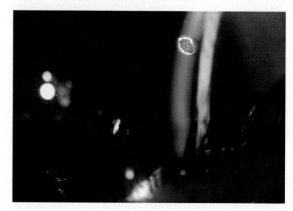

FIGURE 1.143. Coats' ring represents remnants of a foreign body. The remnants are fine iron deposits in the cornea. This benign condition need not be treated.

Salzmann's Degeneration

Salzmann's degeneration is a noninflammatory, degenerative process appearing in the superficial cornea, usually in the midperiphery. If it occurs in the visual axis, it can cause blurred vision. This was described by Salzmann as a dystrophy, but it is a degenerative change that usually occurs years after some inflammatory condition of the cornea.

Superficial, elevated, grayish opacities replace Bowman's membrane. They are elevated and do not invade the stroma. They may appear in the periphery as single or multiple opacities, or they may spread to the central cornea (Fig. 1.144). There is usually a clear area before the limbus. They are usually unilateral but can be seen in both eyes, appear in all ages, and overlie normal-appearing stroma. Iron lines may be seen around the lesion base, and there is no further extension of these degenerative changes.

When the degenerative Salzmann's changes are in the midperiphery and do not involve the visual axis, no treatment is necessary. For the central appearance of these gray mounds that interfere with vision, superficial keratectomy is indicated.

Band Keratopathy

Deposits of calcium in the cornea in a broad band-like distribution across the middle third of the cornea as a secondary deposition or associated with systemic disorders characterize the degeneration known as band keratopathy.

Band keratopathy may start as areas of light gray opacity adjacent to the limbus nasally and temporally, typically with clear small holes within the opacity. With time, which may be years, the opacities can extend centrally and meet, leading to a band of grayish haze across the cornea (Fig. 1.145). There is an accumulation of hydroxyapatite deposits or calcium carbonate, which accumulate in the epithelium, Bowman's membrane, and superficial stroma.

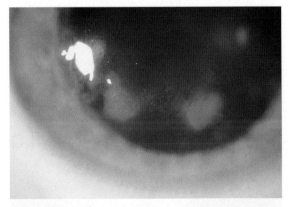

FIGURE 1.144. Salzmann's nodular degeneration. Notice the grayish individual opacities, which sometimes are linked. When these are in the visual axis, they interfere with vision, and the raised abnormalities can cause significant visual distortion. Superficial keratectomy is the treatment of choice when the opacities are in the visual axis.

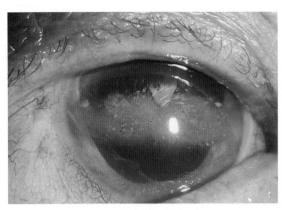

FIGURE 1.145. Band keratopathy. The grayish deposits of calcium in a band-like distribution across the middle one third of the cornea are typical of this disease. These deposits occur secondary to a number of systemic problems and in cases of chronic corneal inflammation and anterior uveitis.

Many systemic conditions that feature hypercalcemia can cause band keratopathy. These include sarcoidosis, vitamin D toxicity, Still's disease, and Fanconi's syndrome. Band keratopathy is also seen secondary to chronic inflammation of the cornea and in cases of anterior uveitis. It may occur secondary to drug toxicity. In the past, the preservative in a commercial pilocarpine preparation was the cause of band keratopathy.

Early cases of band keratopathy, when the calcific degeneration is at the nasal and temporal limbus, do not have to be treated. The deposits of calcium usually are in the region of Bowman's membrane, and the corneal surface is not disturbed. As the deposits move centrally and involve more of the epithelium, there may be irregular astigmatism from the marked surface irregularity. For patients with discomfort from calcific deposits or blurred vision because the calcium deposit is central, the calcium may be removed by using EDTA, a chelating agent. In more severe cases, superficial keratectomy is necessary. Most cases of band keratopathy do not have to be treated.

COMPLICATIONS OF CORNEAL SURGERY

Whorl Keratopathy After Penetrating Keratoplasty

After keratoplasty, some patients may develop a whorl or hurricane vortex of epithelial staining in the newly reepithelialized corneal button. Whorl keratopathy stains with fluorescein or rose bengal and represents a pattern of reepithelialization, with the epithelium growing in from the periphery in a hurricane or whorl-like centripetal pattern (Fig. 1.146). In the more severe cases, this can cause corneal epithelial disturbance and blurred vision. It is more marked after keratoplasty in patients who are sensitive to preservatives in some topical medications. This usually disappears

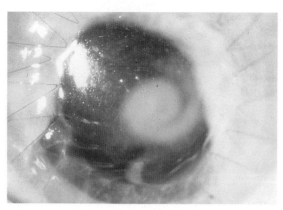

FIGURE 1.146. Whorl keratopathy in a patient who had a corneal transplant. Notice the hurricane-like appearance of this defect, which diffusely stains with fluorescein.

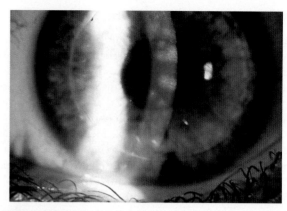

FIGURE 1.147. Subepithelial corneal deposits in the early stage of corneal graft rejection. These deposits are exactly the same as those seen in adenovirus infection, but there is no virus infection in this condition. These deposits can occur individually or grouped, as seen here. They must be treated with topical steroids to prevent more severe forms of rejection.

with time, leaving the corneal epithelium normal and without opacification.

When whorl keratopathy appears in the first week or two after keratoplasty, reducing or eliminating topical medications that contain preservatives can diminish the whorl keratopathy. Artificial tears without preservatives and lubricating ointment at bedtime are helpful. As the condition gradually fades, the corneal epithelium may become opacified in a whorl-like distribution, and epithelial debridement is needed to allow healthy epithelium to grow back in its place. This problem usually does not jeopardize corneal graft clarity.

Subepithelial Corneal Infiltrates in Corneal Graft Rejection

This mild form of graft rejection was described by Krachmer about 15 years ago, and is similar to the subepithelial infiltrates in adenovirus infection. The subepithelial infiltrates appear several weeks to many years after corneal transplantation.

Corneal graft rejection occurs in as many as 25% of corneal transplants. Epithelial or endothelial rejection has been the classic form of corneal transplant rejection. Subepithelial corneal infiltrates may appear weeks or years after transplantation and are also a sign of active graft rejection (Fig. 1.147). They are inflammatory infiltrates beneath Bowman's membrane in the superficial stroma and have the exact appearance of subepithelial infiltrates in adenovirus infection. There is no virus infection of the graft, and these subepithelial infiltrates represent a newly recognized form of graft rejection. They may be associated with epithelial rejection and with endothelial rejection.

Corneal transplants must be observed at each office visit for signs of subepithelial infiltrates. If even one infiltrate appears where there had been none previously, treatment with topical steroids usually is all that is necessary to resolve the infiltrates. The topical steroids should be used more fre-

quently at first QID and then tapered over several weeks to months. These infiltrates may be recurrent.

Endothelial Graft Rejection of Corneal Transplants

Endothelial graft rejection is a serious graft rejection that is first seen as a wavy endothelial line, usually starting at the periphery and going across the back of the new corneal transplant. Epithelial rejection is more common but less serious.

Endothelial graft rejection has been known for many years. Khoudadoust described the linear pattern of the endothelial rejection line that bears his name (Fig. 1.148). This pattern represents a line of sensitized lymphocytes that progresses across the back of the cornea from the host recipient graft edge centrally, until it reaches the other side of the cornea. As this line progresses, new donor endothelial cells are destroyed, but all cells are not destroyed. This line may

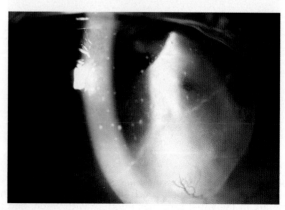

FIGURE 1.148. Endothelial graft rejection with Khoudadoust's line, which is a line of lymphocytes advancing across the back of the cornea. Note also the keratic precipitates.

progress across the cornea, leaving enough viable endothelial cells to maintain graft clarity. In more severe cases of endothelial rejection, corneal stromal edema occurs if enough endothelial cells are damaged as the line progresses.

The use of frequent topical steroids, such as 1% prednisolone, hourly for a few days and then tapering to every 2 hours, every 3 hours, and further, is the treatment of choice. Based on the response of the endothelial rejection line, the treatment is slowly tapered but maintained over a considerable period of time (months to years). If there has been previous rejection or if this is a second graft, some physicians treat endothelial graft rejection with oral or even intravenous cortisone, and in some cases, cyclosporine. Most ophthalmologists treat endothelial rejection with high-frequency topical applications of 1% prednisolone alone.

COMPLICATIONS OF REFRACTIVE SURGERY

Infection in Radial Keratotomy

Infection occurring in the radial keratotomy incisions is an uncommon event. Any appearance of stromal inflammation in one of the radial keratotomy incisions should be treated as a potential corneal infection to prevent spread of the disease and possible endophthalmitis. Recognition of infection in the radial keratotomy incisions should be simple, because the eye is inflamed, and an infiltrate is seen somewhere along the line of the incision (Fig. 1.149).

Treatment of these potential infections requires the frequent application of topical antibiotics in the early phase. Fortified medications to cover gram-positive and gram-negative organisms should be used, or broad-spectrum antibiotics, such as fluoroquinolone drops, should be frequently applied.

Perforation of the Cornea in Radial Keratotomy

Any perforation of the cornea during a radial keratotomy procedure is a potential problem. Microperforations initially were seen in 5% to 10% of cases, but macroperforations were much less common. As the radial keratotomy incision is being made, loss of aqueous in the incision indicates perforation of the cornea. If there is only a bead or small drop of aqueous, many physicians continue the procedure but decrease the blade depth. If there is more than just a bead of aqueous, a macroperforation has occurred.

Microperforations do not require suturing, but a macroperforation with significant softening of the eye requires suturing of the incision and delaying finishing the procedure (Fig. 1.150).

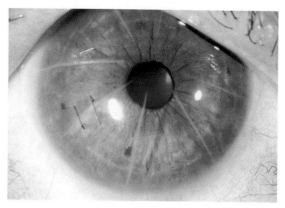

FIGURE 1.150. Radial keratotomy, showing two sutures in the 8-o'clock incision resulting from a macroperforation.

Corneal Haze in Excimer Laser Photorefractive Keratectomy Surgery

Excimer laser photorefractive keratectomy surgery for low degrees of myopia causes little haze of the cornea. For higher amounts of myopia, there may be significant haze that can interfere with vision.

Corneal haze, which occurs after excimer laser photorefractive surgery and phototherapeutic surgery, is located in the superficial stroma and the region of Bowman's membrane. This haze, which occurs fairly frequently for patients with high degrees of myopia, can take many months to 1 year to heal, and in some patients with high degrees of myopia, the haze can be permanent (Fig. 1.151). Fortunately, the haze does not interfere significantly with vision in its milder form, and only when the haze is more apparent is there some visual distortion.

Topical steroids can decrease the haze and even eliminate it, but with use of topical steroids for long periods of time after excimer laser phototherapeutic and photorefractive surgery, there is the risk of lens opacity and glaucoma in steroid responders.

LASIK Complications

Laser in situ keratomileusis (LASIK) is a refractive surgery procedure that involves pressurizing the globe and using a

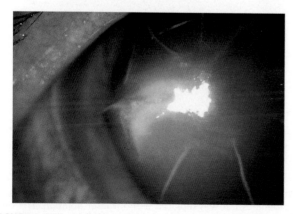

FIGURE 1.149. Radial keratotomy with bacterial infection in the 3-o'clock incision.

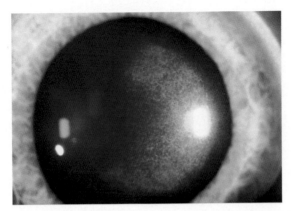

FIGURE 1.151. A superficial haze in the cornea occurred 6 months after excimer laser photorefractive surgery. It was considered a 2+ haze, which produced mild interference with vision.

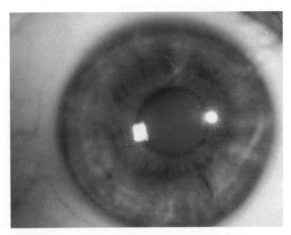

FIGURE 1.152. Epithelial irregularities can be seen paracentrally from the 12- to 1-o'clock and 8- to 9-o'clock positions on postoperative day 1 after a thin irregular laser in situ keratomileusis flap was created secondary to loss of suction during the microkeratome pass. The flap pieces were replaced and bandage soft contact lens used. The vision returned to preoperative levels within a few days.

microkeratome to create a thin corneal flap. A small hinge is left at one edge of the flap to assist in replacing the flap. The flap is lifted and the excimer laser is used to reshape the underlying corneal stroma, after which the flap is replaced and allowed to adhere without sutures. The great majority of the time, the flap fashioned during the LASIK procedure is of perfect quality. It should be well centered, of uniform thickness, without significant epithelial defects and have an adequate hinge.

LASIK Button-hole

Occasionally LASIK flaps are not perfect. Slight decentrations or small epithelial defects are of minimal consequence. If a "free cap" occurs, due to amputation of the hinge, the excimer laser treatment can proceed if the cap is large enough to cover the entire ablation area. If the cap is too small or the flap is not of uniform thickness, the laser treatment should be aborted. Additionally, if the hinge is so large or the flap so decentered that it impinges on a significant portion of the ablation area, the laser treatment should also be aborted. In these cases, the flap or free cap should be placed back in its original position and allowed to heal. Often a bandage soft contact lens aids in stabilizing the flap. After the flap is allowed to heal for at least 3 to 6 months, a repeat LASIK procedure can often be performed by recutting a new, ideally thicker, flap, usually with excellent results. It is possible, however, for the original poor flap to loosen or detach during the second procedure, causing another thin or shredded flap.

A thin, poor quality flap can occur if there is inadequate intraocular pressure elevation during flap creation (Fig. 1.152). A button-hole in the flap may be due to low intraocular pressure, but may also be related to an excessively steep cornea that "dimples" inward when the microkeratome runs across the surface. Corneas with keratometry readings greater than 48 to 49 diopters are at higher risk for button-holes. Corneas with small corneal diameters, for example, less than 11.5 mm, are also at higher risk for button-holes.

LASIK Free Cap

Creation of an excellent flap during the LASIK procedure is critical to obtain a superb refractive result. A "free cap" occurs when the hinge is amputated by the microkeratome pass (Fig. 1.153). This typically occurs in flat corneas, generally with keratometry readings less than 40 to 41 diopters. Large corneas, usually greater than 14.5 mm in horizontal diameter, are also prone to free caps.

If a free cap occurs, it needs to be recognized immediately so it is not lost. It should be carefully removed from the microkeratome head and placed in an antidesiccation chamber with the epithelial side down on a drop of saline. If the area under the free cap is large enough to allow the excimer laser ablation, then the surgeon may proceed with the laser treat-

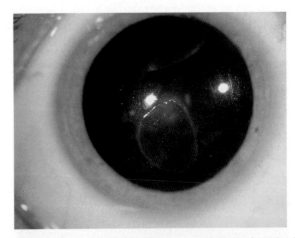

FIGURE 1.153. A small free cap was created during laser in situ keratomileusis. It was replaced without laser ablation. The central edge of the free cap is elevated, causing irregular astigmatism and poor vision.

ment. Whether the laser treatment is performed or not, the cap should be replaced in its original position. It is critical that the epithelial side is up. The preplaced ink marks are used to ensure the cap is right side up and in its natural orientation. A bandage soft contact lens may be used to prevent cap movement.

LASIK Flap Dislocation

During a LASIK procedure, after the flap is resituated in its original position, it is allowed to adhere for several minutes. The eyelid speculum is removed, using care not to touch the flap. The flap is checked at the slit lamp a short time later to ensure good positioning. It is critical that the patient not rub the eye or touch the flap for several days, as the flap can easily dislodge.

Flap dislocations range from mild (Fig. 1.154) to severe (Fig. 1.155). In general, they must be repositioned using an operating microscope. The stromal bed and underside of the flap need to be cleaned of foreign debris and epithelium before the flap is replaced in its original position. An attempt is made to iron out any visible striae. A bandage soft contact lens may be helpful in aiding reepithelialization and securing the flap. If the flap fails to adhere properly to the stromal bed, sutures may be required to secure the flap in position.

LASIK Infection

Infection after LASIK is a rare, but potentially devastating, condition. While sterilized instruments and pre- and postoperative antibiotics are used routinely for LASIK, infection can still occur. Infection can occur in the superficial cornea, at the edge of the flap, or in the flap interface. Mild superficial infections can be treated with topical antibiotics. More

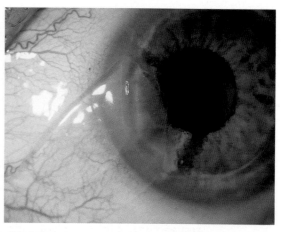

FIGURE 1.155. This flap became totally dislodged 3 months after laser in situ keratomileusis due to being poked in the eye with a stick. The flap is still attached to the cornea at its hinge nasally. It was repositioned under an operating microscope and healed without difficulty.

severe infections require scrapings for smears and cultures and intensive topical antibiotic use. Infections located in the flap interface often require lifting of the flap and obtaining cultures from the interface. At the same time, the stromal bed should be irrigated with antibiotics. Although the usual organisms causing infectious keratitis are often found, there is a higher incidence of unusual organisms, such as atypical mycobacteria (Fig. 1.156).

LASIK Diffuse Lamellar Keratitis

Diffuse lamellar keratitis (DLK) is a condition of inflammation in the LASIK interface that begins within a few days after surgery. It has also been termed Sands of the Sahara syn-

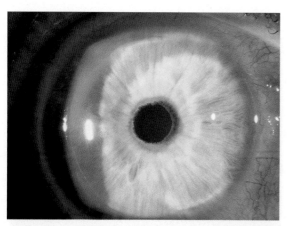

FIGURE 1.154. The flap is slightly dislodged on postoperative day 1. It was associated with "macrostriae" and decreased vision. An epithelial defect is apparent at the flap edge from the 9- to 12-o'clock positions, where there was significant edge misalignment. It was repositioned under the operating microscope with excellent return of vision.

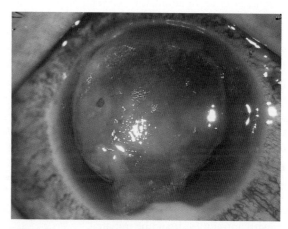

FIGURE 1.156. Five weeks after laser in situ keratomileusis, this flap interface infection has not responded to multiple medical treatments, causing the flap to melt. The flap was surgically amputated to allow better antibiotic penetration to the stroma. The cultures ultimately revealed atypical mycobacteria. The infection eventually responded to additional medical treatment, but the patient was left with a significant corneal scar.

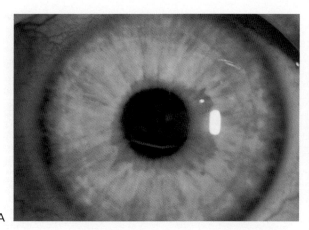 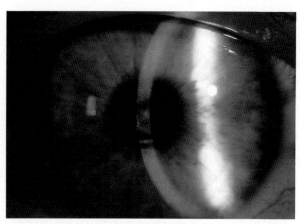

A   B

FIGURE 1.157. A: This eye developed diffuse lamellar keratitis several days after uncomplicated laser in situ keratomileusis. Note the "desert sand" appearance centrally. **B:** In this slit beam view of diffuse lamellar keratitis, the peripheral extent of the granular inflammatory response can be seen. (Courtesy of Irving M. Raber, M.D.)

drome, among other names. Patients notice increased irritation, light sensitivity, glare, and decreased vision within a few days after LASIK. On slit lamp examination, there is little if any conjunctival injection. There is a granular haze in the flap interface, which can be peripheral or central. It may have a "desert sand" appearance (Fig. 1.157A, B). In more severe cases the vision is dramatically affected. The interface opacity can become quite dense, especially centrally. It is differentiated from a bacterial infection by minimal pain, conjunctival injection, and anterior chamber reaction.

The etiology of DLK is most likely multifactorial. It can occur sporadically or in clusters. When DLK has occurred in clusters, there is good evidence that it may be related to bacterial toxins remaining on the instruments and equipment after heat sterilization. It may also be related to lubricating oils from the microkeratome equipment, meibomian secretions, or other inflammatory substances in the flap interface.

The treatment regimen depends on the severity of the inflammation. Mild cases, where the vision is not affected, can be followed closely to monitor for worsening. More severe cases should be treated with intensive topical steroids, such as every 1 to 2 hours, and followed closely. In the most severe cases there is a dense central inflammatory reaction that can lead to stromal necrosis and significant corneal scarring, thinning, and flattening. In such cases, lifting of the flap and irrigation of the inflammatory debris (in addition to intensive topical steroids) may help prevent excessive tissue damage. If an infection cannot be ruled out, the flap should be lifted and scrapings taken for smears and cultures, and treatment with antibiotics should be initiated.

LASIK Epithelial Ingrowth

Corneal surface epithelial cells can grow under a LASIK flap. Epithelial ingrowth typically occurs when an epithelial

defect along the flap edge does not heal properly, allowing a sheet of epithelium to grow under the flap. The epithelium cannot generally be seen until several weeks after surgery, when it looks like a gray-white layer in the flap interface (Fig. 1.158). It often has tongues of epithelial growth and may have a speckled or putty-like pattern (Fig. 1.159). Small islands of epithelial cell growth at the edge of LASIK flaps are common and of minimal concern. When a large sheet of epithelium grows under a flap, it can cause elevation of the flap and irregular astigmatism. Additionally, since it is difficult for nutrients to get from the deep cornea through the sheet of epithelium, and perhaps due to epithelial collagenases, the flap over the epithelial ingrowth can undergo necrosis. Risk factors for epithelial ingrowth include epithelial basement membrane dystrophy, a history of recurrent erosions, advanced age, LASIK enhancement, and flap dislodgment.

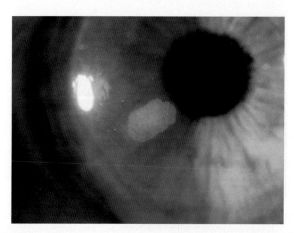

FIGURE 1.158. This dense gray-white plaque of epithelial ingrowth caused punctate staining of the overlying flap along with central irregular astigmatism and decreased vision. It required removal under an operating microscope.

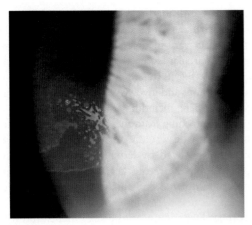

FIGURE 1.159. This putty-like epithelial ingrowth was not causing problems with the health of the flap, but was inducing mild irregular astigmatism and slightly decreased vision.

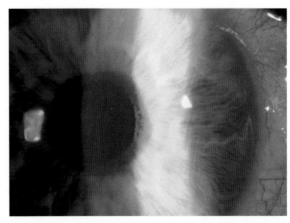

FIGURE 1.161. These "macrostriae" or folds near the flap hinge nasally resulted from a slightly dislodged flap on postoperative day 1 and were associated with decreased vision. The flap was replaced and the vision improved. The striae diminished greatly, but did not completely disappear.

Treatment depends on the extent and severity of the epithelial ingrowth. Mild, peripheral ingrowth measuring less than 1 to 2 mm can be followed. Ingrowth greater than 2 mm, especially if it is thick, requires close follow-up, every 1 to 2 weeks initially, to make sure it doesn't progress or cause damage to the flap. If there is any evidence of flap necrosis or if the ingrowth is causing decreased vision from flap distortion, it should be removed. Removal requires lifting the flap and scraping both the stromal bed and the undersurface of the flap to remove all epithelial cells. The flap is replaced and the epithelial tags at the flap edge are realigned as much as possible to prevent recurrence of the ingrowth.

LASIK Flap Striae

Striae, or folds, in LASIK flaps are often seen. "Microstriae" are common and may result from slight folding in the flaps that are being replaced over a stromal bed that is slightly

smaller than the flap because it has been ablated by the laser (Fig. 1.160). Microstriae do not affect the vision. "Macrostriae," or corneal folds, occur when the LASIK flap is not perfectly aligned (Fig. 1.161). They can affect the vision, especially if they are located centrally, and should generally be ironed out.

LASIK Iron Line

After LASIK for myopia, the central corneal curvature is flatter than before surgery. The tear film distribution is therefore altered, allowing some pooling centrally. This pooling can cause iron deposition in the central epithelium (Fig. 1.162). A similar effect can be seen after steeping of the cornea from treatment of hyperopia. In the case of hyperopia, a pseudo-Fleischer's ring iron deposition can be seen. These iron lines do not affect vision.

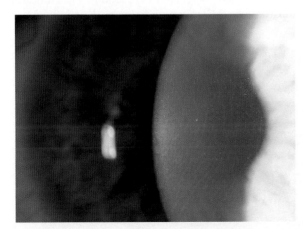

FIGURE 1.160. These "microstriae" are commonly seen after laser in situ keratomileusis and do not affect vision. They probably result from slight folding of the flap, which is being placed into a bed that is slightly smaller due to the laser ablation.

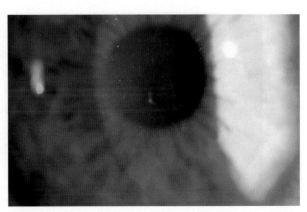

FIGURE 1.162. A small, slightly stellate iron line can be seen centrally in this eye 1 year after myopic laser in situ keratomileusis. It does not affect vision.

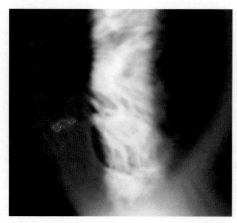

FIGURE 1.163. A tiny fiber fragment is seen in the laser in situ keratomileusis flap interface 5 weeks after surgery. A mild fibrotic reaction around the piece of debris can be seen. Small degrees of interface debris are common and generally do not affect vision.

LASIK Interface Debris

After the flap is replaced during the LASIK procedure, the interface is irrigated with saline to remove debris. The flap is inspected under the operating microscope after irrigation and again at the slit lamp a short time after the procedure. Ideally, minimal to no debris remains in the interface. A small amount of debris is of no consequence. There may be a mild fibrotic reaction around the debris for several weeks to months after surgery (Fig. 1.163). A large amount of debris, especially if it is centrally located, should be removed at the time of surgery. In that case, the flap is refloated, the interface reirrigated, and the flap allowed to readhere.

TUMORS

Limbal Dermoid

A limbal dermoid is a smooth, solid, round mass of tissue containing entities such as hair follicles and fatty deposits. Dermoids are associated with Goldenhar's syndrome, a nonhereditary condition that also includes ear abnormalities such as preauricular skin tags and vertebral abnormalities.

Dermoids can vary in shape and location, but classically, they are white, circular lesions that are several mm in diameter and are elevated (Fig. 1.164A). They typically occur at the inferotemporal limbus and involve the sclera and cornea, but they may occur elsewhere, including centrally (Fig. 1.164B). There may be hairs protruding from the surface of the dermoid.

Dermoids can be visually and cosmetically significant. They may be removed by lamellar keratectomy, lamellar keratoplasty, or penetrating keratoplasty. When lamellar surgery is contemplated, full-thickness corneal tissue should be available, because dermoids can involve the full thickness of the cornea. Depending on the size, shape, and location, surgical removal may or may not improve the visual acuity and cosmetic appearance. *Lipodermoids* are dermoids with a significant lipid component, and consequently, they are more yellow in appearance. They also tend to be more superiorly and posteriorly located than limbal dermoids.

Pyogenic Granuloma

A pyogenic granuloma is a mass of exuberant granulation tissue that develops on the conjunctiva or skin. These can occur secondary to trauma, surgery, a chalazion or hordeolum, a chemical burn, or any necrotizing process. A deep red, highly vascularized, often pedunculated mass arises from the conjunctiva or skin (Fig. 1.165). There may be an associated mucopurulent discharge.

Small, pyogenic granulomas can resolve spontaneously over several weeks. Topical steroids or antibiotic-steroid combinations can also be used to treat pyogenic granulomas. Occasionally, they can require surgical excision.

Conjunctival Intraepithelial Neoplasia

Conjunctival intraepithelial neoplasia is a term used to designate benign and malignant in situ lesions. The clinical and histopathologic differentiation between these lesions is dif-

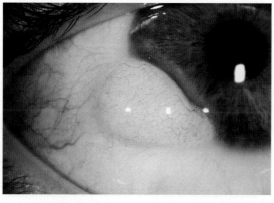
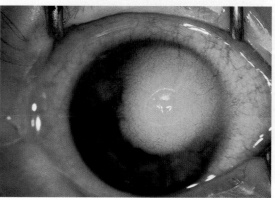

FIGURE 1.164. A: This classic limbal dermoid is smooth, round, white, and in an inferotemporal location. **B:** Central corneal dermoids are much less common and are part of the differential diagnosis of congenital cloudy corneas.

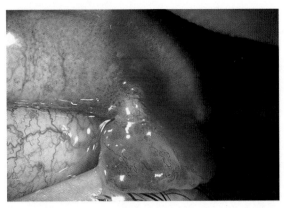

FIGURE 1.165. A large, pedunculated, pyogenic granuloma arising from the conjunctival surface of the upper eyelid is apparent in the area of an old chalazion.

ficult. Conjunctival intraepithelial neoplasia has a typical clinical appearance characterized by a papillomatous lesion beginning at the limbus and extending onto the conjunctiva and cornea (Fig. 1.166A). The presence of vascular fronds in the limbal and conjunctival components is an indication for a wide excisional biopsy for diagnosis and therapy. The corneal component is gray, nonstaining, and slightly raised, with a well-defined geographic or whorl-like border. The conjunctival lesion can also have a gelatinous appearance (Fig. 1.166B). Squamous cell dysplasia and carcinoma in situ have similar clinical appearances but differ histopathologically by the extent of replacement of the conjunctival epithelium with abnormal cells (Fig. 1.166C).

Treatment consists of wide excisional biopsy, cryotherapy of the conjunctival margin, and application of absolute alcohol to the area of corneal involvement in some cases. The prognosis is good. Lesions can recur locally if the margins of excisions are not free of tumor. Invasive disease is uncommon and frequently associated with neglect or immunocompromised hosts.

Malignant Melanoma of the Conjunctiva and Cornea

Malignant melanoma of the conjunctiva can arise from three sources. It can be seen after the development of a primary acquired melanosis, develop from preexisting nevi, or arise de novo. Approximately 75% of cases of conjunctival melanoma arise from primary acquired melanosis.

Malignant melanoma of the conjunctiva occurs equally in men and women, usually in their fifties. It is most often seen in Caucasians, and rarely in persons of African descent.

The clinical manifestations are quite variable, and in many cases, malignant melanoma does not take on any typical appearance (Fig. 1.167A). Melanomas at the limbus

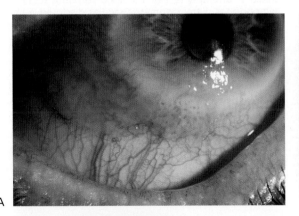

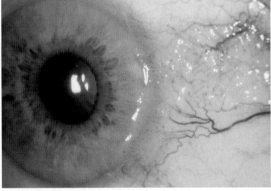

FIGURE 1.166. A: This conjunctival mass with typical vascular fronds and a gray extension onto the cornea was determined to be squamous cell carcinoma in situ by histopathologic analysis. **B:** This gelatinous conjunctival lesion involving the limbus and extending near the caruncle was also a squamous cell carcinoma in situ. **C:** Pathology of this lesion demonstrates the characteristic abrupt transition from normal to diseased conjunctiva. (Courtesy of Ralph C. Eagle, Jr, M.D., Department of Pathology, Wills Eye Hospital.)

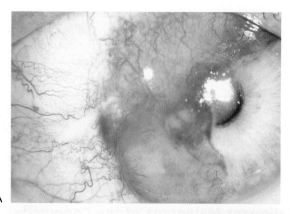

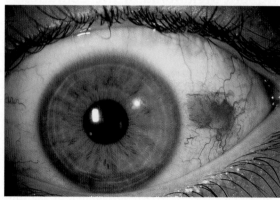

FIGURE 1.167. A: A malignant melanoma of the limbus and cornea had been incompletely excised and recurred. **B:** A conjunctival nevus.

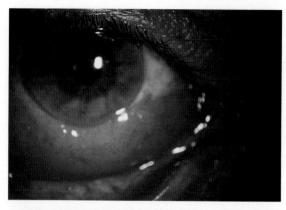

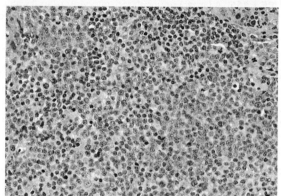

FIGURE 1.168. A: A 45-year-old woman presented with a salmon-colored soft tissue swelling of the inferior bulbar conjunctiva. **B:** Biopsy revealed a monomorphous sheet of atypical lymphocytes. Flow cytometric studies disclosed a monoclonal population of B cells consistent with lymphoma. (Hematoxylin & eosin stain; original magnification ×100.)

usually do not arise from preexisting conjunctival nevi (Fig. 1.167B). Corneal malignant melanomas are rare, with most of these lesions extending from the conjunctival limbus onto the cornea. Increased vascularity and nodular thickening with fixation to underlying tissue may indicate change from primary acquired melanosis to malignant melanoma.

Complete surgical excision is the ideal treatment of conjunctival, limbal, and corneal malignant melanomas. Because it is difficult to be certain that all of the lesions have been removed on the conjunctival side, cryotherapy should be applied to the surrounding conjunctiva and the lesion base. The recurrence rate for conjunctival melanoma is approximately 25%.

Lymphomatous Infiltration

The conjunctiva may be involved by several benign and malignant lymphoid infiltrative processes, including hyperplasia, lymphoma, pseudotumor, and leukemia.

The typical lymphomatous lesion involving the conjunctiva presents as a salmon-colored, soft, fleshy elevation without an inflammatory reaction (Fig. 1.168). Benign and malignant lesions are often difficult to differentiate clinically. Biopsy with a histopathologic examination of the specimen and fresh tissue for immunologic marker studies are helpful in making the diagnosis.

Patients with conjunctival lymphoma should have a thorough systemic workup and evaluation by a specialist skilled in this area. Only 10% of these patients have preexisting systemic lymphoma. Local lesions can be excised, and more diffuse lesions can be treated with irradiation. Systemic lymphoma requires treatment and follow-up by an oncologist.

BIBLIOGRAPHY

Berlinger ML. Biomicroscopy of the eye, vol II. New York: Paul B Hoeber; 1949:1091.

Boyd-Monk H, Steinmetz CG. Nursing care of the eye. Norwalk: Appleton & Lange; 1991:13.

Charlton JR, Weinstein GW. Cataract surgery. In: Tasman W, Jaeger EA. Clinical ophthalmology, vol 6. Philadelphia: JB Lippincott; 1994:1.

Cheng KP, Hiles DA, Biglan AW, et al. Management of posterior lenticonus. *J Pediatr Ophthalmol Strabismus* 1991;28:143.

Cogan DG, Kuwabara T. Pathology of cataracts in Mongoloid idiocy. A new concept of pathogenesis of cataracts of the coronary-cerulean type. *Doc Ophthalmol* 1962;16:73.

Cordes FC. Types of congenital and juvenile cataracts. In: Haik GM. Symposium on diseases and surgery of the lens. St. Louis: CV Mosby; 1957:43.

Datiles MB, Kinoshita JH. Pathogenesis of cataracts. In: Tasman W, Jaeger EA. Duane's clinical ophthalmology, vol 1. Philadelphia: JB Lippincott; 1994:1.

Davison JA. Capsule contraction syndrome. *J Cataract Refract Surg* 1993;19:582.

Delamere NA, Paterson CA. The crystalline lens. In: Tasman W, Jaeger EA. Foundations of clinical ophthalmology, vol II. Philadelphia: JB Lippincott; 1994:1.

Gibbs ML, Jacobs M, Wilkie DM, et al. Posterior lenticonus: clinical patterns and genetics. *J Pediatr Ophthalmol Strabismus* 1993;30:171.

Jaffe NS, Jaffe MS, Jaffe GF. Cataract surgery and its complications. 5th ed. St. Louis: CV Mosby; 1990:359.

Kleinman NJ, Worgul BV. Lens. In: Tasman W, Jaeger EA. Foundations of clinical ophthalmology, vol 1. Philadelphia: JB Lippincott; 1994:1.

Kozart DM, Yanoff M. Intraocular pressure statistics in 100 conservative patients with exfoliation syndrome. *Ophthalmology* 1982;89:214.

La Piana FG. Retinal disease. In: Tasman W, Jaeger EA. Duane's clinical ophthalmology, vol 5. Philadelphia: JB Lippincott; 1994:1.

Parks MM, Johnson DA, Reed GW. Long-term visual results and complications in children with aphakia. *Ophthalmology* 1993;100:826.

Rapuano CJ, Luchs JI, Kim T. The requisites in ophthalmology: anterior segment. Philadelphia: Mosby, 2000.

Schotzer-Schrehardt U, Neuman GO. A histopathologic study of zonular instability in pseudoexfoliative syndrome. *Am J Ophthalmol* 1994;118:730.

Skuta GL. Pseudoexfoliation syndrome, pigment dispersion syndrome and the associated glaucomas. In: Tasman W, Jaeger EA. Duane's clinical ophthalmology, vol 3. Philadelphia: JB Lippincott; 1994:1.

Smith SG, Holland E, Peterson J. Peripheral anterior synechiae formation with anterior chamber intraocular lenses. *Ophthalmic Surg* 1992;23:315.

Smith SG, Lindstrom RL. Intraocular lens complications and their management. *Slack* 1988:167.

Spencer WH. Lens. In: Spencer WH. Ophthalmic pathology, an atlas and textbook, vol 1. 3rd ed. Philadelphia: WB Saunders; 1985:423.

Van Heyninger R. Formation of polyols by the lens of the rat with sugar cataract. *Nature* 1959;184:194.

LENS

S. Gregory Smith
Ralph C. Eagle, Jr.
Edward A. Jaeger
William Tasman

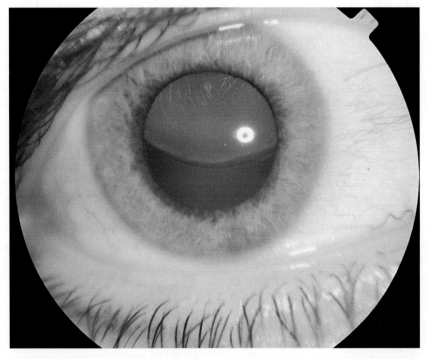

The right eye of a 34-year-old woman with Marfan syndrome shows the typical superior subluxation of the lens. The pupil has been dilated. With a +6.00–7.00 × 180 glass correction, vision was 20/30. A similar condition affected the left eye.

EMBRYOLOGY AND ANATOMY

The crystalline lens is derived embryologically from the surface ectoderm. Early in embryonic life, at about 2 weeks of gestation, the surface ectoderm overlying the optic vesicle (Fig. 2.1A) thickens, forming the lens plate or placode (Fig. 2.1B).

The placode invaginates, forming a hollow ball of cells called the *lens vesicle* as the neuroectodermal optic vesicle concurrently invaginates to form the *optic cup* (Fig. 2.1C, D). The lens vesicle is initially attached to the surface ectoderm, but it separates at about 4 weeks to lie within the anterior portion of the optic cup. The lens vesicle consists of a single layer of cells surrounded by a basal lamina, which becomes the lens capsule.

At about 5 weeks of gestation, the epithelial cells lining the posterior portion of the lens vesicle elongate anteriorly, forming the *primary lens fibers*. The formation of the primary lens fibers obliterates the cavity of the lens vesicle (Fig. 2.1E, F). In the adult lens, these fibers persist as the *central embryonic nucleus*. The layer of epithelium anteriorly continues as a monolayer of cuboidal cells throughout life. Normally, no further cellular proliferation occurs in the posterior portion of the lens, and all new lens cells arise from

a germinative zone located just anterior to the lens equator, where the anterior lens epithelium terminates.

The proliferating equatorial epithelial cells are stimulated to differentiate terminally into mature, highly specialized lens cells, known as *secondary lens fibers* (Fig. 2.2). The secondary lens fibers begin to form at about 7 weeks of gestation. Seven or 8 mm long and hexagonal in cross section, these elongated, strap-like cells are joined together in a remarkably regular array of complex, interdigitating intercellular connections. Mature lens fibers lack nuclei and other organelles, and their homogeneous cytoplasm is filled with a concentrated solution of ordered crystalline proteins. The absence of vessels, lymphatics, nerves, and connective tissue, and the paucity of extracellular space in the lens also contribute to its transparency.

As new secondary lens fibers form, they elongate anteriorly beneath the lens epithelium and posteriorly beneath the capsule to envelope the embryonic nucleus. In the fetal nucleus, the tips of the fibers meet anteriorly and posteriorly, forming the Y-shaped lens sutures. The anterior Y is upright, and the posterior Y is inverted (Fig. 2.2). The Y sutures lie within the fetal nucleus, just beneath the capsule at birth. As new concentric lamellae of secondary lens fibers

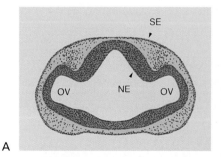
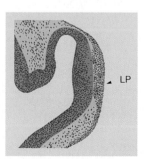
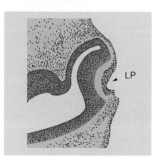

A

B, C

FIGURE 2.1. A: Section through the forebrain of a 4-mm human embryo. The neural ectoderm (NE) is completely internalized, and lateral out-pocketings represent the optic vesicles (OV). The surface ectoderm (SE) is undifferentiated. (Carnegie embryo 6097.) **B:** The surface ectoderm opposite the optic vesicle has thickened to form the lens placode (LP) at the 4.5-mm embryo stage. (Carnegie embryo 8119.) **C:** The lens placode and the internalized neural ectoderm begin to invaginate at about the 7-mm embryonic stage. (Carnegie embryo 7394.) *(continued)*

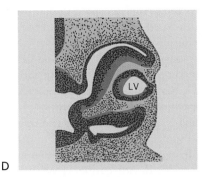 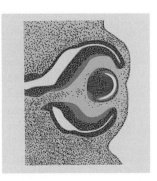 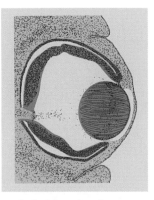

D

E, F

FIGURE 2.1. *Continued.* **D:** At the 10-mm embryonic stage, the lens vesicle (LV) has closed completely and is beginning to separate from the surface ectoderm. The optic cup has developed, but a space remains between the two layers of neural ectoderm. (Carnegie embryo 6517; C–D adapted from Smelser GK. Embryology and morphology of the lens. *Invest Ophthalmol* 1965;4:404, with permission.) **E:** The lens vesicle has separated from the surface ectoderm and lies within the optic cup. The epithelial cells lining the posterior portion of the lens vesicle have elongated anteroposteriorly to form the primary lens fibers at the 15-mm embryonic stage. (Carnegie embryo 6520; adapted from Kleiman NJ, Worgul BV. Lens. In: Tasman W, Jaeger EA. Biomedical foundations of ophthalmology, vol 1. Philadelphia: JB Lippincott; 1994:1; courtesy of Basil V. Worgul, Ph.D., and Victoria Ozamics, New York, NY, with permission.) **F:** At the 18-mm embryonic stage, the lens vesicle is completely filled by the primary lens fibers. These fibers denucleate and will form the embryonal nucleus. (Carnegie embryo 5537; courtesy of Basil V. Worgul, Ph.D., and Victoria Ozamics, New York, NY.)

form after birth, the sutural pattern becomes increasingly complex. A nine-branched stellate pattern is found in the adult nucleus at 20 years of age.

The lens continues to grow throughout life. New con-

centric lamellae of secondary lens fibers successively form in the periphery of the lens in an onion-like fashion. As new cells form, the older cells are sequestered centrally. The newer cells comprise the lens cortex, and the older cells constitute the nucleus (Fig. 2.3). Lines of discontinuity form within the lens and represent the interface between layers. These lines create the typical slit lamp appearance of the adult lens (Fig. 2.4).

Inherent in this normal developmental pattern lies the inevitability of senile nuclear cataract. With the passage of time, the older lens fibers in the nucleus gradually degenerate. Cellular membranes dissolve, and soluble crystalline proteins denature and dehydrate. Yellow-brown urochrome

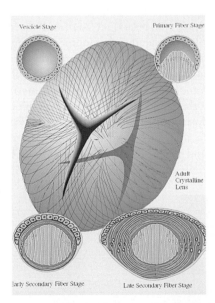

FIGURE 2.2. Lens vesicle development. The *upper left* portion shows closed vesicle stage. In the *upper right* portion, the epithelial cells lining the posterior portion of the lens vesicle have elongated anteriorly to form the primary lens fibers. The *lower left* portion shows the early secondary lens fiber stage. The equatorial cells have elongated into secondary lens fibers and are beginning to engulf the primary fibers. The *lower right* portion demonstrates the advanced secondary fiber stage. The strap-like secondary fibers have enclosed the future embryonal nucleus. Their ends meet to form the Y sutures (*center*) and will eventually comprise the fetal nucleus. (Courtesy of Neal H. Atebara, M.D., Honolulu, HI.)

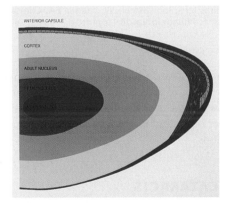

FIGURE 2.3. Schematic drawing of the adult lens showing the nuclear zones, cortex, epithelium, and capsule. New lens fibers are derived from the epithelial cells in the equatorial region. The nuclei remain at the equator, and the cytoplasm extends anteriorly and posteriorly. (From Hogan MJ, Alvarado JA, Weddel JE. Histology of the human eye. Philadelphia: WB Saunders; 1971:642, with permission.)

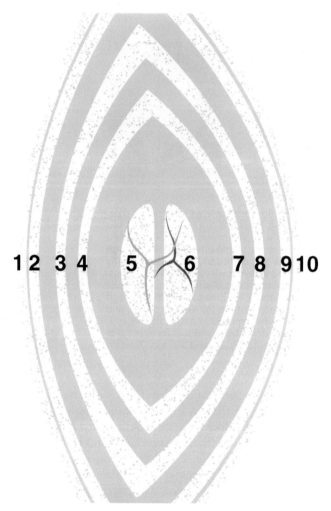

FIGURE 2.4. Schematic optical section of the normal adult lens. (1, anterior capsule; 2, anterior line of disjunction between the lens epithelium and the cortex; 3, anterior surface of the adult nucleus; 4, anterior surface of the fetal nucleus; 5, anterior half of the fetal nucleus, containing the anterior Y suture; 6, posterior half of the fetal nucleus, containing the posterior Y suture; 7, posterior surface of the fetal nucleus; 8, posterior surface of the adult nucleus; 9, posterior line of disjunction; 10, posterior capsule. From Phelps CD. Examination and functional evaluation of the crystalline lens. In: Tasman W, Jaeger EA. Clinical ophthalmology, vol 1. Philadelphia: JB Lippincott; 1994:2, with permission.)

pigment accumulates, and densification of the nucleus increases its index of refraction. These changes are evident clinically as nuclear sclerosis. The former Y suture lines tend to fade later in life and may not be visible after nuclear sclerosis develops.

ADULT CATARACTS

Classification and Pathophysiology

There has been considerable variation in and some degree of confusion about the terminology used to identify cataracts. The older literature tended to be descriptive in that opaci-

ties were labeled according to their appearance, such as cerulean (i.e., blue), stellate, spear, cupuliform (i.e., saucer shaped). Latin-based phraseology was often used, such as cataract pisciformis (i.e., fish-like cataract). Many of these terms are no longer commonly used, and cataracts tend to be described according to their anatomic location: cortical, nuclear, and subcapsular. Frequently, more than one area of the lens is opacified in the same patient.

This section is not intended to be a compendium of lens opacities, but some of the more common varieties are illustrated. Specific types of lens opacities often have been associated with specific disease entities. Included in this group are the blue dot cortical opacities and posterior subcapsular cataract (PSC) of myotonic dystrophy, the PSC of atopic dermatitis, and the discrete white cortical opacities associated with hypocalcemia. Snowflake opacities located in the anterior and posterior subcapsular cortex have been associated with diabetes mellitus and Down syndrome (Fig. 2.5). Cortical wedges caused by lens fiber swelling may be seen in acute-onset diabetes. More commonly, age-related cataract types occur earlier and more frequently in diabetics (particularly PSC) and Down syndrome patients and progress at a faster rate. Retinal degenerations, such as retinitis pigmentosa and gyrate atrophy, are usually associated with PSCs.

A category of "presenile" cataracts has been described in which age-related cataracts occur prematurely. Lens opacities may occur earlier in life than "normal" because of genetic defects, other ocular and systemic diseases, certain medications, trauma, and idiopathic causes.

Much research has been directed toward determining the pathophysiology of cataract development. Extensive studies in animal models have revealed information regarding the fundamental cataractous process, but much still remains a mystery. Datiles and Kinoshita have summarized current thinking on this subject. There is no single process that results in the formation of lens opacities. A wide variety of precipitating factors, including nutritional, environmental, metabolic, and genetic elements, are involved. However, ac-

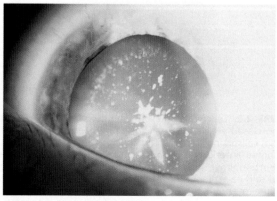

FIGURE 2.5. Discrete flakes in the anterior and posterior cortex in a 26-year-old man with Down syndrome. An incomplete, cortical, star-shaped opacity is also evident.

cording to Datiles and others, there appear to be two fundamental processes that lead to lens opacification. One process occurs in the lens cortex and is characterized by an electrolyte imbalance. The normal lens contains a low-sodium, high-potassium content. The reverse is true in a cortical cataract, leading to increased membrane permeability and hydration of the cortex. The second process occurs in the nucleus, where modification of lens fiber proteins occurs, resulting in higher-molecular-weight protein aggregates. There is no significant change in the electrolyte balance. Oxidation, proteolysis, glycation, and deamidation may be responsible for these changes.

This is a gross oversimplification of a complex and poorly understood process, and interested readers should explore the extensive research reports available throughout the literature. Much work remains to be done in this area.

The diabetic cataract presents a better understood pathophysiologic process. Twenty-five years ago, Van Heyninger reported the finding of polyol sorbitol in the lenses of diabetic rats. Sorbitol forms from the reduction of glucose by the enzyme aldose reductase. Because sorbitol does not pass freely through cell membranes, an osmotic pressure gradient forms, resulting in an influx of water into the cell and swelling. Hydration of the cell leads to opacification.

Types of Cataracts

Flecks, Dots, Flakes, and Clubs

When examining the lens with the slit lamp, a wide variety of opacities in the form of multiple white, grayish, or blue dots, flecks, or clubs may be seen (Fig. 2.6).

Clinical Features. These opacities may appear in the anterior or posterior cortex. These may be congenital or develop in the transition to the adult lens. If they occur in a ring configuration near the lens equator, the term *coronary cataract* has been applied (Fig. 2.7). Their cause remains speculative. They may result from a degeneration of the cytoplasm of lens cells over which normal lens fibers were sub-

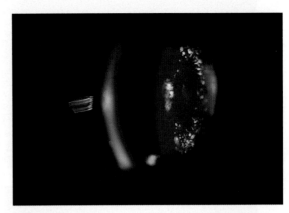

FIGURE 2.7. A coronary cataract is characterized by dot- and club-shaped opacities in a wreath-like configuration in the anterior and posterior cortex.

sequently formed. Cogan and Kuwabara suggested that these were the result of wart-like excrescences that developed on the back surface of the anterior lens capsule. These eventually degenerate and are displaced inward by newly formed fibers.

These opacities do not affect vision, and their relation to the development of any subsequent age-related cataract remains speculative.

Cortical Cataract

A cortical cataract is characterized by spoke-like opacifications in the periphery of the lens that radiate toward the center (Fig. 2.8).

Clinical Features. These radial opacifications may remain peripheral but often coalesce and encroach on the visual axis. They can occur anterior or posterior to the nucleus. Water clefts and vacuoles, clear areas within the cortex, are frequently observed in the early stages of cataract formation (Fig. 2.9).

Patients with cortical cataracts may become visually symptomatic under bright light conditions. The clinical course is usually one of slow progression, and good visual acuity can be maintained for years.

Management. The decision to recommend cataract removal depends on subjective visual functional impairment, objective measures of visual function, density of the opacity, presence of other ocular disease, and the patient's health.

Nuclear Sclerosis

Nuclear sclerosis is characterized by hardening and yellowing of the lens nucleus.

Clinical Features. Typically a brownish yellow discoloration of the lens is seen centrally (Fig. 2.10). In its more advanced forms, the lens may become reddish, and in the most severe form, it may become black. Patients with nuclear sclerosis may have complaints of monocular diplopia

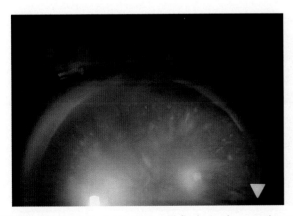

FIGURE 2.6. Discrete dots, clubs, and flecks in the anterior cortex.

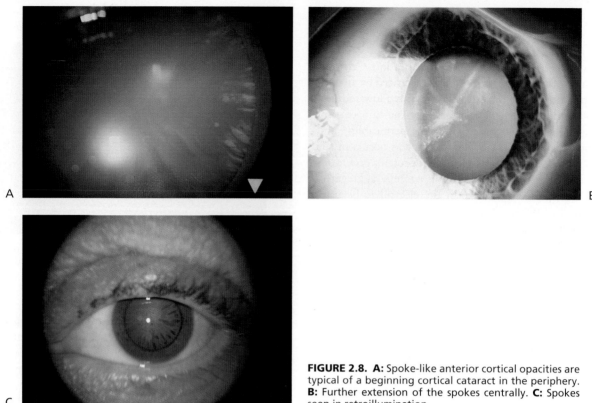

FIGURE 2.8. **A:** Spoke-like anterior cortical opacities are typical of a beginning cortical cataract in the periphery. **B:** Further extension of the spokes centrally. **C:** Spokes seen in retroillumination.

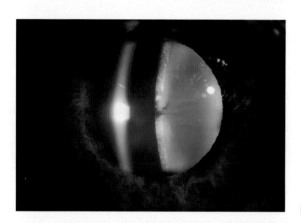

FIGURE 2.9. Water clefts *(clear areas)* in the anterior cortex.

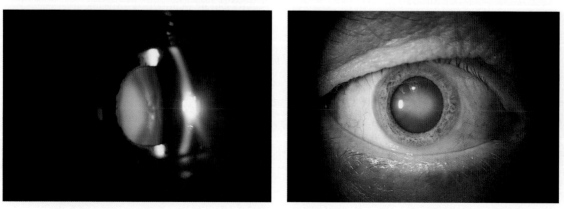

FIGURE 2.10. Yellowish brown discoloration of the nucleus is typical of nuclear sclerosis. Slit lamp cross-sectional view **(A)** and direct view **(B)**, in which the discoloration is more gray.

and glare. Typically, patients with nuclear sclerotic cataracts have worsening of their symptoms at night or under low levels of light. Nuclear sclerosis increases the refractive index of the lens, resulting in progressively more myopia or less hyperopia. Although patients may initially have good near vision, as the cataract matures, they may have increasing difficulty reading for extended periods because of multiple images from irregular hardening and refraction of the lens nucleus.

Management. Change in the refractive index of the lens results in a myopic shift and frequently requires a change in the distance prescription. However, the glass change may make the middle range or near vision worse, requiring a detailed explanation by the refractionist. When the best refraction does not provide adequate visual function, surgery is indicated.

Posterior Subcapsular Cataract

Posterior subcapsular cataract is characterized by a proliferation of cells on the posterior capsule of the lens, usually accompanied by opacification of the adjacent posterior cortex.

Clinical Features. The posterior capsular opacification is frequently located in the visual axis but may occur outside of it as well (Fig. 2.11). The affected area appears irregular and looks like the surface of the moon on slit lamp examination. Its growth is often rapid. Fortunately, this is the least common of the three main cataract types. This cataract can be seen in the presence of other types of cataracts and may be associated with uveitis, prolonged steroid use, irradiation, and diabetes. The symptoms of these patients worsen in bright light, and decreased reading vision is an early symptom.

Management. It is important to test the patient's vision under normal and bright light conditions. Initially, the patient has good vision under scotopic testing conditions but later has difficulty under bright light conditions. The indications for cataract surgery are similar to those for other forms of lens opacity.

Mature Cataract

In a mature cataract, the lens is white, and no iris shadow is seen on oblique penlight examination.

Clinical Features. Complete opacification of the cortex results in the white appearance of the lens (Fig. 2.12). Sometimes, a sclerotic nucleus can be seen through the cortex on slit lamp examination. The fundus cannot be adequately examined ophthalmoscopically. Typically, this type of cataract is acquired over a long period.

Management. Before cataract surgery, some assessment of retinal function is necessary. The pupils should be checked for an afferent defect. Two-point light discrimination and light projection in each quadrant can be tested. Other tests of macular function include blue field entoptic phenomena and the use of a potential acuity meter and laser interferometry. Unfortunately, these tests are not totally reliable in cases of very dense cataracts. B-scan ultrasonography should be done to rule out other posterior segment pathology. Care is necessary during the anterior capsulotomy, because cortical material may leak out and blur the view. If surgery is deferred for any reason, these patients should be followed regularly. Leakage of lens material into the anterior chamber may result in phacolytic glaucoma, or further swelling of the lens may induce angle closure.

Hypermature or Morgagnian Cataract

A hypermature or morgagnian cataract is a further deterioration of a mature cataract in which the cortex has liquefied.

Clinical Features. The lens is totally opaque and no fundus reflex is visible. The brownish nucleus drops into a dependent position and may be detected inferiorly through the milky cortex on slit lamp examination (Fig. 2.13). The nucleus undergoes partial reabsorption and is smaller than normal.

The lens may spontaneously rupture, allowing liquid cortex to permeate the anterior chamber and resulting in phacolytic glaucoma.

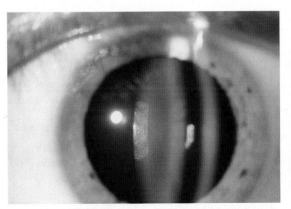

A

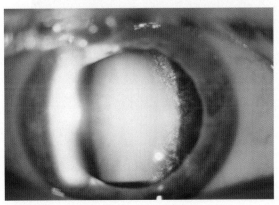

B

FIGURE 2.11. Posterior subcapsular cataract (PSC) is characterized by opacification of the posterior capsule and adjacent posterior cortex. **A:** Early PSC and **(B)** more advanced opacification along with nuclear sclerosis. (Courtesy of Stephen B. Lichtenstein, M.D., Philadelphia, PA.)

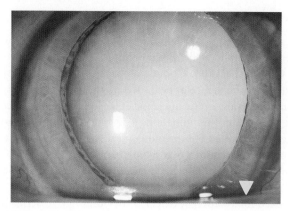

FIGURE 2.12. Mature cataract with complete opacification of the lens.

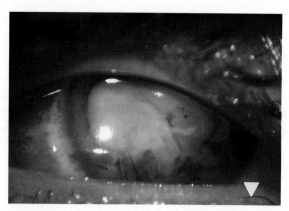

FIGURE 2.14. Traumatic cataract with opacification of the cortex and disruption of the iris due to a penetrating injury.

Management. B-scan ultrasound should be done to rule out retinal detachment or intraocular tumor, and the previously described tests can be attempted to assess visual potential. Cataract extraction presents some technical difficulties. The anterior capsule is usually thin, and once incised, it may be obscured by the milky cortex. Because visualization is poor, care must be taken to ensure that the capsulotomy does not extend posteriorly. A manual extracapsular technique is probably the procedure of choice. The nucleus can often be removed with an irrigating vectis through a 7-mm incision. If phacoemulsification is used, a second stab incision should be made to provide a second instrument for manipulation of the nucleus. In the absence of formed cortex, the nucleus is forced directly against the posterior capsule, increasing the risk of a capsular tear.

Plaques and fibrosis are common on the posterior capsule, which may be difficult to remove. Care must be exercised not to rupture the capsule. In most cases, a posterior chamber lens can be placed in the bag.

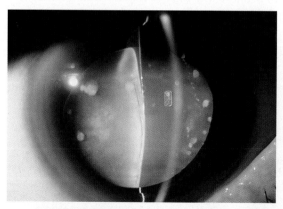

FIGURE 2.13. Hypermature (i.e., morgagnian) cataract. The cortex has liquefied, and the brownish nucleus has dropped into a dependent position. (Courtesy of Jamie E. Nichols, Philadelphia, PA.)

Traumatic Cataract

A traumatic cataract occurs when the lens capsule is perforated by a foreign object but may also occur secondary to severe blunt trauma.

Clinical Features. In the initial few days after the trauma, the lens may remain clear, and in some cases, the area of perforation can spontaneously seal. If it does not seal, fluid imbibition occurs, and rapid swelling and opacification of the lens ensues, markedly decreasing vision (Fig. 2.14). Lens opacification associated with blunt trauma can develop months or years after injury.

Management. Surgery is indicated when the lens opacity becomes visually significant, particularly if there is rapid swelling, which may compromise the anterior chamber angle. In doing cataract surgery, care must be taken to identify the original tear in the anterior capsule, and a capsulotomy should be performed in such a way that prevents tearing into the posterior capsule. An initial incision in the anterior capsule with a Vannas scissors often works well, and a can-opener type capsulotomy may be necessary to perform an adequate anterior capsulotomy. In a young patient, the nucleus is usually soft, and phacoemulsification can be readily performed. The lens may need to be placed in the sulcus if the capsular bag is inadequate.

Complicated Cataract

Complicated cataract develops as a result of longstanding intraocular disease, such as chronic uveitis, retinal detachment, prolonged hemorrhage, or tumor.

Clinical Features. Chronic iridocyclitis is the most common cause of complicated cataract. Typically, chronic inflammation and the use of steroid medication result initially in a posterior subcapsular type of opacity. After prolonged inflammation, cortical changes develop that can progress to a mature cataract (Fig. 2.15). Posterior synechiae often are present.

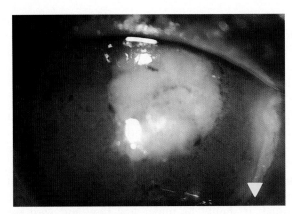

FIGURE 2.15. This complicated cataract was characterized by extensive opacification of the cortex and iris atrophy in a patient with longstanding sarcoid uveitis.

Management. Control of the inflammation or other underlying pathology often arrests the cataract development. If vision is significantly decreased and retinal function has not been affected, cataract surgery can be considered. In the case of uveitis, the inflammation may recur after surgery.

Cataract Associated With Medication

Certain drugs, usually administered over a long period, have been associated with cataract formation.

Corticosteroid-Related Cataract
Clinical Features. Corticosteroids given topically or systemically are the most commonly encountered group of drugs causing cataracts. These lesions begin as axially positioned posterior subcapsular opacities (Fig. 2.16). They are dose and duration related, and they rarely begin before 1 year of steroid therapy is completed.

Management. Cessation of the drug may stop or retard lens opacification. In some patients, continued steroid therapy is necessary, resulting in further cataract development. Surgical removal is judged on the basis of the degree of interference with visual function.

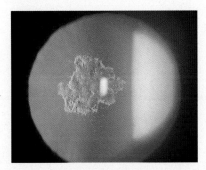

FIGURE 2.16. Posterior subcapsular cataract seen in retroillumination in a 32-year-old patient with severe steroid-dependent asthma. (Courtesy of Stephen B. Lichtenstein, M.D., Philadelphia, PA.)

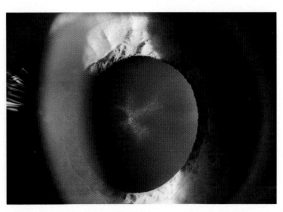

FIGURE 2.17. Stellate anterior subcapsular lens opacity in a patient with a history of high-dose, long-term treatment with a phenothiazine medication for psychiatric dysfunction. (Courtesy of Kit Johnson and M. Lisa McHam, M.D., Boston, MA.)

Phenothiazine-Related Cataract
Clinical Features. The phenothiazine class of antipsychotic drugs (e.g., chlorpromazine, thioridazine) is frequently used in the treatment of patients with chronic psychiatric conditions. Bilateral stellate anterior subcapsular lens opacities have been associated with phenothiazine therapy (Fig. 2.17). Other ocular findings associated with toxicity include pigment dusting of the corneal endothelium, atrophy of the retinal pigment epithelium, and associated pigmentary retinopathy. The ocular findings seen with phenothiazine toxicity appear to be duration and dose related.

Management. The lens opacities usually do not result in serious visual dysfunction. The pigmentary retinopathy is more of a concern. The ocular findings usually persist even after the cessation of therapy.

Topical Miotic-Related Cataract
Lens opacities have been associated with long-term use of topical miotics for the treatment of esotropia in children. Echothiophate and demecarium bromide have been reported to cause anterior subcapsular vacuoles, as well as posterior cortical and nuclear changes. Cessation of the therapy stops or even reverses the opacities.

OTHER DISEASES OF THE LENS
Pseudoexfoliation Syndrome

Pseudoexfoliation syndrome (PXS) appears as whitish blue dandruff-like deposits on the anterior lens capsule and pupillary margin. It is found primarily in the elderly, and incidence increases with increasing age.

Clinical Features. Pseudoexfoliation is appreciated best with the pupil dilated. The deposits on the front surface of the lens usually form a target-like configuration. The central bull's-eye corresponds to the diameter of the undilated pupil (Fig. 2.18). Surrounding the central disc is an intermediate

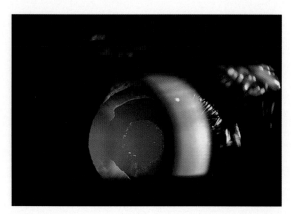

FIGURE 2.18. Typical appearance of the anterior surface of the lens capsule in a patient with pseudoexfoliation syndrome. (Courtesy of Robert Bailey, M.D., Philadelphia, PA.)

clear area that is presumably wiped clean by movement of the juxtapupillary iris. Some of the deposit areas may exhibit curled edges or strands. Sheet-like granular areas with curled edges are peripheral to the clear zone. There can be considerable variation in this clinical appearance. Additional deposits occur on the back of the cornea, angle, zonules, and ciliary processes in addition to the pupil margin. Increased iris pigment dispersion occurs in PXS, and iris transillumination defects may be found. The accumulation of pigment anterior to Schwalbe's line is known as Sampaolesi's line and is characteristic of PXS.

The zonules are weakened in PXS. Rarely, subluxation of the lens occurs in the case of a mature cataract and longstanding PXS (Fig. 2.19). Exfoliation material is produced by the lens epithelium and the nonpigmented epithelium of the ciliary processes. Evidence suggests the PXS may be the ocular manifestation of an otherwise benign disorder of elastic tissue.

An increased prevalence of open-angle glaucoma is associated with PXS. Presumably, this is the result of deposition of the material and pigment within the drainage system. Although figures vary widely, one study reported that 15% of patients with PXS also had elevated intraocular pressure. The longer the duration of PXS, the more likely is the development of increased intraocular pressure.

Management. Patients with PXS should be followed periodically for the development of glaucoma. Cataract surgery must be approached with caution in patients with PXS. The iris is more rigid, and the pupil does not dilate well, making surgery more difficult. The zonules are weakened and are more prone to rupture during cataract extraction, resulting in vitreous loss. If phacoemulsification is preformed, it should be under low flow and with rotary movements of the nucleus. The lens can be safely removed without disinserting of the capsular bag in most cases.

Subluxation of the Lens

Weakening or rupture of a segment of the zonules results in displacement of the lens (i.e., ectopia lentis) in a direction opposite to the disinsertion. Many diseases and trauma are associated with lens subluxation.

Clinical Features. All degrees of subluxation may be seen. Classically, iridodonesis is seen on slit lamp examination with eye movement. Phakodonesis may also be observed. The body of the lens is displaced, and stretched or absent zonules may be noticed in the affected segment when the pupil is dilated. In severe cases, the lens may be displaced into the vitreous cavity or anterior chamber.

The most common causes of subluxation of the lens are Marfan syndrome, homocystinuria, and trauma. Subluxation occurs in 80% of those with Marfan syndrome, and typically, the lens is displaced superiorly (Fig. 2.20). In homocystinuria, the zonular weakness is generalized rather than segmental, resulting in a gravity-induced downward displacement of the lens. Other systemic abnormalities that have been associated with ectopia lentis include Weill-

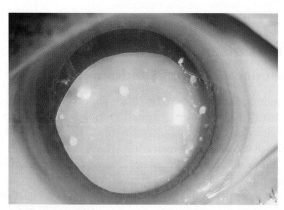

FIGURE 2.19. Inferior subluxation of the lens in an 82-year-old patient with longstanding pseudoexfoliation and a mature cataract. (Courtesy of Jamie E. Nichols, Philadelphia, PA.)

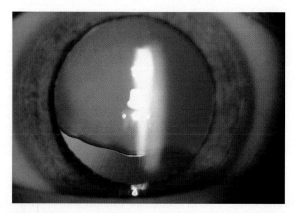

FIGURE 2.20. Superior subluxation of the lens in a 32-year-old woman with Marfan syndrome. Notice the irregular inferior border of the lens created by variable zonular traction. (Courtesy of Robert Bailey, M.D., Philadelphia, PA.)

Marchesani syndrome, sulfite oxidase deficiency, and syphilis.

Management. A conservative approach is indicated in the management of patients with subluxation of the lens. In particular, patients with Marfan syndrome may be followed for many years, even though the observer is uncomfortable with the degree of subluxation. Periodic refraction and observation are necessary. If the lens is subluxated into the vitreous, observation alone still may be indicated, and the patient fitted with a soft contact lens. Subluxation into the anterior chamber may result in an acute glaucoma. Sometimes, if the pupil is dilated and the patient placed in a supine position, the lens returns to the posterior chamber, in which case pilocarpine should be instilled. In other cases, it may be wise to remove the lens at this time. Any eye sustaining blunt trauma should be examined for zonular rupture and lens subluxation.

If cataract surgery must be undertaken, the surgeon must pay close attention to the zonules, because they may further disinsert during the extraction. An anterior vitrectomy is often necessary. Because the capsular support is often lacking, the surgeon should be prepared to suture a posterior chamber lens to the sulcus or the iris, use an anterior chamber lens, or consider contact lens aphakic correction.

Microspherophakia

Microspherophakia is characterized by a small, round lens.

Clinical Features. The dilated examination reveals the entire lens and supporting zonules to be within the pupillary space (Fig. 2.21). Patients with microspherophakia frequently develop a pupillary block-type glaucoma caused by anterior prolapse of the lens. This commonly occurs at nighttime, causing pain and discomfort. The situation is usually relieved by placing the patient in a supine position, permitting the lens to fall back into the posterior chamber. However, progressive peripheral anterior synechiae may form.

Microspherophakia is commonly associated with Weill-Marchesani syndrome, in which the lens is displaced superior temporally. Other features of this syndrome include small stature, brachydactyly, deafness, and a high degree of myopia.

Management. Patients with microspherophakia should undergo gonioscopy to determine whether peripheral anterior synechiae are present. A peripheral laser iridotomy should be considered to prevent repeated attacks of pupillary block glaucoma and progressive closure of the filtration angle by peripheral anterior synechiae. The zonules are loose, and the lens may eventually disinsert, resulting in dislocation. If cataract surgery is undertaken, the surgeon should be prepared to suture the intraocular lens to the iris or sclera. An anterior chamber lens is usually contraindicated in these patients because of peripheral anterior synechiae.

Anterior Lenticonus

The term *lenticonus* refers to a developmental anomaly in which the surface of the axial portion of the lens protrudes like a cone. If this localized protrusion is spherical, the term *lentiglobus* is used.

Clinical Features. Anterior lenticonus is a rare condition in which the front surface of the lens is conically shaped (Fig. 2.22). The lens capsule thins or even disappears at the apex of the cone. This abnormal lens shape may result in a high degree of lenticular myopia. Focal opacification of the lens may develop within the area of the cone. The condition may be discovered because of poor vision on a screening examination, strabismus, or a distorted fundus reflex.

Anterior lenticonus has been associated with Alport's syndrome, a hereditary disorder of basement membrane collagen that is transmitted as an autosomal dominant condition with variable penetrance. Other features of this syndrome include hemorrhagic nephritis and nerve deafness. Anterior polar cataracts and an albipunctatus-like fundus appearance have been associated with this syndrome.

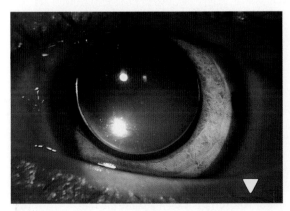

FIGURE 2.21. In microspherophakia, the entire lens appears within the dilated pupil and has been displaced into the anterior chamber.

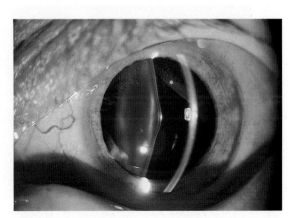

FIGURE 2.22. Localized cone-like protrusions of the lens surface occur in anterior lenticonus. (Courtesy of Stephen B. Lichtenstein, M.D., Philadelphia, PA.)

Management. Visual symptoms depend on the degree of distortion and anisometropia created by the cone. If minimal and discovered early, significant amblyopia may be avoided. Frequent refraction is necessary. If the lens opacity becomes significant, it is managed as any other developmental cataract.

Posterior Lenticonus

Posterior lenticonus is an uncommon abnormality in which the back surface of the lens undergoes progressive posterior bowing. The condition begins in early infancy and is usually unilateral and sporadic, although bilateral and familial cases have been reported. The cause is unknown, but trauma, traction from the hyaloid system, and inflammation have been suggested.

Clinical Features. Posterior lenticonus is seen initially as a transparent, usually axial, conical, posterior projection of the posterior lens in a normal-sized eye. If the projection is more generalized, the term lentiglobus has been used. The initial clinical findings are an oil droplet appearance in the central red reflex on ophthalmoscopy and a pathognomonic scissors movement on retinoscopy (Fig. 2.23A). The axial refraction is markedly myopic, and the peripheral error may be hyperopic.

Anisometropia or optical distortion may result in amblyopia. Strabismus affects a significant percentage of patients. Cataracts develop in the most severe cases, beginning with opacification of the posterior cortex, which may obscure the underlying defect (Fig. 2.23B).

Management. Amblyopia detected in the oil droplet, clear lens stage or found postoperatively should be managed in the usual fashion. Significant lens opacification presents all of the therapeutic challenges of unilateral congenital cataract. Management techniques have included lens extraction with refractive correction by intraocular lens implantation, a contact lens, aphakic glass correction, or epikeratoplasty. Visual results may be reasonably good (i.e., 49% achieved 20/20 to 20/40 in one series) if the condition is detected early.

COMMON COMPLICATIONS OF CATARACT SURGERY

Wound Gape and Dehiscence

Clinical Features. On slit lamp examination, a space is seen between the anterior and posterior edges of the wound; the space results from inadequate suturing techniques, excessive cautery, or overheating during phacoemulsification (Fig. 2.24A). Iris tissue can become incarcerated in the wound (Fig. 2.24B). Wound gape may be noticed immediately after surgery or may occur after minor trauma during the wound healing process. The patient often notices a decrease in vision as a result of the development of plus cylinder astigmatism at 180 degrees. The wound leak can also lead to the development of a flat or shallow anterior chamber and choroidal detachment. The patient is also at greater risk for the development of endophthalmitis and epithelial downgrowth. A wound leak is thought to be an inciting factor in the development of pupillary block. These complications were much more common after intracapsular cataract extraction. Although they may occur in extracapsular-type procedures, particularly in complicated cases with vitreous loss, the advent of small-incision surgery has greatly reduced their incidence.

Management. Seidel's test should be done to rule out the presence of a wound leak. With the patient looking downward, a fluorescein strip wetted with a topical anesthetic should be used to "paint" the incision area. Under a cobalt light, the leak produces a bright ribbon of the dye flowing downward. Keratometric and refractive readings should be obtained. If the Seidel's test result is positive, the iris is exposed, or the astigmatism marked, resuturing of the wound should be considered.

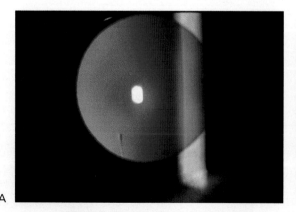
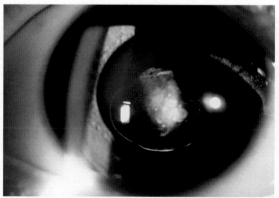

FIGURE 2.23. A: "Oil droplet" appearance of the posterior lens surface is seen against the red fundus reflex on slit lamp examination in a 4-year-old boy with posterior lenticonus. **B:** Axial opacification in the posterior cortex is seen in the other eye of the same patient. (Courtesy of Jonathan S. Myers, M.D., Philadelphia, PA.)

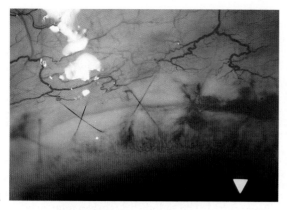
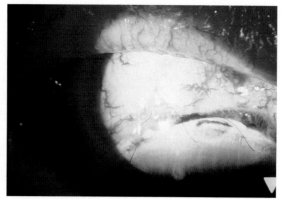

A

B

FIGURE 2.24. A: A gap can be seen between the wound edges. **B:** Brownish tissue indicates the inclusion of iris in the wound.

Iris Prolapse

Clinical Features. An iris prolapse appears as a dark brown bulge of tissue through the cataract wound (Fig. 2.25). This may be the result of faulty wound closure but more frequently results from increased intraocular pressure during the immediate postoperative period. Direct trauma may also cause iris prolapse.

Management. Continued exposure of the iris increases the risk of intraocular infection or persistent low-grade inflammation, which can result in cystoid macular edema. The intraocular pressure should be controlled. In most cases, surgical management consists of excising the prolapsed iris, constricting the remaining iris with Miochol, and resuturing the wound.

Wound Bleb

Clinical Features. A bleb may form with a limbal or fornix-based flap if the conjunctival wound has sealed and a scleral wound leak remains. It is rare in modern small-incision surgery. Initially, the conjunctiva may appear edematous over the area of wound dehiscence. With continued leakage, the bleb may enlarge, producing conjunctival thinning (Fig.

2.26). Blebs may develop later in the wound-healing process as well. If large, the bleb itself may result in a scratchy, foreign body sensation, and it may induce refractive changes. More importantly, the patient needs to be observed for all of the complications associated with wound leak previously mentioned.

Management. Seidel's test should be done. Sometimes, a wound leak detected in the immediate postoperative period can be treated by a pressure patch and Diamox to reduce aqueous secretion. If the bleb remains small, observation may be indicated. However, continued evidence of leakage or hypotony dictates surgical repair of the wound.

Blebs that develop late or are of long duration present more difficult problems. If asymptomatic in a quiet eye, no action is necessary. If the bleb is large and thinning and if leakage or chronic inflammation is present, more aggressive action is indicated. Cryotherapy applied to the bleb may thicken the conjunctiva and shrink the bleb. The application of trichloroacetic acid to the bleb has been used in the past. Autologous blood has been injected into the bleb to try to initiate scar formation. Surgical repair is difficult because the wound leak has formed a fistula with an endothelial cell lining. Creation of a scleral flap to cover the wound has been

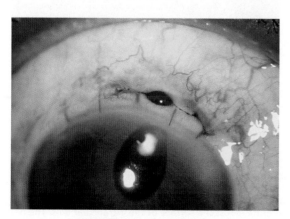

FIGURE 2.25. Iris prolapse.

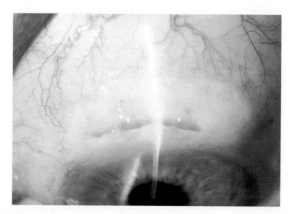

FIGURE 2.26. Conjunctival bleb resulting from a wound leak. (Courtesy of Stephen B. Lichtenstein, M.D., Philadelphia, PA.)

tried. The most definitive treatment involves the use of a lamellar patch of donor corneal tissue. A 5-mm trephine is used to create a one-third depth bed over the fistula. A similar button is obtained from the donor cornea and sutured in place.

Corneal Edema and Bullous Keratopathy

A decrease in the integrity of the corneal endothelium may result in persistent corneal edema or bullous keratopathy after cataract surgery.

Clinical Features. The endothelium is a single cell layer that does not have the ability to reproduce, although the existing cells can expand to maintain the integrity of the layer. Cataract surgery results in a decrease in the corneal endothelial cell count. Endothelial cell loss rates of 8% or less during surgery have been reported. A critical cell count may be reached (400 to 600 cells/mm^2), at which point the cellular pump mechanism is insufficient to preserve the proper electrolyte and fluid balance, and the cornea becomes edematous. This situation may occur in the immediate postoperative period or take many years to develop.

The edema can begin in a focal area in the peripheral or central cornea with thickening of the stroma and bedewing of the epithelium. Symptoms include decreased vision, intermittent pain, a scratchy sensation, tearing, and sensitivity to lights. As the edema becomes widespread, symptoms increase, and vision becomes blurred. The cornea loses its luster, thickens, and appears cloudy (Fig. 2.27). The epithelium becomes edematous, with areas of breakdown and subepithelial fluid accumulation. This condition is called *bullous keratopathy.*

Cataract surgery is the most common precipitating factor leading to the development of corneal edema. If an implant has been inserted, the term *pseudophakic bullous keratopathy* is used. Conditions that predispose to bullous keratopathy include preoperative corneal disease (such as cornea guttata), poor surgical technique, excessive irrigation and ma-

nipulation, vitreous touch, prolonged postoperative inflammation, and anterior chamber lenses.

Management. In the early stages of bullous keratopathy, the patient can be maintained on hyperosmotic drops and ointment. Any elevation of intraocular pressure should be controlled. If the edema becomes generalized and the vision compromised, corneal transplant and lens exchange should be considered. The decision to proceed should be based on the patient's desires, general health, life expectancy, absence of other ocular pathology, and status of the other eye.

An anterior chamber lens should be removed if peripheral anterior synechiae are present and corneal decompensation has occurred. The endothelial cells can migrate off the peripheral anterior synechiae and touch the lens material. In these eyes, a sutured posterior chamber lens should be considered.

Residual Cortical and Nuclear Fragments

Occasionally, remnants of the lens cortex or nuclear fragments remain in the eye after cataract surgery (Fig. 2.28A, B).

Clinical Features. Cortical remnants may appear small or

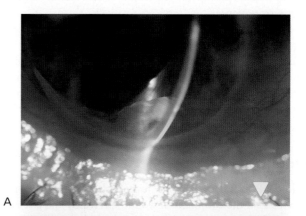

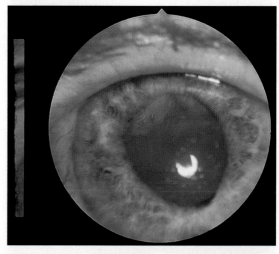

FIGURE 2.28. A: A residual fragment of nucleus seen in the anterior chamber after a complicated cataract extraction. **B:** A patient demonstrating residual cortical material that is starting to proliferate across the surface of the intraocular lens. The patient complained of glare at nighttime.

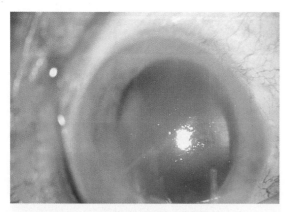

FIGURE 2.27. Pseudophakic bullous keratopathy associated with a closed loop anterior chamber lens developed 4 years after cataract surgery.

may be hidden by the iris at the time of surgery but swell into larger, fluffy, white opacities in the postoperative period. They often migrate into the anterior chamber. However, cortex in the anterior chamber is relatively benign and usually dissolves in several weeks. Cortex that is located between the intraocular lens and the posterior capsule or between the peripheral anterior and posterior capsule takes longer to be reabsorbed and may result in early opacification of the capsule or a Soemmering's ring. Cortex in the vitreous also takes longer to resolve. Increased inflammatory reactions sometimes develop in these eyes.

Nuclear fragments in the anterior chamber or vitreous may remain for an extended period and cause marked inflammation. One of the most dreaded complications is the rupture of the posterior capsule, with loss of the entire nucleus or a large fragment into the vitreous (Fig. 2.29).

Management. Most cortex in the anterior chamber reabsorbs. The inflammatory reaction and any elevation of intraocular pressure can usually be controlled medically. Excessive cortex between the intraocular lens and the capsule may need to be removed surgically.

The management of nuclear fragments depends on their size and associated reaction. Fragments in the anterior chamber frequently damage the corneal endothelium and are very slow to dissolve. The patient should be followed with periodic cell counts. If decreasing, the fragment should be removed. Small nuclear fragments in the vitreous can be observed, but larger ones should be removed by a retinal surgeon. Many surgeons think that a lens can be inserted at the time of surgery even if the nucleus cannot be completely removed.

Peaked Pupil

The peaked pupil is not round but appears peaked or shaped like a teardrop, with the apex pointed toward the cataract wound.

Clinical Features. A peaked pupil may result from a variety of intraoperative circumstances. Adhesion to or en-

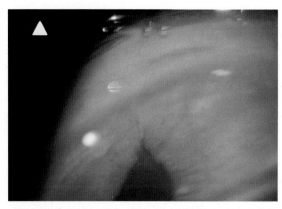

FIGURE 2.30. Gonioscopic view of a peaked pupil caused by a strand of vitreous extending to the wound.

trapment of the iris in the wound can result in an updrawn, peaked pupil. The inclusion of vitreous strands, cortical fragments, and capsular fragments in the wound can produce a similar appearance (Fig. 2.30). Adhesions of the posterior iris surface to the underlying capsule, intraocular lens positioning hole, or haptic loop with subsequent contracture can tent the pupil. Sphincter tears during manual delivery of the nucleus and inadvertent inclusion of the iris in the phacoemulsification tip can result in iris distortion.

Tenting was a relatively common phenomenon associated with closed-loop anterior chamber lenses. The haptic loop compressed the last roll of the iris against the ciliary sulcus (Fig. 2.31). The resulting vertical distortion of the pupil often became progressive over many years as peripheral anterior synechiae continued to form.

Management. Meticulous attention to detail, especially wound hygiene, during cataract surgery is the key to preventing a peaked pupil. This is especially true if capsule disruption has occurred. Small strands of vitreous, cortex, and capsule are difficult to see during surgery. Weck sponge cleaning can detect unseen strands. Irregularities in the pupil before and after pharmacologic miosis should arouse a high degree of suspicion. The wound should be swept inter-

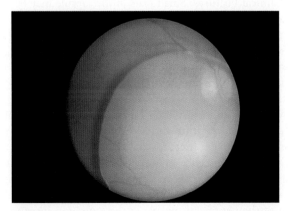

FIGURE 2.29. The entire nucleus has fallen into the vitreous cavity during cataract surgery. (Courtesy of Terry Tomer, Philadelphia, PA.)

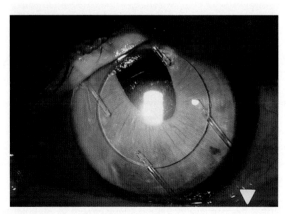

FIGURE 2.31. The closed loop anterior chamber lens has compressed the superior iris against the angle.

nally from a side port incision at the conclusion of a complicated case.

The peaked pupil is usually a benign condition, but associated low-grade inflammation and cystoid macular edema may occur. Isolated strands can be severed with the yttrium-argon-garnet (YAG) laser if the pupil is cosmetically a problem or cystoid macular edema is persistent. Vitrectomy may be necessary in cases of severe and persistent cystoid macular edema.

Atonic Pupil

Postoperatively, the pupil may remain semidilated and weakly reactive to light.

Clinical Features. The postoperative atonic pupil most frequently occurs in cases in which the pupil does not dilate well preoperatively because of iris sphincter fibrosis or chronic miotic therapy. At surgery, the sphincter is stretched during manual nuclear expression or during phacoemulsification, resulting in muscle tears. Sometimes, multiple marginal sphincterectomies are performed to enlarge the pupil and facilitate removal of the nucleus. The resulting pupil is enlarged and has an irregular margin (Fig. 2.32). Rarely, the pupil may remain enlarged and poorly reactive postoperatively even after uneventful surgery. In these cases, interruption of the vascular or nerve supply to the iris may be causative factors.

Management. An atonic pupil seldom requires definitive action. If the enlargement exposes the optic edge or a positioning hole, the patient may notice glare or related visual symptoms. If necessary, pilocarpine may partially constrict the pupil.

Pupillary Capture

In pupillary capture, part of the optic edge of a posterior chamber lens lies anterior to the iris and has been "captured" by the iris (Fig. 2.33).

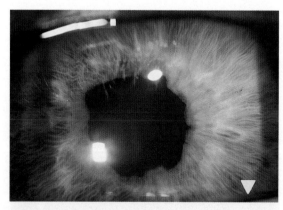

FIGURE 2.32. The atonic pupil is characterized by an enlarged, irregular, and poorly reactive pupil after cataract extraction. This frequently occurs in patients on long-term miotic therapy.

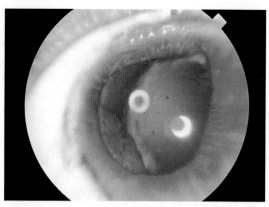

FIGURE 2.33. Pupil capture. A portion of the optic edge of a posterior chamber lens lies anterior to the iris.

Clinical Features. This condition can occur at the time of surgery if the intraocular lens is not positioned properly and the iris remains dilated. Pupil capture is more likely to occur when one haptic loop is in the bag and the other is in the sulcus. Pupil capture also can develop if the integrity of the posterior capsule has been compromised and vitreous forces a portion of the optic anteriorly. Trauma in the immediate postoperative period can result in pupil capture.

Management. The condition usually is benign, although the pupil distortion may be a cosmetic concern. There is an increased risk of cystoid macular edema. Occasionally, the condition can be treated by dilating the pupil, placing the patient in a supine position that permits the lens to fall back into the posterior chamber, and constricting the pupil with pilocarpine. If surgical repositioning is to be done, it should be done early, before adhesions between the iris and posterior capsule develop.

Posterior Capsule Disruption

The integrity of the posterior capsule may be disrupted during surgery. This can result from a tear in the capsule or a rupture of the zonules attaching the capsule to the ciliary body (i.e., zonular dehiscence).

Clinical Features. Small tears in the capsule may be difficult to recognize at the time of surgery, but the edges of the tear usually can be seen against the red retinal reflex. Absence of the normal circular light reflex created by slight posterior pressure with the irrigation and aspiration tip on an intact capsule is another indication of capsule disruption. If the tear extends, linear folds develop at the edge. Tears may result from inclusion of the capsule in the phacoemulsification, the irrigation and aspiration instruments, or excessive capsule polishing.

Zonular dehiscence may result from excessive pressure during manual nucleus expression, excessive nuclear manipulation during phacoemulsification, or unrecognized inclusion of the peripheral capsule in the aspiration instrument during cortical cleanup. Typically, the folds are seen at the edge of the remaining capsule (Fig. 2.34).

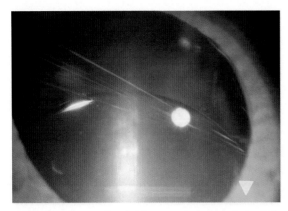

FIGURE 2.34. In zonular dehiscence, rupture of the inferior zonules has resulted in the typical folds seen at the edge of the remaining attached capsule. The intraocular lens is decentered inferiorly, resulting in the appropriately named sunset syndrome.

Management. It is essential to recognize the presence and extent of capsule disruption at the time of surgery to avoid inserting a posterior chamber lens without adequate support. In some cases, a posterior lens may still be inserted into the remaining capsular bag, but in others, the lens should be placed in the sulcus. If capsule support is totally inadequate, other options include a posterior chamber lens sutured to the sclera or iris, an anterior chamber lens, or no intraocular lens and subsequent aphakic contact lens correction.

Optic Decentration

The optic edge of a posterior chamber lens may become decentered with respect to the visual axis. This may be caused by one haptic loop being placed in the bag and one in the sulcus. As the capsular bag contracts, the implant is pulled to one side. More commonly, a tear in the posterior capsule or a segmental dehiscence of the zonules is involved. The haptic may be placed inadvertently through the capsular tear. Contracture of the remaining capsule and unopposed pull of the zonules result in displacement of the optic edge.

Clinical Features. If the decentration is minor, no symptoms may be experienced. Glare from the lens edge or images from a positioning hole in the optic edge may be noticed if these elements fall within the pupillary space. As the lens further decenters, monocular diplopia is experienced, and marked blurred vision occurs when the optic disappears from the visual axis. Frequently, as the lens progressively decenters, increased ocular inflammation becomes evident.

Sunrise Syndrome

When the optic edge decenters superiorly, the condition is referred to as a sunrise syndrome.

Clinical Features. This condition develops when the lens is placed in the bag and a zonular dehiscence is present inferiorly, or the superior haptic is through a superior capsular

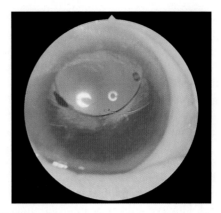

FIGURE 2.35. In this case of sunrise syndrome, the posterior chamber lens was placed in the capsular bag, but the inferior zonules had ruptured; with subsequent contracture of the capsule, the optic edge was decentered superiorly.

tear. As the capsule contracts, the lens is drawn superiorly (Fig. 2.35). The same decentration may occur, but to a lesser extent, if the vertically oriented inferior loop is in the bag and the superior loop is in the sulcus.

Sunset Syndrome

In the sunset syndrome, the intraocular lens is displaced inferiorly.

Clinical Features. In addition to zonular dehiscence and capsule contraction, gravity also is a factor (Fig. 2.36). Any inferior capsular tear or a zonular rupture inferiorly in which the loop is vertically oriented and not in the bag also results in a sunset syndrome.

East-West Decentration

Nasal or temporal displacement of the intraocular lens can occur.

Clinical Features. The same circumstances that result in a vertical malposition of the lens also may cause horizontal

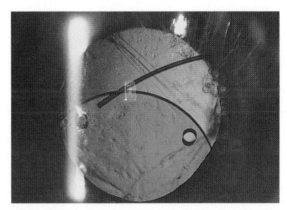

FIGURE 2.36. In this case of sunset syndrome, the inferior portion of the posterior capsule has been disrupted, and the optic edge has decentered inferiorly.

displacement (Fig. 2.37). A temporal zonular dehiscence with in-the-bag, horizontally oriented loops results in a nasally displaced optic. The lens also may be pushed nasally if there is a nasal capsular tear and the haptic loop is forced through the opening.

Management. Definitive action depends on the severity of the associated symptoms, degree of displacement, and persistent inflammation. If the symptoms are minor, the patient may be treated medically with pilocarpine. Frequently, this is not sufficient, and surgical repositioning or replacement of the lens is necessary.

If sufficient capsular support is possible, the lens may be repositioned. However, it may be more advantageous to remove the original lens and replace it with a sulcus-fixated, large (7-mm) optic lens. Usually, fibrosis has fused the peripheral anterior and posterior capsular flaps.

If the capsular support is inadequate, consideration should be given to anchoring the lens with an iris fixation (i.e., McCannel's) suture or a scleral suture, or to replacing the lens with an anterior chamber variety. Removal of the lens with visual correction by contact lens is also an option.

Posteriorly Dislocated Intraocular Lens

Posterior chamber intraocular lenses may dislocate into the vitreous at the time of surgery or sometime later because of the loss of capsular support (Figs. 2.38, 2.39).

Clinical Features. Dislocation into the vitreous may occur suddenly or gradually. Often, one haptic loop is hung up on residual peripheral capsule, creating a hinge-like situation. Vision is blurred as the intraocular lens disappears from the visual axis. Although the lens may remain inert in many cases, some exhibit chronic inflammation.

Management. Dislocated intraocular lenses may be retrieved from the surface of the retina and removed by vitreo-retinal surgical techniques. Perfluorocarbon liquids are sometimes helpful in elevating the intraocular lens from the retinal surface. A posterior chamber lens can be sutured into the sulcus, or an anterior chamber lens can be inserted.

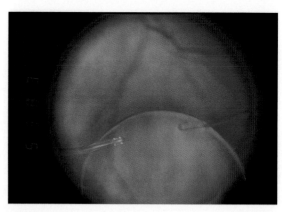

FIGURE 2.38. The intraocular lens has been lost in the vitreous and can be seen outlined on the retinal surface. (Courtesy of Terry Tomer, Philadelphia, PA.)

Clinical Features. Subluxated posterior chamber lenses still do occur even with incision surgery. We have recently seen a case in which an acrylic lens was used in a patient with 4+ nuclear sclerotic cataract, small pupil, and PXS. The posterior capsule was torn during the procedure and because of the tear and the extent of the tear, it was elected to put the foldable acrylic lens in the ciliary sulcus. The patient recovered 20/20 vision and did well for 3 months but then presented with sudden loss of vision in that eye. At this point, he was found to have the lens subluxated into the vitreous. No posterior capsule was now visible within the pupil. The intraocular lens had one haptic still attached to the capsular bag remnant and was just barely visible inferiorly with the indirect ophthalmoscope.

Management. With repair of this type of problem, it is important that the patient undergo specular microscopy to determine the health of the corneal endothelium prior to the repair. It is also important that the retina be thoroughly evaluated. These surgeries should be performed with two surgeons available: one skilled in posterior vitrectomy, and the other skilled in anterior segment surgical techniques such as suturing in a posterior chamber lens. Both sets of skills are

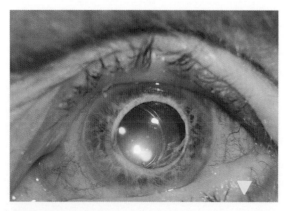

FIGURE 2.37. East-west decentration. The posterior chamber lens was inadvertently placed through a tear in the capsule nasally, resulting in medial decentration of the optic.

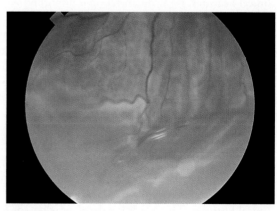

FIGURE 2.39. A posterior chamber lens has dislocated into the vitreous, resulting in associated retinal detachment. (Courtesy of Brian P. Connolly, Philadelphia, PA.)

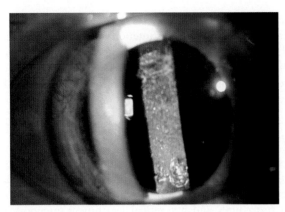

FIGURE 2.40. Opacification of the posterior capsule. (Courtesy of Stephen B. Lichtenstein, M.D., Philadelphia, PA.)

necessary as the intraocular lens may appear to be retrievable when the patient is vertical at the slit lamp; however, when the patient is in the supine position, the intraocular lens will drop down into the vitreous and may prove impossible for the anterior segment surgeon to easily retrieve. Once the intraocular lens has been retrieved, our recommendation is to suture a new implant into position. The haptics will sometimes deform after being in the eye and this will contribute to another subluxation if the same lens is used. A variety of suturing techniques can be used for suturing in the intraocular lens, and a list of references is shown below.

Posterior Capsule Opacification

After extracapsular cataract extraction, proliferation of lens epithelial cells can lead to posterior capsule opacification (Fig. 2.40).

Clinical Features. Posterior capsule opacification occurs in 50% of patients within 5 years of surgery with some IOL types. The posterior capsule can become opacified as a result of continued proliferation of lens cells from the residual anterior lens epithelium or from residual fibrosis that could not be removed at the time of surgery. Blurred vision and in-

creasing glare are the primary symptoms. Sometimes, tension striae develop in the capsule and become symptomatic. Other causes of blurred vision, particularly macular pathology, must be ruled out. The clarity of the examiner's direct ophthalmoscopic view of the fundus is a clinical indicator of the effect of the capsular opacification.

Management. A YAG laser capsulotomy should be done when the patient is symptomatic (Fig. 2.41A). The improvement in visual acuity is often dramatic. The patient must be observed for an increase in intraocular pressure, which is usually transient. There is an increased risk of retinal detachment, particularly in myopic patients, after YAG capsulotomy. Retinal detachment has occurred in 1% to 3% of patients. Pitting of the intraocular lens may occur because of difficulty in focusing the laser beam. Although this may be bothersome to the surgeon, it seldom interferes with vision (Fig. 2.41B).

Cortical Pearl Formation

Clinical Features. Cortical pearl formation used to be very frequent in the time of extracapsular cataract surgery with no intraocular lens. With the use of smaller anterior capsulotomies, this problem has started to resurface. The small anterior capsulotomy results in cortical proliferation that can extend across the posterior surface of the intraocular lens even after a YAG capsulotomy previously has been performed. As a cortical proliferation at the edges progresses, the patients will often complain of glare, particularly at night.

Management. The treatment for cortical pearl formation is to use the YAG laser and disrupt the cortical proliferative material. This usually resolves the problem; however, in time, it may recur. In our experience, the rate of recurrence is approximately 3 in 1,000.

Capsule Contraction Syndrome

Capsule contraction syndrome is characterized by a progressive reduction in the diameter of the anterior capsulotomy after cataract surgery (Fig. 2.42).

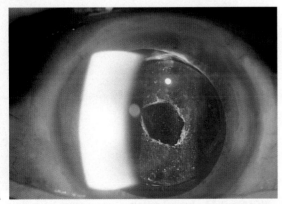
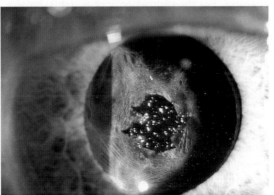

FIGURE 2.41. A: YAG laser capsulotomy. **(B)** Pitting of the lens can occur during YAG laser capsulotomy. (Courtesy of Stephen B. Lichtenstein, M.D., Philadelphia, PA.)

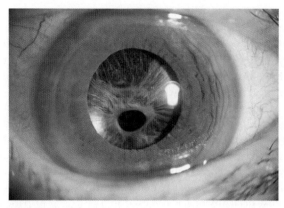

FIGURE 2.42. Capsule contraction syndrome. The anterior capsule has contracted over the lens and displaced the remaining opening inferior to the visual axis. (Courtesy of James A. Davison, M.D., Marshalltown, IA.)

Clinical Features. Most cases are associated with a capsulorrhexis-type anterior capsulotomy. Davison surmised the reduction of the anterior capsule opening to be the result of the contraction of residual lens epithelial cells that have undergone fibrous dysplasia. The contraction may occur in the weeks immediately after surgery or at a later time. In Davison's experience, contraction occurred more frequently in eyes with pseudoexfoliation, poorly dilated pupils, small capsulorrhexis, and chronic uveitis.

Capsule contraction may greatly reduce the size of the opening, displace the opening from the visual axis, and result in a malposition of the intraocular lens. Cases of zonular rupture as a result of bag contracture have been reported.

Management. If the capsular contracture is recognized early, YAG laser radial anterior capsulotomies may reduce the sphincter effect. A larger capsulorrhexis or can-opener–type capsulotomy with a deliberate superior radial tear may be considered at the time of surgery for predisposed patients. The use of an intraocular lens with a large optic and more rigid haptic may help oppose capsule contraction forces.

Nonencapsulated Anterior Capsular Flaps

Clinical Features. For the vast majority of patients, having an anterior capsular flap present within the pupillary space does not cause any difficulty. However, we have recently seen a patient who underwent topical clear corneal cataract extraction in the left eye. An anterior capsular tear was encountered, which extended to the edge of the posterior capsule. An intraocular lens was still implanted in the capsular bag, and postoperatively this patient had pain and mild cystoid macular edema. There was no vitreous to the wound, but a portion of the anterior capsule was visible within the pupillary space. This anterior capsule was freely moveable. With pupil constriction, the capsule seemed to offer very little resistance. The patient's visual acuity, however, did drop to the 20/60 level because of cystoid macular edema.

Management. The patient's eye was dilated and the YAG

laser was used to cut the anterior capsule flap completely from the remainder of the anterior capsule. This flap then fell into the anterior chamber and appeared to have vitreous attached to the capsular flap itself. The patient's symptoms resolved completely with no discomfort, and visual acuity returned to the 20/20 level.

Cystoid Macular Edema

Cystoid macular edema is a condition in which fluid accumulates within the sensory retina in the macular area. It may occur after intraocular surgery, such as cataract and filtration procedures, and after retinal detachment surgery. Many other conditions, including diabetes, peripheral uveitis, retinitis pigmentosa, and angiomatous retinae, are associated with cystoid macular edema.

Clinical Features. The patient complains of decreased or hazy vision. Refraction may show a hyperopic shift, and fine macular detail is hazy ophthalmoscopically. However, the classic characteristic of cystoid macular edema is a petaloid appearance caused by leakage of the fluorescein dye in the outer plexiform layer (Fig. 2.43). The cause is still obscure, but there is evidence suggesting that inflammation plays a role. This hypothesis is reinforced by the more frequent occurrence of cystoid macular edema when complications of intraocular surgery, such as a vitreous wick, have occurred, and by cases associated with peripheral uveitis.

Management. Where there have been no surgical complications, cystoid macular edema after cataract surgery may frequently improve, even without treatment. The use of topical antiinflammatory drops may prove helpful, but after treatment is discontinued, cystoid macular edema may return. When there has been vitreous incarceration in the wound, a vitrectomy may be necessary.

Pseudophakic Retinal Detachment

Patients are at higher risk for retinal detachment after cataract surgery.

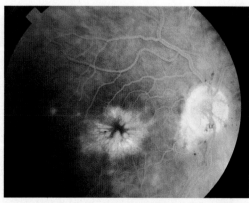

FIGURE 2.43. Typical petaloid appearance of cystoid macular edema caused by leakage of the fluorescein dye during angiography.

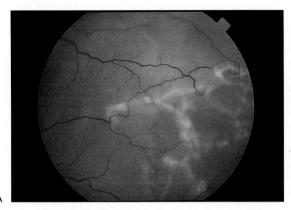 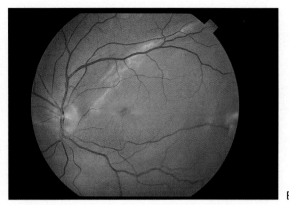

FIGURE 2.44. Pseudophakic retinal detachment at **(A)** the temporal periphery and **(B)** the posterior pole.

Clinical Features. Symptoms and findings of pseudophakic retinal detachment are similar to those in phakic patients (Fig. 2.44). Retinal detachment is more common when complications of surgery such as vitreous loss have occurred, or after YAG laser capsulotomy. Patients at greatest risk for retinal detachment after YAG laser capsulotomy are those with high degrees of myopia, lattice degeneration, or a history of retinal detachment in the fellow eye.

Management. Most pseudophakic retinal detachments are caused by small breaks above the horizontal meridian near the ora serrata. Multiple breaks are common. Occasionally larger equatorial breaks occur (Fig. 2.45), and rarely a giant retinal break may be noted.

Endophthalmitis

Clinical Features. Patients with endophthalmitis occurring within the first week after intraocular surgery may present with or without pain. Early cases are characterized by inflammation and minimal hypopyon. The fundus may still be visualized. In these instances, it is difficult to differentiate between a purely inflammatory process and an infectious one. The level of discomfort, degree of injection and chemosis, and presence or absence of vitreous cells are factors that may help make this distinction. In mild cases, hourly steroids may be tried to determine if the condition improves. Close observation is essential. If the patient has more severe pain and there is fibrin on the anterior surface of the implant with a hypopyon, the condition is probably infectious (Fig. 2.46). A view of the retina may be difficult because of vitreous involvement.

One of the most frequent pathogens encountered in postoperative endophthalmitis is *Staphylococcus epidermidis*. This organism is less virulent than others, and many of these patients usually do well. When the organism is more virulent, such as *Staphylococcus aureus* or a gram-negative rod, the prognosis is considerably more guarded.

Management. When the first edition of *Atlas of Clinical Ophthalmology* was published, endophthalmitis after in-

traocular surgery was usually treated with vitrectomy accompanied by culture of the vitreous and anterior chamber aspirates. Since that time, the results of the Endophthalmitis Vitrectomy Study Group (EVS) were published. The study showed that for patients with hand motion or better vision,

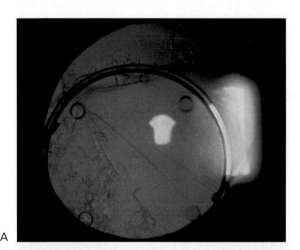

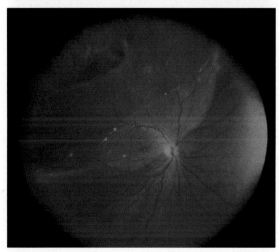

FIGURE 2.45. A: Pseudophakia and **(B)** large equatorial break with retinal detachment.

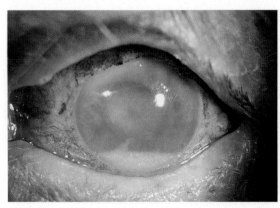

FIGURE 2.46. Acute endophthalmitis is characterized by hazy cornea, hypopyon, and exudative reaction over the implant surface in a patient 6 days after cataract surgery.

there was no difference in outcomes between immediate three ports pars plana vitrectomy versus anterior chamber and vitreous taps followed by injection of intravitreal antibiotics. However, when visual acuity presentation was light perception only, better visual results were obtained when a vitrectomy was done. The EVS treatment outcomes demonstrated no difference in final visual acuity or media clarity outcomes whether or not systemic antibiotics were used.

BIBLIOGRAPHY

Berliner ML. Biomicroscopy of the eye, vol II. New York: Paul B. Hoeber; 1949:1091.

Boyd-Monk H, Steinmetz CG. Nursing care of the eye. Norwalk: Appleton & Lange; 1991:13.

Charlton JR, Weinstein GW. Cataract surgery. In: Tasman W, Jaeger EA. Clinical ophthalmology, vol 6. Philadelphia: JB Lippincott; 1994:1.

Cheng KP, Hiles DA, Biglan AW, et al. Management of posterior lenticonus. *J Pediatr Ophthalmol Strabismus* 1991;28:143.

Cogan DG, Kuwabara T. Pathology of cataracts in Mongoloid idiocy. A new concept of pathogenesis of cataracts of the coronary-cerulean type. *Doc Ophthalmol* 1962;16:73.

Cordes FC. Types of congenital and juvenile cataracts. In: Haik GM. Symposium on diseases and surgery of the lens. St. Louis: CV Mosby; 1957:43.

Datiles MB, Kinoshita JH. Pathogenesis of cataracts. In: Tasman W, Jaeger EA. Duane's clinical ophthalmology, vol 1. Philadelphia: JB Lippincott; 1994:1.

Davison JA. Capsule contraction syndrome. *J Cataract Refract Surg* 1993;19:582.

Delamere NA, Paterson CA. The crystalline lens. In: Tasman W, Jaeger EA. Foundations of clinical ophthalmology, vol II. Philadelphia: JB Lippincott; 1994:1.

Endophthalmitis Vitrectomy Study Group. Results of the Endophthalmitis Vitrectomy Study. *Arch Ophthalmol* 1995;113:1479.

Gibbs ML, Jacobs M, Wilkie DM, et al. Posterior lenticonus: clinical patterns and genetics. *J Pediatr Ophthalmol Strabismus* 1993;30:171.

Jaffe NS, Jaffe MS, Jaffe GF. Cataract surgery and its complications. 5th ed. St. Louis: CV Mosby; 1990:359.

Kleiman NJ, Worgul BV. Lens. In: Tasman W, Jaeger EA. Foundations of clinical ophthalmology, vol 1. Philadelphia: JB Lippincott; 1994:1.

Kozart DM, Yanoff M. Intraocular pressure statistics in 100 conservative patients with exfoliation syndrome. *Ophthalmology* 1982;89:214.

La Piana FG. Renal disease. In: Tasman W, Jaeger EA. Duane's clinical ophthalmology, vol 5. Philadelphia: JB Lippincott; 1994:4.

Parks MM, Johnson DA, Reed GW. Long-term visual results and complications in children with aphakia. *Ophthalmology* 1993;100:826.

Schotzer-Schrehardt U, Neuman GO. A histopathologic study of zonular instability in pseudoexfoliative syndrome. *Am J Ophthalmol* 1994;118:730.

Skuta GL. Pseudoexfoliation syndrome, pigment dispersion syndrome and the associated glaucomas. In: Tasman W, Jaeger EA. Duane's clinical ophthalmology, vol 3. Philadelphia: JB Lippincott; 1994:1.

Smith SG, Holland E, Peterson J. Peripheral anterior synechiae formation with anterior chamber intraocular lenses. *Ophthalmic Surg* 1992;23:315.

Smith SG, Lindstrom RL. Intraocular lens complications and their management. *Slack* 1988:167.

Spencer WH. Lens. In: Spencer WH. Ophthalmic pathology, an atlas and textbook, vol 1. 3rd ed. Philadelphia: WB Saunders; 1985:423.

Van Heyninger R. Formation of polyols by the lens of the rat with sugar cataract. *Nature* 1959;184:194.

CHAPTER 3

GLAUCOMA

George L. Spaeth
Augusto Azuara-Blanco
Jeffrey D. Henderer
L. Jay Katz
Marlene R. Moster
Jonathan S. Myers
Douglas J. Rhee
Annette K. Terebuh
Richard P. Wilson

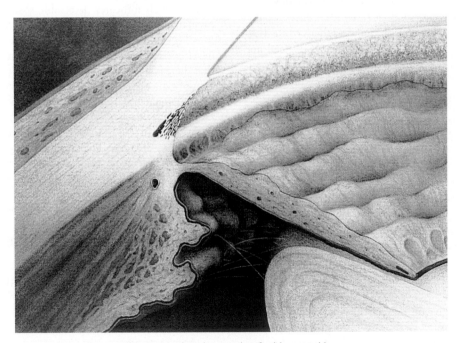

A normal anterior chamber angle of a blue-eyed human eye.

WHAT IS GLAUCOMA?

We define glaucoma in this chapter as **the process of ocular tissue damage caused at least partially by intraocular pressure (IOP)**. Note that "elevated" IOP by itself is not a criterion for diagnosing glaucoma. Note also that, while IOP plays a pathogenetic role in every glaucoma, IOP need not be elevated in the sense of being above average. Glaucoma can be associated with IOP as low as 10 mm Hg or perhaps even lower than that. (See sections on IOP, pages 97,125–126).

A second consideration is whether glaucoma can occur without tissue damage. Tissue damage can occur without being detected by current methods. For example, many optic neurons must become nonfunctional before visual field loss is detectable. Also, certain levels of IOP are so certain to cause damage that it would seem sensible to use the label glaucoma. However, these arguments are not sufficient: first, if damage cannot be detected it is not certain that it will occur; and second, there is great variability in the level of IOP that can be tolerated. We limit the definition of glaucoma, then, to situations in which tissue damage is detectable. If it seems virtually certain that the person will develop glaucoma damage, we use the term **preglaucoma**. If there is a question about whether tissue damage has occurred, the phrase **glaucoma suspect** is employed.

Glaucoma is a group of conditions. Even entities characteristically considered as specific diagnostic groups, such as primary open-angle glaucoma (POAG), are usually composites of different conditions.

To repeat, then, **glaucoma is the process of ocular tissue damage caused at least in part by IOP.**

CLASSIFICATION: TERMINOLOGY AND RISK FACTORS

The broad classification used in this chapter includes **glaucoma**, which indicates detectable tissue damage (Fig. 3.1); **preglaucoma**, which indicates some finding (e.g., IOP of 80 mm Hg) that makes it virtually certain that the patient will develop tissue damage; and **glaucoma suspect**, which means that there is something about the patient that raises the suspicion of glaucoma, but does not denote with certainty whether tissue damage has occurred. Glaucoma suspects are individuals in whom the development of glaucoma is considered to be more likely than in individuals who possesses none of the risk factors for glaucoma. The glaucoma suspect is further categorized as an individual who has a suspicious finding, such as an optic disc asymmetry, or an individual with a presumed predisposition to glaucoma because of some risk factor, such as a positive family history or pigment dispersion syndrome.

Stage, Stability, and Treatable Factors

This chapter is employing a different classification scheme than has been traditional (Table 3.1). Glaucoma can be clas-

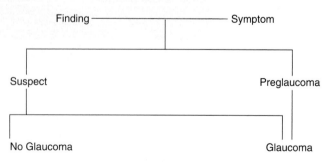

FIGURE 3.1. Classification of glaucoma.

TABLE 3-1. MANAGEMENT CONSIDERATIONS: FACTORS THAT INFLUENCE THE TYPE AND VIGOR OF THERAPY

Stage of Disease	Stability and Rate of Change
Suspected	Condition improving
Early	Condition stable
Disease	Condition worsening
Worsening disease	Condition uncertain

Life Expectancy
Consider age of patient
Obtain family history
Ask for details of the patient's lifestyle
Assess general health
Take blood pressure and weight measurements

Treatable Conditions
Anterior chamber angle configuration (peripheral iridectomy)
Intraocular pressure (argon laser trabeculoplasty, medicine, surgery)
Neovascularization (panretinal photocoagulation)
Vasospasm (calcium channel blocker)
Malnutrition (supplements as needed)
Hypotension (prevention)
Hypertension (weight loss, exercise)

sified by the *stage* of the condition, the *stability* of the condition, and the *treatable factors* of the condition, including whatever is affecting the control of IOP. This newer classification recognizes that the treatment of glaucoma is based on attempts to avoid or minimize tissue damage. However, the mechanism for damage of the optic nerve in conditions as apparently similar as focal and POAG or primary angle-closure glaucoma varies. In POAG, the damage may be solely mechanical or almost solely vascular. In primary angle-closure glaucoma, in which the patient has low-grade recurrent attacks of angle-closure, the mechanism for optic nerve damage may be a mechanical change similar to that in POAG, but in the cases in which the elevation of IOP is extremely marked, the mechanism of damage is an acute ischemic optic neuropathy. Because treatment of the many conditions called glaucoma depends on the stage of the condition and the stability of the condition, those elements are stressed.

Stage

The stage of glaucoma refers to amount of damage. Although this refers typically to the optic nerve, it also applies to the health of other tissues, such as the cornea.

In the earliest stage, the diagnosis is *suspected* but not definite. There is only a suspicious finding, such as an IOP above 30 mm Hg or moderate disc asymmetry. The patient has no ocular symptoms and no evidence of definite damage. The physician may be suspicious that damage has occurred or may occur but cannot ascertain this at the time of the evaluation. The second stage is *early glaucoma*. In early glaucoma, the patient is still asymptomatic, but there is definite damage, such as an unmistakable nasal step in the visual field, a notch in the optic nerve, a hemorrhage on the optic nerve, or a minimal but definite afferent pupillary defect. The third stage is *glaucomatous disease*. The patient has some symptoms. He or she notices the field loss, is aware of halos or pain, or notices something else that interferes with visual function. The fourth stage is *worsening disease*. The patient notices functional impairment and is aware that the functional impairment is worsening.

Stability

The stability of the glaucoma must also be assessed (Fig. 3.2). The patient's condition may be improving such that the symptoms or even the visual field or optic nerve head is improving. The patient's condition may be stable, with no detectable change on repeated evaluations of the objective or the subjective aspects of the patient's condition. The patient does not think that he or she is changing or worse, and the physician notices no change in the results of the physical evaluation. If the stability of the patient's condition is worsening, the symptoms are getting worse, or the optic disc or visual field is worsening. Sometimes, the stability of the condition is uncertain. When a patient is first evaluated, it may not be possible at that point to establish the stability of the patient's condition. Repeated evaluations of the history or the findings are usually necessary to determine the stability of the condition. If it cannot be determined, physicians must be honest about this difficulty and not mislead themselves or the patient.

The determination of stability is influenced by the patient's life expectancy. Many physicians cringe at this idea and feel that they are "playing God." However, a fairly accurate estimate of life expectancy is not difficult to determine. Life insurance companies do a good job of anticipating life expectancy, and physicians can as well. Life expectancy can be determined by obtaining a thorough family history, including the ages at death of the parents and the health of siblings. Added to this is information about the patient's lifestyle. Does the patient smoke cigarettes, drink excessively, use drugs, or in some other way abuse his or her body? Is the patient overweight? Does the patient eat well? Does the patient exercise regularly? An estimate of the patient's general health is essential. This information can be obtained with relative ease; it must be known to make sense of the information related to the stability of the condition and the rapidity with which that stability is changing.

On the vertical axis of the graph in Figure 3.3 is the visual function, from normal to totally nonfunctional. On the horizontal axis is the duration of the patient's life, from birth to death; because this varies among individuals, it is not given in terms of years. The stability of the patient's condition and the rapidity with which that stability is changing are reflected by the slope of the line that describes

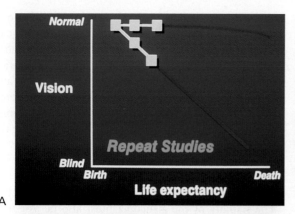

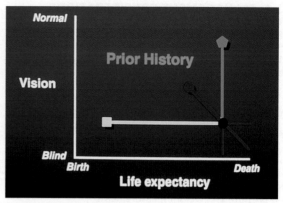

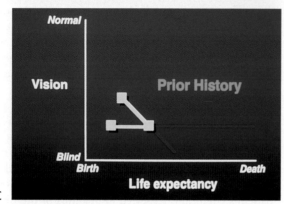

FIGURE 3.2. A: Stability of the glaucomatous disease is a factor in management. **B:** A careful history may be the only clue to the rate of change when the diagnosis is made late in the glaucomatous disease process. **C:** A patient diagnosed with advanced glaucoma but with a long life expectancy may demand vigorous treatment.

the course of the patient's glaucoma. For example, Patient 1 (Fig. 3.2A) has early glaucoma and a long life expectancy. This early-stage glaucoma would need minimal treatment if its stage were changing slowly (top line), but because of the patient's long life expectancy, it requires vigorous treatment if the stability is changing rapidly. In contrast, Patient

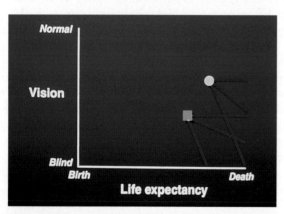

FIGURE 3.3. Two patients demonstrate the different rates of change in glaucoma. One patient has more advanced disease and a longer life expectancy. Even if the rate of deterioration is "slow," this patient will become blind before death. The other patient, who has less severe disease and a shorter life expectancy, will retain vision until death, although the rate of deterioration is the same as that in the other patient. If the rate of deterioration is rapid, both patients would become blind before death.

2 (Fig. 3.3) has a short life expectancy. If such a patient had early-stage glaucoma, treatment would be justified only if the rate of change were fairly rapid. If the patient had an advanced stage of glaucoma, as is shown on the graph, treatment must be vigorous, even if the rate of change is relatively slow.

The stability of the patient's condition is affected by how rapidly the stage is changing. The development of a graph indicating this phenomenon can help the physician and the patient (Fig. 3.2A). In the first or second stages of glaucoma, the most important way of determining the rapidity of change is by repeating meticulous evaluations of the optic nerve. The optic nerve should be drawn carefully at every visit to determine whether change is occurring. Photographs or image analysis methods may be helpful. The visual field needs to be repeated sufficiently frequently to notice any early defect that may develop or any change that may occur. If it becomes apparent that the optic disc is worsening within a period of 3 months and still worse 3 months later, the condition is rapidly worsening. However, if a patient has an early visual field defect that shows only a tiny deterioration over 15 years, the rate of worsening is extremely slow.

It is essential to determine the rate of change in the patient's stability, because it is the rate of change that determines the vigor of therapy that is appropriate. When the glaucoma is advanced (Fig. 3.2B), a careful history is the best method for determining the rate of change. Consider the patient whose condition is graphed in Figure 3.2C. The person has a long life expectancy and has already lost much vision (i.e., stage 3 or 4). If the condition is unchanging, the patient can expect to continue to see until he dies; if the condition is changing rapidly or even relatively slowly, vision will be lost before death. The importance of stability for prognosis and for determining the needed therapy is demonstrated in Figure 3.3, in which the different slopes depict different clinical outcomes. However, the clinical course is rarely linear, and there may be sudden downturns or plateaus in an extended graph of the disease.

Intraocular Pressure

Traditional classifications of glaucoma have been based on the mechanism for pressure elevation, but the pressure need not be elevated for glaucoma to develop. However, pressure is a factor, and the mechanism for pressure regulation is essential to understand, because alteration of the IOP is the major way in which the course of glaucoma can be altered.

Treatable Factors

Determining which factors are treatable is the next step in the management of the patient considered to have glaucoma or to be at significant risk for developing glaucoma (Table 3.2). An anterior chamber angle that is narrow enough to be occluded, or one in which occlusion has been proven because of the presence of peripheral anterior synechiae of the type that are seen in primary angle-closure glaucoma, is usually a sufficient justification for a peripheral iridotomy, assuming that damage to the optic nerve or other ocular disease is not present.

The method of lowering IOP is directed at the mechanism responsible for the control of IOP. In virtually all patients, this may involve medical or surgical therapy. In those with idiopathic POAG, the pigment dispersion syndrome, and the exfoliation syndrome, argon laser trabeculoplasty (ALT) is appropriate to consider as adjunctive or primary treatment. Surgical correction of an interference with aqueous flow is often appropriate if such a blockage is the primary problem.

Factors other than IOP can be treated. Methods of evaluating the adequacy of blood flow to the optic nerve are still rudimentary, but it seems likely that treatments that affect blood flow, especially those that limit vasospasm, will become a standard part of the treatment of patients with glaucoma. Certain aspects of a patient's lifestyle affect the patient's glaucoma, and it is appropriate to direct attention toward some of these. Patients with low-tension glaucoma who have a sedentary lifestyle have a more rapid progression of their glaucoma than patients who exercise. Exercise can lower IOP by about 4 mm Hg. In Japan, obesity was found to correlate strongly with progressive glaucomatous nerve damage. Malnutrition sensitizes the nerve to further damage. Systemic hypertension should be avoided, as should sudden decreases in blood pressure.

Risk Factors

Glaucoma is a progressive disease. However, the rate at which it progresses varies markedly from person to person. It was once believed that the only important factor to be controlled was the IOP, but it has become clear that many other factors affect the course of the disease (Table 3.2). Because the major damage that occurs in most persons with glaucoma is deterioration of the optic nerve, the most important risk factor is the ability of the optic nerve to resist damage. Because most glaucomas are chronic conditions and because they are usually responsive to treatment, the ability of the patient to manage his or her own life is a critical factor in determining whether the patient's glaucoma deteriorates. The patients with the best prognoses are those who know how to develop a relationship with the physician in which the physician acts as a junior partner, who take primary responsibility for their health, and who do those things most likely to keep them healthy.

Intraocular Pressure and Glaucoma

For many years, IOP was considered the definition of glaucoma. Persons with pressures two standard deviations above the population norm (usually 21 mm Hg) had the disease, and those that fell within the "normal" range did not. In more recent years, this view has steadily lost favor as several lines of evidence indicate that glaucoma can exist at "normal" levels of IOP and persons with elevated levels of pressure may not have the disease. Yet there is compelling evi-

TABLE 3-2. RISK FACTORS FOR GLAUCOMA

Classic Factors	Nutritional Factors
Race	Malnutrition
Heredity	
Myopia	**Lifestyle**
Pigment dispersion	Self-management ability
Exfoliation syndrome	Exercise
Angle configuration	Obesity
Angle recession	Diet (?)
	Smoking
Cardiovascular Factors	
Hypotension	
Hypertension	
Diabetes mellitus	
Migraine	
Exercise	
Raynaud's phenomenon	
Hyperviscosity	
Ocular ischemia	
Obesity	

dence to indicate that IOP is somehow related to this disease, even for persons who have glaucomatous damage with a "normal" IOP. In fact current thinking views glaucoma as ocular tissue damage related in some way to IOP, and IOP is a risk factor, perhaps even the most important risk factor, for developing glaucoma.

Evidence for IOP as a component of the pathogenesis of glaucoma comes from several directions. First, population-based glaucoma surveys indicate that the prevalence of glaucoma and the probability of glaucoma increase as the level of IOP increases. Second, in population studies of ocular hypertension, the incidence of conversion to glaucoma rises with increased IOP. This has been demonstrated in different racial groups and in different locations around the world (Table 3.3). Third, persons who acquire a pressure asym-

metry in both eyes, if they develop glaucoma, tend to develop it in the eye with the higher pressure. Fourth, investigators have repeatedly demonstrated in controlled randomized clinical trials of glaucoma therapy that persons being treated for glaucoma seemed to do worse if their pressures were elevated compared to those who pressures were reduced. Persons who had their pressures reduced had lower rates of progression, and if the IOP could be lowered to the low-normal range (usually considered less than 15 mm Hg), the rate of progression was slowed markedly. Finally, the "Normal Tension Glaucoma," a randomized, prospective, clinical trial, more conclusively demonstrated the role of IOP in glaucoma. This landmark clinical trial indicated that an IOP reduction of 30% could significantly reduce the rate of progression of so-called "normal-tension glaucoma." This

TABLE 3-3. NATURAL HISTORY OF OCULAR HYPERTENSION

Author (year)	Number of Patients	Follow-up (years)	Initial IOP (mm Hg)	Incidence of POAG (%)	Total Incidence of POAG (%)
Becker (1966)	50	4 to 5	19 to 29		14
Linnér (1976)	152	5	21.9 to 25.8		1.9
Graham (1969)	195	4	≥21		0.5
Armaly (1969)	90 eyes	10	24 to 29		1.1
Norskov (1970)	72 eyes	5	20 to 25		0
Perkins (1973)	124	5 to 7	>21		3.2
Walker (1974)	58	11	21 to 24	10	11 ("chronic simple glaucoma")
	39	11	24 to 29	7	
	12	11	≥30	17	
Wilensky (1974)	50	5	22		6
Pohjanpe Ito (1974)	211	2 to 5	25 to 29	7	28
			30 to 34	14	
			35 to 39	52	
			40 to 44	61	
			45 to 49	73	
			≥50	79	
Linnér (1976)	92	10	23		0
Kass (1976)	31	3 to 7	<24	10	29
			≥24	64	
Kitazawa (1977)	75	9.5	21 to 25	5.7	9.3
			26 to 30	0	
			>30	25	
David (1977)	48 eyes	1 to 11	21 to 25	0	4.5
	16 eyes		26 to 30	12.5	
	3 eyes		≥31	33	
David (1978)	25 black	1 to 12	21 to 25	0	18.1
			26 to 30	11.7	
			≥31	50	
	47 white	1 to 12	21 to 25	2.9	5.4
			26 to 30	11.1	
			≥31	16.6	
Sörensen (1978)	55	15	≥20		5.6
Armaly (1980)	5000	5	<20	1.5	
			≥20	6.7	
Quigley (1994)	647	6.2	>21		10.5
Leske (1997)	3155	4	>21		5.8

IOP = intraocular pressure; POAG = primary open-angle glaucoma.

finding has provided the most convincing clinical evidence to indicate that IOP is a component of glaucoma.

However, despite the importance of IOP, there is likely more to the pathogenesis than pressure. Evidence for this comes from the fact that IOP above the population norm is not uncommon, and yet the vast majority of those with elevated IOP do not have, and will never develop, glaucoma (Table 3.3). There is still no consensus on how to approach patients with elevated IOP and no evidence of glaucoma. Evidence both for withholding and starting treatment has been published. A large multicenter, prospective, randomized, controlled trial is currently underway to investigate whether there is any benefit to IOP reduction in this class of patient. Further evidence comes from clinical experience that indicates that despite pressure reduction, even very significant pressure reduction, some patients continue to worsen. Additionally, persons with a history of migraine headache and Raynaud's syndrome who have presumed vasospastic disease may be at increased risk for open-angle glaucoma. Certainly genetics is related to glaucoma and may or may not be related to IOP. The optic nerve itself may be susceptible to injury secondary to problems with glial cells and the extracellular matrix. Myopia may be a risk factor as well, and is unlikely to be related to IOP.

Our current understanding of the relationship between IOP and glaucoma has evolved considerably and is still evolving. Convincing evidence has finally arrived to implicate IOP in the pathogenesis of the disease, yet clinical experience indicates that IOP is not the whole story. Genetic defects, blood flow defects, optic nerve structural defects or problems related to ocular neurotoxins and neurotrophic growth factors may yet be found to be important in the pathogenesis of glaucoma. Important animal research and human clinical trials investigating novel non–pressure-related treatments of glaucoma are currently underway. For now, however, despite this shift in thinking, the fact that IOP remains an important component of glaucoma means that, from a treatment standpoint, the goal is still a reduction of IOP.

EVALUATION OF THE ANTERIOR CHAMBER ANGLE

Evaluation of the anterior chamber angle is essential for the diagnosis and management of glaucoma. It is important for the practitioner to recognize the normal anterior chamber angle (Fig. 3.4A–D) and to use a consistent method for grading the anterior chamber angle (Figs. 3.5 through 3.7). The angle shown in the photograph in Figure 3.4D is wide open, with no pigmentation of the posterior trabecular meshwork. It is graded E40c. This includes an estimate of the place where the iris "inserts" onto the inner wall of the eye, of the depth of the peripheral an-

terior chamber angle, and of the peripheral curvature of the iris. All three of these factors must be evaluated if a meaningful description of the angle configuration is to be obtained. These measurements can be easily and rapidly recorded using the system described.

Narrow Angles and Optically Closed Angles

Figure 3.8A shows an optically closed angle (i.e., Goldmann lens). Figure 3.8B shows the angle opened by indentation gonioscopy. A narrow angle viewed through the Zeiss lens is seen in Figure 3.9A. The posterior trabecular meshwork is just barely visible. With Zeiss lens indentation gonioscopy, the angle can be deepened; extensive adhesions are present and can now be seen (Fig. 3.9B).

Angle Grading System

The exact nature of the angle configuration is easily described using the grading system shown in Figures 3.4 through 3.9. The angle shown in Figure 3.10 is partially optically closed. The parenthetic designation describes the deepest structure visible before indentation. The capital D refers to the site of adhesions between the iris and the inner wall of the eye.

Angle Pigmentation

The amount and character of pigment in the anterior chamber angle must also be determined, because it helps to provide an accurate diagnosis and is critical in deciding on appropriate treatment (Fig. 3.11). The examiner should determine whether the pigment is brownish, which is characteristic of the pigment in the normal angle (Fig. 3.11A) or that seen in the pigment dispersion syndrome, or black, which is more characteristic of the pigment in the exfoliation syndrome. The pigment in the pigment dispersion syndrome is phagocytized and is more characteristically limited to the trabecular meshwork (Fig. 3.11B), but in the exfoliation syndrome, the pigment is more prominent inferiorly than superiorly and tends to spread over the angle recess and up onto Schwalbe's line, where inferiorly it is seen as the highly characteristic Sampaolesi's line (Fig. 3.11C). Sampaolesi's line is a scalloped line of pigment on or anterior to Schwalbe's line and is diagnostic of the exfoliation syndrome.

Patients with minimal pigmentation of the posterior trabecular meshwork do not respond well to ALT, but patients with 2+ (on a scale of 0 to 4+) pigmentation or more in the trabecular meshwork are more likely to have a beneficial effect from ALT. Figure 3.11D shows an angle with 3+ pigmentation after ALT, with disappearance of the pigment in treated areas.

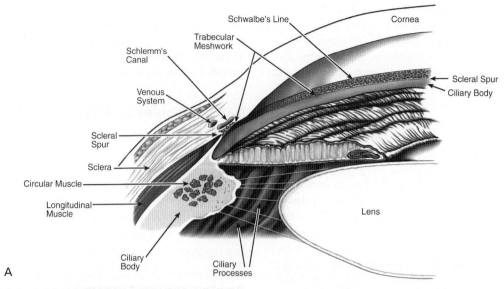

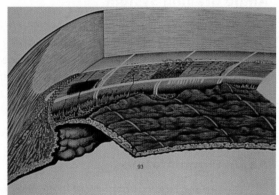

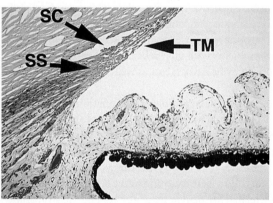

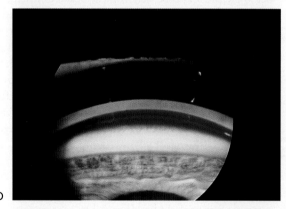

FIGURE 3.4. A: Aqueous pathway and anatomy of the angle. The production of aqueous humor is the result of a complex sequence of events that occurs in the ciliary processes. Secretion involves active transport and hydrostatic pressure that forces fluid, electrolytes, and small molecules through the fine capillaries and loosely connected cells of the double-layered epithelium (i.e., pigmented and nonpigmented) of the *ciliary body* and into the posterior chamber. Aqueous passes between the iris and the lens and into the anterior chamber and is responsible for supplying nutrients and removing metabolic waste from the nonvascularized structures of the anterior segment of the eye. The *angle* refers to the junction of the cornea and the iris, and contains the drainage pathway for 90% of the aqueous. This area cannot be seen directly; a contact lens or mirror must be used for visualization (i.e., gonioscopy). *Schwalbe's line* is considered the posterior limit of the cornea. The *trabecular meshwork* consists of a network of beams and interconnecting spaces and fibers that extends from Schwalbe's line to the iris insertion or *scleral spur*. The trabecular meshwork is actually a double layer of interlacing fibers; the innermost layer is the uveal trabecula, and the outermost layer is the corneoscleral trabecula. The trabecular meshwork is normally translucent, although it frequently contains pigment in its posterior portion. The scleral spur is a short extension of the sclera anteriorly and appears shiny white on gonioscopy. It serves as a point of insertion for the corneoscleral trabecular fibers and separates the meshwork from the anterior portion of the ciliary body, which is seen as a darker band in the posterior angle on gonioscopy. The trabecular meshwork is the most important structure to identify properly at the time of gonioscopy, because its nature (e.g., amount of pigment, presence of a neovascular membrane, closed angle, iris adhesions) determines the level of intraocular pressure (IOP) and the direction of therapy. The trabecular meshwork can best be recognized by noticing that it has depth, unlike any of the other angle structures. The examiner can see into the trabecular meshwork. *Schlemm's canal* lies outward from the trabecular meshwork and is not normally visible. However, sometimes the canal fills with blood during gonioscopy, and this can serve as a valuable landmark in identifying angle anatomy. Aqueous passes through the trabecular meshwork into Schlemm's canal and then to the episcleral venous circulation. **B:** An open angle showing normal variations in the pigmentation

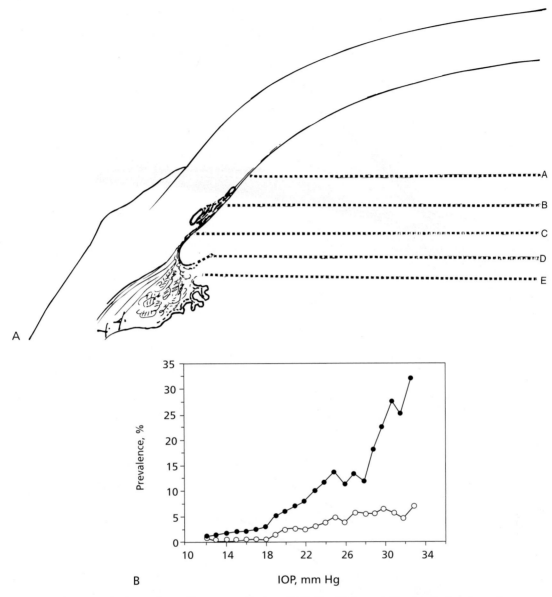

FIGURE 3.5. A: Angle grading system. Each capital letter (A through E) refers to the place where the iris attaches to the wall of the eye. **B:** Prevalence of primary open-angle glaucoma (POAG) in relation to screening intraocular pressure (IOP). The curve is smoothed using a running mean with window width of 7 mm Hg. (Caucasian American subjects, n=5,700 eyes [open circles]; African American subjects, n=4,674 eyes [closed circles].) (Reproduced from Alfred E. Sommer, M.D. Relationship between intraocular pressure and POAG among white and black Americans. *Arch Ophthalmol* 1991;109:1090, with permission. Copyright 1991, American Medical Association.)

of the trabecular meshwork, iris processes, and configuration of the "last roll" of the iris. The dark, rectangular window *(left)* is the ideal position for a trabeculectomy excision for uncontrolled IOP. **C:** Histologic section of the normal angle. (SC, Schlemm's canal; SS, scleral spur; TM, trabecular meshwork.) (Courtesy of Ralph C. Eagle Jr., M.D., Philadelphia, PA.) **D:** Gonioscopic view of an open angle. The brown line just anterior to the iris is the anterior portion of the ciliary body. The remainder of the trabecular meshwork is devoid of pigmentation and barely visible.

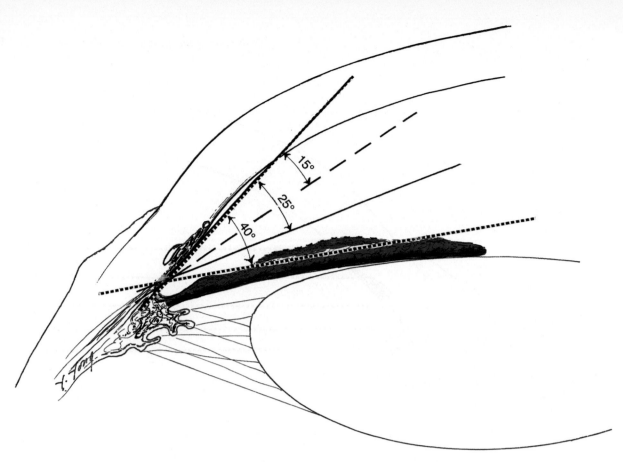

FIGURE 3.6. Angle grading system. The number of degrees refers to the depth of the peripheral anterior chamber.

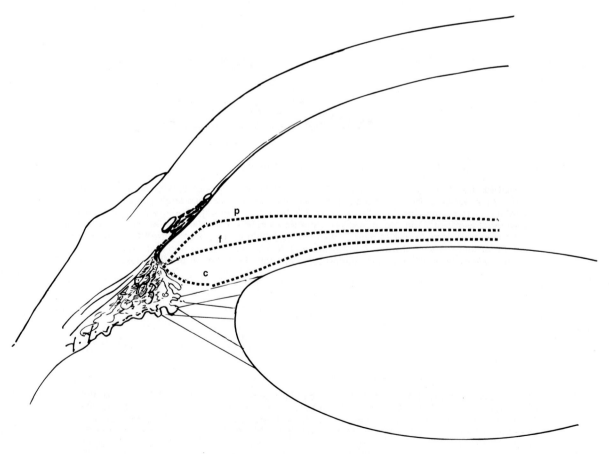

FIGURE 3.7. Angle grading system. Each lower-case letter refers to an estimate of the peripheral curvature of the iris.

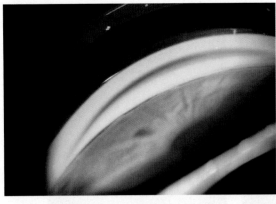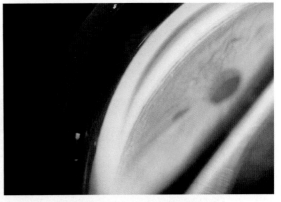

FIGURE 3.8. A: An optically closed angle as seen through a Goldmann three-mirror lens during gonioscopy. **B:** The same angle partially opened by the indentation during gonioscopy.

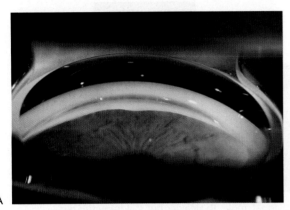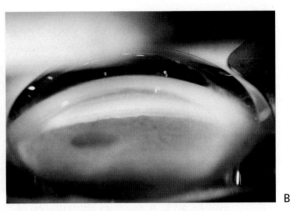

FIGURE 3.9. A: A narrow angle viewed through the Zeiss lens. The posterior trabecular meshwork is barely visible. **B:** During indentation, the angle is deepened, and adhesions can be seen.

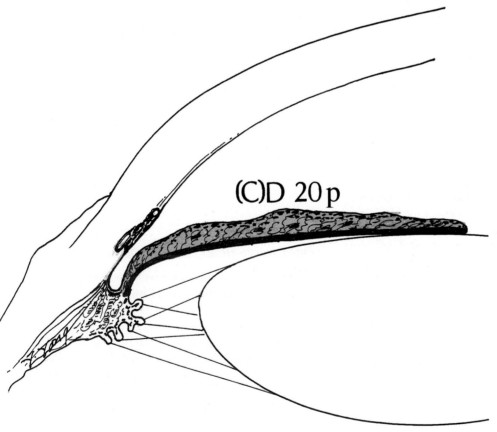

FIGURE 3.10. A partially closed angle that would be graded (C)D 20p. The (C) refers to the deepest structure visible before indentation, and the D refers to the actual site of adhesions between the iris and the inner wall of the eye.

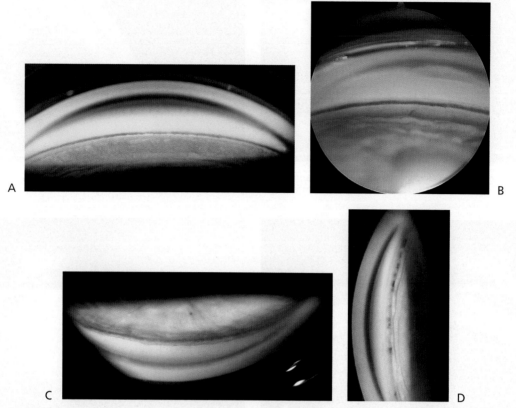

FIGURE 3.11. A: Brownish pigmentation of the normal angle. **B:** Heavier but still brownish pigmentation in a patient with pigment dispersion syndrome. **C:** Pigmentation of the inferior angle in a patient with pseudoexfoliation syndrome. The pigment tends to be darker and is spread over the angle recess. A distinct black line is seen inferiorly at the level of Schwalbe's line and is known as Sampaolesi's line. **D:** An angle with 3+ pigmentation after argon laser trabeculoplasty and disappearance of pigment in treated areas.

EVALUATION OF THE OPTIC DISC AND NERVE FIBER LAYER

Introduction

Optic nerve head (ONH) evaluation is integral to the diagnosis and management of glaucoma for several reasons. Glaucoma causes characteristic, although not pathognomonic, defects in the ONH, which aids in the diagnosis. Glaucoma also causes progressive changes in the ONH that occur slowly, typically over months to years. Therefore, serial observation and recording of appearance are good indicators for overall disease management. Because documenting the ONH does not require the patient to perform the test, it is more objective than perimetry. However, ascertaining progression of the ONH by clinical examination and photography involves subjective interpretation by the clinician, which is susceptible to intra- and interobserver variability. Newer imaging techniques attempt to limit this variability to increase the sensitivity of detecting subtle change.

Defects in the retinal nerve fiber layer (RNFL) occur in patients with glaucoma. Recent evidence suggests that RNFL defects may predate visual field or ONH changes. Changes as small as 10 to 20 μm may indicate disease progression before visual field changes are noted. RNFL imaging technology's potential for earlier diagnosis and finer sensitivity to disease progression is actively being evaluated. Its exact clinical role has not yet been established.

Optic Nerve Head

Optic Nerve Head Changes Occurring in Glaucoma

Progressive Thinning of the Rim

The only change that is completely diagnostic of glaucomatous damage is a progressive change in the appearance of the optic nerve: thinning of the neural rim (Fig. 3.12). This may occur concentrically (Figure 3.12A, B) or focally (Figure 3.12C). A large cup by itself, however, is not diagnostic of glaucoma; Figures 3.12A and B, for example, could be photographs

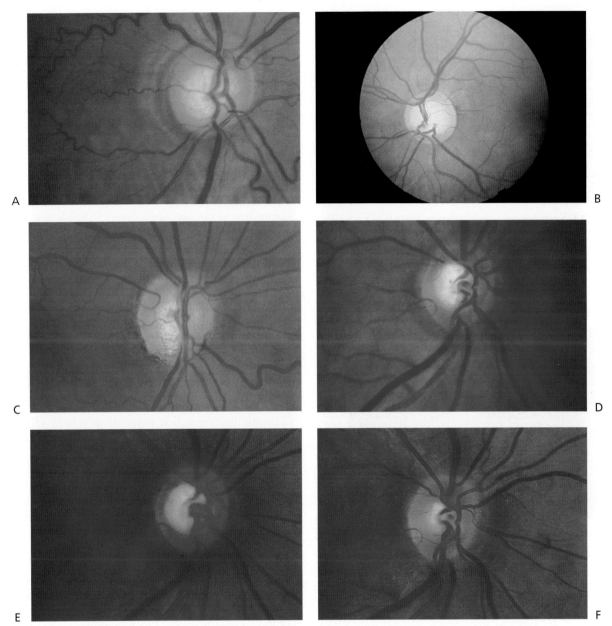

FIGURE 3.12. A: Slight concentric enlargement in the cup is present in a patient with early glaucoma. No visual field loss would be present here. **B:** More extensive concentric cup enlargement is seen in a patient with more advanced glaucoma. No visual field loss would be present here. **C:** Inferior, "focal" extension of the cup. **D:** Concentric enlargement of the cup. **E:** Further enlargement of the cup in the same patient with inadequate control of the intraocular pressure. **F:** Improvement in disc appearance in the same patient after trabeculectomy.

of normal optic nerves. Only by documenting that the cup was once smaller can these discs be considered glaucomatous. Figures 3.12D and E show worsening of the disc before surgery, and Figure 3.12F shows improvement after surgery.

Cupping With No Rim Remaining

Though large cups are less frequent in normal persons than are small cups, the size of the cup does not rule out or confirm glaucoma. If there is no rim, the nerve is abnormal (Fig.

3.13), but cup-to-disc ratios of 0.3 or less do not rule out the presence of glaucoma (Fig. 3.12F), and cup-to-disc ratios of 0.7 or larger are not always indicative of glaucoma (Fig. 3.12B).

Focal Glaucoma

The appearance of the nerve is often helpful in determining whether it is glaucomatous. An acquired pit of the optic nerve is virtually diagnostic of glaucoma damage (Fig. 3.14).

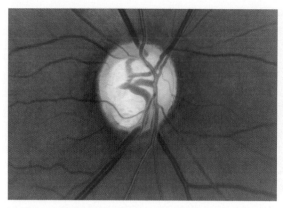

FIGURE 3.13. Enlarged cup with a thin temporal rim but normal intraocular pressure and marked visual field loss.

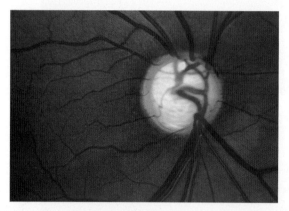

FIGURE 3.14. Acquired pit of the inferior portion of the optic nerve rim (at 6:30). This is diagnostic of glaucoma.

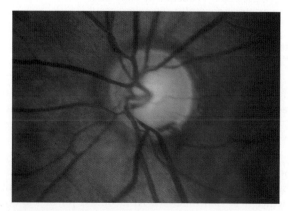

FIGURE 3.15. Striate hemorrhage at the inferior disc margin. This finding frequently indicates that the glaucoma is not well controlled.

These pits are usually at the 5:30 or 6:30 position and less frequently found at the 1:30 or 11:30 position. They are found at the outer edge of the optic nerve.

Hemorrhage

A superficial hemorrhage crossing the optic nerve edge is highly characteristic of glaucoma, and this should be specifically looked for by the examiner (Fig. 3.15). These hemorrhages are uncommon, occurring in a small percentage of patients. However, they are almost always a sign that the glaucoma is uncontrolled.

Disc Asymmetry

Asymmetry of the two optic nerves is highly suggestive of an acquired change, alerting the examiner to the possible presence of glaucoma nerve damage. In the patient illustrated, neither eye shows much damage, but tissue loss is more apparent in the left eye (Fig. 3.16B) than in the right eye (Fig. 3.16A). Myopic eyes tend to have larger scleral rims than hyperopic eyes, and cup asymmetry may in some cases be accounted for by anisometropia. (Also see page 144, Fig. 3.88).

Clinical Evaluation of the Optic Nerve Head

Historical Perspective

The optic nerve was first observed *in vivo* in 1851 when Hermann von Helmholtz (1821 to 1894) invented the direct ophthalmoscope. Edward von Jaeger (1818 to 1884) published the first ONH drawing from a patient with glaucoma in 1854. He used Helmholtz's direct ophthalmoscope with a candle as the illumination source; a single disc drawing required 80 to 120 hours. Both he and Albrecht von Graefe (1828 to 1870), confused by the two-dimensional view of the direct ophthalmoscope, believed that the optic nerve in glaucoma was elevated. In 1855, Adolf Weber (1829 to 1915), a student of von Graefe, suggested that the optic nerve was instead depressed, which was later confirmed by the German anatomist Heinrich Muller (1820 to 1864) in 1858. The first photographs of the human fundus were published by Howe in 1886. Nordenson modified a Zeiss camera to create the first stereoscopic camera in 1925.

Clinical examination remains the mainstay for evaluation of the ONH. It is inexpensive, quick to perform, and highly sensitive and specific. The direct ophthalmoscope gives a very magnified, direct view of the ONH, but it is a two-dimensional image. The slip lamp biomicroscope using a Hruby, 60 diopter (D), 78 D, or 90 D lens offers a three-dimensional view. The indirect ophthalmoscope gives a very minified image of the ONH, which makes a detailed evaluation of the ONH difficult.

Photographic Techniques

The most basic ONH imaging technique is a simple two-dimensional photograph. However, cupping can only be in-

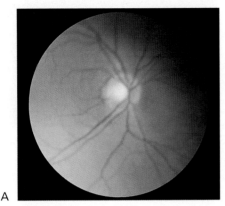 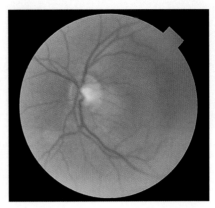

FIGURE 3.16. Disc asymmetry is present in a 55-year-old patient with an elevated pressure in the right eye associated with the exfoliation syndrome. The cup in the right eye **(A)** is larger than that in the left eye **(B)**. (Also see page 144, Fig. 3.88).

ferred indirectly by observations of color and vessel course. Stereoscopic photography allows a three-dimensional perception of the ONH. There are two methods of obtaining a stereoscopic pair of ONH photos—sequential, which captures two separate images photographed consecutively, and simultaneous, which creates the stereoscopic pair from a single image reflection. Simultaneous methods provide greater reproducibility of disc assessments. Figure 3.17 shows images obtained simultaneously.

The next advancement involved digitization of the photographic image and using a computer program to create a topographic map of the ONH. Examples of this include the Nidek 3Dx (Nidek Technologies, Inc., Pasadena, CA) and the Topcon TRC-SS2 (Topcon Instrument Corp. of America, Paramus, NJ). The computer relies on a ratio of distances between the same reference point that appears in each stereo photo to generate this map. In one comparison, the Topcon system was twice as sensitive at detecting vessel shift as conventional stereo disc photos. This system is no longer commercially available. In other studies, the Nidek system was more reproducible than images from a Zeiss camera using a sequential photo technique, and less variable in disc assessments than conventional simultaneous photos us-

ing a Donaldson camera. The Nidek 3Dx generally estimates a smaller horizontal cup-to-disc (c/d) ratio than the Topcon.

The Discam (Marcher Enterprises Ltd., Hereford, England) utilizes a digital camera and stereochronoscopy with alternation flicker to generate a stereopair of images (Fig 3.18A). In addition to measuring horizontal and vertical c/d ratios, this system looks for neuroretinal rim loss along a "chevron," which uses the supero- and inferotemporal aspects of the cup as the axes (Fig. 3.18B). However, the placement of the chevron and determination of the location of the neuroretinal rim rely on human interpretation. This method provides reproducible inter- and intraobserver estimates of optic disc measurements.

In summary, the conventional photographic cameras have the same degree of image resolution. The Zeiss camera using a sequential technique is still probably the most common method for obtaining stereo disc photos despite evidence in the literature that simultaneously acquired photos may have an advantage.

Confocal Scanning Laser Ophthalmoscopy (CSLO)

CSLO is another imaging technique that also generates topographic maps of the ONH. Conventional photography uses broad spectrum white light and captures the reflected light from the entire area of interest. CSLO uses a diode laser, focused on a very small point, and captures light in a collector focused only on that very spot. The amount of time it takes to receive the reflected light is used to calculate the distance to the surface. This information is then used to create the topography map. The cup is defined as the area below a reference plane set 50 μm below the surface of the optic nerve head. There are several manufacturers of confocal scanning laser ophthalmoscopes—Heidelberg Retina Tomograph (HRT, Heidelberg Engineering, Heidelberg, Germany), Topographic Scanning System (TopSS, Laser Diagnostic Technologies, San Diego, CA), and the Zeiss Laser Topographic Scanner (LTS, Zeiss Instruments, Thornwood, NJ—no longer commercially available). When the HRT and Topcon TRC were compared, the Topcon measured the rim

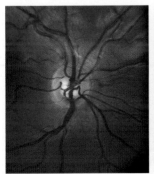 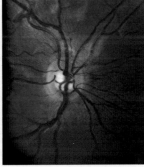

FIGURE 3.17. Optic nerve head simultaneous stereoscopic pair using a Topcon.

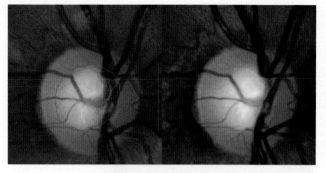 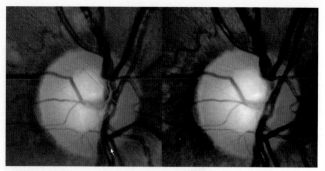

FIGURE 3.18. A: Two-dimensional photo and stereoscopic pair with **(B)** chevron drawn. (Courtesy of Donald L. Budenz, M.D., Miami, FL.)

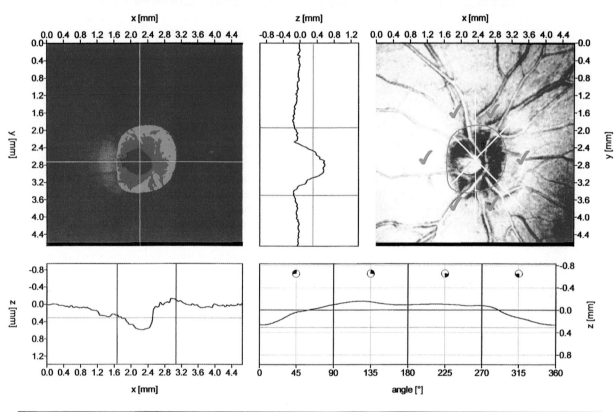

Stereometric Analysis ONH		
Disk Area	1.862	mm²
Cup Area	0.316	mm²
Rim Area	1.546	mm²
Cup Volume	0.046	cmm
Rim Volume	0.477	cmm
Cup/Disk Area Ratio	0.170	
Horizontal Cup/Disk Ratio	0.526	
Vertical Cup/Disk Ratio	0.291	
Mean Cup Depth	0.172	mm
Maximum Cup Depth	0.587	mm
Cup Shape Measure	-0.277	
Height Variation Contour	0.427	mm
Mean RNFL Thickness	0.315	mm
RNFL Cross Sectional Area	1.526	mm²
Reference Height	0.309	mm

Comments:

Date: 10/25/99 Signature: _____

Classification: Within normal limits (*)

(*) Moorfields regression classification (Ophthalmology 1998;105:1557-1563).
Classification based on statitstics. Diagnosis is physician's responsibility.

FIGURE 3.19. Confocal scanning laser ophthalmoscopy of the same patient using the **(A)** Heidelberg Retina Tomograph and **(B)** Topographic Scanning System machines. *(continues)*

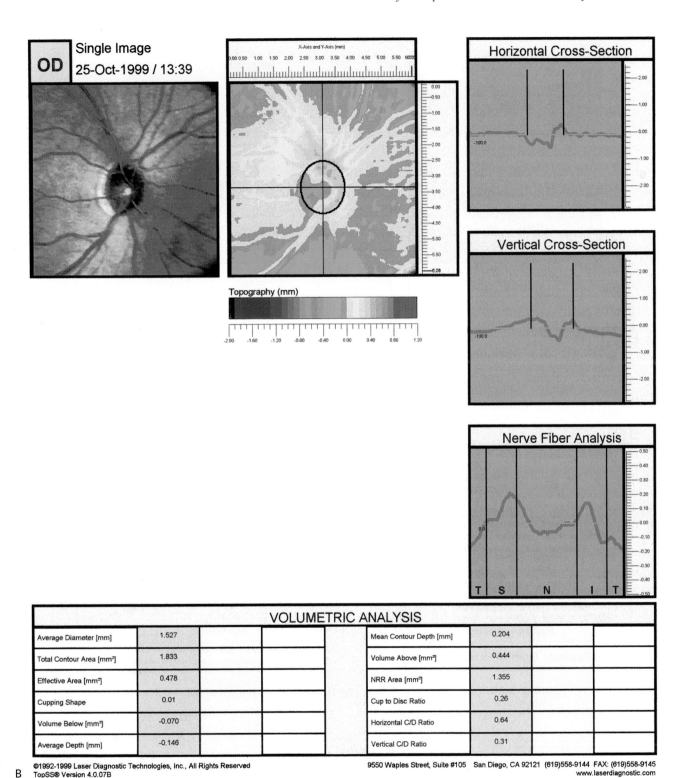

FIGURE 3.19. *Continued.*

area and cup volume to be larger, but the c/d ratio was the same. Additionally, the HRT was more reproducible regarding disc parameters than the Topcon System. Serial HRT analysis may be able to detect conversion from ocular hypertension to glaucoma before automated achromatic perimetry.

One study comparing the ability of HRT, optical coherence tomography (OCT), and scanning laser polarimetry (SLP) (note: OCT and SLP are ways of measuring RNFL thickness—see below) to detect patients with glaucoma found HRT to be the most sensitive and specific method. Figure

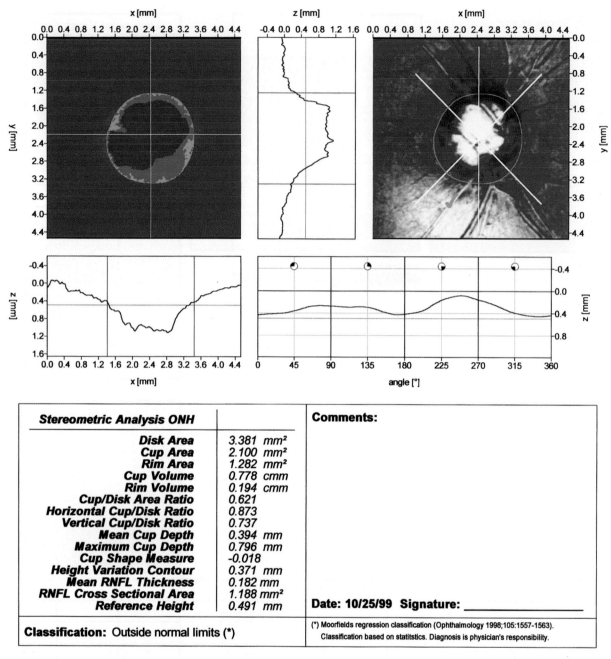

Stereometric Analysis ONH	
Disk Area	3.381 mm²
Cup Area	2.100 mm²
Rim Area	1.282 mm²
Cup Volume	0.778 cmm
Rim Volume	0.194 cmm
Cup/Disk Area Ratio	0.621
Horizontal Cup/Disk Ratio	0.873
Vertical Cup/Disk Ratio	0.737
Mean Cup Depth	0.394 mm
Maximum Cup Depth	0.796 mm
Cup Shape Measure	-0.018
Height Variation Contour	0.371 mm
Mean RNFL Thickness	0.182 mm
RNFL Cross Sectional Area	1.188 mm²
Reference Height	0.491 mm

Comments:

Date: 10/25/99 Signature: _____

Classification: Outside normal limits (*)

(*) Moorfields regression classification (Ophthalmology 1998;105:1557-1563).
Classification based on statitstics. Diagnosis is physician's responsibility.

FIGURE 3.20. Confocal scanning laser ophthalmoscopy using a Heidelberg Retina Tomograph from a patient with glaucoma.

3.19A, B shows an example of CSLO of the same patient using two different machines. Figure 3.20 is an example of CSLO in a patient with glaucoma using the HRT.

RETINAL NERVE FIBER LAYER

Introduction

The RNFL is composed of ganglion cell axons, neuroglia, and astrocytes. The RNFL becomes thicker as one ap-proaches the optic nerve head. The superior and inferior poles are thicker than the nasal and temporal poles; this gives the classic "double hump" seen in graphic representations of RNFL thickness (Fig 3.21). (See also "double hump" in Figure 3.15.) The presence of RNFL defects may aid in the diagnosis of glaucoma, but RNFL photography lacks the reproducibility to be more useful than ONH eval-uation or perimetry for monitoring progression of disease. Newer technologies indirectly measure the actual thickness of the RNFL.

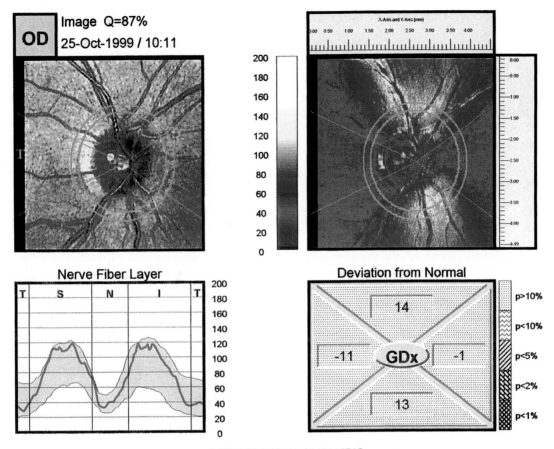

NERVE FIBER ANALYSIS

	Act. Value	Status	Probability		Act. Value	Status	Probability
Symmetry	1.04	Within Normal		The Number	7		
Superior Ratio	2.95	Within Normal		Average Thickness	67	Within Normal	
Inferior Ratio	2.84	Within Normal		Ellipse Average	73	Within Normal	
Superior/Nasal	2.47	Within Normal		Superior Average	90	Within Normal	
Max. Modulation	1.95	Within Normal		Inferior Average	86	Within Normal	
Ellipse Modulation	3.08	Within Normal		Superior Integral	0.225	Within Normal	

Comment:

©1992-1999 Laser Diagnostic Technologies, Inc., All Rights Reserved
GDx® Version 2.0.09

9550 Waples Street, Suite #105   San Diego, CA 92121 (619)558-9144 FAX: (619)558-9145
www.laserdiagnostic.com

FIGURE 3.21. Graphic representation of retinal nerve fiber layer thickness results from scanning laser polarimetry GDx of the same normal patient seen in Figure 3.20. One sees the "double-hump" appearance. (T, temporal; S, superior; N, nasal; I, inferior.)

Clinical Evaluation of the Retinal Nerve Fiber Layer

Historical Perspective

Clinical examination of the nerve fiber layer was first described by Vogt in 1917. The first published photograph of the nerve fiber layer was taken by Behrendt and Wilson in 1965. Examination of the RNFL was repopularized by Hoyt and Newman in the early 1970s.

Scanning Laser Polarimetry (SLP)

This technology exploits the birefringent nature of the RNFL to change the polarization of reflected light from the retina and RNFL. Assuming that the rotation of the polarized light is proportional to the RNFL thickness, the amount of rotation observed can be used to quantitatively measure RNFL thickness—termed "retardance" (Fig. 3.22). The only SLP machine currently available is the GDx (Laser Diagnostic Technologies, Inc., San Diego, CA). Patients with glaucoma have a thinner RNFL (Fig. 3.23), which is reflected in a flattening of the "double hump."

Optical Coherence Tomography

Optical coherence tomography (OCT; Zeiss-Humphrey Inst., San Leandro, CA) uses low coherence interferometry and measures the time it takes for light to be reflected from the different structures to generate its images. This is analogous to A-mode ultrasound, which instead uses sound waves. OCT can differentiate between patients clinically diagnosed as normal, ocular hypertensive, or glaucomatous, and glaucomatous versus nonglaucomatous eyes. In a direct comparison, OCT had a higher correlation between RNFL structure and visual function than SLP; however, further study is needed. Like SLP, OCT shows RNFL thinning in glaucomatous eyes (Fig. 3.24) compared to normals (Fig. 3.25).

VISUAL FIELD LOSS

Glaucoma causes the loss of visual function. The evaluation of the effects of the glaucomatous process on visual function is essential in the diagnosis and management of the condition. In some patients, interference with other functions may be more marked; contrast sensitivity, dark adaptation, color vision, and the ability to discriminate flicker are all affected to some extent by the glaucomatous process. However, for tests to be clinically useful, they must be sensitive and specific. A clinically useful test must be able to find the condition (i.e., have few false-negative results) and must not be positive for other conditions (i.e., have few false-positive results). Of all the tests of visual function investigated, evaluation of the visual field combines the highest level of specificity and sensitivity. It is the best standardized of all the tests and continues to be clinically the most useful method of evaluating visual function in patients with glaucoma. And, perhaps most importantly, it is the only test currently available that can somewhat objectively assess the subjective experience of the patient's visual function.

Confrontation Fields

Determining the visual field by confrontation methods can often provide extremely useful information, and the value of the test should not be forgotten. Confrontation fields are underused as methods of evaluating visual function in patients with glaucoma. For patients with very poor vision from cataract, for example, it may be the only practical test possible. For patients with extremely poor vision, the unshielded light of a penlight is a useful method, and for patients with slightly less impaired vision, covering the penlight with a finger so that a red glow is produced is a useful method of evaluating the field. For patients with good vision, a small, colored object, such as the red top on a bottle of a cycloplegic agent, can be used to determine a color field by confrontation. To evaluate the field in the setting of large central nervous system (CNS) disease such as stroke, finger counting may be used as well.

With any of these methods, the patient is first asked to fixate upon the examiner's nose, eye, or face. For patients with very poor vision, fixation can be maintained upon the source of the examiner's voice. The examiner monitors fixation during the subsequent testing phase. Next, the object is moved in from the periphery, and the patient is requested to indicate when he or she first sees the object or, in the case of the red top bottle, can see the red as a clear red color. The four quadrants corresponding to superonasal, superotemporal, inferonasal, and inferotemporal are tested. A nasal step is specifically sought by moving the object vertically on the nasal side of the patient's visual field, asking the patient to state whether the object changes in brightness or color as it crosses the horizontal line through the visual axis. Scotomas can be mapped in a similar fashion. The red object can be moved from a scotoma into a visible location and vise versa to define the extent of the lesion.

One very useful confrontation technique is a modification of the Tangent screen to test for functional visual field loss. Tunnel vision is a typical pattern of functional field loss and can be readily demonstrated by mapping the field while sitting a few feet from the patient. Typically, there will be an extremely constricted field. The examiner then increases the distance between himself or herself and the patient. The field is retested, and failure to find an overall expanded field is indicative of tunnel vision.

The results of the confrontation field test should be charted as exactly as possible, providing a baseline for future reference to determine whether the field is changing.

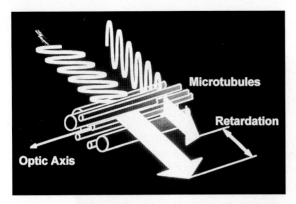

FIGURE 3.22. Graphic representation of retardance. (Reprinted from Schuman JS, Noecker RJ. Imaging of the optic nerve and nerve fiber layer in glaucoma. *Ophthalmol Clin North Am* 1995;8:259, with permission.)

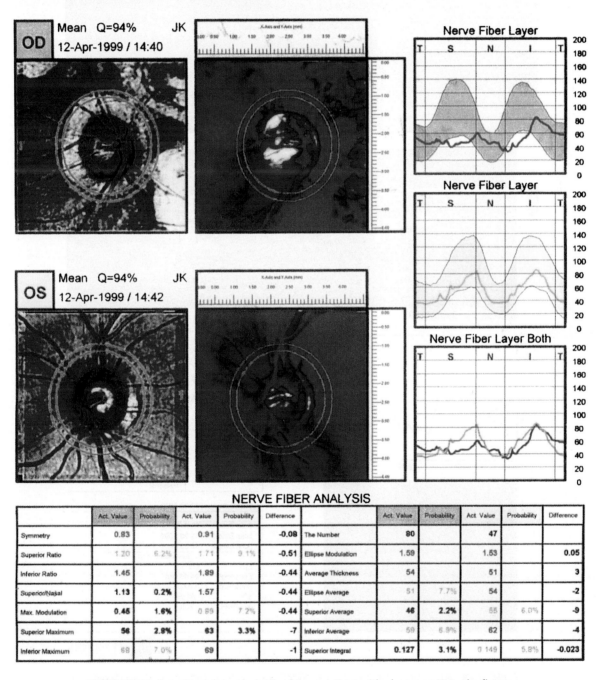

NERVE FIBER ANALYSIS

	Act. Value	Probability	Act. Value	Probability	Difference		Act. Value	Probability	Act. Value	Probability	Difference
Symmetry	0.83		0.91		-0.08	The Number	80		47		
Superior Ratio	1.20	6.2%	1.71	9.1%	-0.51	Ellipse Modulation	1.59		1.53		0.05
Inferior Ratio	1.45		1.89		-0.44	Average Thickness	54		51		3
Superior/Nasal	1.13	0.2%	1.57		-0.44	Ellipse Average	51	7.7%	54		-2
Max. Modulation	0.45	1.6%	0.89	7.2%	-0.44	Superior Average	46	2.2%	55	6.0%	-9
Superior Maximum	56	2.8%	63	3.3%	-7	Inferior Average	59	6.9%	62		-4
Inferior Maximum	68	7.0%	69		-1	Superior Integral	0.127	3.1%	0.149	5.8%	-0.023

FIGURE 3.23. Scanning laser polarimetry from a patient with glaucoma. Note the flattening of the double hump on the graphic representation of the retinal nerve fiber layer. (Courtesy of Laser Diagnostics.)

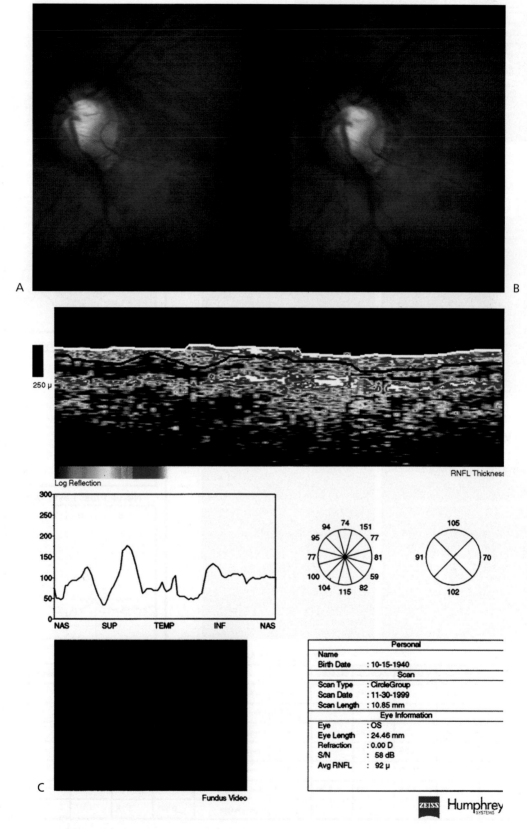

FIGURE 3.24. A: Optic nerve head with Nidek 3Dx from a patient with glaucoma. **B:** Corresponding achromatic visual field. **C:** Optical coherence tomography image from the same glaucomatous patient demonstrating retinal nerve fiber layer thinning in a glaucomatous eye. (Courtesy of Joel S. Schuman, M.D., Boston, MA.)

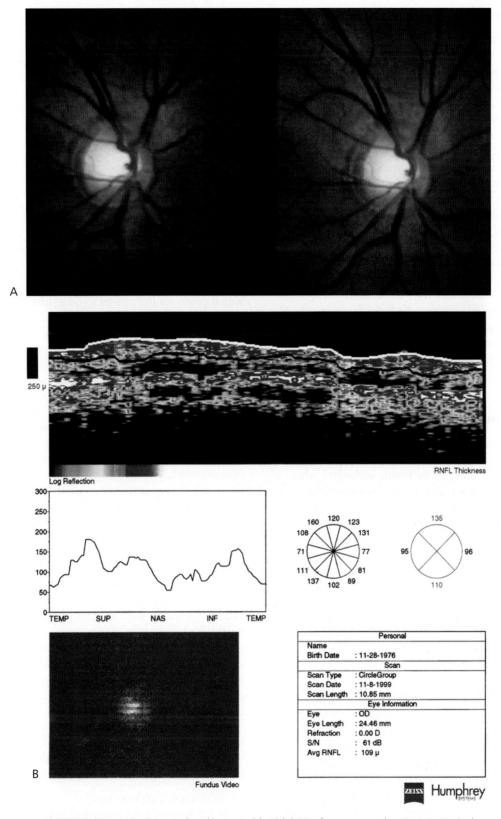

FIGURE 3.25. A: Optic nerve head image with Nidek 3Dx from a normal patient. **B:** Optical coherence tomography image from the same patient of a normal retinal nerve fiber layer. (Courtesy of Joel S. Schuman, M.D., Boston, MA.)

Kinetic Perimetry

The visual field has been described by Traquair as an island of vision in a sea of blindness. The central portion of the island is peaked, and this corresponds to the most sensitive portion of the field to light. The peripheral portion is less sensitive to light and is therefore lower in elevation, like the shores of the island. In order to create a two-dimensional map of this three-dimensional island, a topographic map must be made. The basis of kinetic perimetry is to take a stimulus of fixed intensity and size and move it across the visual field to create a "ring" that, identically to a contour interval on a topographic map, defines where that stimulus is seen. The stimulus intensity is then reduced to test the more sensitive parts of the field (the peak of the island) or increased to test the less sensitive parts of the field. Eventually, a map of the island of vision is created.

The Goldmann kinetic perimeter is the most well known example of kinetic perimetry. Until automated static perimetry was developed, it was the best way to test the visual field. Although static perimetry has now replaced it as the test of choice for glaucoma, the Goldmann kinetic perimeter remains a viable option for certain patients who cannot perform static perimetry.

Computerized Static Perimetry

The most widely accepted method of evaluating the visual field is computerized perimetry, using a technique known as static perimetry. In contrast to kinetic perimetry where a stimulus of fixed intensity is moved in the visual field, static perimetry maps the island of vision by varying the intensity of the stimulus in a fixed location. This is akin to a mountain climber taking altitude measurements at various fixed locations all over the island of vision. The advantage is that not only can computers perform the testing, thereby permitting standardization, reproducibility, and statistical analysis, but the very fine changes in stimulus intensity that can be performed also permit very sensitive maps of the island of vision, and glaucomatous defects can be detected earlier than they become apparent using kinetic perimetry.

The most commonly used automated perimeters are Humphrey or Octopus instruments. Full threshold tests, such as the Humphrey 24-2 examination, provide a high level of sensitivity and specificity. However, these levels are not absolute. A "normal" visual field examination, which is a test in which no defect is found, does not mean that the patient does not have glaucoma. Repeated visual field tests that show no apparent deterioration do not prove that the patient's glaucoma is not deteriorating. Many neurons must be lost before a field defect is evident, and many more neurons must be lost before a visual field defect progresses.

Additionally, the visual field may demonstrate a visual field defect that is not due to glaucoma. Droopy lids, small pupils, refractive error, opacities in the media, retinal disease, and CNS disease all can cause visual field defects. Even age, with its accompanying smaller pupil and hazy lens, typically causes loss of sensitivity in the peripheral field. These changes may mimic the changes that occur as glaucoma gets better or worse. Additionally, changes in testing strategy, such as switching from one machine to another, or even different testing strategies on the same machine, can demonstrate changes in the field that may, or may not, be real. The astute examiner must be aware of the changes that can cause an apparent improvement or, more commonly, a deterioration of the field, and must consider those possibilities when interpreting the visual field examination.

Most of the new instruments provide software analyses of the hardware results. These analyses provide much useful information for the practitioner trying to decide whether the field is normal or abnormal, stable or changing. The individual points on the patient's visual field are compared with the age-matched controls to determine what is abnormal about the field, and then a subtraction technique is used to attempt to eliminate the factors that may decrease the overall sensitivity of the field as a result of opacities in the media. These statistical calculations attempt to highlight localized abnormal areas of the field that are in excess of any generalized depression and so may be buried in overall darkness of the field. Such localized defects are more typical of glaucoma. Additional tests are built into the automated examination to investigate the intratest reliability. Fixation losses, false-positives, and false-negatives are routinely calculated. On some testing protocols, certain defined points in the field are retested in an attempt to measure the patient's internal consistency. This measure of "short-term fluctuation" provides an estimate of the reproducibility of the data and assists the interpreter by providing a useful method of estimating the reliability of the test.

It is essential for those interpreting visual field examinations to understand the difference between reliability and validity. A visual field evaluation may be highly reproducible and, therefore, may be reliable. However, that reliable visual field may not be a valid indicator of the patient's visual field. For example, when tests are repeatedly done with the correcting lens too far from the eye, there is a reproducible peripheral contraction, but the peripheral contraction is not a valid indicator of the patient's field.

When interpreting the visual field, we recommend a systematic approach. We believe this will provide that examiner the best opportunity to interpret the field correctly. We recommend that a seven-step strategy be followed:

1. Which test was performed?
2. Is the patient's demographic and clinical information correct?
3. Is the field reliable?
4. Is the field abnormal?

5. What is the pattern of the abnormality?
6. Is the current examination different (worse) than previous examinations?
7. Is the abnormality or worsening due to disease or artifact?

Each strategy will be examined in some detail using the Humphrey perimeter as the model. This is not the only perimeter that can be used, but is the most widely used and is the one used at the Wills Eye Hospital. See Figure 3.28 for a typical Swedish interactive threshold algorithm (SITA) single-field printout.

The test that was performed is indicated at the top of the printout. This is important, not only because it will determine how to interpret that field, but also because for patients who have undergone multiple field examinations, a change in testing protocol can alter the appearance of the field. We believe that a consistent approach of using the same testing protocol over time is often best. Patients who are switched to one of the newer, faster test protocols may require two or more fields to be performed to establish a new baseline.

The patient demographic information is critical. Care must be taken with persons with the same name, and extreme care must be taken to ensure that the age of the patient and the refraction used for the examination are correct. Problems in either of these areas will often greatly affect the results of the test.

Reliability of the field is best assessed by examining the fixation losses (or the gaze tracker on the newer Humphrey Field Analyzer [HFA] II), false-positives, false-negatives, and short-term fluctuation. Fixation losses are a measure of how attentive the patient was in looking at the fixation target during the test. Generally speaking, a high number indicates unreliability, but in certain cases where the remaining reliability parameters are normal, this can be acceptable. False-positives measure times that the patient indicated a stimulus was seen even when no stimulus was presented. Such errors tend to make the field look "better" than it actually is and can seriously confound interpretation. We consider more than two false-positives (or 10% to 15% on a SITA exam) to be concerning. False-negatives measure the patient's lack of response to a retest with a stimulus that was previously seen in a certain location. High false-negatives generally result in making the field appear "worse" than it is, but can be understood and even expected in patients with pathologic defects in their fields due to fluctuation inherent in a scotoma. Therefore, a high number may not be terribly concerning if the overall field is poor. Short-term fluctuation is calculated by retesting certain defined points in the field and determining the difference in sensitivity for the two tests. This is a useful measure of reliability and can even represent the first change in glaucoma or glaucomatous progression. However, it takes time and has been abandoned on the newer SITA testing algorithms.

Abnormality of the visual field is best demonstrated on the total deviation plot. This plot is a comparison of each point in the field with a database of normal age-matched controls and represents the deviation from the normal expected value for each point in the field. A statistical calculation is then performed to indicate the level of abnormality and is indicated by various shaded boxes.

The real interpretation work begins with deciding if there is artifact in the field and what pathology the pattern of field loss indicates. Extensive atlases of visual field artifacts are available, and a thorough discussion of these is beyond the scope of this text. Suffice it to say that knowledge of nonphysiologic (such as lens-rim artifact) and nonglaucomatous (such as ptosis) patterns of field loss is essential to proper interpretation. To aid the interpreter who is interested in testing for glaucoma, the Humphrey printout contains a plot called the pattern deviation plot. This plot is a subtraction plot based on the total deviation plot and is designed to normalize an island of vision that has been diffusely depressed, typically by media opacity or small pupil size. It should reveal the focal areas of depression in excess of the generalized background depression that may indicate glaucoma is present. Statistical measures of the amount of deviation from normal are also presented. Note that this plot cannot adjust for other causes of field loss, such as retinal or CNS, that may simulate the focal losses of glaucoma. A correlation of the visual field and the clinical examination is required to confirm which disease process is present.

There is no universally accepted definition of what constitutes a glaucomatous defect; however, there are three major patterns of visual field loss that are characteristic of glaucoma: a diffuse decrease in sensitivity, primarily peripherally; an ocular scotoma involving the area about 15 degrees from fixation (i.e., arcuate); and a dense paracentral scotoma that starts nasal to fixation. There are probably other patterns that have been less well established. These three separate patterns can occur individually or in various combinations. The diffuse type of decreased sensitivity tends to be typical of ischemic, high-pressure glaucomas, while the arcuate type of defect is characteristic of chronic, moderate pressure elevation glaucomas, and the paracentral type of defect is more typical of the glaucomas that occur with normal levels of IOP.

Arbitrary classification schemes have been developed to attempt to classify glaucomatous visual field defects according to their level of severity. For the most part, these are complicated research tools and are not useful in clinical practice. One scale, however, is relatively simple and can be used to classify defects for use in deciding treatment strategies. The Hodapp-Parrish-Anderson Scale (Hodapp, 1993) requires that certain minimal abnormalities be present before a field is called glaucomatous, and then classifies defects as early, moderate, or severe. The definitions (and our own modifications for SITA testing) are based on a Humphrey perimeter equipped with STATPAC 2 and are found in

Table 3.4. See Figures 3.26, 3.27, and 3.28 for examples of the Hodapp Interpretation Scale applied to a visual field. At Wills, we have devised our own arbitrary grading scale that divides field abnormalities into seven stages of progressively more and more damage. It is based upon the Humphrey visual field pattern deviation plot, but can be relatively easily adapted to other perimeters. This method simply counts the number of depressed points on the plot and assigns a point value. Although there is no allowance made for a glaucoma hemifield test or clusters of points in typical glaucomatous regions, there is some adjustment made for location as the central four points, if depressed, count for triple value. This scale is designed for use in conjunction with a new optic nerve staging scale that we have also developed in order to arrive at a Glaucoma Likelihood Score (GLS) that seeks to estimate the chance that a patient has glaucoma. The visual field scale is seen in Table 3.5, and examples of visual fields are seen in Figures 3.26, 3.27, and 3.28.

Determining if the current examination differs from previous examinations may be even harder than deciding if the field is abnormal in the first place. In glaucoma, typically the field is followed over time to assess if it is stable or worsening. A series of visual fields in which there is no apparent change does not necessarily indicate stability of the patient's condition, and a series of visual fields indicating progressive change does not always indicate instability of the patient's glaucoma. Confounding factors such as pupil size, developing cataract, fatigue, improperly performed tests, and long-term fluctuation must always be considered and ruled out

before concluding that a change in a visual field is a valid indicator of a change in the patient's status. Once again, there are no universally accepted criteria for what determines if one field is different from another, but again, there are three patterns of glaucomatous progression: a new scotoma developing in a previously normal area; deepening of an existing scotoma; and enlargement of a preexisting scotoma. Scales to determine progression, much like scales to determine abnormality, are arbitrary and generally very complex and used only for research. The Hodapp-Parrish-Anderson criteria are relatively easy and readily applicable. The criteria for a new scotoma are identical to those discussed above. For deepening of an existing scotoma, two points must be depressed by 10 dB from baseline, and for enlargement of an existing scotoma, three points must be depressed by 10 dB from baseline. An additional criterion is if the mean deviation declines at a rate of $p < 5\%$ (about 1 dB per year) on the Humphrey glaucoma change analysis plot. This criterion is less specific for glaucoma, but may serve to identify the less common group of patients that demonstrate progression not by focal change, but by diffuse change in the visual field. Whichever criteria are used, the most important factor to remember is the effect of long-term fluctuation. Recent data indicate that the vast majority of visual fields that appear to have worsened will normalize (or return to baseline) upon repeat testing. Treatment decisions based upon the worsening of a single visual field, especially in the setting of other subjective and objective signs of stability, may be unnecessarily hasty.

TABLE 3-4. HODAPP-PARRISH-ANDERSON VISUAL FIELD GRADING SCALE (HODAPP, 1993)

Grade (need to meet only ONE of the definitions to be of a given grade)	Definition
Minimal	1. Abnormal glaucoma hemifield test 2. Corrected PSD depressed at the $p < 5\%$ level (or PSD of $p < 5\%$ on a SITA field) 3. A cluster of 3 nonedge points (for a 30-2 field) in an expected location for glaucoma, all of which are depressed on the pattern deviation plot at the 5% level (or greater) and at least one of which is depressed at the 1% level (or greater)
Early	1. Mean deviation < -6 dB 2. No point at 5 degrees from fixation is less than 15 dB 3. The total number of points depressed at the 5% level or worse on the pattern deviation plot is less than 1 quadrant, while the number of points depressed at the 1% level or worse is less than ½ quadrant, or ⅛ field
Moderate	1. Mean deviation between -6 dB and -12 dB 2. One point at 5 degrees from fixation measures less than 15 dB 3. The total number of points depressed at the 5% level or worse on the pattern deviation plot is less than 2 quadrants, while the number of points depressed at the 1% level or worse is less than 1 quadrant
Severe	1. Mean deviation > -12 dB 2. One point at 5 degrees from fixation of 0 dB 3. One point in each hemifield at 5 degrees from fixation measuring less than 15 dB 4. The total number of points depressed at the 5% level or worse on the pattern deviation plot is greater than 2 quadrants, while the number of points depressed at the 1% level or worse is greater than 1 quadrant

PSD, pattern of standard deviation; SITA, Swedish interactive threshold algorithm.

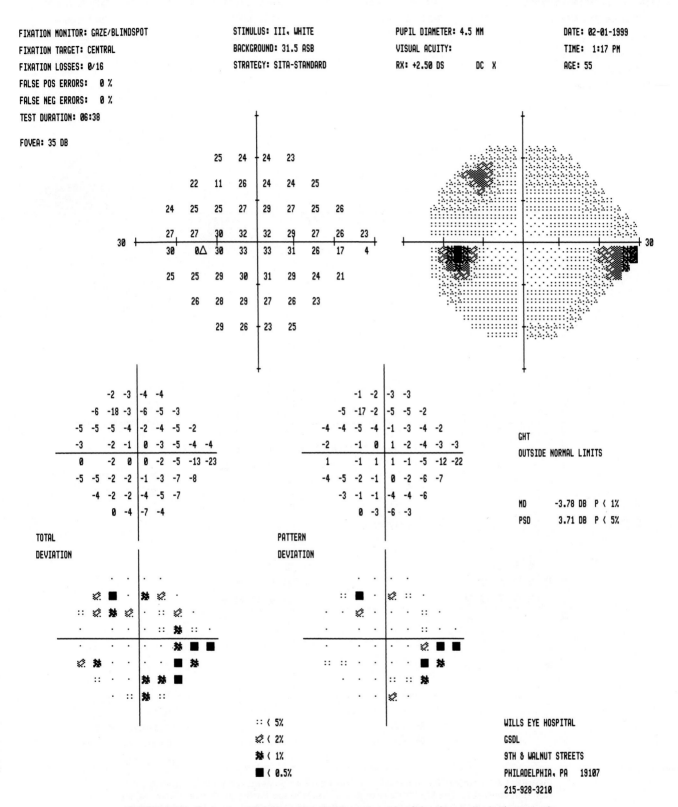

FIXATION MONITOR: GAZE/BLINDSPOT

FIXATION TARGET: CENTRAL

FIXATION LOSSES: 0/16

FALSE POS ERRORS: 0 %

FALSE NEG ERRORS: 0 %

TEST DURATION: 06:38

FOVEA: 35 DB

STIMULUS: III, WHITE

BACKGROUND: 31.5 ASB

STRATEGY: SITA-STANDARD

PUPIL DIAMETER: 4.5 MM

VISUAL ACUITY:

RX: +2.50 DS   DC X

DATE: 02-01-1999

TIME: 1:17 PM

AGE: 55

GHT

OUTSIDE NORMAL LIMITS

MD   -3.78 DB P < 1%

PSD   3.71 DB P < 5%

TOTAL DEVIATION

PATTERN DEVIATION

:: < 5%

▨ < 2%

▩ < 1%

■ < 0.5%

WILLS EYE HOSPITAL

GSDL

9TH & WALNUT STREETS

PHILADELPHIA, PA   19107

215-928-3210

FIGURE 3.26. Early visual field loss. This field meets each of the three criteria that constitute the Minimal category of the Hodapp-Parrish-Anderson classification system and should probably be considered in the Early category. According to the Spaeth classification system, this is a stage 2 field (mild) as there are 6 points depressed at the 1% or worse level.

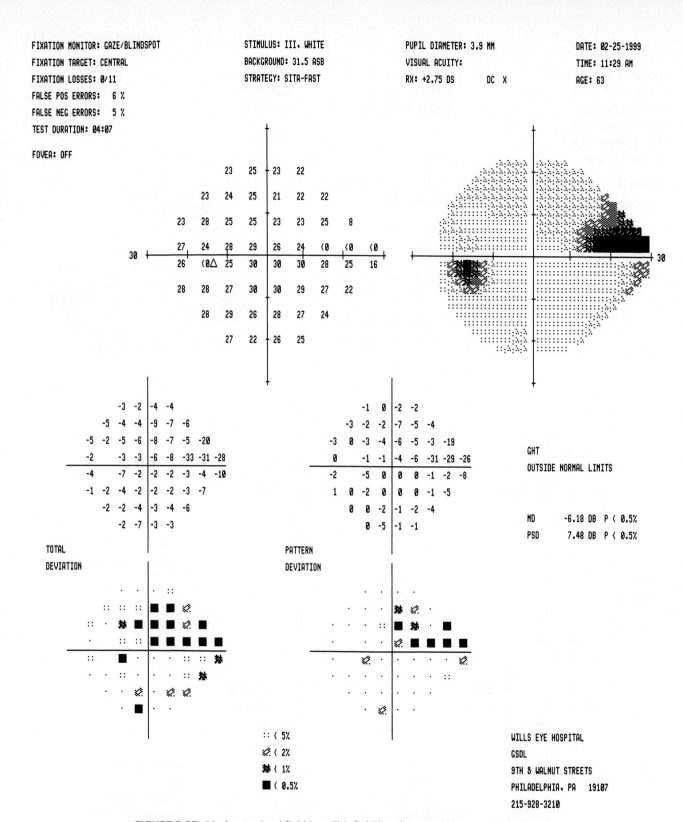

WILLS EYE HOSPITAL

GSDL

9TH & WALNUT STREETS

PHILADELPHIA, PA   19107

215-928-3210

FIGURE 3.27. Moderate visual field loss. This field barely meets the mean deviation criterion that constitutes the Moderate category of the Hodapp-Parrish-Anderson classification system. If the visual field contained more evidence of cataract on the total deviation plot or the foveal threshold, one might consider the mean deviation to be a reflection of more than just glaucoma, and thereby downgrade the field to the Early category. According to the Spaeth classification system, this is a stage 3 (mild-to-moderate) field as there are 8 points depressed at the 1% or worse level. Note that there is a point depressed at the 2% level within 5 degrees of fixation. If this were depressed at the 1% level or worse, then there would be 11 abnormal points (points depressed at this level in this location are counted three times) and the field would still be stage 3.

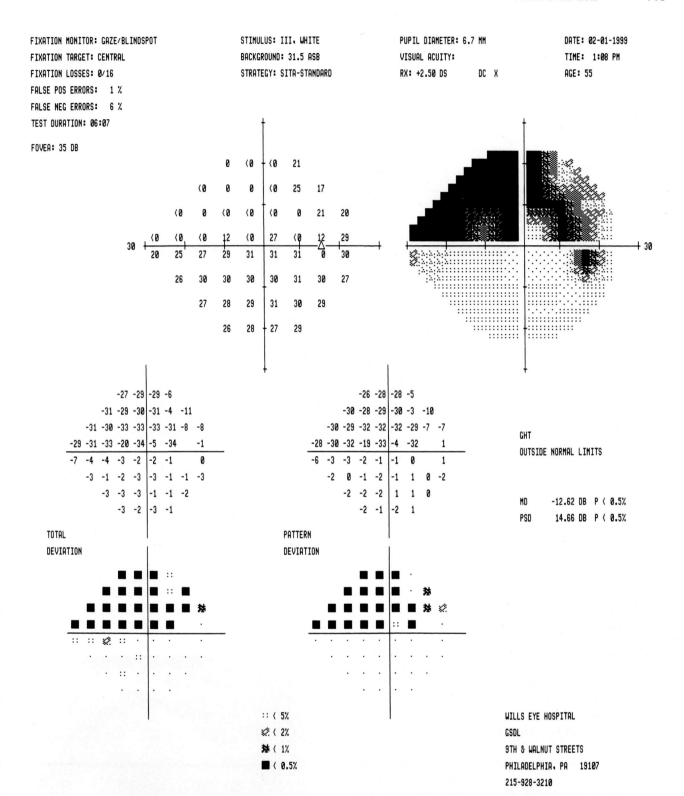

FIXATION MONITOR: GAZE/BLINDSPOT

FIXATION TARGET: CENTRAL

FIXATION LOSSES: 0/16

FALSE POS ERRORS: 1 %

FALSE NEG ERRORS: 6 %

TEST DURATION: 06:07

FOVEA: 35 DB

STIMULUS: III. WHITE

BACKGROUND: 31.5 ASB

STRATEGY: SITA-STANDARD

PUPIL DIAMETER: 6.7 MM

VISUAL ACUITY:

RX: +2.50 DS   DC X

DATE: 02-01-1999

TIME: 1:08 PM

AGE: 55

GHT

OUTSIDE NORMAL LIMITS

MD   -12.62 DB P < 0.5%

PSD   14.66 DB P < 0.5%

TOTAL DEVIATION

PATTERN DEVIATION

:: < 5%

⬚ < 2%

※ < 1%

■ < 0.5%

WILLS EYE HOSPITAL

GSDL

9TH & WALNUT STREETS

PHILADELPHIA, PA   19107

215-928-3210

FIGURE 3.28. Moderate visual field loss. This field contains a point of 0 dB within 5 degrees of fixation, has a mean deviation of more than −12 dB, and the total number of points depressed at the 1% level or greater on the pattern deviation plot exceeds one quadrant. According to the Spaeth classification system, this is a stage 4 field (moderate loss) as there are 20 points depressed at the 1% or worse level (remember to triple the point depressed at the 5 degrees location).

TABLE 3-5. SPAETH VISUAL FIELD GRADING SCALE

Stage	Grading by Visual Field Area	Grading by Number of Abnormal Points
0 (no loss)		0
1 (minimal loss)	Early nasal step	1–3
2 (mild loss)	Less than ½ of 1 quadrant loss	4–6
3 (mild-to-moderate loss)	About 1 quadrant loss	7–12
4 (moderate loss)	About 1 to 2 full quadrants lost	13–22
5 (marked loss)	About 2 to 3 full quadrants lost	23–32
6 (advanced loss)	More than 3 quadrants lost	33–42
7 (far advanced loss)	Residual island <25° or central island <4°	≥43

The visual field standard is the Humphrey 24-2 threshold test. The four points at the upper extreme and lower extreme of the field are ignored for purposes of this staging system.
An abnormal point is defined as a point depressed at the 1% level or more on the corrected pattern standard deviation plot. If any of the central four points is depressed at the 1% level, it is counted three times (tripled).
The worst possible score is 54—42 abnormal points in the peripheral field (remember to ignore the 8 points in the vertical extremes) and 12 for the four central points.

Newer Visual Field Tests

So far, the discussion has centered on the traditional methods of automated perimetry. These employ a white stimulus displayed upon a white background and have the ability to detect scotomas that are completely asymptomatic to the patient. Yet, as more information about the nature of the cellular injuries of glaucoma has become available, tests have been devised to attempt to preferentially target the function of those cells thought to be damaged first in glaucoma. Such special methods of perimetry, including the presentation of a blue stimulus against a yellow background (short wavelength automated perimetry, or SWAP) and frequency-doubling technology, may offer earlier detection of glaucoma than standard white-on-white perimetry. However these methods have not been proven superior and probably are best used only in centers that are investigating their value.

SPECIFIC ENTITIES

Angle-Closure Glaucomas

Angle-closure glaucomas are characterized by temporary or permanent contact of peripheral iris against the trabecular meshwork, resulting in obstruction of aqueous outflow. The clinical presentation can be acute or chronic. It is much less common than POAG.

The most common mechanism of angle-closure glaucoma is relative pupillary block (e.g., primary angle-closure glaucoma). The aqueous cannot flow from the posterior to the anterior chamber because of a functional obstruction between the lens and the iris. The peripheral angle structures are not visible or are partially obscured, and the iris is bowed forward, making contact with the anterior chamber angle. Other possible causes for pupillary block are discussed below.

Angle-closure glaucoma may be related to ocular structures that push the iris forward (e.g., plateau iris syndrome, aqueous misdirection, tumors, cysts) and tissues or membranes that obstruct the outflow directly (e.g., neovascular glaucoma, iridocorneal endothelial [ICE] syndrome, inflammatory debris).

Acute Primary Angle-Closure Glaucoma

Patients with acute angle-closure glaucoma present most often with pain, elevated IOP (often greater than 50 mm Hg), a shallow or flat peripheral anterior chamber, corneal edema, and visual loss (Fig. 3.29). Nausea and vomiting may occur. Predisposed patients are usually older than 50 years, hyperopes, with a shallow anterior chamber, a short axial length of the globe, and a thicker, more anteriorly displaced lens. It is more common in females and there is a familial tendency. Factors than can precipitate an attack include emotional stress, mydriasis, or anticholinergic drugs. Pupillary block is the most common mechanism (Figs. 3.30, 3.31).

Management. Acute angle-closure glaucoma is a medical emergency. The first goals are to break the acute attack, usually with medical therapy, to relieve permanently the

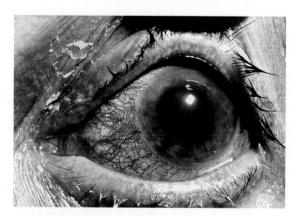

FIGURE 3.29. Typical external appearance of acute angle closure caused by pupillary block, with diffuse hyperemia of the conjunctiva, mid-dilated pupil, and steamy cornea. The intraocular pressure is 64 mm Hg.

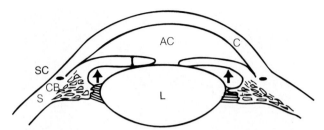

FIGURE 3.30. In pupillary block glaucoma, a physiologic block is created between the iris and the lens, preventing the normal flow of aqueous from the posterior chamber to the anterior chamber. Pressure (*arrows*) within the posterior chamber forces the peripheral iris forward, closing the angle and causing a sudden increase in intraocular pressure. (AC, anterior chamber; C, cornea; CB, ciliary body; I, iris; L, lens; S, sclera; SC, Schlemm's canal.)

pupillary block with neodymium:yttrium-argon-garnet (Nd:YAG) laser iridotomy, and to treat the fellow eye. The urgency of treatment is a factor of the amount of pain present and the likelihood of permanent optic nerve damage. When the optic nerve is already damaged, it is more susceptible to further damage. In such cases, lowering the IOP is urgent. Examination of the optic nerve is an *essential* part of the evaluation of a patient with an angle-closure glaucoma!

Initial medical therapy includes administration of intravenous acetazolamide (500 mg), topical aqueous suppressants (β blocker, carbonic anhydrase inhibitor, α2 agonist), and topical pilocarpine (1% to 2%, twice over 30 minutes). Frequent topical corticosteroids are started. If the attack is not broken, an osmotic agent is given (oral 50% glycerin, oral 45% isosorbide, or intravenous 20% mannitol, 1 to 2 g/kg). In recalcitrant cases, argon laser peripheral iridoplasty (or gonioplasty) or Nd:YAG iridotomy can be tried to break the acute attack. The view is usually suboptimal from corneal edema, and topical glycerin can be helpful.

Permanent relief of pupillary block is achieved with *Nd:YAG laser peripheral iridotomy* (see below). If laser irido-

tomy is not possible, argon laser peripheral iridoplasty (see below) or surgical peripheral iridectomy is necessary. The anterior chamber angle may appear open or show peripheral anterior synechiae of variable extension after the attack. Goniosynechialysis can be effective to open the angle if closure occurred within 12 months of surgical intervention. The fellow eye should undergo prompt prophylactic laser iridotomy to prevent an acute attack.

Chronic Angle-Closure Glaucoma

Some patients describe episodes of ocular discomfort, blurred vision or colored halos around lights that, in the presence of a narrow angle, are suggestive of *subacute angle-closure glaucoma*. These symptoms typically occur at night. Repeated subacute attacks may result in the development of permanent peripheral anterior synechiae and chronic angle-closure glaucoma. The synechiae tend to be broad based, and are most commonly seen in the superior quadrant.

Creeping angle-closure glaucoma is another form of chronic angle-closure glaucoma in which the anterior chamber angle narrows progressively over time. This form of glaucoma is the most common form of angle-closure glaucoma in black patients, especially in those on miotic therapy.

Diagnosis is based on gonioscopy (Fig. 3.32). Indentation gonioscopy (see page 99) is important to differentiate parts of the angle with appositional or permanent/synechial closure.

Management. Laser peripheral iridectomy is the initial treatment of choice. However, if most of the anterior chamber angle is closed, laser iridotomy will not be helpful in controlling the IOP. Long-term aqueous suppressants and, sometimes, filtering surgery, may be required. If more than

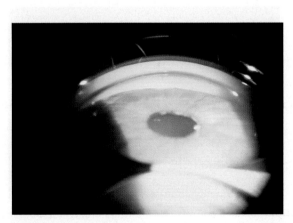

FIGURE 3.31. Gonioscopic view of a closed angle during an acute angle-closure attack.

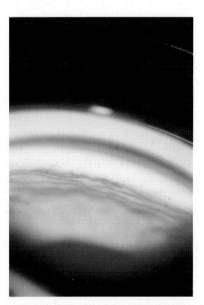

FIGURE 3.32. Gonioscopic view of peripheral anterior synechiae commonly seen in chronic angle closure.

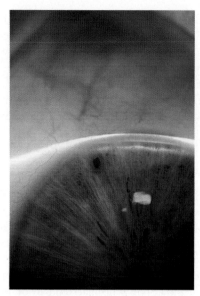

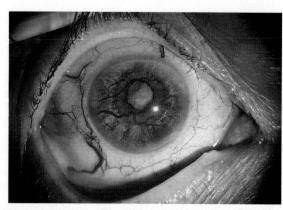

FIGURE 3.34. Neovascularization of the iris with large-caliber vessels on the surface in an 80-year-old diabetic woman. The angle is closed, and the intraocular pressure is 66 mm Hg. Notice the absence of corneal edema as a result of the longstanding duration of the disease.

FIGURE 3.33. Laser peripheral iridectomy successfully reversed the appositional closure.

one quadrant of the anterior chamber angle has appositional closure and opens with indentation gonioscopy, laser iridotomy may be enough to arrest the progression of the disease (Fig. 3.33).

Plateau Iris Syndrome

"Plateau iris *configuration*" refers to a flat iris configuration with an abrupt posterior turn near the iris insertion and, therefore, with a narrow anterior chamber angle. This is graded as a P angle (see page 100). Most eyes with plateau iris configuration have a component of relative pupillary block, and laser iridotomy can widen the anterior chamber angle. Occasionally, however, laser iridotomy does not affect the positioning and shape of the iris and the anterior chamber angle. The term used to describe this condition is "plateau iris *syndrome*," which is due to an anterior position of ciliary processes. Patients with plateau iris may develop acute or chronic angle closure.

Management. All patients with plateau iris should undergo laser peripheral iridectomy. If peripheral iridectomy does not deepen the angle, chronic miotic therapy can be effective to prevent or treat angle closure, although the treatment of choice is laser peripheral iridoplasty (see below).

Neovascular Glaucoma

Neovascular glaucoma occurs when a fibrovascular membrane proliferates from the iris onto the angle structures

(Fig. 3.34, Fig. 3.35). With progression of the disease, the fibrovascular membrane contracts, resulting in secondary angle-closure glaucoma. Fibrovascular membrane growth is related to ocular ischemic microvascular disease such as diabetes and central retinal vein obstruction. Other conditions can lead to neovascularization, such as uveitis, central retinal artery obstruction, branch vein obstruction, and tumors.

Management. Prompt laser panretinal photocoagulation is employed to cause regression of the neovascularization. If the angle is still open, or partially open, effective laser treatment may revert the condition. If the angle is closed, medical treatment with atropine, steroids, and aqueous suppressants can lower the IOP. If this fails, a tube-shunt procedure is usually the procedure of choice, providing there is useful vision. If the eye is blind, then surgery usually should *not* be considered, and treatment with atropine, steroids, and topical glaucoma drops is appropriate.

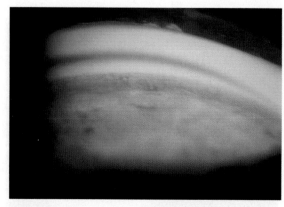

FIGURE 3.35. Blood vessels within the angle in a 64-year-old man 3 months after a central vein occlusion.

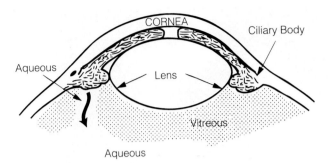

FIGURE 3.36. In aqueous misdirection, aqueous is directed posteriorly into the vitreous cavity, pushing the vitreous, lens, and iris forward; closing the angle; and increasing the intraocular pressure.

Aqueous Misdirection Syndrome

Previously called malignant glaucoma because of its inexorably worsening course and frequently grave outcome, aqueous misdirection syndrome is seen in eyes with small anterior segments. A change in aqueous dynamics brought on by the addition of miotics, surgery, or injury can direct aqueous production posteriorly into the vitreous cavity (Figs. 3.36, 3.37). The increasing volume posteriorly pushes the lens, iris, and hyaloid face forward, progressively making the anterior chamber shallower, closing the angle, and increasing the IOP. Studies with the high-frequency biomicroscope have revealed small, anterior, suprachoroidal effusions in many of the cases examined. The forward rotation of the iris, lens, and ciliary body around scleral spur caused by the effusion could well be the inciting feature in some of the cases with this syndrome. Characteristically, the space between the central cornea and lens is much less than would be expected if the IOP rise were due to angle-closure glaucoma.

Differential Diagnosis:

1. Pupillary block (deeper central anterior chamber, peripheral iridectomy curative)
2. Suprachoroidal hemorrhage (history of pain, visible dark choroidal detachment)
3. Suprachoroidal effusion (visible choroidal detachment, low IOP unless anterior rotation of lens and hyaloid face causes relative aqueous misdirection and pressures in the teens)

Management. The crescendo of flattening anterior chamber and increasing IOP makes medical and, frequently, surgical intervention imperative. Medical treatment consists of maximum aqueous suppression with topical β blockers, α2 agonists, topical and/or systemic carbonic anhydrase inhibitors, maximum cycloplegia with atropine to pull the lens-iris diaphragm posteriorly, and intravenous mannitol every 12 hours to shrink the vitreous maximally and deepen the anterior chamber. Steroids are added to minimize inflammation. If there is access to the anterior hyaloid face, it can be ruptured with the Nd:YAG laser to resolve the misdirection. A capsulotomy often is required in pseudophakes. If no access to the hyaloid face is available, a pars plana anterior vitrectomy is required. Infusion through a corneal paracentesis with pars plana vitrectomy facilitates removal of the anterior vitreous and hyaloid face.

Other Pupillary Block Glaucomas

Conditions than may lead to secondary pupillary block include subluxed or dislocated crystalline lens (Fig. 3.38), iris contact with the anterior vitreous face, a secluded pupil with 360 degrees of posterior synechiae from inflammation (Fig. 3.39, 3.40), and an anterior chamber intraocular lens if there is no patent peripheral iridectomy (Fig. 3.41). There is often a prominent iris bombé, with a billowing of the iris,

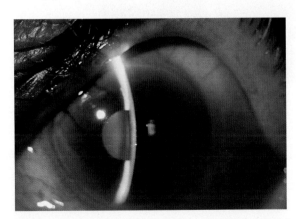

FIGURE 3.37. This posttrabeculectomy patient shows the characteristic features of aqueous misdirection syndrome: low bleb because little aqueous is entering the anterior chamber, shallow to flat central anterior chamber, no choroidal detachments, and elevated intraocular pressure.

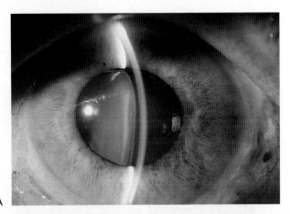

A

FIGURE 3.38. A: Patient with a traumatic subluxation of the crystalline lens that was displaced forward at the superior pole. The zonules were disrupted superiorly, with vitreous presenting through the pupil. *(continued)*

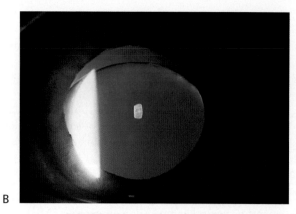
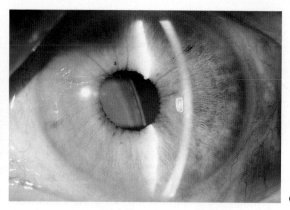

B

C

FIGURE 3.38. *Continued.* **B:** With retroillumination, the lens can be seen below the superior edge of the pupil. The pupil could not be constricted, and the intraocular pressure was markedly elevated. **C:** After laser iridectomy, the anterior chamber deepened, and the pupil constricted promptly with miotics.

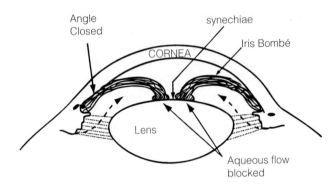

FIGURE 3.39. Posterior synechiae may form between the iris and lens in patients with chronic anterior uveitis, preventing the flow of aqueous into the anterior chamber. An iris bombé is created, closing the angle and increasing the intraocular pressure.

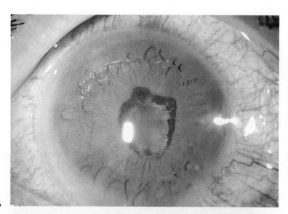
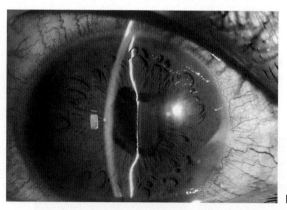

A

B

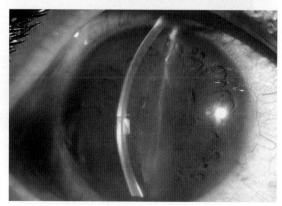

C

FIGURE 3.40. A: Patient with sarcoid uveitis, with 360 degrees of posterior synechiae leading to a secluded pupil. **B:** A patient with chronic uveitis developed posterior synechiae through 360 degrees of the pupil margin. **C:** An iris bombé developed that closed the angle and resulted in an increase in the intraocular pressure.

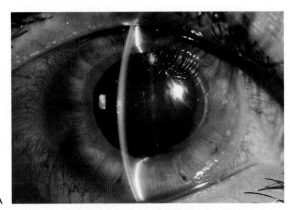
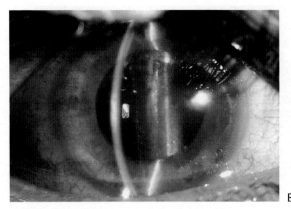

A

B

FIGURE 3.41. A: A pseudophakic patient with a posterior chamber intraocular lens developed a marked iris bombé. An imperforate peripheral iridectomy is evident inferiorly. **B:** A laser iridectomy was performed in several locations, including the imperforate area, and the anterior chamber deepened dramatically. The iris bombé disappeared, and the intraocular pressure was reduced.

especially at the periphery, and coming into direct apposition with the cornea (Fig. 3.40).

Management. Medical treatment is undertaken only as a temporizing measure. By vigorous dilation and the use of aqueous suppressants, the pupillary block may be broken and the IOP lowered. The most effective treatment is an Nd:YAG laser iridectomy or, if not possible, surgical peripheral iridectomy or trabeculectomy.

Tumor-Related Glaucoma

Unilateral secondary glaucoma may result from the presence of a primary or metastatic ocular tumor (Figs. 3.42, 3.43). Several mechanisms may be involved. A ciliary body mass may result in forward displacement of the lens-iris diaphragm or a chronic angle-closure type related to neovascularization and synechial closure of the angle. An iris or ciliary body melanoma may directly infiltrate the trabecular meshwork or liberate cells into the anterior chamber that impair the outflow facility of the trabecular meshwork in an

otherwise open angle (Fig. 3.44). Gonioscopy is essential to establish the mechanism of elevated IOP.

Management. Initial management is medical, with aqueous suppressants. If medical treatment is unable to control the IOP, cyclodestructive procedures or enucleation should be considered. Filtration surgery is usually not recommended because it might facilitate the spread of tumor cells outside the eye.

Open-Angle Glaucomas

The open-angle glaucomas are a heterogeneous group of glaucomas sharing in common the presence of an open anterior chamber angle and pressure-related damage, or the potential for such, to the optic nerve.

Primary Open-Angle Glaucomas

POAG is a condition in which the nerve becomes damaged in association with relatively elevated IOP, but there are no

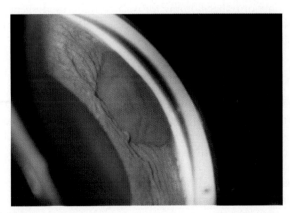

FIGURE 3.42. Melanotic lesion of the iris extending into the angle as seen on gonioscopy.

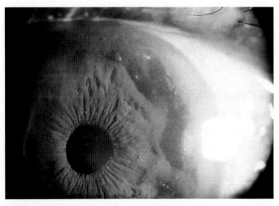

FIGURE 3.43. Diffuse metastatic lesions of the iris resulting in angle closure.

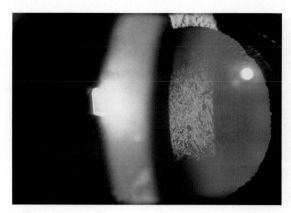

FIGURE 3.44. Deposition of pigmented tumor cells on the anterior lens capsule.

other evident abnormalities on ophthalmic examination. This glaucoma is the most common glaucoma in the United States, affecting over half of all patients with glaucoma. There are probably many entities that lead to POAG, but they are indistinguishable on clinical examination. Current research on the genetic basis of glaucoma holds the promise to identify the underlying pathophysiology of POAG, and reveal the underlying subtypes.

Low-pressure glaucoma, or normal-tension glaucoma, is essentially POAG without elevated IOP. Some clinicians object to the term normal-tension glaucoma because of the arbitrary and judgmental nature of the term "normal," as well as the unnecessarily confusing term "tension" for patients. Others clinicians object to the term "low-pressure" glaucoma, as the pressure is not lower than that found in the general population. Historically, this entity was thought not to exist, and then later a pressure of 22 mm Hg was chosen to distinguish this from POAG. This distinction is now recognized to be completely arbitrary, and most clinicians view primary and low-tension glaucoma as part of an overlapping spectrum of optic nerve damage associated with greater or lesser degrees of pressure-dependent mechanisms of damage, as opposed to other proposed mechanisms, such as vascular, excitotoxic, and growth factor deficiency–related. Certain clinical features are more common at the extremes. For example, reports have linked a greater incidence of paracentral field defects, disc hemorrhages, and vasospastic phenomena to low-pressure glaucoma than to POAG.

Both POAG and low-pressure glaucoma are diagnoses of exclusion. All secondary causes of glaucoma must be excluded before those diagnoses can be made. This requires a thorough ophthalmic examination, including a detailed history, slit lamp examination, gonioscopy, and funduscopic examination. Rarely, additional testing, such as neurologic imaging studies, is required. For low-pressure glaucoma, the history is especially important with regard to possible prior elevated IOP now resolved (e.g., due to oral steroid use in the past), episodes of ischemia (e.g., shock-related optic neuropathy), related vasospastic phenomena (e.g., migraines,

Raynaud's phenomenon), or other neurologic signs and symptoms (e.g., headaches related to an intracranial mass).

POAG and low-pressure glaucoma are treated by reduction of IOP. The Normal Tension Glaucoma Study demonstrated that a 30% reduction from maximal IOP effectively reduces the rate of glaucomatous progression. Some clinicians favor nonvasoactive agents in the medical treatment of low-pressure glaucoma, because of concern regarding already compromised optic nerve blood flow, but increased efficacy of these agents has not been demonstrated. Calcium channel blockers are also employed by some clinicians, but conflicting reports regarding their efficacy have prevented the widespread acceptance of their use in glaucoma.

Developmental Glaucomas

Infantile glaucomas are relatively uncommon, affecting approximately 1 in 10,000 live births. The classic triad of signs is epiphora, photophobia, and blepharospasm. Additional important signs are enlargement of the globe and corneal clouding. Isolated congenital glaucoma is generally sporadic, is bilateral in 75% of the cases, and affects males slightly more than females. Typically, the iris inserts anteriorly and flatly at the trabecular meshwork.

Other conditions presenting with infantile glaucoma include aniridia, Sturge-Weber syndrome, neurofibromatosis, homocystinuria, Lowe syndrome, rubella, retinoblastoma, juvenile xanthogranuloma, Axenfeld's syndrome, Rieger's syndrome, Peters' syndrome, microcornea, microspherophakia, and persistent hyperplastic primary vitreous, among others.

An examination under anesthesia is usually necessary to allow detailed, accurate measurements including IOP (measured immediately after induction of anesthesia, given the pressure-lowering effects of most general anesthetics), corneal diameter, retinoscopy, axial length, and detailed anterior and posterior segment evaluation for associated anomalies, as allowed by the clarity of the media. For the most part, the developmental glaucomas are treated surgically, given the limited success and high potential for side effects of current medications. Most clinicians begin with goniotomy or trabeculotomy for isolated trabeculodysgenesis, which often responds well. It is crucial that refractive and amblyopic issues are addressed promptly.

Secondary Open-Angle Glaucomas

The secondary open-angle glaucomas involve elevated IOPs that are related to pathologic changes. These may be broken down into pretrabecular, trabecular, and posttrabecular mechanisms of outflow obstruction.

Pretrabecular Outflow Obstruction in Secondary Open-Angle Glaucomas

The pretrabecular secondary open-angle glaucomas include neovascular, ICE, epithelial downgrowth, fibrous ingrowth,

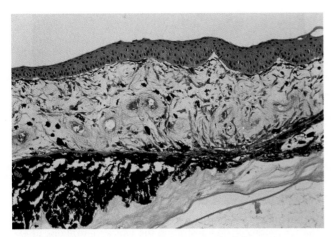

FIGURE 3.45. Epithelial ingrowth. An epithelial membrane covers the anterior iris and the anterior chamber angle recess. (Courtesy of Ralph C. Eagle, Jr., M.D.)

and angle recession glaucomas. The first four of these glaucomas may also produce angle-closure glaucoma with proliferation and contraction of the pretrabecular membranes. Neovascular and ICE syndrome–related glaucomas are discussed later in this chapter.

Epithelial Downgrowth and Stromal Ingrowth.
Perforating injuries create a pathway for epithelial and fibrous connective tissue to grow into the eye. Membranes, often with scalloped edges, may proliferate across anterior chamber structures, including the iris and corneal endothelium (Fig. 3.45). These membranes cover the trabecular meshwork and lead to reduced outflow. The membranes may be identified by argon laser treatment over affected portions of the iris. The laser will create white, rather than brown, spots.

Treatment of these conditions is extremely difficult. Filtering surgeries often fail quickly, even with antimetabo-

lite use, as the internally proliferating membranes close the sclerostomy. Tube shunts have been advocated, but may also fail. Cryotherapy to the cornea and iris has been advocated to destroy the advancing membranes, but may lead to damage to other ocular structures. In selected cases, meticulous surgical removal of the involved areas of iris with membrane peeling from the cornea may be successful.

Angle Recession

Angle recession glaucoma is an important late complication of ocular trauma (Figs. 3.46, 3.47A,B). Angle recession, with or without elevated pressure, is seen in the majority of patients in whom trauma has caused a hyphema. IOPs may remain normal for years to decades before becoming severely elevated. Patients must be strongly advised of the need for lifelong, regular follow-up after significant ocular

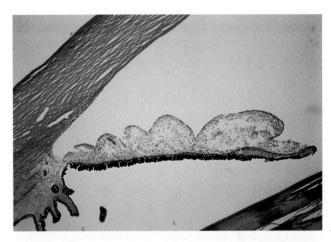

A

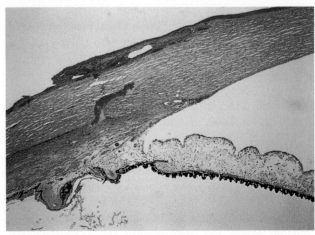

B

FIGURE 3.47. Traumatic angle recession. **A:** Normal anterior chamber angle. A line parallel to the visual axis through the trabecular meshwork crosses the tip of the first ciliary process. **B:** Traumatic angle recession. The iris insertion is moved posteriorly with rotation of the ciliary body. A line parallel to the visual axis through the trabecular meshwork passes internal to the retracted ciliary body processes. (Courtesy of Ralph C. Eagle, Jr., M.D.)

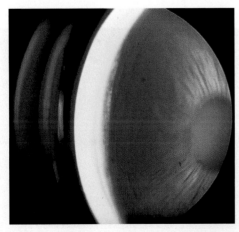

FIGURE 3.46. Traumatic angle recession. Temporally, for 2 clock hours, a widened band of the ciliary body has been exposed, in contrast to the remainder of the angle, where only the anterior portion of the ciliary body is visible.

trauma. Elevated IOP is more likely to occur in eyes with 180 degrees or more of angle recession, and may affect 6% to 20% of eyes with angle recession over a 10-year period. Angle recession must be considered in chronic unilateral glaucomas. Since patients often do not recall the long-past trauma, clinicians must search for clues to the prior trauma, such as facial and corneal scars, pupillary sphincter tears, iris transillumination, iridodonesis, phacodonesis, Vossius' ring, dark brown or black deposits in the inferior angle recess, and localized anterior synechiae as a sign of prior intraocular inflammation, especially at the 6-o'clock position. With time, angle recession may scar, becoming less evident by gonioscopy in apparent severity and extent. The affected areas still have nonfunctioning meshwork, secondary to scarring or their closure by a Descemet's-like membrane. Interestingly, it has been noted that the fellow eye is at significantly increased risk of developing open-angle glaucoma.

Angle recession glaucoma may respond to aqueous suppressants. Miotics and argon laser trabeculoplasty are rarely effective. Long-term success rates for trabeculectomy are worse than for POAG; some surgeons use antimetabolites on primary procedures for this reason.

Glaucoma Associated With the Exfoliation Syndrome

Exfoliative glaucoma was previously called pseudoexfoliative glaucoma to differentiate the syndrome from the splitting off of a layer of the anterior lens capsule exposed to intense heat as seen with glass blowers and blast furnace workers. However, studies have shown the unknown substance found on the lens, zonules, and other intraocular tissues is exfoliated. It is thought to be related to elastic fibers and basement membrane components. Also discovered was the fact that exfoliation in the eye is a local manifestation of a systemic disorder. Transmission electron microscopy has revealed exfoliative fibrils in the connective tissue components of skin, heart, lungs, liver, kidney, and cerebral meninges, suggesting an aberrant connective-tissue metabolism throughout the body. These systemic changes have not been shown to cause an increase in cardiovascular or cerebrovascular mortality.

While exfoliative glaucoma occurs worldwide, its prevalence varies from region to region. Scandinavians and South African blacks are disparate populations who are especially at risk. There is a clear association with age, but males and females are affected equally. An increased prevalence of occludable angles and angle-closure glaucoma has been demonstrated.

The classic appearance of exfoliation is a whitish, dandruff-like material coating the anterior surface of the crystalline lens. The excursions of the pupil over the lens surface have worn off the exfoliative material in a band around a central untouched disc, also leaving the more peripheral material

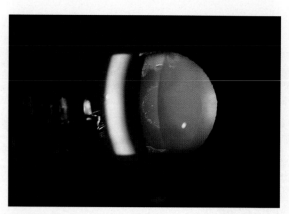

FIGURE 3.48. The anterior lens capsule of a patient with the exfoliation syndrome demonstrating the typical central disc of exfoliative material, clear capsule under the edge of the pupil, and peripheral exfoliative material.

untouched (Fig. 3.48). Constant movement over a rough surface leaves the underside of the pupillary margin worn away in a "saw tooth" pattern, with transillumination of the peripupillary iris and an impaired blood-aqueous barrier. Black pigment exfoliated from the neuroepithelium of the uveal tract and later pigment chafed off the posterior pigment epithelium of the iris is deposited on the anterior iris surface and in the inferior angle. Unlike pigmentary dispersion syndrome, where the pigment is evenly distributed for 360 degrees around the angle, in the exfoliation syndrome the pigment is mostly deposited inferiorly. Gonioscopy in exfoliation patients reveals three distinct lines: pigment in the trabecular meshwork, pigment layered out on Schwalbe's line, and pigment deposited in a serpentine line well anterior to Schwalbe's line (Fig. 3.49). The latter is called Sampaolesi's line and can be especially important when making the diagnosis of exfoliative glaucoma in the presence of a small pupil that cannot be dilated. Other clues are exfoliative material on the pupillary margin, anterior iris surface, corneal

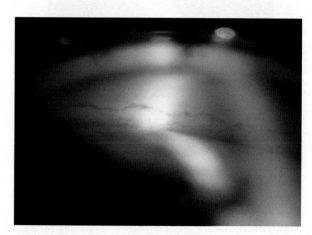

FIGURE 3.49. Inferior angle showing three distinct pigment lines: in trabecular meshwork, on Schwalbe's line, and a serpentine line well anterior to Schwalbe's line.

TABLE 3-6. EXFOLIATION SYNDROME CHARACTERISTICS

Average age, 70 years
Males and females affected equally
Unilateral signals seen in 50% of patients
Glaucoma affects 67% of patients
Cataract affects 75% of patients
Narrow angle found in 20% of patients
Pigmentation of trabecular meshwork tends to be black
Deposits on lens seen in most patients
Central ring seen in most patients
Peripheral ring seen in all patients
Unstable intraocular pressure is usual
Sampaolesi's line seen in many patients

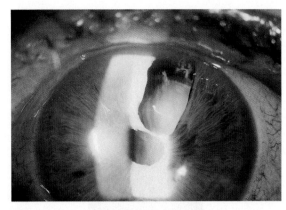

FIGURE 3.50. This peripheral iridectomy allows a look at how exfoliative material forming under the zonular attachment to the lens allows the zonules to pull free of the lens, causing marked phakodonesis in this patient.

endothelium, and anterior vitreous face. When discovered, the exfoliation syndrome is usually unilateral or asymmetric (Table 3.6). Even in fellow eyes with no visible exfoliation, exfoliation material can be detected ultrastructurally and immunohistochemically around iris blood vessels.

Early recognition of the patient with exfoliation syndrome is important in order to foster close follow-up and allow early detection and treatment of glaucoma. At the time of diagnosis, IOP and its diurnal variation are usually higher and the visual field defects greater in exfoliative glaucoma compared to POAG. Exfoliative glaucoma has also been shown to have a poorer prognosis than POAG. Because lowering IOP has been shown to improve visual field prognosis more in exfoliative glaucoma than in POAG, glaucoma progression is felt to be more pressure related in exfoliative glaucoma.

Recognition of the exfoliation syndrome is also crucial in the patient seeking cataract extraction. Because zonules attach to the surface of the lens capsule, exfoliation material forming under the insertion of the zonules into the lens capsule undermines the strength of the zonules and can result

in phakodonesis, lens subluxation, and vitreous loss at the time of surgery (Fig. 3.50).

Management. Treatment of exfoliative glaucoma varies little from that of POAG, with the following exceptions. Of all the sundry glaucomas, argon laser trabeculoplasty works best in exfoliative glaucoma, enhancing its position in the therapeutic armamentarium. Trabecular aspiration, a surgical procedure in which exfoliative material, pigment, and debris are vacuumed from the trabecular meshwork, has been used in Germany with lesser effectiveness in controlling IOP but greater safety than trabeculectomy.

Pigment Dispersion Syndrome and Pigmentary Glaucoma

The pigment dispersion syndrome is characterized by deposition of pigment in the posterior trabecular meshwork (Fig. 3.51A,B), on the endothelial surface of the cornea (Krukenberg's spindle), and on the equatorial surface of the

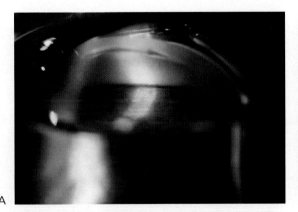
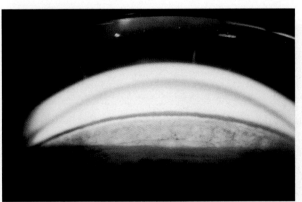

A   B

FIGURE 3.51. A, B: Dense, even pigmentation of the trabecular meshwork over 360 degrees is also a requisite for the diagnosis of pigmentary glaucoma and differentiates this disorder from most of the diseases in the differential diagnosis. The peripheral iris often slopes posteriorly from its insertion, draping over the zonules and, more centrally, over the lens.

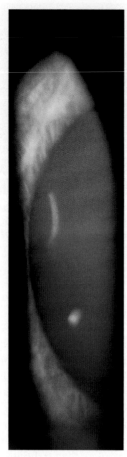

FIGURE 3.52. Pigmentary deposition on the equatorial surface of the lens (Zentmeyer line).

lens (Zentmeyer line) (Fig. 3.52). There is also a characteristic spoke-like loss of pigment from the posterior pigment epithelium in the mid to far periphery of the iris (Fig. 3.53). It is the pigment from the iris that causes the deposits of pigment on the central corneal endothelium in the posterior trabecular meshwork (Fig. 3.51) and on the lens. The anterior surface of the iris may also be involved.

If the pigment deposition and secondary changes to the outflow pathways are sufficient to cause relative blockage of aqueous outflow, the IOP may increase and play a role in the development of optic nerve damage. The combination of the pigment dispersion syndrome with glaucoma is called "pigmentary glaucoma." This type of glaucoma occurs most commonly in myopic individuals between the ages of 20 and 45 years and affects men approximately twice as often as women.

Not all the findings described for the pigment dispersion syndrome are present in every individual. In fact, it is not unusual for some of the findings to be absent. Iris transillumination defects are rarely seen in patients with dark brown irides. In addition, an extraordinarily important aspect of the pigment dispersion syndrome is lattice degeneration of the retina. Patients with the pigment dispersion syndrome are predisposed to retinal detachment, not simply because they are myopic, but also, apparently, as a result of the pigment degeneration itself.

The cause of the pigment dispersion is partly related to "reverse pupillary block." This reverse pupillary block is a phenomenon in which aqueous is pumped anteriorly from the posterior chamber into the anterior chamber, with accommodation or blinking, and the aqueous in the anterior chamber then forces the peripheral, unsupported portion of the iris posteriorly back towards the zonules. The posterior pigment epithelium can then rub against the zonules, which predisposes the pigment epithelium to be released. This "reverse pupillary block" is illustrated in Figure 3.54. If blinking is prevented, the anterior chamber configuration can spontaneously return to normal (Fig. 3.55). This posterior bowing of the iris is called a q iris configuration. The pigment that is lost from the posterior pigment epithelium floats to the trabecular meshwork, where it is phagocytized by the endothelial cells lining the trabecular beams. If overloaded, these cells die, leaving denuded trabecular beams that can no longer rid themselves of further deposition of pigment, glycosaminoglycans, and other debris. Consequently, there is an elevation of IOP.

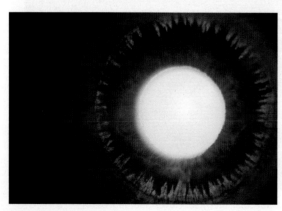

FIGURE 3.53. Midperipheral iris transillumination defects are pathognomonic of pigmentary glaucoma and reveal the source of the malady.

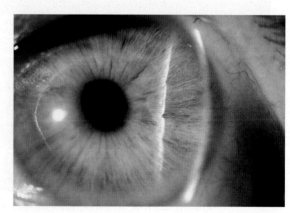

FIGURE 3.54. Reverse pupillary block. The iris is pushed back against the lens and zonules during normal blinking in this eye with loose zonules.

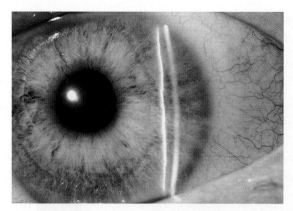

FIGURE 3.55. The same eye as in Figure 3.54 after 1 minute without blinking.

Pigmentary glaucoma may be especially serious in some individuals, at least partially because of the tendency of myopes to develop optic nerve damage more easily than emmetropes or hyperopes.

Some authors comment on the tendency of the pigment dispersion syndrome and pigmentary glaucoma to become less severe with increasing age. They point out that as the individual ages the pupil becomes smaller and the lens enlarges, as a result of which there is an increase in the degree of relative pupillary block. This results in elimination of the q configuration and development of an actual anterior convexity, decreasing the contact between the posterior pigment epithelium and the zonules, and therefore decreasing the amount of pigment release. While this phenomenon is probably real, it is probably also of little clinical significance. It is unwise to think that a patient who has pigmentary glaucoma will have a disappearance of the glaucoma with increasing age.

The differential diagnosis of pigmentary glaucoma is shown in Table 3.7.

Management. Two methods have been recommended by some authors to stop or lessen the pigment dispersion syndrome in patients with pigmentary glaucoma who have elevated IOP characterized by posterior bowing of the peripheral iris. Miotics can cause increased lens-iris apposition and therefore increase the amount of relative anterior pupillary

TABLE 3-7. DIFFERENTIAL DIAGNOSIS OF PIGMENTARY GLAUCOMA

1. Exfoliation (exfoliative material on lens, pigment heavier inferiorly, patients older, no Zentmeyer line)
2. Trauma, including surgery (signs of injury)
3. Uveitis (anterior chamber reaction, posterior or peripheral anterior synechiae)
4. Melanoma (pigment thicker and less homogeneous, iris or choroidal lesions)
5. Megalocornea
6. Irradiation trauma
7. Siderosis bulbi

block. This can, as mentioned above, decrease the contact between the posterior pigment epithelium and the zonules, decreasing the amount of pigment release. However, miotics also predispose to retinal detachment, a condition to which patients with pigment dispersion syndrome and pigmentary glaucoma are strongly predisposed. Consequently, if miotics are to be considered, they should only be used after a meticulous examination of the peripheral retina. Additionally, because miotics cause a marked myopic shift in individuals below the age of 40, they are usually not well tolerated. Administering pilocarpine through a sustained-release system such as the pilocarpine "Ocusert" has the advantage that the constant release of a small amount of pilocarpine causes less accommodative spasm, allows for a constant refraction, and therefore may allow the pilocarpine to be tolerated, even by younger individuals. However, the pilocarpine "Ocusert" can sometimes malfunction, allowing a sudden release of pilocarpine, predisposing the patient to retinal detachment. Additionally, the long-term use of miotics results in small, rigid pupils in a condition that makes the use of miotics undesirable in most patients. A different method of reducing the pigment release has been suggested by authors who recommend peripheral iridotomy. The peripheral iridotomy can decrease the "reverse pupillary block." However, the long-term benefit of peripheral iridotomy has not been demonstrated. Additionally, patients who develop marked pigment release with exercise do not appear to be significantly helped with peripheral iridotomy. The benefit, then, is not proven, but there is a risk, specifically, a pressure elevation that may push the marginally compensated individual into a need for a glaucoma filtering procedure.

Argon laser trabeculoplasty is usually highly effective in patients with the pigment dispersion syndrome, even relatively young individuals. The amount of energy needs to be reduced, in view of the intense pigmentation of the posterior trabecular meshwork, and powers of 400 mW or sometimes even less are usually adequate.

Aphakic and Pseudophakic Glaucomas

Increased IOP is a potential complication of cataract extraction. Many etiologies lead to postoperative pressure elevations and are best considered by time of onset.

Within the first week, many of the materials dispersed during surgery can lead to elevated pressures. α-Chymotrypsin frequently resulted in pressure spikes in the first 2 days following intracapsular cataract extraction. Retained viscoelastic material is a source of trabecular obstruction manifesting in the first postoperative day. Increased IOPs are seen with all current viscoelastics; no definitive difference in incidence has been shown among them. Meticulous removal at time of surgery may reduce the frequency of this complication. Hyphema following surgery also blocks outflow and can lead to elevated IOP. Debris, inflammation, and trabecular edema may also play roles in acutely

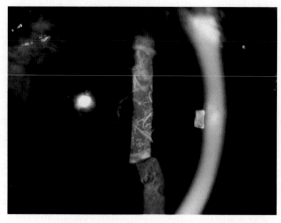
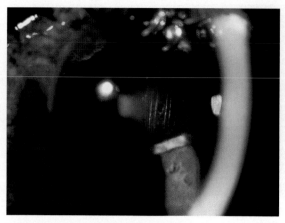

FIGURE 3.56. Fibrin clot over posterior chamber intraocular lens with elevated intraocular pressure (IOP) following combined guarded filtration procedure and cataract extraction **(A)**. Same eye **(B)** following intracameral injection of tissue plasminogen activator. Visual acuity improved dramatically and IOP dropped from 38 to 10 mm Hg, and remained well controlled.

elevated pressures postoperatively. Preexisting glaucoma increases the frequency and severity of acute postoperative pressure elevations. These complications are best treated medically with aqueous suppressants and topical steroids.

Fibrin clots may be treated with intracameral injection of tissue plasminogen activator (Fig. 3.56A, B). Surgical evacuation of viscoelastic or blood is reserved for pressures that do not respond to medical therapy and threaten the optic nerve.

After the first week, other factors may lead to glaucoma. Vitreous in the anterior chamber may reduce aqueous outflow. Hyphema related to wound construction or intraocular lens position may occur. Ghost cell glaucoma results from longstanding hyphema or vitreous hemorrhage leading to degenerated erythrocytes that are less flexible and block trabecular channels. Retained lens particles become hydrated and more prominent, blocking the trabecular meshwork. Postoperative inflammation related to retained lens particles,

intraocular lens position, vitreous traction, and surgical trauma may become more evident. Corticosteroid induced glaucoma must be considered as a common source of increased IOP in postoperative patients on topical steroids. Discontinuation of steroids or a therapeutic challenge of the fellow eye with topical steroids often will aid in the diagnosis.

Late pressure elevations, occurring months to years following surgery, may also be secondary to inflammation and hemorrhage. *Propionibacterium acnes* endophthalmitis may lead to chronic inflammation with increased pressures. Intraocular lenses may be a source of inflammation and hyphema in the UGH (uveitis, glaucoma, hyphema) syndrome (Figs. 3.57A,B; 3.58A,B). Anterior chamber lenses may directly damage the trabecular meshwork. Vitreous in the anterior chamber may still block outflow. Following YAG laser capsulotomy, inflammation may lead to quite significant pressure elevations whose frequency is greatly reduced by pretreatment with apraclonidine.

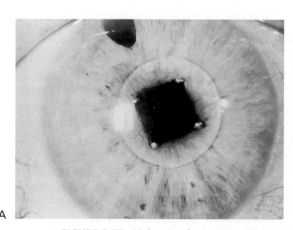
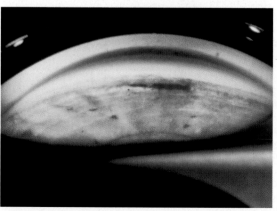

FIGURE 3.57. Right eye of a patient with intraocular lenses and the uveitis, glaucoma, hyphema syndrome in both eyes. This patient had multiple hyphemas over a period of years. In some instances, the inflammation was readily apparent, but the hyphema was only appreciated on gonioscopy. **A:** Iris-supported intraocular lens. **B:** Gonioscopy reveals small hyphema.

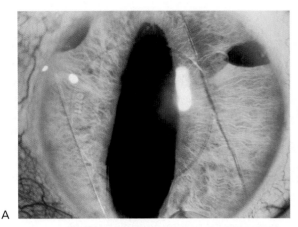
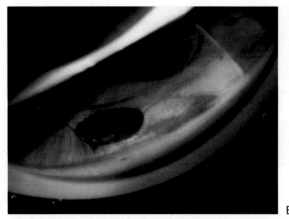

A   B

FIGURE 3.58. Left eye of the same patient seen in Figure 3.57. **A:** Solid one-piece anterior chamber intraocular lens. **B:** Gonioscopy shows haptic through iridectomy abutting ciliary body.

Angle-closure glaucoma may be seen throughout the postoperative course, related to inflammation, pupil block, or shallow chambers. Malignant glaucoma is a relatively uncommon but important cause of postoperative glaucoma. Epithelial downgrowth is another rare cause of late postoperative glaucoma that represents a severe threat to the eye.

Cyclodialysis Cleft Closure

Traumatic cyclodialysis clefts divert aqueous away from the trabecular meshwork, and may lead to hypotony (Fig. 3.59). These clefts may be caused by trauma or may occur during intraocular surgery, such as cataract extraction. The unused trabecular meshwork becomes less permeable to aqueous. Months or years later, spontaneous closure of the cyclodialysis cleft may lead to dramatic elevations of IOP. Patients present with sudden onset of ocular pain, headaches, and reduced vision. Slit lamp and gonioscopic evaluation differentiates this entity from the similar presentation of acute an-

gle-closure glaucoma. Aqueous suppressants are often effective in reducing IOP chronically, or until the trabecular meshwork recovers and better outflow facility resumes. Miotics are avoided as they may reopen cyclodialysis clefts. An exception to this is the sudden closure of a longstanding cleft with prior good IOP control. In this situation, immediate use of a strong miotic, such as pilocarpine 4%, may open and reestablish the cleft. Occasionally, filtering surgery may be necessary in cases of persistently elevated pressures.

Corticosteroid-Induced Glaucoma

The use of corticosteroids in any form may lead to the development of a secondary open-angle glaucoma. Increased IOP has been demonstrated with topical, periocular, inhalational, and systemic steroids, as well as with increased endogenous steroids in adrenal hyperplasia and Cushing's syndrome (Figs. 3.60, 3.61). Past steroid use and glaucoma may simulate the presentation of normal-tension glaucoma.

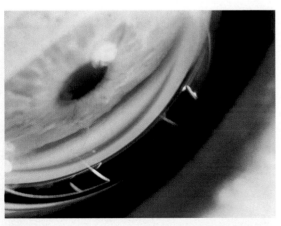

FIGURE 3.59. Two small areas of cyclodialysis just able to be visualized in hypotonus eye. Intracameral injection of viscoelastic may aid in the gonioscopic examination.

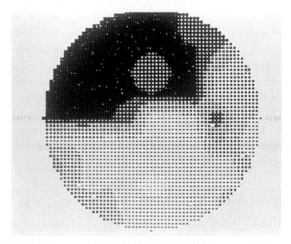

FIGURE 3.60. Advanced visual field loss in a doctor who self-prescribed topical steroids for vernal conjunctivitis for many years without eye examinations.

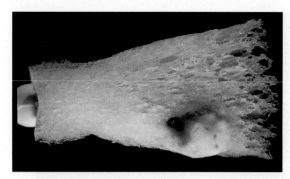

FIGURE 3.61. For 5 months following vitrectomy, intraocular pressures were elevated to as high as 44 mm Hg, despite medications in a patient without previous glaucoma. The subconjunctival steroid depot, shown here, was excised and the glaucoma resolved completely in 1 month.

Topical steroids are more likely to elevate IOP than systemic steroids. IOPs rise more frequently and more severely with the more potent steroids and with greater dosing. Pressure elevation typically manifests 2 to 6 weeks after the initiation of steroids. Patients with POAG respond much more frequently and severely to steroids with elevated IOP. Depending on steroid dose, duration, and diagnostic criteria, over 90% of patients with POAG may have pressure elevations with steroids compared to 5% to 10% of normals. Other risk factors for steroid responsiveness include ocular hypertension, angle recession glaucoma (in either eye), primary relative of patient with POAG, pigmentary glaucoma, myopia, diabetes, and history of connective tissue disease, but not exfoliative glaucoma.

Corticosteroids result in the accumulation of glycosaminoglycans in the trabecular meshwork, reducing outflow facility. Theories for the mechanism of this accumulation of glycosaminoglycans include increased production and reduced clearance, mediated either by nuclear steroid receptors or by membrane stabilization.

The diagnosis may be made either by withdrawing steroid therapy and observing reduced pressures or by challenging the fellow eye in topical steroid cases. IOPs usually may begin to drop in days and return to baseline within 1 to 2 months, but sometimes remain high in patients who have been on steroids for long periods of time. Elevated pressures following periocular injection of steroids may require the excision of depot steroids. Aqueous suppressants and miotics can be effective in treating the elevated pressure. Argon laser trabeculoplasty may be useful, although less effective than in POAG, pigmentary glaucoma, and exfoliative glaucoma.

Posttraumatic Glaucomas

Nonpenetrating injuries of the eye secondary to blunt trauma are usually related to the anterior-to-posterior compression of the eye with secondary equatorial stretching. This stretching may result in pupil sphincter tears, irido-

dialysis, angle recession, cyclodialysis, trabecular dialysis, disruption of the lens zonule, and retinal dialysis or detachment.

Tears in the face of the ciliary body, usually between the circular and longitudinal muscles, may disrupt the major arterial circle of the iris and the arterial and venous connections of the ciliary body, resulting in hyphema. Severity may range from a microhyphema, in which the slit-lamp microscope is necessary to appreciate the presence of blood in the anterior chamber, to total hyphema, in which the anterior and posterior chambers are entirely filled with blood (Figs. 3.62; 3.63A,B).

IOP may be elevated or reduced, depending on the balance of several factors. Aqueous secretion may be acutely reduced; uveoscleral outflow may be increased by an accompanying cyclodialysis; blood may obstruct an injured and inflamed trabecular meshwork. Although red blood cells normally pass through the pores in the meshwork, acute inflammation and swelling of the meshwork combined with excessive amounts of red blood cells and debris may overwhelm the meshwork's capacity. Aqueous suppressants are effective in many cases. Steroids help to reduce inflammation. Miotics are generally avoided as they may predispose to posterior synechiae, further compromise the blood aqueous barrier, and reduce uveoscleral outflow. Patients with hyphema are generally kept at bedrest and treated with mydriatics and topical steroids. Aminocaproic acid, an antifibrinolytic agent, is also used in some centers to reduce the incidents of rebleeds, which may be severe.

Prolonged elevation of IOP may require surgical evacuation of the blood. Timing is dependent on the ability of the nerve to withstand elevated pressures; otherwise, healthy nerves may tolerate pressures of up to 50 mm Hg for several days. Evacuation may also be necessary because of the development of blood staining, especially in those at risk for amblyopia (Fig. 3.64). Surgical evacuation is ideally performed near the fourth day posttrauma. This is past the peak incidence of rebleeding and allows time for the anterior

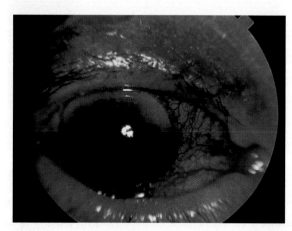

FIGURE 3.62. Traumatic hyphema. Two fluid levels exist as the red blood cells settle and clot.

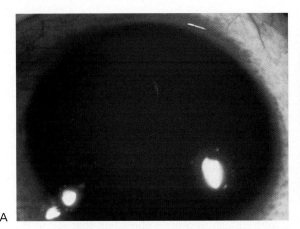
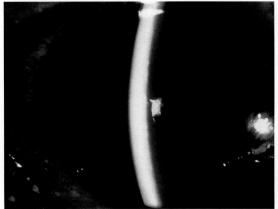

A   B

FIGURE 3.63. Total hyphema **(A)**. The incidence of elevated intraocular pressure increases with the amount of blood in the anterior chamber. More than half of those with total hyphemas have significant pressure elevations; with "blackball" or "eight-ball" hyphemas **(B)** this approaches 100%. Patients with sickle cell disease may suffer severe pressure elevations with relatively minor hyphemas.

chamber blood to clot and retract somewhat from ocular structures, facilitating removal.

Patients with sickle cell disease are at greater risk for complications from hyphemas. Significant IOP elevations may occur with even small hyphemas. Sickling has been demonstrated in the anterior chamber blood; this may reduce clearance and increase IOP. Central retinal arterial obstruction may occur at lower pressures following hyphemas in these patients. Carbonic anhydrase inhibitors are avoided in sickle cell disease as they may worsen sickling and reduce clearance of blood by increasing aqueous ascorbic acid and by promoting systemic acidosis. Black patients with hyphemas should be screened for sickle cell hemoglobin; positive patients should undergo hemoglobin electrophoresis. All available therapies should be used to keep IOPs below 25 mm Hg.

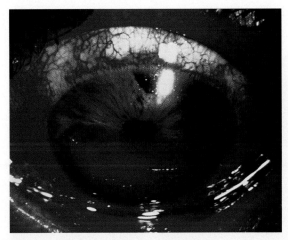

FIGURE 3.64. Corneal blood staining following a traumatic hyphema. These generally clear over weeks to months, starting at the periphery, following hyphema resolution. In patients in the amblyopic age group, incipient blood staining may require surgical evacuation of the blood.

Trauma may also lead to angle-closure glaucoma through a variety of mechanisms. Clots may cover the pupil, leading to pupillary block and angle closure. Dislocated lenses may cause pupillary block. Posttraumatic inflammation may lead to extensive peripheral anterior and posterior synechiae. Shallow anterior chambers with penetrating trauma also may create extensive anterior synechiae.

Trauma may also lead to retinal detachments. A rare cause of open-angle glaucoma in the setting of a retinal detachment is Schwartz's syndrome.

Schwartz's Syndrome

Schwartz's syndrome is elevated IOP secondary to obstruction of the trabecular meshwork by photoreceptor outer segments. These photoreceptor outer segments are released from a chronic retinal detachment through a tear in the retina (Fig. 3.65). The retinal detachments are often low lying and peripheral and may be easily overlooked. The photoreceptor outer segments may be mistaken for white blood cells and the glaucoma erroneously diagnosed as uveitic. Pressures may fluctuate widely depending on the balance of trabecular meshwork outflow obstruction and increased outflow through the retinal detachment. The retinal pigment epithelium has a pumping function that normally evacuates subretinal fluid, keeping the retina firmly attached to the pigment epithelium. In the case of a retinal detachment, this pumping function helps to lower IOP. This can very rarely lead to the iris retraction syndrome, in which patients with Schwartz's syndrome and extensive posterior synechiae show iris retraction when placed on aqueous suppressants. The theory is that the reduced inflow from aqueous suppression, coupled with the reduced flow into the anterior chamber and increased outflow through the retinal detachment, leads to hypotony and an exceptionally deep anterior chamber.

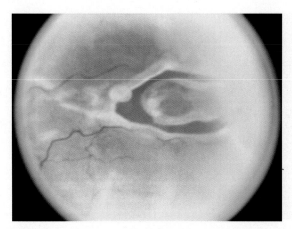

FIGURE 3.65. Peripheral horseshoe tear of the retina. Retinal tears with detachments can release photoreceptor outer segments. In Schwartz's syndrome these segments may clog the trabecular meshwork and increase intraocular pressure.

Ghost Cell Glaucoma

Ghost cells are degenerated red blood cells whose leaky membranes have allowed much of the cell's hemoglobin to escape. Residual, degenerated hemoglobin precipitates on inner cell walls in the form of Heinz bodies. These spherical cells are much less pliable than red blood cells and cannot pass through the intertrabecular spaces, leading to pressure elevations at relatively lower concentrations than expected with normal red blood cells.

The formation of ghost cells requires the sequestration of red blood cells in the vitreous for several weeks. The source of vitreous hemorrhage does not matter—a bleed from diabetic neovascularization of the retina, hemorrhage secondary to trauma, or a postsurgical hyphema with spill-over into the vitreous through a compromised vitreous face may evolve into a secondary glaucoma. After several weeks, the degenerated cells migrate back into the anterior chamber

through a defect in the vitreous face, surgical or traumatic, and obstruct the trabecular meshwork. Tan or khaki-colored cells are seen in the anterior chamber, the anterior vitreous, and the trabecular meshwork, and may also form a pseudohypopyon (Fig. 3.66A,B). If the vitreous face is intact, the ghost cells do not reach the anterior chamber and no glaucoma results.

Several other blood-related elevations of IOP may be differentiated from ghost cell glaucoma. Hyphemas may result in acutely elevated pressure, especially in patients with sickle cell disease. This is secondary to obstruction of the meshwork by red blood cells in the first days following the hyphema. Rarely, an eight-ball, total hyphema may persist long enough to contain ghost cells that add to the trabecular obstruction. Hemolytic glaucoma occurs when the contents of ruptured red blood cells are ingested by macrophages that then obstruct the meshwork. Hemolytic glaucoma is also typically seen in the first days to weeks following the initial hemorrhage. Hemosiderotic glaucoma, in which iron-containing blood breakdown products stain and poison the cells of the trabecular meshwork, occurs much later, often years after the hemorrhage.

Aqueous suppressants often control the IOP. Miotics are rarely helpful as the meshwork is obstructed; similarly, argon laser trabeculoplasty is not indicated. Anterior chamber lavage with balanced salt solution may resolve the glaucoma. If unsuccessful, or too great a reservoir of ghost cells remains in the vitreous, total vitrectomy, removing as much hemorrhagic material as possible, is usually effective in resolving the glaucoma.

Inflammatory Glaucomas

Inflammation within the eye alters aqueous humor dynamics and can lead to increased IOP. Acute inflammation may reduce aqueous secretion and increase uveoscleral outflow, reducing IOP. However, inflammatory material, consisting

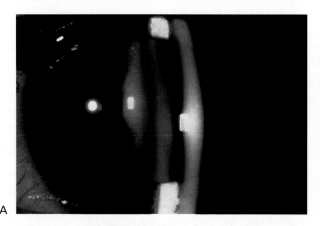

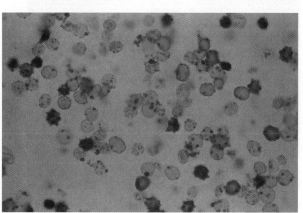

A   B

FIGURE 3.66. This patient with ghost cell glaucoma had 2+ anterior chamber khaki-colored cells and marked khaki-colored cells in the anterior vitreous **(A)**. Vitrectomy specimen showed ghost cells **(B)**.

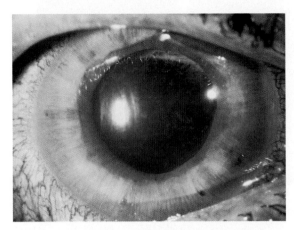

FIGURE 3.67. Idiopathic uveitis resulting in secondary glaucoma with closed- and open-angle components. Note the multiple laser peripheral iridotomies for previous acute iris bombé. Following resolution of acute attacks, patient had persistent elevation of intraocular pressure in spite of large of areas of anterior chamber angle on gonioscopy.

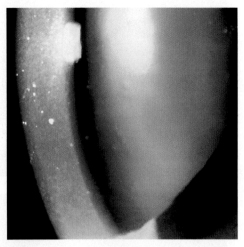

FIGURE 3.68. Glaucomatocyclitic crisis (Posner-Schlossman syndrome). Unilateral involvement consisting of fine keratic precipitates in a patient with minimal anterior chamber reaction and markedly elevated intraocular pressure (IOP). Following multiple similar attacks, patient developed chronically elevated IOP and optic nerve damage requiring trabeculectomy.

of white blood cells, macrophages, and proteins, may obstruct the trabecular meshwork. Chemical mediators of inflammation may further compromise trabecular function, as may trabeculitis, inflammation of the trabecular meshwork itself. Trabecular dysfunction may be transient, clearing with resolution of the inflammation, or may persist, with permanent structural changes reducing trabecular outflow facility.

Additionally, inflammatory scarring may lead to peripheral anterior synechiae and posterior synechiae, resulting in angle-closure glaucoma. Chronic uveitis may lead to neovascularization and neovascular glaucoma. Patients may manifest some or all of these findings, the balance dictating the nature of the glaucoma. For example, a patient may present acutely during a uveitic episode with uveitic hypotony, progress to a secondary open-angle glaucoma as white blood cells block the meshwork, develop an angle-closure component as synechiae form, and then be left with a chronic mixed mechanism secondary glaucoma with residual synechiae and scarring of the meshwork.

Virtually all sources of ocular inflammation can lead to glaucoma. Idiopathic uveitis (Fig. 3.67), glaucomatocyclitic crisis (Fig. 3.68), Fuch's heterochromic cyclitis (Fig. 3.69), lens-related uveitis (Fig. 3.70), herpes (Fig. 3.71), and sarcoidosis (Fig. 3.72) may all result in increased IOP. Other uveitic glaucomas include HLA-B27–related uveitides, pars planitis, sarcoidosis, juvenile rheumatoid arthritis, Behçet's disease, Crohn's disease, syphilis, toxoplasmosis, coccidioidomycosis, mumps, rubella, leprosy, sympathetic ophthalmia, Vogt-Koyanagi-Harada syndrome, and other less common entities.

Treatment strategies are similar for these entities. Resolution of inflammation is the first goal, which may require topical or systemic steroids, antibiotics for infectious diseases, and lens extraction in lens-related conditions.

Increased IOP secondary to steroid therapy or to increased aqueous production with resolving inflammation may confuse the clinical picture. Cycloplegics are effective through many mechanisms. Dilation prevents the formation of a small secluded pupil and relieves the discomfort of ciliary spasm. Cycloplegics also improve uveoscleral outflow and stabilize the blood-aqueous barrier. Topical and systemic aqueous suppressants are effective. Miotics are avoided as these agents further reduce the blood-aqueous barrier and reduce uveoscleral outflow. Similar concerns argue against the use of prostaglandin analogs, although limited data are available. Argon laser trabeculoplasty is generally ineffective

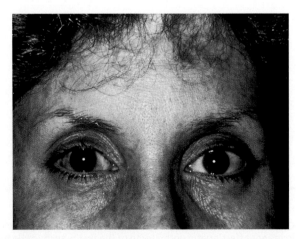

FIGURE 3.69. Fuch's heterochromic cyclitis. Note the much lighter iris color in the involved eye. The triad of heterochromia, uveitis, and cataract typically appears in the third to fourth decade. The uveitis is asymptomatic. Open-angle glaucoma is common, increasing with duration of the disease. Friable angle vessels may bleed easily with surgery; however, frank neovascularization of the iris and neovascular glaucoma are uncommon.

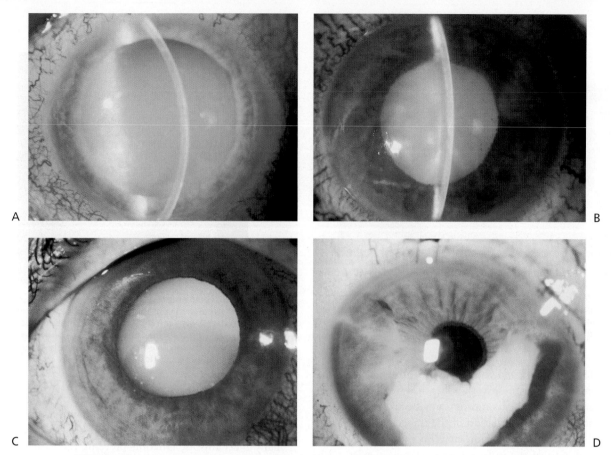

FIGURE 3.70. Lens-related glaucoma. In phacolytic glaucoma, a hypermature lens leaks proteins into the anterior chamber through a grossly intact capsule **(A)**; these proteins and ingesting macrophages block the trabecular meshwork. A swollen, mature cataract may also lead to pupillary block in phacomorphic glaucoma; note the narrow angle present in a patient with phacolytic glaucoma in **(B)**. A hypermature cataract with liquefied cortex and dense nucleus may also lead to phacolytic glaucoma **(C)**. Retained lens cortex **(D)** following cataract extraction may increase in size with hydration and lead to glaucoma through trabecular obstruction by lens material. Phacoanaphylaxis exists when lens material is present outside the capsule following surgery or trauma and leads to granulomatous inflammation. A previous history of trauma to the lens or cataract surgery in the fellow eye is typical. Phacoanaphylaxis often leads to significant pressure elevation.

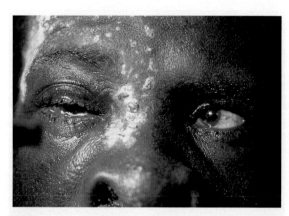

FIGURE 3.71. Herpes zoster ophthalmicus with characteristic skin lesions affecting the dermatome of the first branch of the facial nerve. The tip of the nose is involved, a harbinger of ocular involvement (Hutchinson's sign). Marked conjunctival injection and a granulomatous uveitis are present. Glaucoma is a frequent complication in herpes zoster and herpes simplex uveitis.

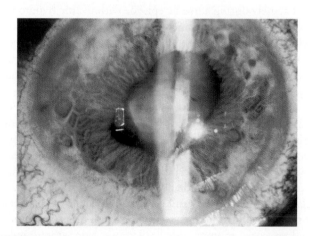

FIGURE 3.72. Sarcoid uveitis with posterior synechiae and cataract. Up to half of the patients with sarcoid suffer from uveitis at some point during the disease process. Granulomatous anterior uveitis is a common manifestation, frequently becoming bilateral, recurrent, and chronic. Sarcoid nodules on the iris (Busacca nodules in the crypts, Koeppe nodules at the pupillary margin) may be seen. Secondary open- and closed-angle glaucoma is common. As the disease is more common in blacks, clinicians must be wary of steroid-induced glaucoma as a complication of treatment.

and increases inflammation. Filtering surgery is less successful in these patients, especially during acute attacks. Adjunctive use of antimetabolites such as 5-fluorouracil (5-FU) and mitomycin-C may improve results. Drainage tube implants may also be effective. Cyclodestructive procedures can be used in refractory cases, but contribute to intraocular inflammation and pose significant risks to vision.

Glaucoma Associated With Ocular Tumors

Benign and malignant intraocular tumors may cause glaucoma by a variety of mechanisms. Direct infiltration of the trabecular meshwork can block aqueous outflow. Free-floating tumor cells may obstruct the meshwork. Hemorrhage may produce a secondary open-angle glaucoma. Tumor-related neovascularization of the iris and angle produces glaucoma in some cases. Large posterior masses sometimes may press the iris and lens anteriorly, resulting in angle closure. Tumor-related glaucomas are typically unilateral. Treatment of the glaucoma without diagnosis of the tumor may have serious consequences for the patient. A thorough examination will reveal most intraocular malignancies, especially for clinicians alert to such tip-offs as a sentinel vessel, a prominent episcleral vessel overlying a choroidal tumor.

Uveal melanomas are the most common intraocular malignancy in adults, and are the most common cause of tumor-related glaucoma. Iris melanomas may obstruct the trabecular meshwork by direct invasion or by hemorrhage (Fig. 3.73). Ciliary body melanomas may be more difficult to detect, remaining hidden until relatively large. Glaucoma most often results from the tumor pushing the iris anteriorly to close the anterior chamber angle. Glaucoma may also result due to direct extension of the tumor into the trabecular meshwork, iris neovascularization, hyphema, or tumor necrosis causing obstruction of the meshwork by cells and debris (Fig. 3.74). Choroidal melanomas less commonly cause glaucoma. Mechanisms of glaucoma in choroidal melanomas include iris and angle neovascularization most commonly, as well as angle closure, hemorrhage, and necrosis.

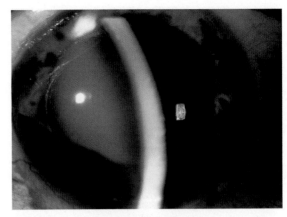

FIGURE 3.74. Hyphema causing secondary open-angle glaucoma in a patient with uveal melanoma.

Histologically benign tumors of the iris may also cause glaucoma. Diffuse uveal melanomas may block the meshwork with melanoma cells or pigment. Melanocytomas, most commonly found on the optic disc but also seen in the iris or ciliary body, can produce glaucoma. These tumors have a propensity to undergo necrosis and fragmentation, blocking the trabecular meshwork with debris, producing the so-called melanomalytic glaucoma. Differentiation of these tumors from their malignant counterparts is a crucial step in treatment, often requiring histopathologic study.

Intraocular metastases are typically to the uveal tissues. Glaucoma is found more frequently in metastases to the iris and ciliary body (64% and 67%, respectively) than in metastases to the choroid (2%). Common primary tumors include those of the breast and lung, as well as tumors of the gastrointestinal tract, kidney, thyroid, and skin. Efforts to identify the primary neoplasm are not always successful. Friable metastases often seed the anterior chamber angle, obstructing the trabecular meshwork (Figs. 3.75, 3.76). Pseudohypopyons and ring infiltrates are sometimes seen.

Benign reactive lymphoid hyperplasia can directly invade the trabecular meshwork. Large cell lymphoma (reticulum cell sarcoma, histiocytic lymphoma) and leukemia may also infiltrate the meshwork and lead to glaucoma.

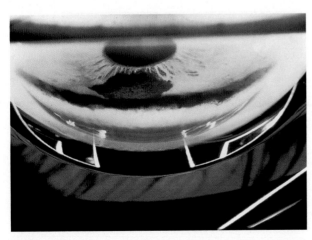

FIGURE 3.73. Iris melanoma with involvement of the trabecular meshwork.

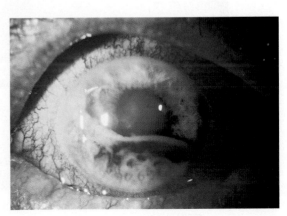

FIGURE 3.75. Metastatic tumor from primary tumor in lung to iris.

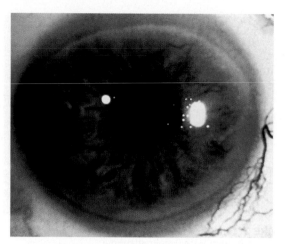

FIGURE 3.76. Multiple myeloma invading iris.

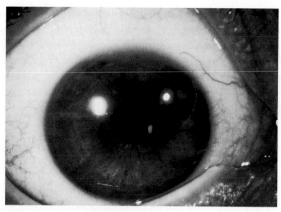

FIGURE 3.78. Neurofibromatosis type 1 with Lisch nodules, most prominently superonasal. Lisch nodules, variably pigmented collections of melanocytic spindle cells, are seen bilaterally in all patients over age 16 with neurofibromatosis type 1. Nodules are rare and unilateral in neurofibromatosis type 2.

Retinoblastoma is the most common intraocular malignancy of childhood. Glaucoma is not uncommon, occurring in 17% of cases in one study. In that study of 303 eyes, the glaucoma was thought to be secondary to iris neovascularization with or without hemorrhage in 72%, angle closure in 26%, and tumor seeding in 2% (Fig. 3.77A, B). The less common but benign medulloepithelioma may also cause glaucoma secondary to iris neovascularization, as well as direct invasion of angle structures or obstruction of the meshwork by hyphema and tumor-related debris.

Various ocular tumors are manifested by the phakomatoses. Unilateral glaucoma, congenital or later onset, may be seen in neurofibromatosis of both types (Fig 3.78). Half of all eyes with plexiform neuromas of the upper lid develop glaucoma. The glaucoma associated with encephalotrigeminal angiomatosis (Sturge-Weber syndrome) is discussed along with other causes of increased episcleral venous pressure. Congenital glaucoma may also be seen. Oculodermal melanocytosis (nevus of Ota) has been reported to have an incidence of glaucoma of 10%, including angle-closure, open-angle, and congenital varieties.

Posttrabecular Outflow Obstruction in Secondary Open-Angle Glaucomas

Increased Episcleral Venous Pressure

The Goldmann equation,

$$Po = F/C + Pev$$

where Po is IOP, F is aqueous production, C is outflow facility, and Pev is episcleral venous pressure, describes a direct relation of IOP to episcleral venous pressure. Normal episcleral venous pressure is between 9 and 10 mm Hg. Increases in episcleral venous pressure lead to increases in IOP. Experimentally, this relationship is slightly less than 1:1, possibly due to decreased aqueous inflow or increased uveoscleral outflow with increased IOP. However, any cause of increased episcleral venous pressure may increase IOP.

The aqueous outflow pathway may be summarized as follows:

Anterior chamber; Schlemm's canal; aqueous veins; epi-

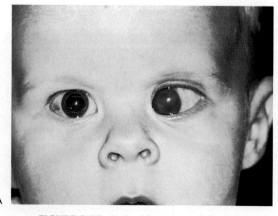

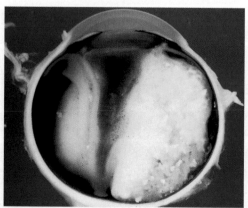

FIGURE 3.77. Retinoblastoma causing glaucoma. **A:** External photo. **B:** Gross pathologic specimen.

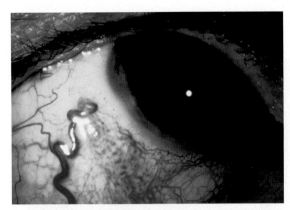

FIGURE 3.79. Sturge-Weber syndrome with glaucoma. Note dilated conjunctival vessel and episcleral hemangioma.

scleral veins; anterior ciliary veins; superior ophthalmic vein; cavernous sinus; internal jugular vein.

Some conjunctival veins also carry aqueous via the facial vein to the external jugular vein.

Obstruction of venous drainage along any of these pathways may lead to increased episcleral venous pressure and increased IOP. Dilated vessels are seen beneath the conjunctiva that do not blanch with epinephrine. Blood may be seen in Schlemm's canal on gonioscopy. Orbital congestion in thyroid ophthalmopathy may increase episcleral pressure and IOP; this may be responsive to steroids, radiation, and decompression. Thrombosis of an orbital vein or the cavernous sinus can produce similar findings. Retrobulbar tumors, jugular vein obstruction, and superior vena cava syndrome also lead to increased episcleral pressure.

Arteriovenous anomalies, by exposing the venous system

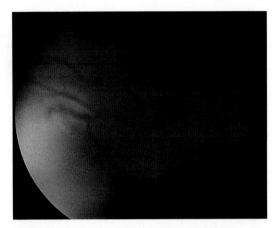

FIGURE 3.81. Resolving suprachoroidal hemorrhage following trabeculectomy in a patient with Sturge-Weber syndrome. Although prophylactic partial-thickness scleral windows with full-thickness sclerostomies were performed, a moderately large hemorrhage still occurred.

to the greater pressures of the arterial system, result in increased episcleral venous pressure. Sturge-Weber syndrome (Figs. 3.79, 3.80, 3.81), carotid cavernous fistulas (Fig. 3.82A,B), and orbital varices can in this manner produce

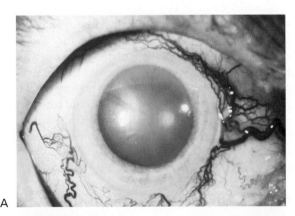

A

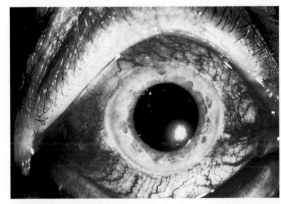

B

FIGURE 3.82. Dilated and tortuous episcleral vessels in patients with increased intraocular pressure secondary to **A:** carotid cavernous fistula and **B:** dural cavernous fistula. Although typically dural cavernous fistulas have a less dramatic appearance, this is not the case in these two patients. These patients are also at risk for ocular ischemia leading to neovascular glaucoma, uveal effusions with angle closure, and central retinal arterial and venous obstruction.

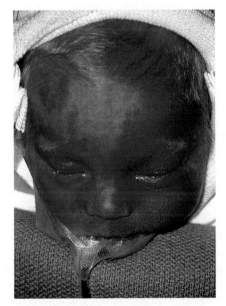

FIGURE 3.80. Infant with Sturge-Weber syndrome undergoing examination under anesthesia. Intraocular pressure was normal. Glaucoma is more common with upper lid involvement by the hemangioma.

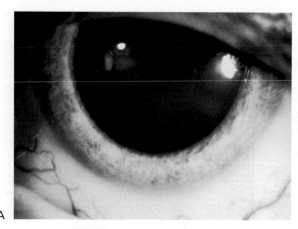
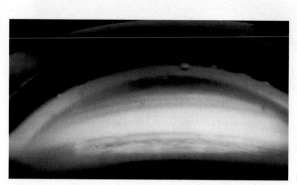

A   B

FIGURE 3.83. Patient with sporadic, idiopathic elevated episcleral venous pressure shows mildly dilated episcleral vessels **(A)** and blood in Schlemm's canal on gonioscopy **(B)**. A familial form of idiopathic elevated episcleral venous pressure exists as well.

glaucoma. Idiopathic cases of increased episcleral venous pressure exist as well (Fig. 3.83A,B).

Treatment of the underlying cause of increased venous pressure is ideal but not always possible or worthwhile. Embolization of carotid cavernous fistulas carries significant risk of CNS vascular accident; many close spontaneously. Aqueous suppressants often are helpful. Miotics and argon laser trabeculoplasty are not often useful, given the typically normal facility of outflow. Trabeculectomy is effective as it bypasses the elevated episcleral venous pressure, but has a higher incidence in these patients of serous and hemorrhagic choroidal detachments. Prophylactic partial thickness scleral flaps with full thickness sclerostomies have been advocated.

MEDICAL THERAPY FOR GLAUCOMA

The goal of treatment of a patient with glaucoma or suspected of having glaucoma is enhanced health. That goal is achieved by preserving vision, helping the individual develop a better understanding of what health is and how to achieve it, and, importantly, avoiding doing those things that are likely to make the person feel unhealthy. These three issues will all be briefly discussed in reverse order.

Avoidance of Actions That Make the Person Unhealthy

Merely telling a person he or she has glaucoma decreases the person's quality of life. Consequently, physicians need to be circumspect in this regard. To label a person as having "glaucoma" requires that the person have definite signs of damage. Even though certain genes have now been found to be associated with the diagnosis of glaucoma, it is still im-

possible on the basis of a laboratory test to determine with certainty whether or not a person has this entity. However, there are relative degrees of certainty, and when the findings are sufficiently intense or characteristic, it is possible to say with relative certainty that the person does, indeed, have glaucoma.

At the present time, the two most important indicators of the presence or absence of glaucoma are the nature of the optic nerve and the nature of the visual field. Clues suggesting the presence of glaucoma are indicated in Table 3.8 (Figs. 3.84; 3.85; 3.86; 3.87A, B; 3.88A–F; 3.89A, B).

The likelihood of an optic nerve being glaucomatous can be estimated based on a scale of disc damage (Fig 3.90). Note that what is determined here is the width of the neuroretinal rim. This is at least a partially subjective determination. However, by the width of the rim, we mean that portion of the optic nerve that appears to be on about the same plane as the retina. The internal edge of the rim is defined as that point where there is a sudden change in the curvature of the disc. Some discs have rims that slope so gradually toward the center that it is virtually impossible to determine with certainty the point at which the "neuroretinal rim" starts and stops. When considering these optic nerves, it is probably best to "admit defeat" rather than make a spurious estimate as to the width of the alleged neuroretinal rim.

The rim width is utilized rather than the cup/disc ratio. A cup/disc ratio may be small, such as perhaps .2, but may be highly pathologic if eccentrically placed. This problem also relates to rim width but is of less concern.

In staging the optic nerve, the area of thinnest rim width is chosen. When the examiner cannot determine with reasonable certainty whether the rim is at a particular figure or slightly smaller, the number chosen is always the larger. For example, if a rim width is considered to be about .2, but the

TABLE 3-8.* FEATURES OF THE OPTIC NERVE HEAD IN GLAUCOMA

Optic Disc Feature	Certainty That It Represents Glaucoma
Loss of rim tissue	
Notching (focal extension)	Highly suggestive
Acquired pit of the optic nerve (pseudopit)	Definite
Documented diffuse thinning of neuroretinal rim	Definite†
Changes of optic cup	
Documented concentric enlargement of cup	Definite‡
Asymmetry between eyes	Highly suggestive§
Vertical extension	Highly suggestive
Cup/disc ratio greater than 0.6	Moderately suggestive
Overpass cupping	Moderately suggestive
Temporal unfolding	Mildly suggestive
Nasal extension of the cup	Mildly suggestive
Alterations of the lamina cribrosa	Nonspecific
Localized pallor of the optic disc	Moderately suggestive
Vascular changes	
Localized hemorrhage crossing the disc	Highly suggestive
Bayoneting sign	Highly suggestive
Nasal shift of disc vessels	Nonspecific
Baring of circumlinear vessels	Mildly suggestive
Progressive vascular loops on the optic disc	Mildly suggestive
Cilioretinal veins	Mildly suggestive
Dilated retinal veins	Mildly suggestive
Narrowing of retinal vessels	Mildly suggestive
Peripapillary atrophy near thin rim	Moderately suggestive

*From Eid TM, Spaeth GL. The glaucomas: Concepts and fundamentals. Philadelphia: Lippincott Williams&Wilkins; 2000:45, with permission.
†Definitely pathogenic; may rarely be caused by other conditions.
‡Enlargement of the cup is due to thinning of the rim; the two are reverse sides of the coin, and the same qualifications apply to both.
§Highly suggestive when there is no specific cause for asymmetry, such as anisometropia.

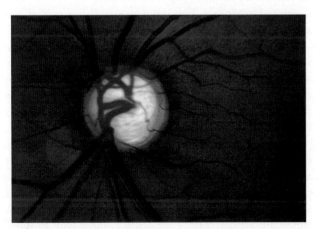

FIGURE 3.84. This optic nerve shows an acquired pit of the optic nerve, pathognomonic of glaucoma.

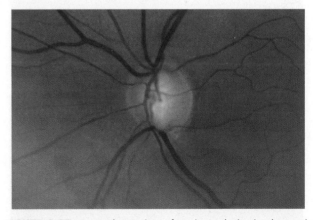

FIGURE 3.85. A notch consists of an irregularity in the optic nerve in which there is a change in the curvature of the rim localized to an area of less than 2 clock hours. The notch may extend all the way to the edge of the rim, or may be only partial. Both are highly indicative of the presence of a glaucomatous process.

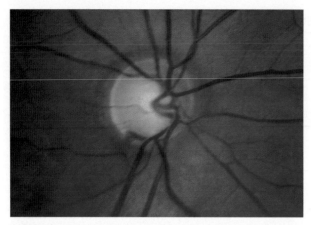

FIGURE 3.86. A flame-shaped hemorrhage crossing the rim of the optic nerve is highly suggestive of glaucoma. A similar finding may be seen rarely in patients with systemic hypertension or following a posterior vitreous detachment.

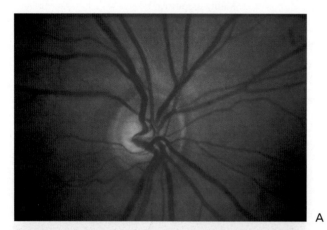

A

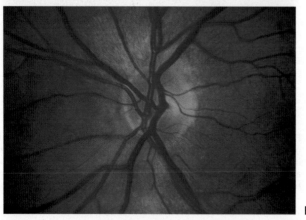

B

FIGURE 3.87. A, B: This patient with an essential iris atrophy has a significantly thinner rim in the left eye than in the right, without any other apparent cause for the asymmetry except asymmetry of intraocular pressure. The discs are the same size. The asymmetry is highly suggestive of glaucoma damage.

examiner thinks it may be slightly smaller than that, the figure chosen is .2.

It is essential to determine the disc size when using the Disc Damage Score. Indeed, it is essential to examine the disc size whenever evaluating the optic disc in a meaningful way. This can be readily done with a slit lamp using a lens with a strong dioptric power such as a 60, 66, 78, or 90 D lens. With good illumination and excellent fixation, and with the oculars properly adjusted so as to be parfocal for the examiner, the vertical height of the optic disc is measured from the pole at 12 o'clock to the pole at 6 o'clock. It is important to make sure that one does not measure peripapillary atrophy or the scleral ring, and that one measures from the outer edge of the rim to the outer edge of the rim. It is helpful if the illumination is reduced slightly, and if the width of the beam is such that it extends very slightly beyond the nasal and the temporal edges of the optic disc. Thus, the examiner uses a rectangle to isolate the optic nerve and estimate the vertical disc diameter. This diameter is then read directly from the graticule of the slit lamp and the appropriate correction factors made. These correction factors are shown in Table 3.9. There are advantages to using a Volk 66 D lens as no correction needs to be made. The measured size on the slit lamp is multiplied by the appropriate correction factor. This applies only to eyes with refractive errors less than +5 D. The optic nerve will appear spuriously small in eyes with more than 5 D of hyperopia and spuriously large in those with more than 5 D of myopia. The exact correction factors for these amounts of refractive error have not been determined, but it has been suggested that a correction can be made by multiplying the disc size by 1.1 for each diopter of myopia or dividing by 1.1 for each diopter of hyperopia. This is not an established method and is mentioned only as a rough method of estimating disc size.

For purposes of estimating the amount of disc damage with our staging system, discs are divided into small, average, and large discs. Small discs are those with vertical disc diameters less than 1.50 mm; large discs, those with vertical disc diameters greater than 2.0 mm; and average, in between (1.50 to 2.00 mm).

The stage of disc damage is determined by estimating the thinnest rim width, measuring the vertical disc diameter, and then using the nomogram to assign a disc stage. From a practical point of view, this becomes quite easy for discs with an average size if one remembers that discs with a thinnest-rim-width greater than .2 are grade 1, those with thinnest-rim-width slightly smaller than .2 are grade 2, and those with extremely thin rims are grade 3. The final four stages, 4, 5, 6, and 7, are utilized when there is *an area of the disc in which no rim is present.* Stage 4 indicates that rim is absent for less than 45 degrees; stage 5, absent between 45 degrees and 90 degrees; stage 6, absent between 90 degrees and 180 degrees; and stage 7, absent over more than 180 degrees.

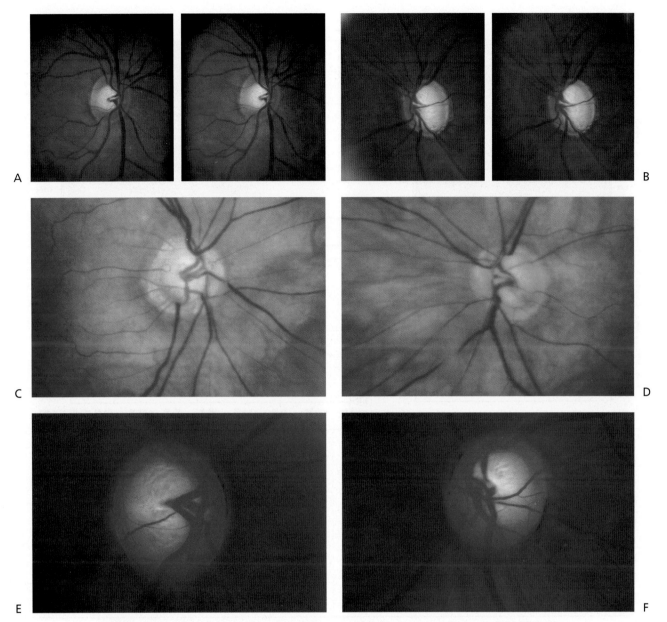

FIGURE 3.88. A–F: In this patient, the optic nerve with the narrower rim is considerably larger than the optic nerve with the wider rim. The difference in the width of the rim is due to the size of the optic disc, not to the damaging effect of glaucoma.

The likelihood that glaucoma damage is present is small for discs of grade 0 or 1, intermediate for discs of grade 2, and virtually certain for discs of grades 3 and higher (Table 3.10).

The other primary estimate of glaucoma damage is visual field loss. This is discussed elsewhere in this section. A simple grading system intended to be used in conjunction with the Disc Damage Score is shown on page 148. This ranges from 0, indicating no apparent visual field loss, to 7, denoting advanced field loss. Staging visual fields is even more problematic than staging optic disc damage, because the

field test is more subjective, more variable in the way it is administered, and more dependent upon the methodology of testing and the response of the patient. These grades, then, are highly approximate.

A relatively complete estimate of the likelihood of glaucoma damage can be obtained by adding the Disc Damage Score and the Visual Field Damage Score. A total score of 2 or less would strongly suggest that the patient did not have significant glaucoma damage, whereas a total score of 5 or more would be highly indicative of the presence of actual

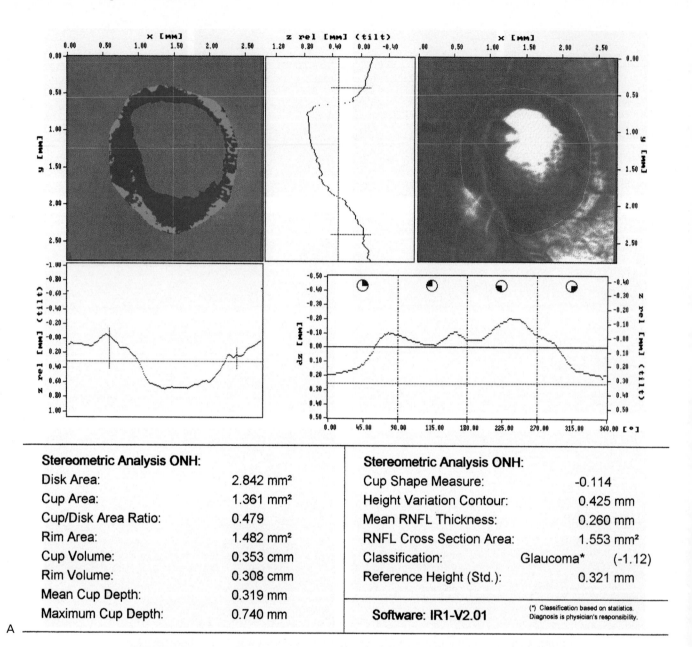

Stereometric Analysis ONH:

Disk Area:	2.842 mm²
Cup Area:	1.361 mm²
Cup/Disk Area Ratio:	0.479
Rim Area:	1.482 mm²
Cup Volume:	0.353 cmm
Rim Volume:	0.308 cmm
Mean Cup Depth:	0.319 mm
Maximum Cup Depth:	0.740 mm

Stereometric Analysis ONH:

Cup Shape Measure:	-0.114
Height Variation Contour:	0.425 mm
Mean RNFL Thickness:	0.260 mm
RNFL Cross Section Area:	1.553 mm²
Classification:	Glaucoma* (-1.12)
Reference Height (Std.):	0.321 mm

Software: IR1-V2.01

(*) Classification based on statistics.
Diagnosis is physician's responsibility.

A

FIGURE 3.89. A, B: These plots of the Heidelberg Retinal Tomograph show a large disc and a small disc. It is likely that the disc with the narrower rim has a narrower rim simply because the disc is larger, and not because of glaucoma. *(continued)*

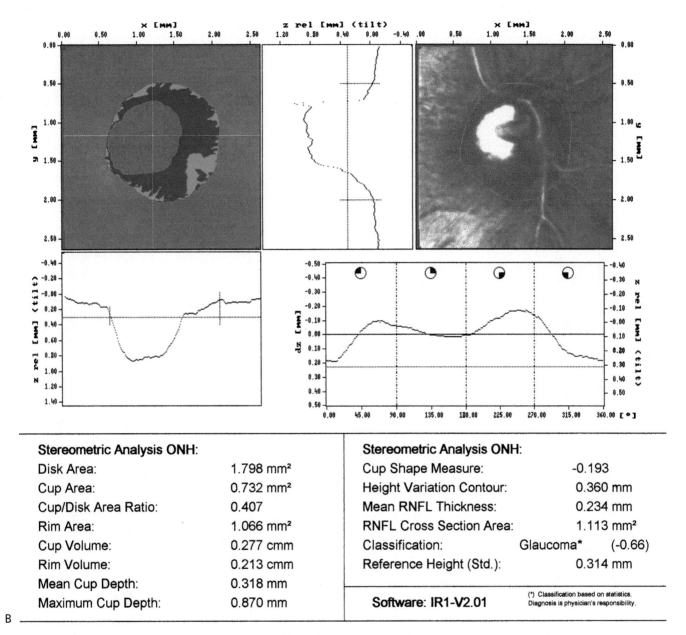

Stereometric Analysis ONH:		Stereometric Analysis ONH:	
Disk Area:	1.798 mm²	Cup Shape Measure:	-0.193
Cup Area:	0.732 mm²	Height Variation Contour:	0.360 mm
Cup/Disk Area Ratio:	0.407	Mean RNFL Thickness:	0.234 mm
Rim Area:	1.066 mm²	RNFL Cross Section Area:	1.113 mm²
Cup Volume:	0.277 cmm	Classification:	Glaucoma* (-0.66)
Rim Volume:	0.213 cmm	Reference Height (Std.):	0.314 mm
Mean Cup Depth:	0.318 mm		
Maximum Cup Depth:	0.870 mm	**Software: IR1-V2.01**	(*) Classification based on statistics. Diagnosis is physician's responsibility.

B

FIGURE 3.89. A, B: *Continued.*

glaucoma damage. The Glaucoma Damage Likelihood Score (GDLS) is indicated in Table 3.11. This refers, of course, only to the eye under consideration, not to the person.

The reader will note that these scales deal with glaucoma damage. There is a period of time when the glaucomatous process is advancing, but before glaucoma damage can be detected. The most important factor known to influence the likelihood that glaucoma damage will occur is IOP. The nature of the person's constitution, that is the genetic structure and family history, also plays a role. Consequently, in estimating the likelihood that a person will develop damage in the future, it is useful to include a measure of IOP and a

consideration of the family history. However, the most important consideration is the actual presence of damage. Where damage is already present, it is likely to progress. Consequently, in estimating the likelihood that a person has the glaucomatous process, that is, a condition in which the optic nerve deteriorates over time, it is helpful to include an estimate of IOP, family history, and the amount of damage believed already present. These three criteria make up the Glaucoma Probability Score, as indicated in Table 3.12. **The Glaucoma Probability Score, then, provides an estimate of the likelihood that the individual is affected with the glaucomatous process, whereas the Glaucoma Damage**

THE DISC DAMAGE LIKELIHOOD SCALE – DDLS

DDLS	For Small Disc <1.50 mm	Thinnest width of rim (rim/disc ratio) For Average Size Disc 1.50 – 2.00 mm	For Large Disc > 2.00 mm	DDLS Stage	EXAMPLES Small Optic Nerve	Average Optic Nerve	Large Optic Nerve
0a	.5	.4 or more	.3 or more	0a	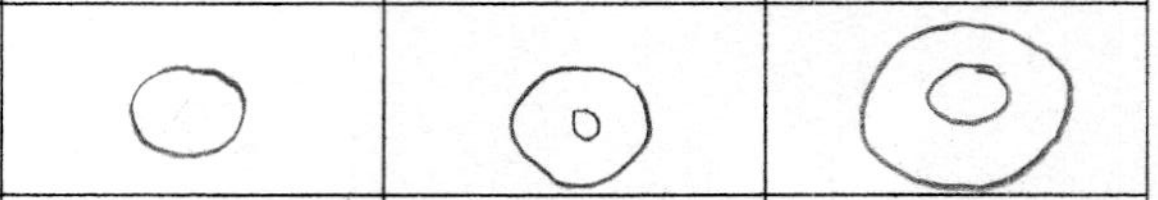		
0b	.4 to .5	.3 to .4	.2 to .3	0b	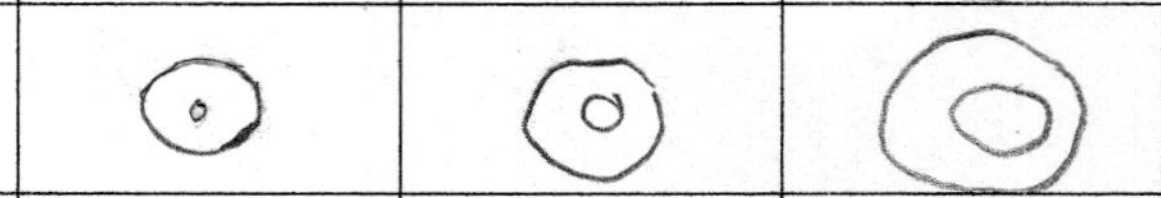		
1	.3 to .4	.2 to .3	.1 to .15	1	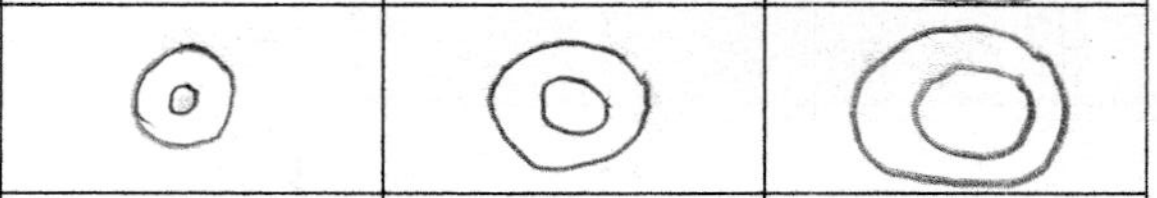		
2	.2 to .3	.1 to .2	.05 to .1	2	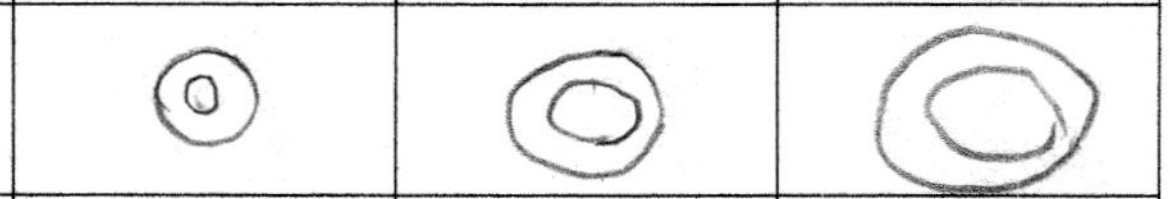		
3	.1 to .2	less than .1	.01 to .05	3	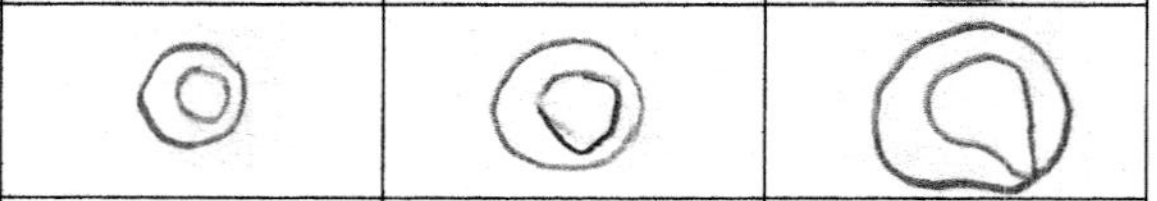		
4	less than .1	$0 < 45^0$	0 for 45^0	4	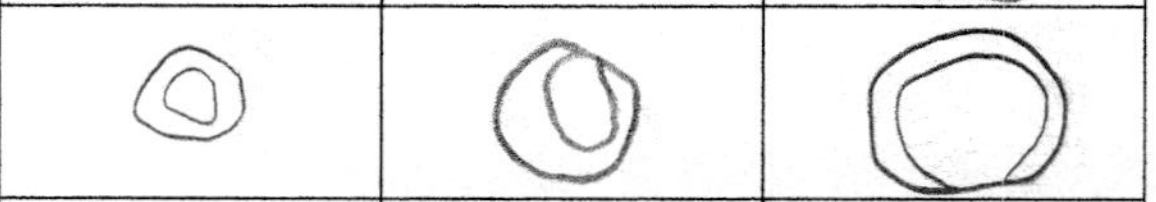		
5	0 for $< 45^0$	0 for 45^0 to 90^0	0 for 45^0 to 90^0	5	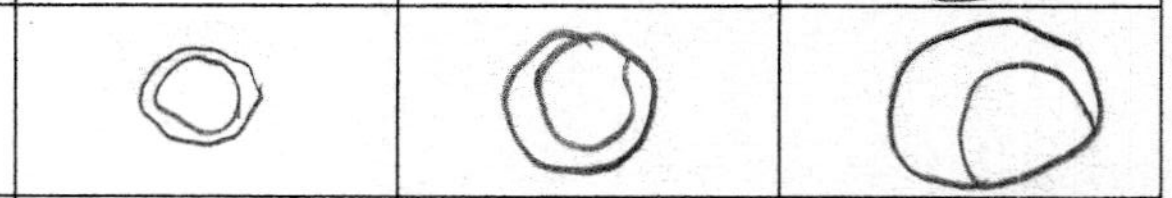		
6	0 for 45^0 to 90^0	0 for 90^0 to 180^0	0 for 90^0 to 180^0	6	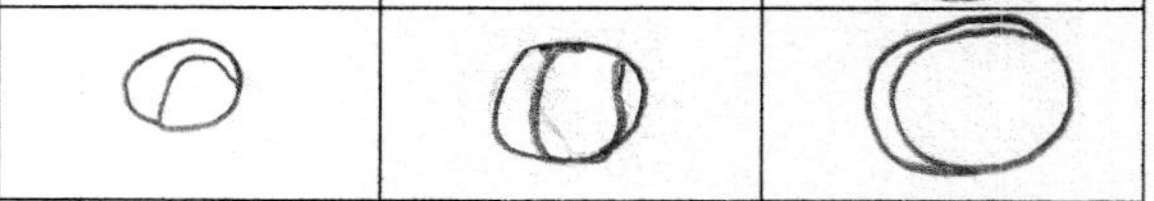		
7	0 for more than 90^0	0 for more than 180^0	0 for more than 180^0	7	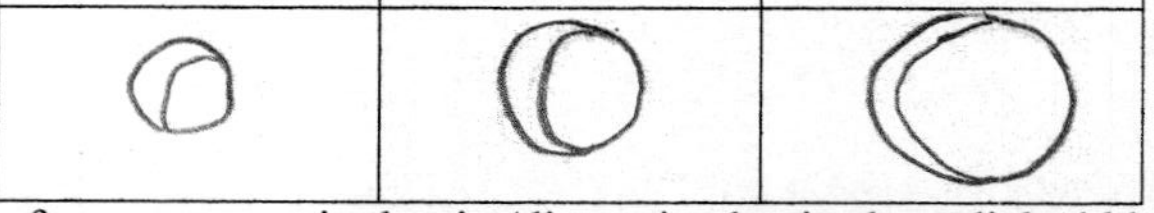		

Legend: The DDLS is based on the radial width of the neuroretinal rim measured at its thinnest point. The unit of measurement in the rim/disc ratio, that is, the radial width of the rim compared to the diameter of the disc in the same axis. When there is no rim remaining the rim/disc ratio is 0. The circumferential extent of rim absence (0 rim/disc ratio) is measured in degrees. Caution must be taken to differentiate the actual absence of rim from sloping of the rim as, for example, can occur temporally in some patients with myopia. A sloping rim is not an absent rim. Because rim width is a function of disc size, disc size must be evaluated prior to attributing a DDLS stage. This is done with a 60D to 90D lens with appropriate corrective factors. The Volk 60D lens minimally underestimates the disc size. Corrective factors for other lenses are: Volk 60D x .88, 78D x 1.2, 90D x 1.33. Nikon 60D x 1.03, 90D x 1.63.

FIGURE 3.90. The Disc Damage Scale.

TABLE 3-9. APPROXIMATE CORRECTION FACTORS OF ESTIMATING DISC SIZE WITH A SLIT LAMP

Lens	Nikon	Volk
90 D	1.6	1.3
78 D	1.3	1.1
66 D	1.1	0
60 D	1.0	.9

TABLE 3-10. DISC DAMAGE SCORE: LIKELIHOOD THAT ONE HAS OPTIC NERVE DAMAGE DUE TO GLAUCOMA

0	1	2	3	4	5	6	7
Low		?			Likely		

least likely←likelihood that damage is present→most likely

TABLE 3-11. GLAUCOMA DAMAGE SCORE: LIKELIHOOD THAT AN EYE HAS GLAUCOMA BASED ON THE SUM OF THE SCALES INDICATING DISC AND FIELD DAMAGE

0	1	2	3	4	5	6	7	8	9	10	11	12	13	14
Low			?			Probable								High

← least likely————————————————most likely →

The higher the score, the greater the likelihood that glaucoma is present. When the score is less than 2, the likelihood of glaucoma damage being present is low, and above 4, high.

TABLE 3-12. GLAUCOMA PROBABILITY SCORE: LIKELIHOOD OF THE PRESENCE OF THE GLAUCOMATOUS PROCESS

Factors Considered	Range of Scores
Glaucoma damage likelihood score	0–4
Disc damage score	0–7
Field damage score	0–7
Asymmetry of GDLS*	0–1
IOP score†	0–9
IOP asymmetry score‡	0–1
Genetics score§	0–1
Ethnic origin score‖	0–½
Refraction score¶	0–½

GDLS, glaucoma damage likelihood score; IOP, intraocular pressure. Interpretation: <4 = glaucomatous process unlikely; 4–5 = glaucomatous process suspect; 6–7 = glaucomatous process likely; ≥8 = glaucomatous process certain.
*GDLS asymmetry score = the difference between the two eyes >+2.
†Intraocular pressure (IOP) score: 10–19 mm Hg = 1; 20–29 mm Hg = 2; 30–39 mm Hg = 3; 40–49 mm Hg = 5; 50–59 mm Hg = 7; 60 or higher = 9.
‡IOP asymmetry score: IOP >5<10 mm Hg = ½; IOP ≥10 mm Hg = 1.
§Genetic score: family history of visual loss = ½; gene for glaucoma = 1.
‖Ethnic origin score: black African origin = ½.
¶Refraction score: myopia >5 D = ½; Hyperopia >5 D = ½.

Score indicates the likelihood that the person actually has glaucoma damage already present.

Examples:

1. IOP=37 mm Hg with no visual field loss and with slightly suspicious optic discs, which are symmetrical.
   - GDLS=2
   - GDLS asymmetry=0
   - IOP=3
   - IOP asymmetry=0
   - Ethnic origin=0
   - Genetic score=0
   - Refraction=0
   - GPS=5
   - Interpretation: Glaucomatous process suspect

2. Presence of a probable early notch in both eyes, making the discs highly suspicious, with IOP of 22 mm Hg in one eye and 16 mm Hg in the other in a black patient with a family history of glaucomatous visual loss.
   - GDLS=3
   - GDLS asymmetry=0
   - IOP=2
   - IOP asymmetry=1
   - Ethnic origin=½
   - Genetic score=½
   - Refraction =½
   - Total=GPS=7½
   - Interpretation: Glaucomatous process likely

3. Patient with healthy-appearing optic discs and visual fields, with IOP of 58 mm Hg in one eye and 49 mm Hg in the other, and 10 D of myopia in both eyes.
   - GDLS=1
   - GDLS asymmetry=0
   - IOP=7
   - IOP asymmetry=1
   - Ethnic origin=0
   - Genetic score=0
   - Refraction =½
   - Total=GPS=9½
   - Interpretation: Glaucomatous process certain

4. Definite visual field loss with probable optic nerve damage, IOP of 17 mm Hg in a Caucasian patient.
   - GDLS=5
   - GDLS asymmetry=0
   - IOP=1
   - IOP asymmetry=1
   - Ethnic origin=0
   - Genetic score=0
   - Refraction=0
   - Total=GPS=7
   - Interpretation: Glaucomatous process likely

These two scores are discussed in detail because one wishes to avoid the damaging effects of treatments where possible. Every treatment for glaucoma has some damaging

TABLE 3-13. LIKELIHOOD THAT A PERSON WILL HAVE SYMPTOMS AS A RESULT OF GLAUCOMATOUS OPTIC NERVE DAMAGE*

0	2	4	6	8	10	12	14	16	18	20	22	24	26	28
Low				Mod						High				

*Sum of the glaucoma damage scores of the right and left eyes.

effect. This may simply be cost or inconvenience. It is more often a topical or systemic side effect. Consequently, one needs to have a relative degree of certainty that the person in question will actually become damaged by the glaucomatous process before there is justification for initiating any type of treatment.

To repeat: One needs to have a relative degree of certainty that the person in question will actually become damaged by the glaucomatous process before there is justification for initiating any type of treatment.

The likelihood that an eye will become damaged can be estimated by using a graph that considers three aspects of the eye's condition: first, the stage of glaucoma; second, the duration that it is anticipated the glaucoma will exist; and third, the rate of change of this stage of glaucoma. The stage

of glaucoma can be estimated by using either the Disc Damage Scale or preferably the Glaucoma Damage Likelihood Scale, which includes both the Disc Damage Scale, and the Visual Field Damage Scale.

This graph refers to one eye only. The likelihood that a person will have symptoms as a result of glaucoma damage is highly complex. It depends upon the type and intensity of field loss, the visual awareness and needs of the person, and the person's psychological make-up. A rough indication of the likelihood that a person will have symptoms from glaucoma, however, can be gathered by combining the Glaucoma Damage Likelihood Score for the two eyes, as shown in Table 3.13.

The Glaucoma Graph

The Glaucoma Graph (Fig. 3.91) is a way of determining and understanding the clinical course of glaucoma in an individual patient.

On the y axis of the graph is the stage of the glaucoma, and on the x axis is the life expectancy. The slope and the curve of each of the individual lines are determined and graphed in different ways:

Dotted lines indicate that the slope and the curve have

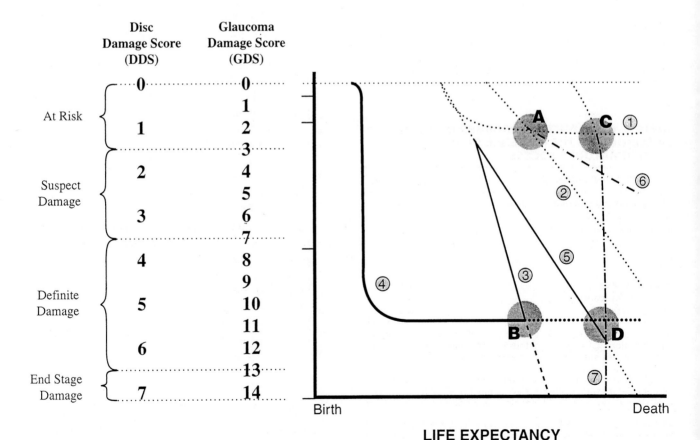

FIGURE 3.91. The Glaucoma Graph.

been determined by plotting the results of serial studies, such as repeated disc photographs taken yearly or repeated visual field examinations.

Solid lines depict the clinical course as described in the patient's history.

Dashed lines are extrapolations that are presumed to represent what will happen in the future. These hypothetical, extrapolated future courses are based on the nature of the previous courses and on knowledge of what has happened since a known point in time.

This illustration shows the courses of seven different patients with different manifestations of glaucoma:

A patient at point "A" has minimal glaucoma, and about one third of his or her life still to live.

A patient at point "B" has advanced glaucoma and has about one third of his or her life still to live.

A patient at point "C" has very early glaucoma and only a few years to live.

A patient at point "D" has advanced glaucoma and only a few years to live.

Patient 1, considered at point "A," has one third of his or her life to live and is in an early stage of glaucoma. About one third of his or her life earlier, this patient was noted to have elevated pressure and followed without treatment. The patient continued to be followed without treatment and no damage to the optic nerve or visual field was ever noted. It is reasonable to assume that, if the patient continues to have IOPs around the same level as those noted initially, he or she will probably follow the course described by line 1, and will die without any evidence of glaucoma damage.

Patient 2 is also considered at point "A," ie, having minimal damage with one third of his or her life left to live. In this case, however, the patient's IOP rose continuously, and the patient was noted to develop early disc and field damage, which then continued at the rate depicted by the dotted line 2. This patient, if untreated, would develop definite asymptomatic damage. However, the patient would have no functional loss at the time of his or her death.

Patients 3 and 4 are at point "B." Both have advanced glaucoma and one third of their lives left to live. However, Patient 3 is deteriorating rapidly and will be blind long before he or she dies, whereas Patient 4, who had a blow to the eye as a child and lost vision to a steroid-induced glaucoma at that time, has had stable vision for most of his or her life, and it is reasonable to expect that it will continue to be stable.

Patients at points "C" and "D" both have only a few years to live, but those at point "C" (like Patients 1 and 2 at point "A") have minimal damage, and those at point "D" (like Patient 4 at point "B") have marked damage.

Patient 5 started with a clinical course similar to that of Patient 3 (advanced glaucoma and deteriorating rapidly), but around the midpoint of his or her life, the glaucoma became less severe. Nevertheless, this patient will be blind at the time of his or her death unless there is effective intervention. Compare Patient 4, who at point "D" has the same

life expectancy and the same amount of damage as Patient 5 (only a few years to live and advanced glaucoma). Patient 4, however, has a stable clinical course and does not appear to need a change in therapy. In contrast, Patient 5 needs lowering of IOP urgently.

Patient 6, at around point "C," also has only a few years of life remaining, but has a glaucoma that is getting worse a little bit more slowly than that affecting Patients 2 and 5. However, since Patient 6 has so little damage to start with, no treatment is necessary, even though he or she is getting worse. Even without treatment, he or she will not have enough damage or visual loss due to glaucoma at the time of death that he or she will have any awareness of being ill, and will have no limitation in function.

Patient 7, at point "C," has only a few years left to live, but has a type of glaucoma that is deteriorating so rapidly that even though he or she has only a short period of time to live, he or she will be blind well before the time of death.

Using the Glaucoma Graph to define and characterize the nature of the clinical course helps the physician and patient to understand that:

Patients 1, 4, and 6 do not need any treatment at all; Patient 1 will never develop damage, Patient 4 has marked damage but it is not getting worse, and Patient 6 is getting worse so slowly that it will not interfere with his or her life.

Patients 3, 5, and 7 can be seen to need treatment urgently in order to prevent them from becoming totally blind prior to the time of their deaths.

In Patient 2, the need for treatment is controversial. Since this patient would never develop glaucoma, perhaps he or she should not be treated at all. But since he or she would develop some damage, those who want to prevent any damage at all would advise therapy.

The Glaucoma Graph is used by locating the individual on the vertical axis based on the Disc Damage Score or the Glaucoma Damage Score, and on the horizontal axis based on estimated life expectancy. Life expectancy cannot be estimated with certainty of course, but meaningful estimates can be made. Without an estimate, one cannot rationally decide upon treatment. Factors that help arrive at a meaningful estimate of life expectancy are indicated in Table 3.14.

The evaluation of the optic disc and the visual field are repeated at appropriate intervals between 3 and 6 months, depending upon the suspicion that the individual is getting worse. The new scores are plotted on the graph and given an estimate of the stability or rate of change (improvement or deterioration) of the patient's condition. Once enough points have been established to develop a meaningful line, then the line can be extrapolated so that one gets an estimate of the likelihood that the patient will pass into the field of symptomatic damage prior to his or her death.

The less the amount of damage, the less the justification for starting treatment. The greater the damage, the greater the need to start treatment, as even slow amounts of deteri-

TABLE 3-14. FACTORS AFFECTING LIFE EXPECTANCY

A. Genetic factors
1. Age and cause of death of the person's parents and siblings
2. Known health problems (nature *and* seriousness of any illness) of the person:
   - Heart disease
   - Lung disease
   - Bleeding disease
   - Cancer
   - Disease of the nervous system
   - Inherited diseases
   - Depression
   - Diabetes mellitus
   - Chronic infectious disease
   - Severe allergies
   - Current use of medications
   - Other problems
3. Person's height and weight, and whether they are proportionate and are in a roughly average range
4. Blood pressure and pulse, and whether appropriate for age

B. Lifestyle characteristics
- Cigarette smoking
- Amount of alcoholic beverage usage
- Use of any drugs except for medicinal use
- Amount and intensity of exercise
- Yearly physical examinations
- Travel or recreation associated with increased risk (travel to countries with epidemic or endemic diseases; automobile racing; etc.)

C. Occupational exposures
- Commute by car greater than 10 miles/day
- Frequent trips by plane or boat
- Travel to countries with endemic or epidemic disease
- Hazardous occupations, such as police officer, firefighter, soldier, etc.

oration will result in the patient becoming symptomatically worse.

The likelihood of the patient developing an attack of angle-closure glaucoma or developing some other type of glaucoma is not included in the system just described. However, it is important when counseling a person who has an occludable anterior chamber angle not to say that the person has glaucoma. Indeed, the person does not yet have glaucoma, but merely has the predisposition to glaucoma. That is an important predisposition that usually indicates the need for therapy. The treatment, then, is preventive. It is important for patients to understand the distinction between the prevention of glaucoma and the actual treatment of glaucoma. There are justifiable reasons for trying to prevent glaucoma from occurring, either the angle-closure type of glaucoma or the glaucoma that occurs as progressive optic nerve damage. Thus, simply because a person does not yet have glaucoma does not mean that therapy is not indicated. Therapy is indicated when the likelihood is suffi-

ciently great that the individual's life will be affected in a harmful way by the glaucomatous process.

Enhancing the Patient's Health

The major goal of any treatment is to preserve or enhance the patient's health. This can be done in glaucoma by helping an individual understand what it means to have a chronic disease or the likelihood of the development of an acute disease. It is not known exactly how much a person's glaucoma benefits from improving the general state of health. There is fairly good evidence that losing weight and exercising can lower IOP in some individuals, perhaps by about as much as 4 mm Hg. There is also reason to believe that avoiding systemic hypertension may prevent a microvascular disease that could accelerate the progress of glaucoma. Some studies have suggested that cigarette smoking and obesity are risk factors for glaucomatous deterioration. Telling patients that their glaucoma will be benefited by measures that enhance their general health is probably too strong a statement. On the other hand, there are sufficient indicators that abnormalities of blood flow play a role in the development of glaucoma that it seems prudent to try to maintain cardiovascular fitness. If maintaining one's general health is beneficial from the point of view of glaucoma, that is certainly a plus. If it is not beneficial to the glaucoma, it is at any rate beneficial to the person who adopts a lifestyle that is conducive to maintaining a good state of health. This will clearly vary from person to person and includes the full spectrum of factors that affect health: diet, exercise, lifestyle, attitudes, and emotional characteristics. The goal is physical, social, emotional, and spiritual health. All of those interrelate, and complete health requires wholeness in all areas. Assisting patients to develop healthier lifestyles, more positive attitudes, better socialization, and more meaningful spiritual lives is one of the responsibilities and the joys of every physician, including those involved in caring for patients with glaucoma or suspected of having glaucoma.

Alternative therapies for glaucoma have been suggested. Some ophthalmologists use agents such as ginkgo to try to improve blood flow or some of the calcium channel blockers. Antioxidants have been suggested by others. When considering any of these agents, the potential risks need to be measured against the potential benefits. Because at this time there is little convincing demonstration of any real benefits to the glaucomatous eye of alternative therapies, and because all agents have some risk, the risk/benefit ratio of all therapies must usually be unfavorable. There is some evidence that a subgroup of patients with progressive glaucoma and low IOPs who have abnormal regulation of the vasculature as demonstrated by provocation with perturbation of blood gases may benefit from calcium channel blockers. This is not established, and unless one is willing to utilize the appropriate studies, the use of the calcium channel blockers should be considered experimental.

Lowering Intraocular Pressure

The only treatment that to date has been proven to prevent development of progressive optic nerve damage in patients with glaucoma is lowering IOP. It is not known whether this effect is due to absolute lowering of IOP, or to stabilization of IOP. Either or both may be true. It appears that, for a considerable number of patients with glaucoma, it is necessary to lower the IOP by approximately 30% if one is to obtain a meaningful alteration in the clinical course of the disease. However, it has not been established that it is necessary to lower the pressure by 30% in every individual, nor has it been established that lowering IOP by 30% will be beneficial in every individual. Nevertheless, the 30% figure is a guideline that has some evidence to support it. Having said that, however, it seems clear that IOP needs to be lowered by a greater percentage in people whose IOPs are initially low in order to have a beneficial effect than in people whose IOPs are initially high. Zeyen has suggested a method of arriving at a target pressure that takes into account this variability. He suggests that a reasonable approach is to try to lower the IOP by a percentage that is equal to the IOP at which the optic nerve is being damaged. Thus, if an individual has an IOP of 40 mm Hg, at which pressure the optic nerve is being damaged, then it would be reasonable to lower the pressure 40%, that is, by 16 mm Hg, and set a target pressure of around 24 mm Hg. In contrast, in the person who is getting worse with a pressure of 15 mm Hg, it may be appropriate to lower the IOP 15% of 15 mm Hg, or slightly more than 2 mm Hg. An estimate of a suitable target pressure in such a patient may be around 12 mm Hg.

Some ophthalmologists believe that when the optic nerve is already damaged it is more prone to subsequent damage. This has not been established, but has a ring of logic to it. It may simply be that those individuals who develop marked damage are those individuals whose optic discs are very sensitive to damage, and that the likelihood that patients with advanced damage will progress is not related to the advanced damage but rather to the nature of the underlying disease. Nevertheless, it seems prudent to be slightly more vigorous in those individuals in whom disc damage is advanced. As such, the ophthalmologist may wish to add or subtract 1 or 2 mm Hg from the target pressure described by Zeyen in those individuals in whom there is far advanced damage.

Target Pressure Range

There are benefits to both the physician and the patient to set a target pressure. However, for both the physician and the patient, it should be clear that the target pressure represents merely a range. If the target pressure can be easily reached without inducing troublesome symptomatology, then it seems prudent to continue to try to keep the IOP around the same level as the selected target pressure. However, where the target pressure is not able to be reached with ease, then the ophthalmologist must consider carefully the risks of pushing therapy more vigorously. By and large, it is helpful to think of a target range. Thus, the ophthalmologist may indicate on the chart and tell the patient that the goal is to get the IOP down to a range of between x and y mm Hg (Table 3.15). For example, x could be 10 and y 15, or, perhaps, x 25 and y 30 mm Hg.

Initiation of Therapy on the Basis of Risk/Benefit Ratio

Risks of Therapy

Whether to start the patient on medicinal, laser, or surgical therapy depends upon the diagnosis and the risk/benefit ratio of the intended therapy. The Glaucoma Graph is of great assistance in this regard. Risks of therapy include topical and systemic considerations. They exist for medicinal, laser, or surgical treatments. It is extraordinarily difficult to try to balance the relative risks of these modes of therapy because the onset and permanence of the risks is so different. For example, the risk to ocular and systemic health in association with the use of a topical carbonic anhydrase inhibitor is initially so small as to be barely measurable. However, the risks are cumulative, and with many years of use the risk becomes a real factor. In contrast, the risk to sight or general health in association with a surgical procedure is largely related to the time immediately around the procedure itself. Thus, considering the relative importance of immediate and long-term risks (and benefits) is essential in trying to establish a meaningful risk/benefit ratio. It is, of course, not sufficient merely to consider the risks of treatment; one must also consider the risks of not utilizing treatment, that is, what is the expected clinical course in the absence of therapy. This has been discussed in detail on pages 149–152. Table 3.16 provides rough guidelines about the relative effect of various types of therapeutic approaches to glaucoma.

Factors that influence whether to start with medicinal therapy or an argon laser trabeculoplasty are suggested in Table 3.16. An argon laser trabeculoplasty is especially appropriate in elderly individuals with a clear-cut diagnosis of a primary type of open-angle glaucoma and marked pigmentation of the posterior trabecular meshwork, and is probably the treatment of choice in such individuals. Additionally, argon laser trabeculoplasty has a role in those individuals in whom problems of systemic health introduce concerns with regard to the use of the medicinal agents.

TABLE 3-15. ESTIMATING TARGET PRESSURE RANGE

TPR = IOP − [IOP × IOP/100] + FF

FF, fudge factor (when damage is marked, field loss is close to fixation, and deterioration is rapid, target range is usually lowered); IOP, intraocular pressure at which deterioration occurs; TPR, target pressure range.

Choice of Medications Used to Treat Glaucoma

Two different considerations are of major help in deciding upon which agent is most appropriate for a particular individual. The first has to do with the characteristics of the drug, and the second, the characteristics of the patient. The challenge is to match the two as perfectly as possible. Table 3.17 categorizes patients into groups. Agents are categorized as either usually inappropriate, occasionally appropriate, or usually a good choice for each of the patient groups. The way to use the table is to consider all those characteristics that describe the patient under consideration, and find which agent or agents are most likely to fit that particular

TABLE 3-16. RELATIVE EFFECTS OF VARIOUS THERAPEUTIC METHODS FOR TREATING GLAUCOMA

Medicines

1. IOP level	15% ↓ (variable)
2. IOP variation	Mild decrease
3. IOP duration	6 hours to 1 month
4. Other eye	Minimal
5. Vision	Mild (60%) to severe (10%)
6. Health	Mild to fatal

Argon laser trabeculoplasty

1. IOP level	25% ↓ primary open-angle glaucoma
	2+ posterior trabecular meshwork
	30% ↓ pigmentary glaucoma or exfoliation syndrome
2. IOP variation	Definite decrease
3. IOP duration	Average of 5 years in favorable case
4. Other eye	0
5. Vision	0
6. Health improved	0

YAG peripheral iridotomy

1. IOP level	0+
2. IOP variation	0
3. IOP duration	Permanent
4. Other eye	0
5. Vision	Ghost image
6. Health	0

Guarded filtration procedure

1. IOP level	15 mm Hg (>30%)
2. IOP variation	Flat
3. IOP duration	20 years
4. Other eye	Sympathetic ophthalmia rare
5. Vision	Always, better to much worse
6. Health	0+

Guarded filtration procedure with 5-fluorouracil

1. IOP level	14 mm Hg (>30%)
2. IOP variation	Flat
3. IOP duration	20+ years (?)
4. Other eye	Sympathetic ophthalmia possible
5. Vision	As per guarded filtration procedure, but more concern and more severe
6. Health	0+

Guarded filtration procedure with mitomycin C

1. IOP level	11 mm Hg (>40%)
2. IOP variation	Flat
3. IOP duration	20 years (?)
4. Other eye	Sympathetic ophthalmia possible
5. Vision	As per guarded filtration procedure, but much more concern
6. Health	0 (?)

Tube shunt procedure

1. IOP level	19 mm Hg (?)
2. IOP variation	Moderate decrease
3. IOP duration	5 to 10 years
4. Other eye	Presumedly slight
5. Vision	Moderate
6. Health	0+

IOP, intraocular pressure.

TABLE 3-17. FACTORS THAT SUGGEST A TOPICAL DRUG IS PARTICULARLY INAPPROPRIATE OR APPROPRIATE FOR USE IN A PATIENT WITH GLAUCOMA

Patient Characteristics	Should Almost Never Be Used	May Be Appropriate	May Be a Good Choice
Person needs maximum intra-ocular pressure lowering	Epinephrine	β Blockers, carbonic anhydrase inhibitors, α agonists	Prostaglandin analogs, combined agents*
Age			
≥10 years	α Agonists	β Blockers	Topical carbonic anhydrase inhibitors
10–39 years		Pilocarpine	Dipivefrin°, epinephrine
40–49 years		No particular problem	No particular preference
50–69 years		Pilocarpine	β Blockers, α agonists, carbonic anhydrase inhibitors
≥70 years		β Blockers	Carbonic anhydrase inhibitors
Ease of administration important	Ocusert		Systemic carbonic anhydrase inhibitors, β blockers, prostaglandin analogs
Compliance likely to be a problem	Any agent requiring use 3 or more times a day		Long-acting timolol, echothiophate iodide, latanoprost, combined agents*
Expense a major factor			Pilocarpine, epinephrine
High myopia, lattice degeneration, or predisposition to retinal detachment	Echothiophate iodide, dimacarium bromide	Any miotic	β Blockers, α agonists, carbonic anhydrase inhibitors, prostaglandin analogs
Avoidance of macular problems important		Prostaglandin analogs, pilocarpine	β Blockers, carbonic anhydrase inhibitors
Cataract present	Miotics		β Blockers, α agonists, carbonic anhydrase inhibitors, prostaglandin analogs
Aphakia		Epinephrine compound, prostaglandin analogs	β Blockers, $\alpha 2$ agonists, carbonic anhydrase inhibitors
Pseudophakia		Epinephrine	β Blockers, α agonists, $\alpha 2$ agonists, carbonic anhydrase inhibitors, prostaglandin analogs
Uveitis	Miotics	Prostaglandin analogs	β Blockers, carbonic anhydrase inhibitors, α agonists
Angle recession glaucoma		Miotics	β Blockers, α agonists, carbonic anhydrase inhibitors, prostaglandin analogs
Reaction to preservatives	All agents with preservatives		Preservative-free timolol or pilocarpine, systemic carbonic anhydrase inhibitors
Severe irritation of eyes probably related to topical medications		All eyedrops	Systemic anhydrase inhibitors
Neovascular glaucoma	Miotics, prostaglandin analogs		β Blockers, carbonic anhydrase inhibitors, α agonists
Asthma, chronic cough, emphysema	Nonselective β blockers	Betaxolol, echothiophate iodate	α Agonists, carbonic anhydrase inhibitors, prostaglandin analogs
Congestive heart failure	β Blockers, α agonists		Carbonic anhydrase inhibitors, prostaglandin analogs, miotics
Irregular heartbeat		β Blockers, α agonists, epinephrine	Carbonic anhydrase inhibitors, prostaglandin analogs, miotics
Renal failure	Systemic carbonic anhydrase inhibitors	Topical carbonic anhydrase inhibitors	β Blockers, α agonists, prostaglandin analogs, miotics
Irritable bowel syndrome	Miotics	Carbonic anhydrase inhibitors	β Blockers, α agonists
Sickle cell disease	Systemic carbonic anhydrase inhibitors	Topical carbonic anhydrase inhibitors	α Agonists, β blockers, miotics, prostaglandin analogs
Myasthenia gravis		β Blockers	
Patient very apprehensive about toxic side effects of medications		Carbonic anhydrase inhibitors, β blockers, α agonists, prostaglandin analogs	Dipivefrin
Concern about possible cosmetic blemish		Prostaglandin analogs, α agonists, miotics	β Blockers, carbonic anhydrase inhibitors
Athlete, serious exerciser		β Blockers, α agonists	Carbonic anhydrase inhibitors, miotics, prostaglandin analogs
Low blood pressure		β Blockers	Carbonic anhydrase inhibitors, prostaglandin analogs, α agonists, miotics
High blood pressure		α Agonists	Carbonic anhydrase inhibitors, prostaglandin analogs, miotics, β blockers
Frequent urination		Miotics, systemic carbonic anhydrase inhibitors	
Prostatic hypertrophy or problem initiating urination		α Agonists, systemic carbonic anhydrase inhibitors	
Pregnancy	Carbonic anhydrase inhibitors, prostaglandin analogs	α Agonists†	β Blockers,† miotics†
Nursing mothers	β Blockers		

*Combination of timolol plus latanoprost, or timolol plus dorzolamide.
†No drugs should be used during pregnancy, especially during the first trimester, unless essential.

TABLE 3-18. CLASSES OF SIDE EFFECTS AND AGENTS MOST LIKELY TO CAUSE THEM*

Fatigue
    Systemic carbonic anhydrase inhibitors
    β Blockers
    α Agonists
    Topical carbonic anhydrase inhibitors
    Prostaglandin analogs (rare)

Irregular heartbeat
    Epinephrine
    α Agonists
    β Blockers

Slow heartbeat
    β Blockers

Changes in blood pressure
    β Blockers
    α Agonists

Blurred vision
    Miotics
    β Blockers

Upset stomach
    Carbonic anhydrase inhibitors

Diarrhea or frequent urination
    Carbonic anhydrase inhibitors
    Miotics

Red eyes
    Epinephrine†
    α Agonists†
    Prostaglandin analogs

Dark vision
    Miotics
    α Agonists

Achy bones and joints
    Prostaglandin analogs

Confusion or forgetfulness
    β Blockers

Weight loss
    Carbonic anhydrase inhibitors

Hair loss
    β Blockers
    Carbonic anhydrase inhibitors

Ringing in the ears
    Carbonic anhydrase inhibitors

Congestion
    Miotics
    Prostaglandin analogs

Depression
    Carbonic anhydrase inhibitors
    β Blockers

Sexual dysfunction
    β Blockers

Poor appetite
    Carbonic anhydrase inhibitors

Numbness and tingling in the hands and feet
    Carbonic anhydrase inhibitors

Stomach cramps
    Miotics
    Carbonic anhydrase inhibitors

*Agents most likely to cause side effects are listed first, and those least likely are listed last. Listing an agent does not indicate that it always or even frequently causes the side effect. Agents that are not listed can cause the side effects that are listed.
†α Agonists and epinephrine frequently make the eyes white immediately after placement in the eye; redness develops hours later.

patient with those particular characteristics. Clearly, these are merely guidelines. Finally, Table 3.18 lists classes of side effects and agents most likely to cause them.

SURGICAL THERAPY FOR GLAUCOMA

Principles of Glaucoma Surgery

The objective of lowering or stabilizing IOP with surgery for glaucoma involves either improving aqueous outflow or reducing aqueous inflow. Lasers have proven to be invaluable for glaucoma therapy. They have not replaced but rather only complemented incisional operations. Individualized assessment for each eye of each patient will help direct the proper sequence of surgical intervention if medical therapy proves insufficient or is deemed inappropriate. The goal must be clear. In other words, is the treatment for pain relief from high IOP in a blind eye, or is it for maintaining vision in the patient's only seeing eye? With informed consent, the patient will also have the opportunity to voice his or her preference.

Lasers

Laser Peripheral Iridectomy

Goal
    A peripheral iridectomy can prevent or alleviate a lens pupillary block leading to angle-closure glaucoma.
    Indications

- narrow angle capable of angle closure
- primary angle closure leading to chronic or acute angle closure
- iris bombé (posterior iris-lens synechia)
- dramatic/spontaneous lens subluxation
- microspherophakia
- phacomorphic glaucoma

    Technique
    Nd:YAG lasers are typically preferred over the argon or diode laser because of the relative ease with which the iridotomy can be performed.
    Preoperative Care
    Pilocarpine to constrict the pupil and an α agonist (apraclonidine or brimonidine) to minimize bleeding and blunt any IOP spike.
    Contact Lens
    Abraham off-center button lens or similar magnifying lens (CC-I 1.4).
    Location of Treatment
    11 o'clock or 1 o'clock (12 o'clock may lead to bubbles that obscure viewing). A lower location may increase the likelihood of ghost images. The far periphery is ideal, as the iris is thinnest in those regions.

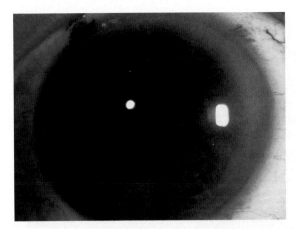

FIGURE 3.92. Biomicroscopic confirmation of iridotomy.

Power
6.0 mJ
Bursts
1 to 3
Total Number of Shots
1 to 6 on average (brown greater than blue)
End Point
Posterior pigment blows into the anterior chamber. Special situation with a bleeding diathesis (aspirin or Coumadin), for example: Pretreat with the argon laser to coagulate and protect against potential bleeding. The argon settings are: power, 400 to 800 mW; size, 50 to 100 μm; number, 20 to 40; duration, 1.0 seconds.

Patient must look to side to avoid macular burn.

Potential Complications

- corneal abrasion
- hyphema
- uveitis
- IOP spike
- ghost image

Postoperative Care
α Agonist pre- and posttreatment. Topical steroid or nonsteroidal antiinflammatory agent four times a day for 4 days.
Measurement of Success
Gonioscopic confirmation that angle is deeper. Transillumination is an unreliable means of confirming iridotomy patency. Must be able to see the iridotomy is full thickness (Fig. 3.92).

Laser Trabeculoplasty

Goal
Reduction of intraocular pressure by enhancing outflow through the trabecular meshwork.
Indications
Open angle with clear visualization of angle structures, good prognosis. Diagnosis of POAG, "low-tension glaucoma," pigmentary glaucoma, or pseudoexfoliation glaucoma. Age: the older the better, the exception being with pigmentary glaucoma. Trabecular meshwork pigmentation, heavy, greater than light.
Technique
Argon laser predominates, although diode- and frequency-doubled Nd:YAG laser also have been found to be equally effective.
Preoperative Treatment
α Agonists.
Lens
Single or three-mirrored Goldmann lens or a Ritch lens.
Location
Spots at the junction of pigmented trabecular meshwork with 180 degrees or 360 degrees of angle being treated at one sitting—360 degrees in most cases, 180 degrees in high-risk cases (Fig. 3.93A, B).
End Point
Mild blanching of trabecular meshwork.

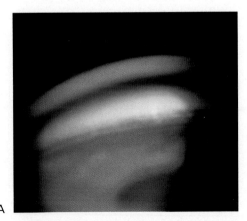

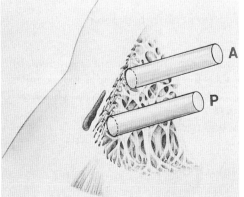

FIGURE 3.93. A: Spots at the junction of pigmented trabecular meshwork with 180 degrees or 360 degrees of angle being treated. **B:** Location of anterior (A) and posterior (B) beam placement.

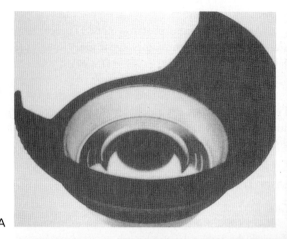

A

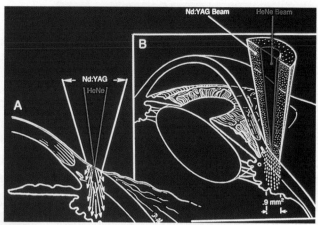

B

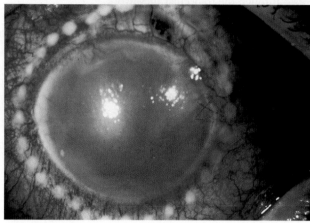

C

FIGURE 3.94. A: Shields lens. **B:** Focus of beam on ciliary body. **C:** External appearance of eye after cyclophotocoagulation.

Power
200 to 800 mW.
Size
50 μm.
Number of Shots
Total of 70 to 100 over 360 degrees.
Potential Complications

- corneal abrasion
- IOP spike
- hyphema
- uveitis
- discomfort (inadvertent ciliary body shots)

Postoperative Care
α Agonists posttreatment, topical steroid or nonsteroidal agent four times a day for 4 days. Examine at 1 week and 4 weeks.
Measure of Success
Determined at 4 to 6 weeks after the laser.

Cyclophotocoagulation

Goal
IOP reduction by partial ciliary body ablation, which slows aqueous production.

Indications
Eyes with limited visual potential, or those that are not candidates for laser trabeculoplasty or filtering surgery, such as those with neovascular glaucoma or multiple intraocular surgeries.

Technique
Three commonly used delivery systems:

1. Slit-lamp delivery (YAG laser on thermal mode)
   Lens: Shields lens (Fig. 3.94A–C)
   Power: 4 to 6 J
   No. shots: 30 to 40 over 360 degrees
2. Contact probe (diode G probe) (Fig. 3.95A–C)
   Power: 5 to 7 W, 1 to 2 seconds
   No. shots: 18 over 360 degrees
3. Endoscopic (diode or argon) limbal incision with intraocular probe (Fig. 3.96)
   Power: 400 to 800 mW, 1 second
   No. shots: 30 to 40 over 360 degrees

Potential Complications

- uveitis
- phthisis
- sympathetic ophthalmia
- vitreous hemorrhage

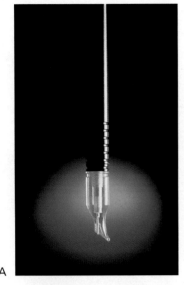
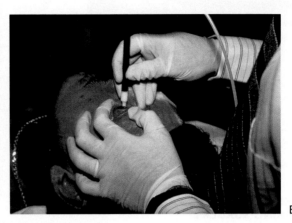
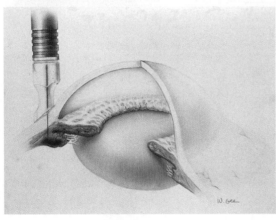

FIGURE 3.95. A: Diode G probe. **B:** Placement of G probe. **C:** Artist's side view of G probe application.

- globe perforation, especially in thin scleral regions that appear blue
- endophthalmitis (for the endoscopic delivery system)
- cataract

Measure of Success

It usually takes 4 to 6 weeks to evaluate the full effect of treatment. If it is inadequate, additional applications of cyclophotocoagulation can be tried.

Postoperative Care

Cycloplegic and topical steroids given over 1 to 3 months.

Incisional Surgery

Guarded Filtering Surgery

Goal

Create an alternative pathway for aqueous into the subconjunctival space, which leads to a filtering bleb.

Indications

Whenever medication and/or laser treatment has proven ineffective or is not indicated. Adequate conjunctival tissue

at the limbus is required for procedure. Table 3.19 lists the risk factors for failure of guarded filtering surgery.

Technique

Guarded filtering surgery (trabeculectomy) has replaced full-thickness operations such as thermosclerostomy or posterior lip sclerectomy because of the lower complication rate, such as flat anterior chambers and suprachoroidal hemorrhages.

1. Conjunctival flap (Fig. 3.97A, B). A limbal- (A) or fornix-based (B) conjunctival flap may be used with comparable success rates, although with different bleb morphologies, in that a limbal flap has more localized bleb, and a fornix flap has a more diffuse, flatter bleb.
2. Antimetabolite use. Risk factor assessment helps determine the need and extent of antimetabolite use to minimize conjunctival scarring (see Table 3.20).
3. Scleral flap (Fig. 3.98). A one-half-thickness flap is raised with the hinge at the limbus. The size, shape, and thickness of the scleral flap have not proven to be critical determinants of success.
4. Paracentesis. Using a 25-gauge needle, a clear corneal paracentesis tract is created.

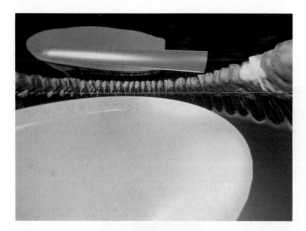

FIGURE 3.96. Endoscopic limbal incision with intraocular probe.

TABLE 3-19. RISK FACTORS FOR FAILURE OF GUARDED FILTERING SURGERY

- African-American
- Pseudophakic or aphakic
- Uveitis
- Previous filtering surgery
- Previous eye surgery such as retinal detachment or pars plana vitrectomy
- Regression of neovascular glaucoma
- Noncompliance
- Multiple eyedrop regimens; long-term eyedrop use
- Severe glaucomatous injury requiring a very low intraocular pressure
- Age less than 20 years

5. Sclerectomy. The sclerectomy is placed eccentrically, close to the edge of the scleral flap (Fig. 3.99). This ensures a good amount of flow into the subconjunctival space of the region. The corneoscleral bloc can be excised free hand, or it can be "punched out" with a scleral punch on the inferior wound edge.

6. Peripheral iridectomy. A generous iridectomy prevents iris plugging up the sclerostomy site.

7. Scleral flap sutures. Sutures are placed into the scleral flap with the intent of cutting or releasing the sutures in the postoperative period to encourage further subconjunctival filtration. There are two ways suture may be cut preoperatively:

TABLE 3-20. SUGGESTED ANTIMETABOLITE USE DEPENDING ON DEGREE OF RISK OF FAILURE

Risk for Failure	Antimetabolite Use
1. Low	None
2. Some	5-fluorouracil soak for 2 minutes
3. Moderate	5-fluorouracil soak for 5 minutes
4. Considerable	Mitomycin soak for 1 minute
5. High	Mitomycin soak for 3 minutes

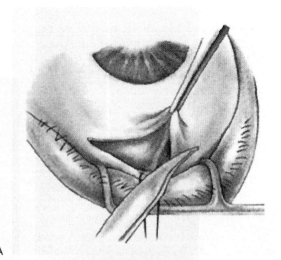

A

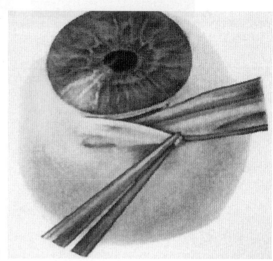

B

FIGURE 3.97. A: Limbal-based conjunctival flap in guarded filtration procedure. **B:** Fornix-based conjunctival flap.

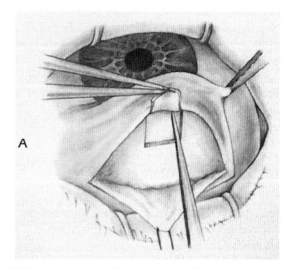

A

FIGURE 3.98. Scleral flap in guarded filtration procedure.

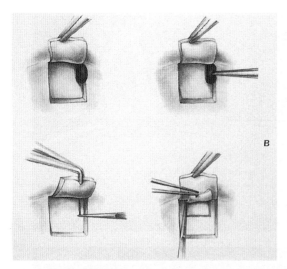

FIGURE 3.99. The sclerectomy is placed eccentrically, close to the edge of the scleral flap.

i. *Laser suture lysis* using argon or diode laser. Lens: Hoskins (Fig. 3.100) or a Ritch compression lens. Setting: .05 seconds. Power: 200 to 800 mW. Spot size: 75 μm. Special situation: If the conjunctiva is hemorrhagic, then a diode is preferred because of less heat absorption into the subconjunctival tissue, which may lead to a hole and possible leak.

ii. *Releasable externalized sutures* (Fig. 3.101A–D). Sutures may be preplaced so that they can be easily retrieved and removed to release the scleral flap at that position. A commonly used releasable suture is one in which a slipknot is placed prior to the suture being exteriorized into the cornea and passed in such a fashion that only the elbow of the suture is exposed. In this way, that elbow can be grasped in the post-

operative period and pulled, releasing and opening up the scleral flap in that region.

8. Assessment of outflow irrigating through the paracentesis tract. The anterior chamber is reformed and a slow leakage should be evident at the trabeculectomy site.

9. Conjunctiva closure (Fig. 3.102A, B). Using an absorbable suture, such as 8-0 Vicryl, the conjunctiva is closed in a locking, running fashion for Tenon's layers and in a running, nonlocking, manner for the conjunctiva. A vascular needle tip is preferred when available, so as to minimize the chance of creating a hole in the conjunctiva that may lead to a bleb leak.

10. Evaluating bleb integrity. Upon irrigating through the paracentesis tract through the anterior chamber, three events ideally should occur: (1) the eye should firm up slightly before softening spontaneously; (2) the anterior chamber should deepen and not shallow after reformation; and (3) the bleb should form and remain elevated.

Potential Complications

Intraoperatively: suprachoroidal hemorrhage, subconjunctival buttonhole. Postoperatively: suprachoroidal hemorrhage, bleb infection—endophthalmitis, flat anterior chamber with choroidal attachments, bleb failure, hypotony maculopathy (Table 3.21).

Postoperative Care

Laser suture lysis or release. Timing: with no antimetabolite may be up to 2 weeks; with 5-FU, up to 1 month; with mitomycin C, 2 months or longer, will still often give an adequate response.

Measure of Success

IOP at desired target level with a functioning limbal filtering bleb without visual loss or discomfort.

Postoperative Care

Cycloplegia and topical antibiotic. Topical steroids are given on a tapering schedule over a 4- to 8-week period.

Tube Shunts (See Table 3.22)

Goal

Lowering IOP by shunting aqueous from the anterior chamber into the subconjunctival space.

Indications

- refractory glaucoma not amenable to trabeculectomy
- neovascular glaucoma
- previously failed guarded filtering procedure
- uveitis
- contact-lens wearer with a fear of limbal bleb infection
- extensive limbal scarring from previous ocular surgery

Technique (using the Baerveldt shunt as an example)

1. Conjunctival incision (either a fornix-based or conjunctival flap can be fashioned) (Fig. 3.103)

2. Preparation of the tube ligature. A 4-0 nylon suture is placed inside the lumen of the tube (Fig. 3.104). An external 6-0 Vicryl suture is tied externally around the tube. If the tube is totally occluded, a 1- to 2-mm vent-

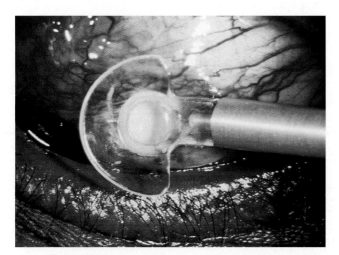

FIGURE 3.100. Laser suture lysis with a Hoskins lens.

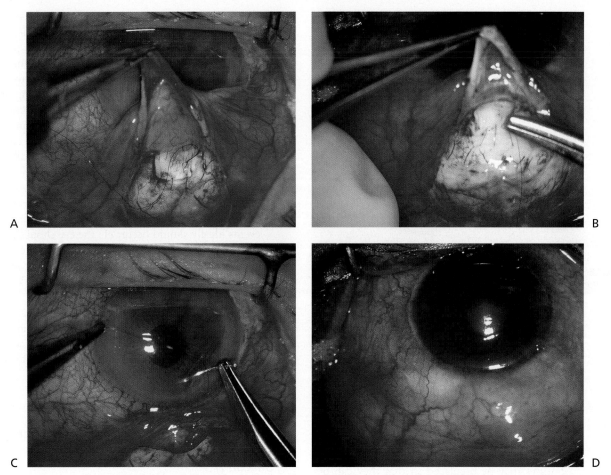

FIGURE 3.101. A–D: Four steps in placement of releasable externalized sutures.

ing slit may be put in the proximal portion of the tube with a Sharp blade. These vents act as "pseudovalves." Alternatively, the external ligature tension can be adjusted to titrate outflow rather than totally obstructing it.

3. Superotemporal quadrant optimal location. Superior and lateral recti are identified with a muscle hook. The reservoir is placed, with the wings of the reservoir un-

derneath the recti. The reservoir is secured to the globe with two 6-0 Mersilene sutures.

4. The tube is trimmed to desired length and placed in the anterior chamber through the paracentesis tract previously made by a 23-gauge needle. The placement of the tube should leave 1 to 2 mm of the distal end in the anterior chamber, with no iris or corneal touch (Fig. 3.105).

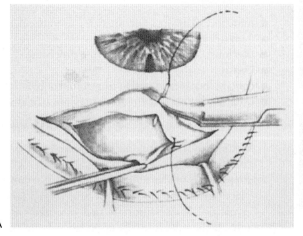 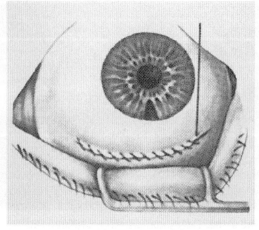

FIGURE 3.102. A, B: Two steps in conjunctiva closure in guarded filtration procedure.

TABLE 3-21. TROUBLESHOOTING LIST POSTOPERATIVELY

Intraocular Pressure	Bleb	Anterior Chamber Depth	Problem
Elevated	Flat	Deep	Failure of trabeculectomy flap
		Shallow	Aqueous misdirection or suprachoroidal hemorrhage
Low	High	Deep or shallow	Overfiltration
Low	Flat	Shallow or deep	Bleb leak
Low	Low	Shallow	Choroidal detachment

TABLE 3-22. TUBE SHUNTS CURRENTLY AVAILABLE

Type	Size (mm²)	Valve
Molteno		
Single plate	135	No
Double plate	270	No
Baerveldt	250, 350, 425	No
Krupin	185	Yes
Ahmed	185	Yes

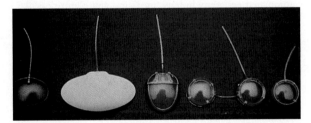

FIGURE 3.103. Conjunctival incision for placing the Baerveldt shunt.

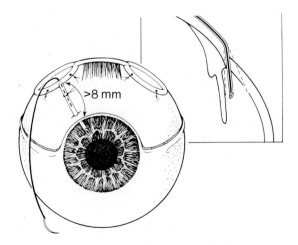

FIGURE 3.104. A 4-0 nylon suture is placed inside the lumen of the Baerveldt shunt tube.

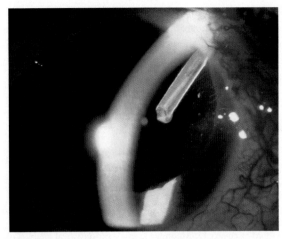

FIGURE 3.105. Placement of the tube leaves 1 to 2 mm of the distal end in the anterior chamber, with no iris or corneal touch.

5. The donor patch graft (either cadaver or autologous sclera, pericardium, or fascia lata) is placed over the tube to prevent later tube erosion through the conjunctiva (Fig. 3.106).
6. The conjunctiva is closed with an absorbable suture such as Vicryl.

The Ahmed tube shunt placement is similar to that of the Baerveldt with two exceptions: (1) the valve is primed by injecting fluid through the tube, which opens up the valve, composed of two adjacent membranes; and (2) the reservoir is placed between the two recti muscles rather than underneath them.

Potential Complications

- suprachoroidal hemorrhage
- aqueous misdirection
- flat anterior chamber
- choroidal detachments
- choroidal edema
- tube erosion—extrusions
- tube retraction from the anterior chamber

Postoperative Care

Cycloplegics and antibiotics for 1 to 2 weeks. A topical steroid may be used for 2 months. It is prudent to defer

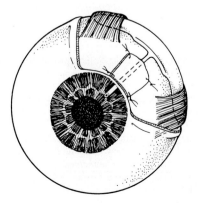

FIGURE 3.106. Donor patch graft is glaced over the tube.

pulling the intraluminal suture until conditions are ideal, usually 1 month postoperatively. It is removed by making a small cut down in the conjunctiva to externalize the distal end of the suture, grabbing the suture with a forceps and gently pulling it out.

BIBLIOGRAPHY

Anderson DR, Cynader MS. Glaucomatous optic nerve cupping as an optic neuropathy. *Clin Neurosci* 1997;4:274.

Anderson DR, Patella VM. Automated static perimetry. 2nd ed. St. Louis: Mosby; 1999:278.

Armaly M. Ocular pressure and visual fields. *Arch Ophthalmol* 1969;81:25.

Armaly M, Krueger D, Maunder L, et al. Biostatistical analysis of the Collaborative Glaucoma Study. *Arch Ophthalmol* 1980;98:2163.

Azuara-Blanco A, Spaeth GL, Nicholl J, Lanzl M, Augsburger JJ. Comparison between laser scanning tomography and computerized image analysis of the optic disc. *Br J Ophthalmol* 1999;83:295.

Azuara-Blanco A, Harris A, Cantor LB. Reproducibility of optic disk topographic measurements with the Topcon Imagenet and the Heidelberg Retina Tomograph. *Ophthalmologica* 1998;212:95.

Becker B, Morton W. Topical epinephrine in glaucoma suspects. *Am J Ophthalmol* 1966;62:272.

Behrendt T, Wilson LA. Spectral reflectance photography of the retina. *Am J Ophthalmol* 1965;59;1079.

Boes DA, Spaeth GL, Mills RP, Smith M, Nicholl JE, Clifton BC. Relative optic cup depth assessments using three stereo photograph viewing methods. *J Glaucoma* 1996;5:9.

Bowd C, Weinreb RN, Williams JM, Zangwill LM. The retinal nerve fiber layer thickness in ocular hypertensive, normal, and glaucomatous eyes with optical coherence tomography. *Arch Ophthalmol* 2000;188:22.

Brusini P, Busatto P. Frequency doubling perimetry in glaucoma early diagnosis. *Acta Ophthalmol Scand Suppl* 1998;227:23.

Campbell DG. Pigmentary dispersion and glaucoma. A new theory. *Arch Ophthalmol* 1979;79:1667.

Cartwright MJ, Anderson DR. Correlation of asymmetric damage with asymmetric intraocular pressure in normal-tension glaucoma (low-tension glaucoma). *Arch Ophthalmol* 1988;106:898.

Chauhan B, Drance S, Douglas G. The effect of long-term intraocular pressure reduction on the differential light sensitivity in glaucoma suspects. *Invest Ophthalmol Vis Sci* 1988;29:1478.

Collaborative Normal-Tension Glaucoma Study Group. Comparison of glaucomatous progression between untreated patients with normal-tension glaucoma and patients with therapeutically reduced intraocular pressures. *Am J Ophthalmol* 1998;126:487.

Collaborative Normal-Tension Glaucoma Study Group. The effectiveness of intraocular pressure reduction in the treatment of normal-tension glaucoma. *Am J Ophthalmol* 1998;126:498.

Daubs J, Crick R. Effect of refractive error on the risk of ocular hypertension and open-angle glaucoma. *Trans Ophthalmol Soc UK* 1981;101:121.

Davanger M, Ringvold A, Blika S. The probability of having glaucoma at different IOP levels. *Acta Ophthalmol (Copenh)* 1991;69:565.

David R, Livingston D, Luntz MH. Ocular hypertension: a comparative follow-up of black and white patients. *Br J Ophthalmol* 1978;62:676.

Epstein D, Krug J, Hertzmark E, Remis L, Edelstein D. A long-term clinical trial of timolol therapy versus no treatment in the management of glaucoma suspects. *Ophthalmology* 1989;96:1460.

Glaucoma Laser Trial Research Group. The glaucoma laser trial (GLT) and glaucoma laser trial follow-up study: 7. Results. *Am J Ophthalmol* 1995;120:718.

Graham PA. The definition of pre-glaucoma. A prospective study. *Trans Ophthalmol Soc UK* 1969;88:153.

Greenfield DS, Zacharia P, Schuman JS. Comparison of Nidek 3Dx and Donaldson simultaneous stereoscopic disk photography. *Am J Ophthalmol* 1993;116:741.

Haynes WL, Alward WLM, Tello C, Liebmann JM, Ritch R. Incomplete elimination of exercise-induced pigment dispersion by laser iridotomy in pigment dispersion syndrome. *Ophthalmic Surg Lasers* 1995;26:484.

Hernandez MR, Pena JDO. The optic nerve head in glaucomatous optic neuropathy. *Arch Ophthalmol* 1997;115:389.

Hodapp E, Parrish R, Anderson D. Clinical decisions in glaucoma. St. Louis: Mosby-Year Book Inc; 1993.

Hoh ST, Greenfield DS, Mistlberger A, Liebmann JM, Ishikawa H, Ritch R. Optical coherence tomography and scanning laser polarimetry in normal, ocular hypertensive, and glaucomatous eyes. *Am J Ophthalmol* 2000;129:129.

Howe L. Photography of the interior of the eye. *Trans Am Ophthalmol Soc* 1885–7;4:568.

Hoyt WF, Newman NM. The earliest defect in glaucoma? *Lancet* 1972;1:692.

Jacobi PC, Krieglstein GK. Trabecular aspiration, a new mode to treat pseudoexfoliation glaucoma. *Invest Ophthalmol Vis Sci* 1995;36:2270.

Jaeger E. Ueber Staar and Sarroperationen 1854. Verlag von L.W. Seidel.

Jaeger E. Preface to 1869 edition. In: Albert DM. Jaeger's atlas of diseases of the ocular fundus Philadelphia: WB Saunders; 1972:vii.

Jay J, Allan D. The benefit of early trabeculectomy versus conventional management in primary open-angle glaucoma relative to severity of disease. *Eye* 1989;3:528.

Jay JL, Murdoch JR. The rate of visual field loss in untreated primary open angle glaucoma. *Br J Ophthalmol* 1993;77:176.

Johnson CA, Brandt JD, Khong AM, Adams AJ. Short-wavelength automated perimetry in low-, medium-, and high-risk ocular hypertensive eyes. Initial baseline results. *Arch Ophthalmol* 1995;113:70.

Johnson DH. Options in the management of malignant glaucoma. *Arch Ophthalmol* 1998;116:799.

Kamal DS, Vismanathan AC, Garway-Heath DF, Hitchings RA, Poinoosawmy D, Bunce C. Detection of optic disc change with the Heidelberg retina tomograph before confirmed visual field change intraocular hypertensives converting to early glaucoma. *Br J Ophthalmol* 1999;83:290.

Karickhoff JR. Pigmentary dispersion syndrome and pigmentary glaucoma: A new mechanism concept, a new treatment, and a new technique. *Ophthalmic Surg* 1992;23:169.

Kass M, Gordon M, Hoff M, et al. Topical timolol administration reduces the incidence of glaucomatous damage in ocular hypertensive individuals. A randomized, double-masked, long-term clinical trial. *Arch Ophthalmol* 1989;107:1590.

Kass M, Kolker A, Becker B. Prognostic factors in glaucomatous visual field loss. *Arch Ophthalmol* 1976;94:1274.

Katz J, Tielsch JM, Quigley HA, Sommer A. Automated perimetry detects visual field loss before manual Goldmann perimetry. *Ophthalmology* 1995;102:21.

Katz LJ, Spaeth GL, Cantor LB, et al. Reversible optic disc cupping and visual field improvement in adults with glaucoma. *Am J Ophthalmol* 1989;107:485.

Kitazawa Y. Prophylactic therapy of ocular hypertension: a prospective study. *Trans Ophthalmol Soc NZ* 1981;33:30.

Kitazawa Y, Horie T, Aoki S, Suzuki M, Nishioka K. Untreated ocular hypertension. A long term prospective study. *Arch Ophthalmol* 1977;95:1180.

Krohn MA, Keltner JL, Johnson CA. Comparison of photographic techniques and films used in stereophotogrammetry of the optic disc. *Am J Ophthalmol* 1979;88:859.

Kronfeld PC. Glaucoma. In: Albert DM, Edwards DD. The history of ophthalmology. Cambridge, MA: Blackwell Science; 1996:203.

Küchle M, Nguyen NX, Horn F, Naumann GO. Quantitative assessment of aqueous flare and aqueous 'cells' in pseudoexfoliation syndrome. *Acta Ophthalmol* 1992;70:201.

Leske M, Connell A, Wu S-Y, et al. Four-year incidence and progression of open-angle glaucoma—preliminary data from the Barbados Incidence Study of Eye Diseases. *Invest Ophthalmol Vis Sci* 1997;38:S728.

Lichter PR. Variability of expert observers in evaluating the optic disc. *Trans Am Ophthalmol Soc* 1977;74:532.

Liebmann JM, Weinreb RN, Ritch R. Angle-closure glaucoma associated with occult annular ciliary body detachment. *Arch Ophthalmol* 1998;116:731.

Linnér E. Ocular hypertension. I. The clinical course during ten years without therapy. Aqueous humour dynamics. *Acta Ophthalmol (Copenh)* 1976;54:707.

Migdal C, Gregory W, Hitchings R. Long-term functional outcome after early surgery compared with laser and medicine in open-angle glaucoma. Discussion. *Ophthalmology* 1994;101:1651.

Muller H. Ueber niveau-Veranderngen an der eintrittsstelle des sehnerven. *Archiv fur Ophthalmologie* 1858;4:1.

Nakla M, Nduaguba C, Rozier M, Hoffman D, Caprioli J. Comparison of imaging techniques to detect glaucomatous optic nerve damage. *Invest Ophthalmol Vis Sci* 1999;40:S397.

Nicholl JE, Lesk MR, Katz LJ, Spaeth GL, Araujo SV. Comparison of Topcon Imagenet stereometric disc analysis of the Topcon TRC-SS and Nidek 3Dx simultaneous stereoscopic fundus cameras. *Invest Ophthalmol Vis Sci* 1995;36:970.

Nordenson JW. Augenkamera zum stationaren Ophthalmoskop von Gullstrand. *Ber Dtsch Ophthalmol Ges* 1925;45:278.

Norskov K. Glaucoma screening. II. A five-year follow-up carried through in relation to a glaucoma screening among members of the Volunteer Donor Corps of the island of Falster (Denmark). *Acta Ophthalmologica Kbh* 1970;48:418.

Perkins E. The Bedford glaucoma survey. I. Long-term follow up of borderline cases. *Br J Ophthalmol* 1973;57:179.

Perkins E, Phelps C. Open angle glaucoma, ocular hypertension, low-tension glaucoma, and refraction. *Arch Ophthalmol* 1982;100:1464.

Pieroth L, Schuman JS, Hertzmark E, et al. Evaluation of focal defects of the nerve fiber layer using optical coherence tomography. *Ophthalmology* 1999;106:570.

Pohjanpelto P, Palva J. Ocular hypertension and glaucomatous optic nerve damage. *Acta Ophthalmol* 1974;52:194.

Ponte F, Giuffre G, Giammanco R, Dardanoni G. Risk factors of ocular hypertension and glaucoma. The Casteldaccia Eye Study. *Doc Ophthalmol* 1994;85:203.

Quigley HA. Better methods in glaucoma diagnosis. *Arch Ophthalmol* 1985;103:186.

Quigley HA, Duneklberger GR, Green WR. Chronic human glaucoma causing selectively greater loss of larger optic nerve fibers. *Ophthalmology* 1988;95:357.

Quigley HA, Addicks EM, Green WR. Optic nerve damage in human glaucoma. *Arch Ophthalmol* 1982;100:135.

Quigley HA, Duneklberger GR, Green WR. Retinal ganglion cell atrophy correlated with automated perimetry in human eyes with glaucoma. *Am J Ophthalmol* 1989;107:453.

Quigley HA, Enger C, Katz J, Sommer A, Scott R, Gilbert D. Risk factors for the development of glaucomatous visual field loss in ocular hypertension. *Arch Ophthalmol* 1994;112:644.

Ritch R, Liebmann J, Robin A, et al. Argon laser trabeculoplasty in pigmentary glaucoma. *Ophthalmology* 1993;100:909.

Ritch R. Pigmentary dispersion syndrome. *Am J Ophthalmol* 1998;126:442.

Rodrigues MM, Spaeth GL, Sivalingam E, et al. Value of trabeculectomy specimens in glaucoma. *Ophthalmic Surg* 1978;9(2):29.

Rosenthal AR, Kottler MS, Donaldson DD, Falconer DG. Comparative reproducibility of the digital photogrammetric procedure utilizing three methods of stereoscopic photography. *Invest Ophthalmol Vis Sci* 1977;15:54.

Schlötzer-Schrehardt UM, Koca MR, Naumann GOH, Volkholz H. Pseudoexfoliation syndrome, ocular manifestation of a systemic disorder? *Arch Ophthalmol* 1992;110:1752.

Shin D, Kolker A, Kass M, Kaback M, Becker B. Long-term epinephrine therapy of ocular hypertension. *Arch Ophthalmol* 1976;94:2059.

Shrum KR, Hattenhauer MG, Hodge D. Cardiovascular and cerebrovascular mortality associated with ocular pseudoexfoliation. *Am J Ophthalmol* 2000;129:83.

Shuttleworth GN, Khong CH, Diamond JP. A new digital optic disc stereo camera: intraobserver and interobserver repeatability of optic disc measurements. *Br J Ophthalmol* 2000;84:403.

Sommer A, Katz J, Quigley HA, et al. Clinically detectable nerve fiber layer atrophy precedes the onset of glaucomatous field loss. *Arch Ophthalmol* 1991;109:77.

Sommer A, Quigley HA, Robin AL, Miller NR, Katz J, Arkell S. Evaluation of nerve fiber layer assessment. *Arch Ophthalmol* 1984;102:1766.

Sommer A. Doyne lecture. Glaucoma: facts and fancies. *Eye* 1996;10:295.

Sommer A. Intraocular pressure and glaucoma. *Am J Ophthalmol* 1989;107:186.

Sommer A, Miller NR, Pollack I, Maumenee AE, George T. The nerve fiber layer in the diagnosis of glaucoma. *Arch Ophthalmol* 1977;95:2149.

Sommer A, Tielsch JM, Katz J, et al. Relationship between intraocular pressure and primary open angle glaucoma among white and black Americans. The Baltimore Eye Survey. *Arch Ophthalmol* 1991;109:1090.

Sörensen P, Nielsen N, Nörskov K. Ocular hypertension. A 15-year follow-up. *Acta Ophthalmol* 1978;56:363.

Tello C, Chi T, Shepps G, Liebmann J, Ritch R. Ultrasound biomicroscopy in pseudophakic malignant glaucoma. *Ophthalmology* 1993;100:1330.

Tielsch JM, Katz J, Quigley HA, Miller NR, Sommer A. Intraobserver and interobserver agreement in measurement of optic disc characteristics. *Ophthalmology* 1988;95:350.

Trope GE, Pavlin CJ, Bau A, Baumal CR, Foster FS. Malignant glaucoma: clinical and ultrasound biomicroscopic characteristics. *Ophthalmology* 1994;101:1030.

Tsai JC, Barton KA, Mioller MH, Khaw PT, Hitchings RA. Surgical results in malignant glaucoma refractory to medical or laser therapy. *Eye* 1997;11:677.

Varma R, Spaeth GL, Hanau C, Steinmann WC, Feldman RM. Positional changes in the vasculature of the optic disc in glaucoma. *Am J Ophthalmol* 1987;104:45.

Vesti E, Kivel AT. Exfoliation syndrome and exfoliation glaucoma. *Prog Retin Eye Res* 2000;19:345.

Vogt A. Die Nervenfaserstreifung der menschlichen netzhaut mit besonderer berucksichtigung der differentialdiagnose gegenuber pathologischen streifenformigen reflexen (praretinalen faltelungen). *Klin Monatsbl Augenheilkd* 1917:58:399.

Walker W. Ocular hypertension. Follow-up of 109 cases from 1963 to 1974. *Trans Ophthalmol Soc UK* 1974;94:525.

Wang JJ, Mitchell P, Smith W. Is there an association between migraine headache and open-angle glaucoma? Findings from the Blue Mountains Eye Study. *Ophthalmology* 1997;104:1714.

Weber A. Ein fall von partieller hyperamie der choroidea beieinem kanninchen. *Archiv fur Ophthalmologie* 1855;2:133.

Wilensky J, Podos S, Becker B. Prognostic indicators in ocular hypertension. *Arch Ophthalmol* 1974;91:200.

Wilson MR, Hertzmark E, Walker AM, Childs-Shaw K, Epstein DL. A case-control study of risk factors in open angle glaucoma. *Arch Ophthalmol* 1987;105:1066.

Zeyen T. Target pressures in glaucoma. In: Gramer E, Grehn F. Pathogenesis and risk factors of glaucoma. Berlin: Springer; 1999:209.

VITREORETINAL DISORDERS

Carl D. Regillo
William E. Benson
Neal H. Atebara

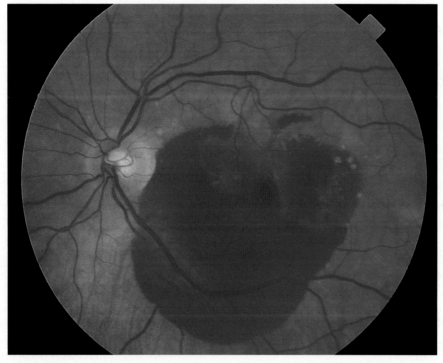

A 67-year-old woman with age-related macular degeneration and sudden visual acuity loss in her left eye. There is subretinal pigment epithelial hemorrhage in the macular from underlying choroidal neovascularization.

ANATOMIC CONSIDERATIONS

Layers of the Retina

The *retinal pigment epithelium* (RPE) is a single layer of melanin-containing cells that extends from the optic nerve to the ora serrata and continues anteriorly as the pigment epithelium of the pars plana (Fig. 4.1A). The RPE is separated from the choriocapillaris by Bruch's membrane. The basement membrane of the RPE forms the inner layer of Bruch's membrane. The layer of rods and cones is formed by the outer and inner segments of the photoreceptor cells (i.e., rods and cones). The outer segments of these cells contain visual pigment molecules that absorb light energy and propagate a nerve impulse.

The *external limiting membrane* is not a true membrane; it is composed of a series of intercellular connections called zonulae adherentes that unite the plasma membranes of adjacent photoreceptors and Müller's cells. This fenestrated membrane separates the outer segments of the rods and cones from their cell bodies and nuclei that form the *outer nuclear layer*.

The axons of the rods and cones and the dendrites of the bipolar cells form, and synapse within, the *outer plexiform layer*, which also includes processes of the horizontal cells and Müller's cells. The bipolar cells receive the visual impulse from the rods and cones and are considered the first-order neurons. The *inner nuclear layer* consists of the cell bodies and nuclei of bipolar, amacrine, Müller's, and horizontal cells.

The *inner plexiform layer* is the zone of synapse between the axons of the bipolar cells and the dendrites of the second-order neurons, the ganglion cells. Processes of amacrine, ganglion, Müller's, and bipolar cells are also contained in this layer. The *ganglion cell layer* contains the cell bodies and nuclei of the ganglion cells. The axons of these ganglion cells form the *nerve fiber layer*. These axons course through the retina and gather to form the optic nerve. The visual impulse initiated in the photoreceptor cells is transferred to the bipolar cells, then to the ganglion cells, and does not synapse again until the lateral geniculate body. The *internal limiting membrane* separates the retina from the vitreous. A true basement membrane, the internal limiting

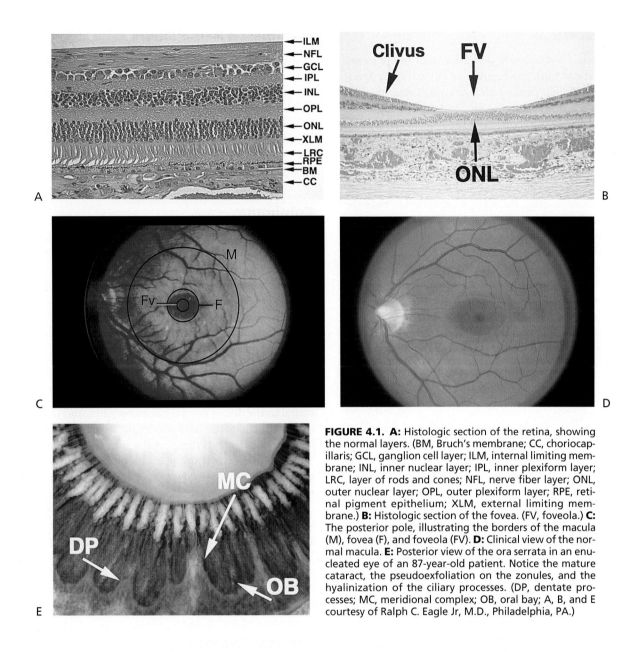

FIGURE 4.1. A: Histologic section of the retina, showing the normal layers. (BM, Bruch's membrane; CC, choriocapillaris; GCL, ganglion cell layer; ILM, internal limiting membrane; INL, inner nuclear layer; IPL, inner plexiform layer; LRC, layer of rods and cones; NFL, nerve fiber layer; ONL, outer nuclear layer; OPL, outer plexiform layer; RPE, retinal pigment epithelium; XLM, external limiting membrane.) **B:** Histologic section of the fovea. (FV, foveola.) **C:** The posterior pole, illustrating the borders of the macula (M), fovea (F), and foveola (FV). **D:** Clinical view of the normal macula. **E:** Posterior view of the ora serrata in an enucleated eye of an 87-year-old patient. Notice the mature cataract, the pseudoexfoliation on the zonules, and the hyalinization of the ciliary processes. (DP, dentate processes; MC, meridional complex; OB, oral bay; A, B, and E courtesy of Ralph C. Eagle Jr, M.D., Philadelphia, PA.)

membrane is derived chiefly from the footplates of the giant glial cells of Müller that extend between the internal and external limiting membranes.

Macula

The Anatomic Macula

There are important anatomic modifications in the macula that subserve the highest level of visual efficiency and color perception. Histologically, the macula is the region of the posterior retina in which the ganglion cell layer is more than one cell layer thick (Fig. 4.1B). This area is about 6 mm in diameter. The central portion of the macula is the *fovea* or pit. It is 1.5 mm wide (i.e., 1 disc diameter) and consists of a sloping area of *clivus* and the *foveola*, which is the floor of the concavity. The foveola is 0.33 mm wide. The RPE cells in the fovea are tall and narrow. In the foveola, the layer of rods and cones and the outer nuclear layer consist entirely of specialized cone cells. These cone cells are tall and narrow, densely packed, and resemble rod cells. Their nuclei are multilayered in the outer nuclear layer. Rod cells and the inner retinal layers are added progressively along the clivus of the fovea. The internal limiting membrane remains intact but thins over the foveola. The outer plexiform layer, also called Henle's fiber layer, is obliquely oriented in the clivus. It is estimated that 10% of the total number of retinal cones are in the foveal area. The center of the fovea is devoid of blood vessels and receives its nutrients from the choriocapillaris. The outer nuclear layer and ganglion cell layer are thickest in the immediate parafoveal area.

The Clinical Macula

The macula is a somewhat ill-defined area of the posterior pole that is about 4 disc diameters wide (6 mm) and extends from the axial center of the retina to a point near the disc margin on the nasal side and to an equal radius temporally (Fig. 4.1C). The central portion of the macula is the *fovea*, which is 1 disc diameter wide. The center or floor of the foveal concavity is the *foveola*. The foveola lies 0.5 mm inferior to a line drawn horizontally through the center of the disc.

Ophthalmoscopically, the fovea appears darker than the surrounding retina because of increased concentration of pigment in the RPE (Fig. 4.1D). A circular light reflex can be seen reflected from the thickened peripheral edge of the fovea in younger individuals, and a central light spot is reflected from the pit of the foveola. The fovea sometimes appears yellowish because of a carotenoid pigment called xanthophyll in the retina. The fine arterioles and venules derived from the central retinal artery form an arcade around the fovea, but the inner portion of the fovea itself is devoid of blood vessels.

Ora Serrata

The ora serrata marks the anterior extension of the neural retina and the junction between the neurosensory retina and the pars plana of the ciliary body (Fig. 4.1E). Because the nasal retina extends farther anteriorly than the temporal retina, the ora serrata lies 6 mm posterior to the limbus on the nasal aspect of the globe and 7 mm temporally. The peripheral retina gradually thins, with a loss of distinct anatomic layers as it approaches the ora. At this point, the multilayered sensory retina becomes continuous with the monolayer of nonpigmented cells that forms the inner half of the ciliary epithelium. The RPE continues as the pigment epithelium of the ciliary body. The internal limiting membrane thins and eventually interweaves with the collagenous filaments of the vitreous base.

The ora is not uniform but is made of alternating *dentate processes* and *oral bays*, which are more prominent nasally. A dentate process is an extension of the hypoplastic peripheral retina into the ciliary body. An oral bay is a posterior extension of the pars plana into the peripheral retina. If a dentate process undergoes hypertrophy, particularly of its glial elements, in a linear configuration, the resulting entity is called a meridional fold. If this fold is contiguous with a ciliary process, the resultant structure is a *meridional complex*.

The vitreous base spans an area of 6 mm, 2 mm anterior and 4 mm posterior to the ora. In this area, vitreous fibers are tightly bound to the internal limiting membrane. This process is particularly prominent in the area of meridional folds. Disruption of the vitreous base from its attachment to the peripheral retina may produce a tear and subsequent retinal detachment.

Myelinated Nerve Fibers

Normally, the myelin covering of the optic nerve fibers stops at the lamina cribrosa (i.e., level of the sclera). Sometimes the myelin continues onto the retina, which can be seen with the ophthalmoscope. Myelinated nerve fibers appear pearly white with feathery edges (Fig. 4.2A) and assume a nerve fiber bundle configuration. They are usually attached to the disc but may appear anywhere in the retina. Scotomatous visual field defects of variable density may be demonstrated.

Coloboma

Clinical Features. Coloboma is a congenital condition that results from a failure of the embryonic fissure to close, and it may involve the optic nerve, retina, and choroid. Anterior segment structures also may be involved. The inner and outer layers of the optic cup are abnormal in this area of faulty closure. The outer layer (i.e., RPE) is usually absent, and the choroid fails to develop. The inner layer, which gives rise to the sensory retina, is often present but attenuated. However, blood vessels often can be seen coursing through the defect.

Retinochoroidal colobomas are located inferior or inferonasal to the disc. They are glistening white and sharply demarcated, and some have patchy pigmentation. They may be isolated or may extend to the inferior periphery (Fig. 4.2B, C). Breaks may occur within or at the edge of the attenuated sensory retina over the coloboma and can result in rhegmatogenous retinal detachment.

Retinochoroidal colobomas are frequently associated with chromosomal abnormalities or multisystem diseases such as trisomy 13 and Goldenhar's syndrome.

Management. No treatment is available for this congenital anomaly or prevention of retinal breaks and detachments. Rhegmatogenous retinal detachments that occasionally develop are repaired with vitrectomy techniques.

Asteroid Hyalosis

Asteroid hyalosis is a degenerative process within the vitreous, characterized by large numbers of whitish, suspended, spherical opacities (Fig. 4.2D and E).

Clinical Features. Viewed through the ophthalmoscope, these vitreous opacities are more numerous and more uniform than those associated with the age-related vitreous liquefaction process. The condition is unilateral in 75% of patients and is more common among those older than 60 years of age. The composition is thought to be consistent with calcium-containing lipid. There is no known cause and no association with systemic or other ocular disease.

Patients occasionally complain of a film in front of their vision but are amazingly asymptomatic considering the debris seen by the ophthalmologist. Asteroid hyalosis almost never causes a significant loss of vision.

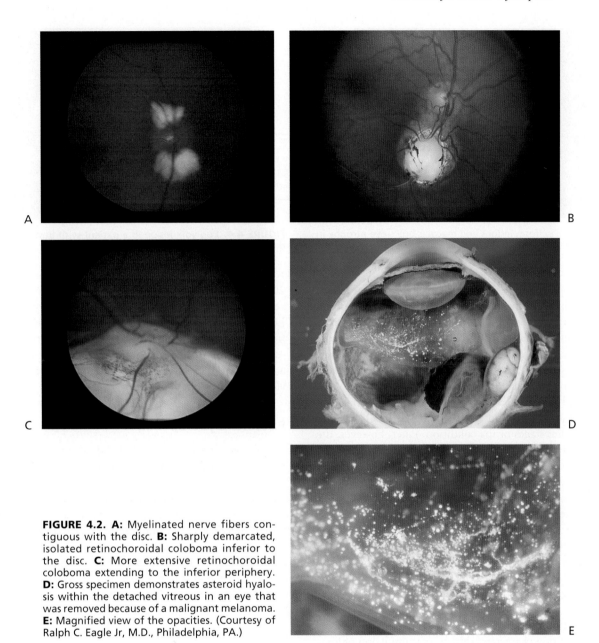

FIGURE 4.2. A: Myelinated nerve fibers contiguous with the disc. **B:** Sharply demarcated, isolated retinochoroidal coloboma inferior to the disc. **C:** More extensive retinochoroidal coloboma extending to the inferior periphery. **D:** Gross specimen demonstrates asteroid hyalosis within the detached vitreous in an eye that was removed because of a malignant melanoma. **E:** Magnified view of the opacities. (Courtesy of Ralph C. Eagle Jr, M.D., Philadelphia, PA.)

Management. No treatment needed as asteroid hyalosis is asymptomatic.

HEREDITARY MACULAR DYSTROPHIES

Stargardt's Disease

Stargardt's disease is an inherited disease in which the quantity of lipofuscin pigment in all RPE cells is markedly increased. The disease is also referred to as fundus flavimaculatus, especially when the yellow flecks dominate the clinical picture (see below). The vast majority of Stargardt's cases are autosomal recessive, and the genetic defect has been traced to mutations in the ABCR gene.

Clinical Features. The onset of the disease occurs between 6 and 20 years of age. The initial symptom is decreased visual acuity. In advanced cases, there may be decreased night vision. When visual acuity is first diminished, the macula may appear normal, and the diagnosis may be extremely difficult to make. Later, mild periforeal pigment epithelial atrophy is detected. Still later, the atrophic changes may progress to a bull's-eye appearance. In some cases, the pigment epithelium is diffusely atrophic.

Focal hyperaccumulations of lipofuscin account for the characteristic pisciform (i.e., fish-like) yellow flecks (Fig. 4.3). These may be localized to the macula, scattered throughout the postequatorial area, or absent. Over time, some disappear, and new ones appear. Fluorescein angiography shows areas of hyperfluorescence that do not neces-

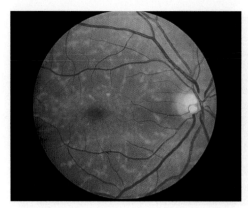

FIGURE 4.3. Pisciform lesions and macular bull's-eye atrophy in patient with Stargardt's disease.

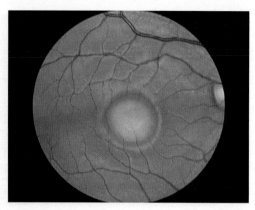

FIGURE 4.4. Egg yolk lesion in a patient with Best's vitelliform dystrophy.

sarily correspond to the flecks seen on clinical examination. Another important finding is that the diffuse pattern of hyperconcentrated lipofuscin in pigment epithelial cells partially blocks the background choroidal fluorescence normally seen on fluorescein angiography. This "dark or silent choroid" is seen in 85% of cases. Some cases are complicated by secondary choroidal neovascularization (CNV).

Electrophysiologic testing typically shows a normal electroretinogram (ERG) and electrooculogram (EOG), especially in earlier stages of the condition. Later, however, the ERG may be mildly to moderately decreased. The visual prognosis is poor. Most patients have a visual acuity of 20/200 or worse by 40 years of age.

Young patients without the flecks are often misdiagnosed as malingerers or hysterics. Cone dystrophy, which is discussed later in the chapter, must be ruled out.

Management. Periodic monitoring, genetic counseling, and support for low vision constitute management.

Best's Vitelliform Dystrophy

Best's vitelliform dystrophy is an autosomal dominantly inherited condition characterized by the accumulation of lipofuscin in RPE cells throughout the fundus and especially in the macula. The genetic defect has recently been shown to be a mutation in a novel retina-specific gene (VMD2) located on chromosome 12. Electrophysiologically, the condition is characterized by diffuse RPE dysfunction (see below).

Clinical Features. The most common fundus finding is the "egg yolk" macular lesion (Fig. 4.4), which is hypofluorescent on fluorescein angiography. It has been observed in patients as young as 1 week of age, but the fundus may be normal until middle age. Some patients have multiple, yellow lesions (i.e., multifocal Best's dystrophy). Most patients' eyes are hyperopic, and many are symptom free, even if the egg yolk appearance is present. With time, the lesion may progress to a "pseudohypopyon" stage. The most common late finding is the "scrambled egg" stage, which may or may not be associated with a CNV.

Unless CNV occurs, the visual prognosis is good (i.e.,

20/50 to 20/100). Best's vitelliform dystrophy is one of a very few conditions in which the ERG is normal but the EOG is abnormal. This condition should be differentiated from adult-onset foveomacular vitelliform dystrophy.

Management. Periodic monitoring, genetic counseling, and support of low vision constitute management of Best's vitelliform dystrophy.

Pattern Dystrophies

The pattern dystrophies include adult-onset foveomacular vitelliform dystrophy, butterfly dystrophy, reticular dystrophy of the pigment epithelium, and coarse pigment mottling in the macula (i.e., fundus pulverulentus). Most forms are inherited as an autosomal dominant trait. A few patients have different patterns in opposite eyes, and some progress from one pattern to another. In some pedigrees, family members express different patterns. For these reasons, it is thought that they all are probably expressions of the same disorder. Mutations in the peripherin/RDS gene have been found in some patients but not others.

Adult-Onset Foveomacular Vitelliform Dystrophy

Adult-onset foveomacular vitelliform dystrophy (AOFVD) is characterized by a slightly elevated, round, yellow lesion at the level of the RPE. The lesion often will have a small, pigmented dot in its center (Fig. 4.5).

Clinical Features. The lesions are usually bilateral and are about one third to one half of the disc diameter. Sometimes, there are adjacent small, yellow flecks. The lesions are hypofluorescent on fluorescein angiography but often have a hyperfluorescent ring. Symptoms such as metamorphopsia or slightly decreased vision usually do not appear until middle age, but many patients remain asymptomatic for life. The prognosis is excellent, except for the occasional case in which CNV develops.

Best's vitelliform dystrophy may closely resemble AOFVD, especially when the AOFVD lesions are large, but the EOG results in AOFVD are normal or only slightly re-

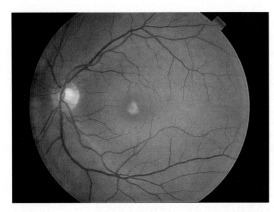

FIGURE 4.5. Central yellow deposit in a patient with pattern dystrophy.

duced. Many patients are misdiagnosed as having a pigment epithelial detachment (PED) caused by age-related macular degeneration (AMD). A fluorescein angiogram can distinguish AOFVD from AMD-related PED as the latter lesion would be expected to be hyperfluorescent.

Butterfly Dystrophy

Butterfly dystrophy is a pattern dystrophy in which there is irregularly branching yellow-gray pigment figure in the macula (Fig. 4.6). Like AOFVD, it is usually bilateral and symmetric and located at the level of the RPE. The visual acuity is normal or only slightly decreased. The ERG is normal, but the EOG is often moderately abnormal, indicating a widespread abnormality in the RPE. Onset may occur between the teens and middle age. As with AOFVD, the fluorescein angiogram shows the pigment figure itself to be hypofluorescent and have a surrounding hyperfluorescent halo.

Reticular Dystrophy of the Retinal Pigment Epithelium

Reticular dystrophy of the RPE is a pattern dystrophy in which the pigment pattern looks like chicken wire, and pigment sometimes extends out of the macular area.

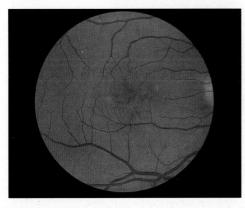

FIGURE 4.6. Deposits at the level of the pigment epithelium in a patient with butterfly dystrophy.

Cone Dystrophy

Cone dystrophy, which is inherited as an autosomal dominant trait or sporadically, is characterized by progressive deterioration of cones.

Clinical Features. The onset of symptoms has a somewhat bimodal distribution; it usually occurs between 4 and 8 years of age or between the late teens and 30 years of age. The chief presenting symptom is decreased visual acuity, but color vision also is abnormal. Photophobia (or hemeralopia) is common. Because rod function is normal or nearly normal, patients see well in dim light, but their vision deteriorates in bright light, in which rod function is suppressed and normal cone function is essential. The prognosis is poor, with most patients deteriorating to 20/200 or worse. In some cases, the condition may progress to cone-rod dystrophy with night blindness in addition to the poor central vision.

Early in the course of the disease, the macula may be normal (Fig. 4.7A) or have only mild RPE depigmentation and be indistinguishable from early cases of Stargardt's disease without pisciform lesions. ERG shows decreased cone function before any decrease in visual acuity or color vision is detected. A sensitive indicator of cone dysfunction is a decreased or flat tracing in response to a 30 cycle per second stimulus (i.e., flicker ERG). Dark adaptation shows a rod phase only. Fluorescein angiography may show small RPE

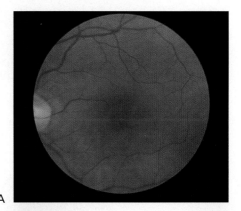

A

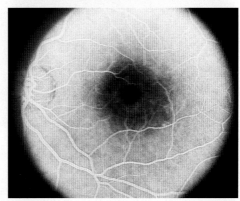

B

FIGURE 4.7. A: The fundus appears almost normal in a patient with cone dystrophy. **B:** Fluorescein angiography reveals a bull's-eye area of depigmentation of the retinal pigment epithelium.

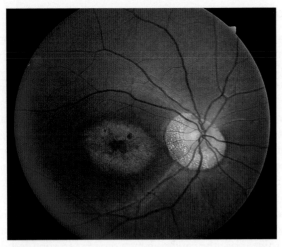

FIGURE 4.8. Severe central macular atrophy in a patient with cone dystrophy.

window-type transmission defects early in the course of the disease and establish the existence of central pigment epithelial degeneration (Fig. 4.7B). Later, there may be a bull's-eye macula, diffuse granular-appearing pigment epithelial atrophy, or geographic atrophy of the macula (Fig. 4.8).

This condition should be differentiated from Stargardt's disease, malingering, and hysteria.

Management. There is no effective treatment. Genetic counseling and low vision support should be suggested.

EXUDATIVE MACULOPATHIES

Central Serous Chorioretinopathy

Idiopathic central serous chorioretinopathy (CSCR) is a condition in which there is a small collection of relatively clear subretinal fluid in the macula (Fig. 4.9).

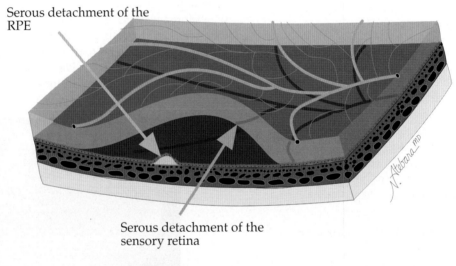

Serous detachment of the RPE

Serous detachment of the sensory retina

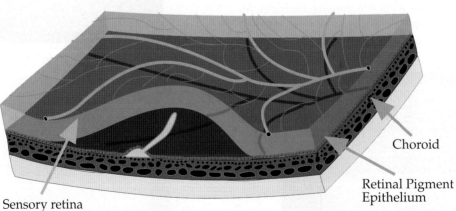

Sensory retina

Choroid

Retinal Pigment Epithelium

FIGURE 4.9. In idiopathic central serous chorioretinopathy, a small serous detachment of the retinal pigment epithelium (RPE) in the macular or paramacular area may be followed by serous detachment of the overlying and surrounding sensory retina *(top)*. Because the fluorescein leaking through the defect in the RPE is lighter than the subretinal fluid, it rises, resulting in the classic smokestack appearance *(bottom)*. (Courtesy of Neil Atebara, M.D., Philadelphia, PA.)

Clinical Features. Symptoms include metamorphopsia, micropsia, decreased color vision, and decreased visual acuity. The visual acuity occasionally is normal. If decreased, it typically improves with a pinhole or with plus lenses.

Eighty percent of cases are men, and most patients are between 30 and 50 years of age. It is rare in persons of African descent. There is no known cause, although some researchers have associated the condition with an aggressive, hard-driving, type A personality. Corticosteroids can exacerbate the condition.

On fundus examination, absence of the foveal reflex and blurring of the choroidal pattern are excellent clues to the presence of subtle subretinal fluid. When the fluid collection is more prominent, a blister-like elevation is readily appreciated with indirect ophthalmoscopy (Fig. 4.10A). By carefully positioning the slit lamp beam through a 90 or 60 diopter lens or through a Goldmann lens, the retinal elevation can be seen, and the clear nature of the subretinal fluid can be appreciated. Outer retinal yellow-white precipitates are common. Granular RPE mottling caused by past attacks may also be noticed.

On fluorescein angiography, 80% of patients show a small dot of hyperfluorescence that slowly expands (Fig. 4.10B, C). Rapid leakage of fluorescein, which rises upward in the characteristic smokestack pattern, is seen in 20% of these patients.

The most common and important differential diagnosis is CNV, which can occur in conditions such as ocular histoplasmosis and AMD. Indirect signs of CNV include hemorrhage and lipid exudate, both of which would not be expected with CSCR. Furthermore, a focal, gray-green pigmented membrane under the retina representing the CNV itself may be directly visible ophthalmoscopically. On fluorescein angiography, the neovascular vessels may be seen in the early phases, and there is usually more leakage than there is in idiopathic CSCR. Less commonly, conditions that cause serous macular detachment, such as eclampsia or Harada's disease, must be ruled out.

Management. Idiopathic CSCR usually is a benign condition. Resolution of the subretinal fluid is expected in most cases, usually within 3 to 4 months. Two thirds of patients recover 20/20 vision, although mild color vision or contrast sensitivity abnormalities may persist. Between 25% and 50% of patients have recurrent attacks. Laser photocoagulation of the leaking spot accelerates resolution of the subretinal fluid, but it does not result in better final visual acuity or better final color vision when performed early in the course of typical CSCR. Also, it does not reduce the rate of recurrence. Furthermore, in rare cases, laser therapy may result in secondary CNV. In general, laser treatment should be reserved for patients who have an occupational need for normal vision, patients with recurrences who have had permanent visual loss from previous episodes, and patients who have had attacks persisting more than 5 months.

Age-Related Macular Degeneration

AMD is a progressive deterioration of Bruch's membrane, the RPE, and the choriocapillaris. It is the leading cause of

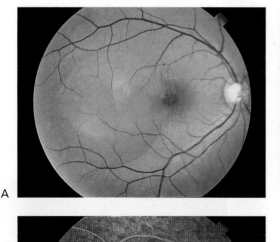
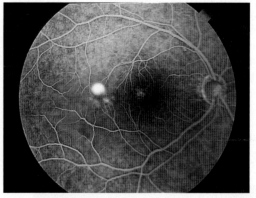

A

B

C

FIGURE 4.10. A: The serous elevation is mostly temporal to but includes the center of the macula in a patient with central serous chorioretinopathy. **B:** The middle phase of the fluorescein angiogram shows a small dot of hyperfluorescence. **C:** The late phase shows additional leakage, with some leakage into the serous elevation of the retina.

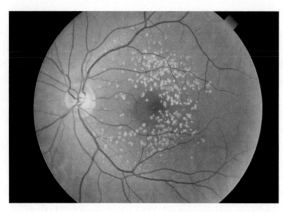

FIGURE 4.11. Multiple, hard drusen in early-stage, age-related macular degeneration.

irreversible, severe central vision loss in people over the age of 50 years in the United States. The clinical hallmark of the disease is drusen (singular: druse) in the macula. Drusen observed ophthalmoscopically represent focal accumulation of undigested products of RPE cells under the basal lamina of Bruch's membrane. Histopathologically, however, AMD is characterized by diffuse thickening of the inner aspect of Bruch's membrane.

There are two basic clinical variants of AMD: the dry, atrophic type and the wet, exudative or neovascular type. The dry type is much more common, accounting for 90% of cases, but it results in only 10% of AMD eyes that suffer severe (20/200 or worse) visual loss.

Clinical Features. "Hard" drusen are small (<64 μm) and well defined (Fig. 4.11). "Soft" drusen are larger and often have mottled overlying pigment epithelium (Fig. 4.12). On fluorescein angiography, both types are hyperfluorescent, representing either a "window defect" in the RPE or a "staining defect." They do not show leakage and, therefore, would not be expected to exhibit increasing brightness or size into the middle and late phases of the angiographic study.

The dry type produces progressive atrophy of the pigment epithelium and the choriocapillaris of varying degrees over time. Large areas of macular RPE-choriocapillaris loss

can result in severe vision loss (if the fovea is involved) and are often referred to as geographic atrophy (Fig. 4.13). Fluorescein angiography may reveal the large choroidal vessels. Again, there is no leakage of dye.

In the wet type, an exudative macular detachment occurs as a result of CNV formation and secondary leakage of fluid, lipid exudate, or blood into the subretinal or sub-RPE space (Fig. 4.14A). Typically, as the CNV grows and leaks over weeks to months, there is progressive visual loss. In most cases, subretinal fibrosis eventually sets in to some degree, and the exudative changes ultimately organize into a so-called "disciform" scar, the end stage of wet AMD (Fig. 4.14B). Larger amounts of exudation and bigger disciform scars involving the fovea usually correlate with poorer visual outcomes.

There are two basic categories of CNV growth patterns on fluorescein angiography, "classic" and "occult." Classic CNV shows up as well-defined, lacy hyperfluorescence in the early phases and demonstrates profuse late leakage (Fig. 4.15). Occult CNV can vary in its appearance but, in general, is characterized by more late-appearing and less intense fluorescein leakage. The borders of occult CNV may be well delineated or poorly delineated and can also be obscured by thick blood or rapid leakage of dye when there is an associated serous pigment epithelial detachment (Fig. 4.16). Indocyanine green angiography can sometimes be helpful as an adjunct to fluorescein angiography in detecting or better delineating the location of occult CNV (Fig. 4.17). Classic CNV tends to grow faster and result in more severe vision loss over a shorter time frame than occult CNV.

The differential diagnosis of dry AMD includes pattern macular dystrophy and old CSCR. For wet AMD, simulating conditions include active CSCR, retinal arterial macroaneurysm, and idiopathic polypoidal choroidal vasculopathy.

Management. There is no treatment for visual loss from dry AMD. Furthermore, there is no proven treatment to slow AMD progression and prevent the dry to wet transformation. There are, however, several different treatment options for wet AMD that can help reduce the risk of severe vi-

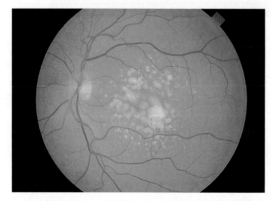

FIGURE 4.12. Multiple, soft, confluent drusen.

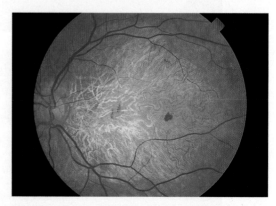

FIGURE 4.13. Dry, age-related macular degeneration with severe atrophy of the pigment epithelium and choriocapillaris.

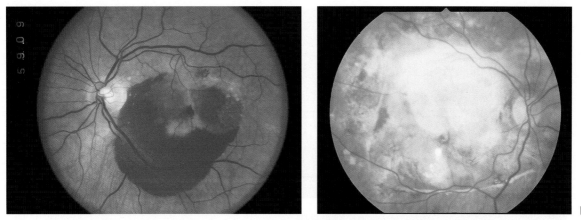

FIGURE 4.14. A: Acute exudative age-related macular degeneration with subretinal hemorrhage. **B:** End-stage exudative macular degeneration with inactive subretinal fibrosis ("disciform scar").

sion loss. Because the best results with these treatments typically come about when CNV is detected early in its development, patients with dry AMD should be monitored regularly. This is especially important for those who have eyes with high-risk features such as numerous soft drusen, focal RPE clumps, and fellow eyes with wet AMD. Patients with these features should self-monitor their central vision with an Amsler grid and be reevaluated should there be any new central visual disturbance.

Treatment of wet AMD depends on the location and

type of CNV (and may also be influenced by the associated exudative features, such as blood). In general, effective forms of treatment currently exist for CNV that is mostly "classic" and well delineated (with minimal associated blood). If the CNV is nonsubfoveal in location, then standard, ablative laser photocoagulation is the treatment of choice (Fig. 4.15). For similar-appearing CNV that has extended through the foveal center, photodynamic therapy is employed. Currently, there is no treatment proven to effectively reduce vision loss in eyes that have wet AMD with

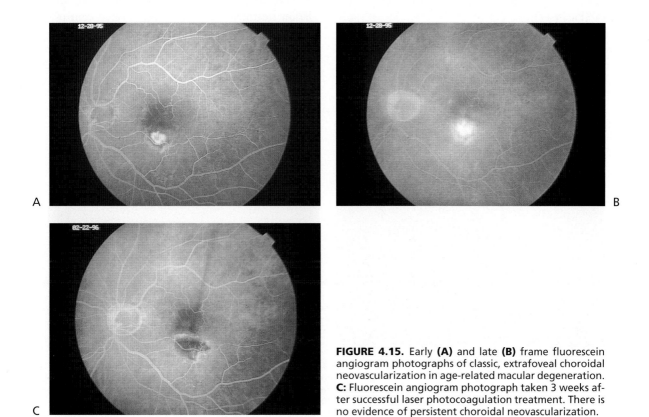

FIGURE 4.15. Early **(A)** and late **(B)** frame fluorescein angiogram photographs of classic, extrafoveal choroidal neovascularization in age-related macular degeneration. **C:** Fluorescein angiogram photograph taken 3 weeks after successful laser photocoagulation treatment. There is no evidence of persistent choroidal neovascularization.

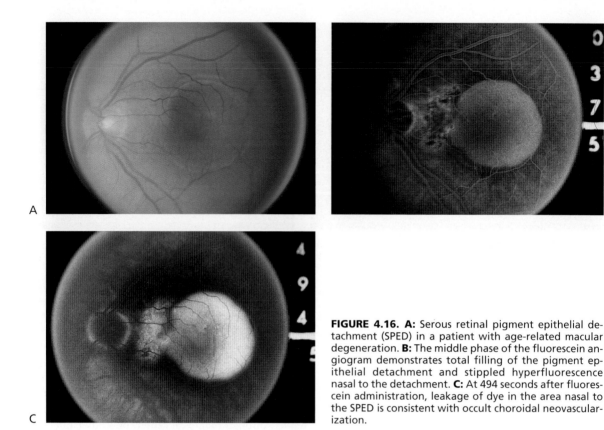

FIGURE 4.16. A: Serous retinal pigment epithelial detachment (SPED) in a patient with age-related macular degeneration. **B:** The middle phase of the fluorescein angiogram demonstrates total filling of the pigment epithelial detachment and stippled hyperfluorescence nasal to the detachment. **C:** At 494 seconds after fluorescein administration, leakage of dye in the area nasal to the SPED is consistent with occult choroidal neovascularization.

CNV that is mostly "occult." Indocyanine green angiography may identify laser-treatable areas in some eyes with "occult" CNV (Fig. 4.17).

The Macular Photocoagulation Study (MPS) showed that eyes with classic CNV located more than 200 μm from the center of the foveal avascular zone ("extrafoveal") and, to a lesser degree, CNV positioned 1 to 199 μm from the cen-

ter of the foveal avascular zone ("juxtafoveal") have about a 50% reduction in severe vision loss with laser photocoagulation treatment compared to untreated control eyes (Fig. 4.18). The treatment results are best in patients whose CNV is adequately initially treated (i.e., confluent laser application over the entire lesion extending 100 μm beyond its border). Despite good treatment, however, CNV recurrence

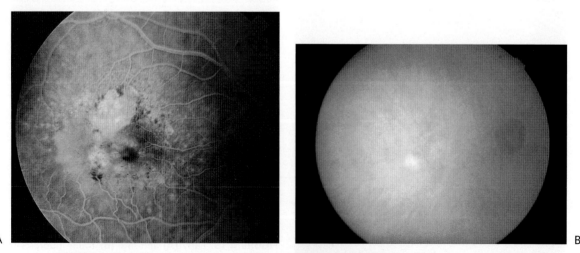

FIGURE 4.17. A: Fluorescein angiogram showing occult choroidal neovascularization adjacent to geographic atrophy. **B:** Corresponding indocyanine green angiogram showing a well-defined spot of hyperfluorescence representing the neovascular focus. (From Regillo CD. The present role of indocyanine green angiography in ophthalmology. *Curr Opin Ophthalmol* 1999;10:189, with permission.)

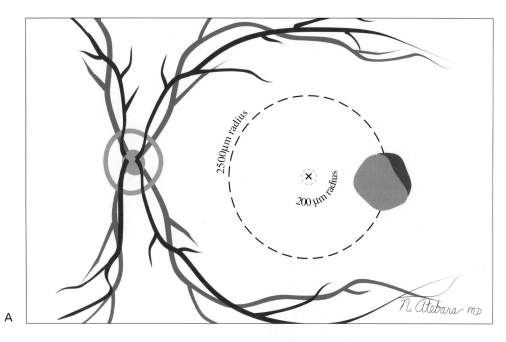

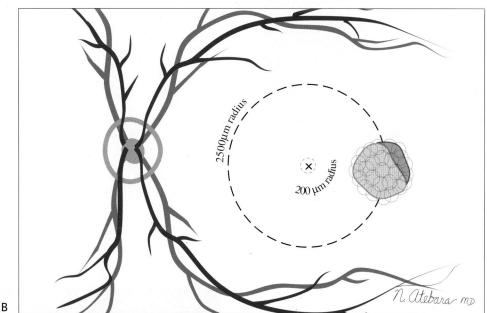

FIGURE 4.18. A: Extrafoveal choroidal neovascularization lies between 200 and 2,500 μm from the center of the foveal avascular zone. The Macular Photocoagulation Study (MPS) found that 41% of untreated eyes suffered six or more lines of visual loss at 1 year, compared with only 24% of the treated eyes. After 5 years, 64% of the untreated eyes suffered severe visual loss, compared with 46% of the treated eyes. **B:** In the MPS, extrafoveal choroidal neovascularization is treated with confluent laser burns that extend 100 μm beyond the choroidal neovascular membrane and adjacent blood or blocked fluorescence.

rates remain high (over 50%), and eyes with recurrent CNV will typically have worse vision outcomes. There is no evidence that any available wavelength (e.g., green vs. red) provides the best treatment results.

For subfoveal CNV that is mostly the classic type, photodynamic therapy (PDT) was recently proven to statistically reduce the risk of vision loss. PDT involves the intra-venous infusion of a photosensitizing dye followed shortly thereafter by the application of a long duration, nonthermal laser light with a wavelength specific for the particular dye in use. Unlike standard photocoagulation, PDT does not destroy the overlying sensory retina and, therefore, is a more selective CNV treatment technique. It is thought to work by promoting temporary thrombosis of CNV. Because there is

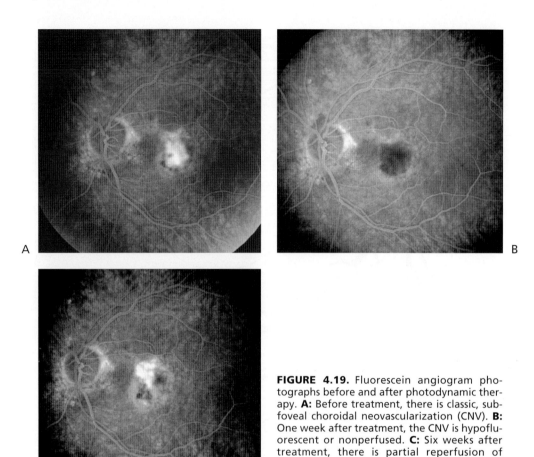

FIGURE 4.19. Fluorescein angiogram photographs before and after photodynamic therapy. **A:** Before treatment, there is classic, subfoveal choroidal neovascularization (CNV). **B:** One week after treatment, the CNV is hypofluorescent or nonperfused. **C:** Six weeks after treatment, there is partial reperfusion of the original CNV lesion. (From Regillo CD. Update on photodynamic therapy. *Curr Opin Ophthalmol* 2000;11:166, with permission.)

often reperfusion of CNV 6 to 12 weeks after treatment, PDT may require retreatment every 3 months for 1 to 2 years to ultimately achieve permanent involution of CNV and complete resolution of exudation (Fig. 4.19).

Other forms of treatment for exudative CNV that are occasionally utilized include macular translocation to treat small, subfoveal CNV; pneumatic displacement or surgical evacuation for large, submacular hemorrhage; and transpupillary thermotherapy to manage occult, subfoveal CNV. Antiangiogenesis drugs are currently in early stages of investigation.

Presumed Ocular Histoplasmosis Syndrome

Presumed ocular histoplasmosis syndrome (POHS) is an acquired condition that appears to develop in certain individuals exposed to the histoplasmosis organism, which, in turn, results in bilateral, focal chorioretinal lesions. There is a high prevalence of POHS in the Ohio/Mississippi River valleys, where histoplasmosis is endemic. The condition is typically detected in young and middle-aged white adults, male or female.

Clinical Features. The classic clinical triad of POHS includes the following signs (Fig. 4.20):

 i. Punched-out chorioretinal scars ("histo spots")
 ii. Peripapillary chorioretinal atrophy
iii. Maculopathy: subretinal fibrosis from CNV

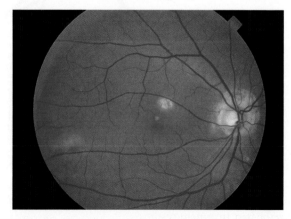

FIGURE 4.20. Presumed ocular histoplasmosis syndrome. Note the peripapillary atrophy and macular "punched-out" chorioretinal scar ("histo spot").

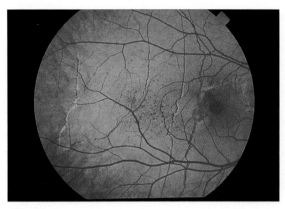

FIGURE 4.21. Peau d'orange in an eye with multiple angioid streaks and two small foci of choroidal neovascularization.

Because POHS is not an active infectious or inflammatory process, anterior chamber or vitreous cells are not present. Over time, one may observe peripapillary atrophy enlargement, histo spots can enlarge, new spots develop (5% to 10% cases), and CNV form in the macula (de novo or from a small macular histo spot).

Vision loss in POHS is almost always the result of macular CNV. The risk of CNV in the eye of a patient whose fellow eye developed CNV in the past varies depending on the following features:

  i. If disk and macula are normal appearing: 1% over 4 years
 ii. If there are peripapillary changes only: 4% over 4 years
iii. If there is a macular scar (i.e., macular histo spots) present: 25% over 4 years

Management. The only proven treatment for POHS-related nonsubfoveal CNV is laser photocoagulation. As with wet AMD, the MPS demonstrated the efficacy of laser (compared to no treatment) with both extrafoveal and juxtafoveal CNV. Persistent or recurrent CNV rates after laser treatment are also relatively high but lower than for laser treatment of AMD-related CNV. For subfoveal CNV,

surgical removal of CNV may be beneficial. The role of surgery is currently being investigated in the Submacular Surgery Trial (SST). PDT is another potential option for subfoveal CNV management.

Angioid Streaks

Angioid streaks are cracks in a thickened, calcified, and brittle Bruch's membrane.

Clinical Features. Angioid streaks can be straight or jagged and may intersect. They are mostly radial but can also be concentric to the optic disc. Fine mottling of the pigment epithelium, called peau d'orange (i.e., orange skin pattern), temporal to the macula is often present (Fig. 4.21). Other associated peripheral findings are focal atrophic spots that resemble "histo spots" and small subretinal crystalline deposits. There is a high risk of subretinal hemorrhage from mild blunt trauma and a high risk of CNV emanating from the streaks (Fig. 4.22).

The most commonly associated systemic condition is pseudoxanthoma elasticum, which can be diagnosed clinically (60% of all patients with angioid streaks) or by scar biopsy (85%). Angioid streaks plus disc drusen are virtually diagnostic of pseudoxanthoma elasticum. Other associated conditions include Paget's disease, sickle cell hemoglobinopathy, and Ehlers-Danlos syndrome. The prevalence of angioid streaks in patients with Paget's disease is somewhat controversial. Paget's disease was found in 10% of a series of patients with angioid streaks, but angioid streaks were found in only one of a series of 70 patients with Paget's disease.

Other causes of CNV must be ruled out. In some patients, the angioid streaks are not prominent and may be overlooked. Fluorescein angiography often will show the streaks more readily appearing as hyperfluorescent lines, and it will be necessary to identify CNV when suspected.

Management. The long-term visual prognosis is relatively poor. In some patients, nonsubfoveal CNV can be treated successfully with laser photocoagulation, but the recurrence rate is high.

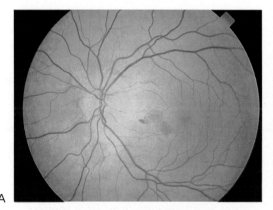
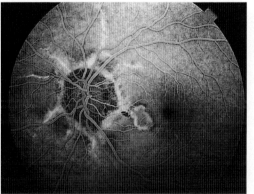

A   B

FIGURE 4.22. A: Subretinal hemorrhage and fluid in a patient with pseudoxanthoma elasticum and angioid streaks. **B:** The fluorescein angiogram shows classic choroidal neovascularization along one of the streaks in the macula.

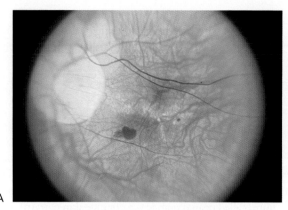
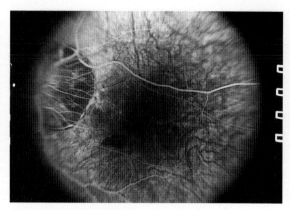

FIGURE 4.23. A: Peripapillary atrophy and a small subretinal hemorrhage in a patient with high myopia. There are a few small lacquer cracks. **B:** Fluorescein angiography shows blockage in the area of submacular hemorrhage. There is no choroidal neovascular membrane.

Myopic Degeneration

In very long eyes, the retina and choriocapillaris are thin, causing myopic macular degeneration.

Clinical Features. The risk of complications increases with increasing axial length of the globe. Early findings include thinning of the macular pigment epithelium, peripapillary atrophy, and tilting of the optic disc. Later complica-

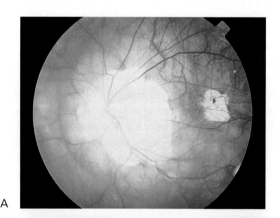

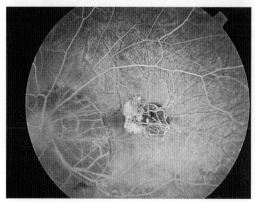

FIGURE 4.24. A: Peripapillary atrophy and a focal area of pigment epithelial atrophy in a patient with high myopia who complained of distorted vision. **B:** Fluorescein angiography reveals classic choroidal neovascularization nasal to the area of pigment epithelial atrophy.

tions include breaks in Bruch's membrane called lacquer cracks (Fig. 4.23), posterior staphyloma, small macular hemorrhages (Fig. 4.23), CNV (Fig. 4.24), and severe macular atrophy. Foerster-Fuchs spots are localized areas of pigment epithelial proliferation. Macular holes may lead to retinal detachment.

Management. Laser photocoagulation of CNV is initially effective, but later enlargement of the laser scar may cause decreased vision. Therefore, laser treatment is recommended only for CNV located ≥100 μm from the foveal center. For subfoveal CNV, PDT appears to be beneficial to decrease the risk of further vision loss. Retinal detachment caused by myopic macular holes is best treated by vitrectomy with gas-liquid exchange or by injection of gas alone. The hole usually does not require laser treatment.

MACULAR HOLE AND PUCKER

Idiopathic Macular Hole

Focal contraction of the posterior hyaloid face can tear the thin central macula, leading to a macular hole. Most occur in elderly women and are spontaneous in nature. Rarely, they result from severe blunt ocular trauma.

Clinical Features. In Gass's classification, a stage I "impending" macular hole is characterized by a localized foveolar detachment, with loss of the foveolar depression and the presence of a yellow macular spot (stage IA) or ring (stage IB) (Fig. 4.25). Visual acuity is minimally affected and usually better than 20/50. Approximately half of stage I eyes progress to stage II, in which the hole begins to develop and, by definition, is small (<400 μm). Typically, vision is in the 20/50 to 20/80 range. Stage III, a completed hole, is larger than a stage II hole (≥400 μm) and often has a cuff (i.e., halo) of subretinal fluid (Fig. 4.26). There also may be an overlying pseudooperculum. Commonly, there are some drusen-like deposits at the base of the hole. The vitreous is

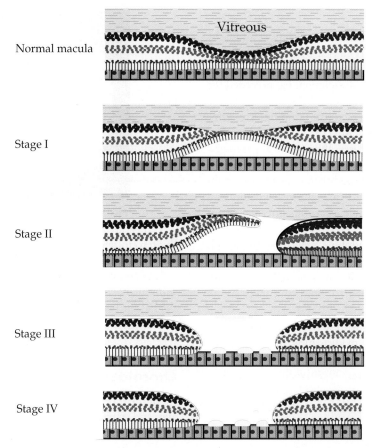

Normal macula

Stage I

Stage II

Stage III

Stage IV

FIGURE 4.25. Stages of macular hole development. In stage I, localized contraction of the perifoveal vitreous causes a traction detachment of the fovea, characterized clinically as a small round yellow spot or ring in the fovea. Stage II is marked by a small full-thickness opening (<400 μm in diameter). The hole gradually enlarges into a fully developed stage III macular hole that is usually approximately one-third disc diameter in size (≥400 μm in diameter). It often has a small rim of subretinal fluid and yellow deposits at the retinal pigment epithelium. A pseudooperculum may or may not be present. A fully developed macular hole with a posterior vitreous detachment is classified as stage IV.

still attached posteriorly at this stage. The visual acuity usually drops to 20/200. In stage IV, there is complete posterior vitreous detachment. The risk of developing a macular hole in a fellow eye is as high as 15%.

Macular pucker with pseudohole and a lamellar macular hole are the entities most commonly confused with macular hole. A lamellar hole does not have a cuff of subretinal fluid, nor is there significant pucker. Clinically, a Watske–Allen test is useful to differentiate a true full-thickness macular hole from a pseudohole. Ocular coherence tomography (OCT) can also be helpful.

Management. Kelly and Wendel were the pioneers in the surgical repair of macular holes. The surgery consists of a standard pars plana vitrectomy, posterior vitreous separation, possible membrane peeling, and injection of a long-acting gas. The patient then remains in a face-down position for 1 to 2 weeks after the operation. Over 90% of the holes can be anatomically closed, and two thirds or more of these eyes will have some degree of improved vision. Both anatomic and functional results are better with holes of less than 2 years in duration and of smaller size (i.e., stage II holes).

After the vitrectomy, most patients develop a cataract within 1 to 2 years that is dense enough to necessitate extraction to ultimately achieve the best potential visual acuity. Retinal detachment and other complications of vitrectomy also occur.

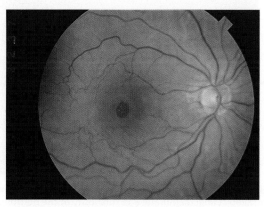

FIGURE 4.26. Photograph of a full-thickness macular hole with a small cuff of subretinal fluid.

Macular Pucker

Macular pucker, also called surface wrinkling retinopathy and cellophane retinopathy, is caused by growth and contraction of an epiretinal membrane over the macular area. In most cases, a posterior vitreous detachment has preceded the membrane formation.

Clinical Features. The characteristic findings are wrinkling of the retina and straightening or zigzagging of retinal vessels (Fig. 4.27). In many cases, fluorescein angiography reveals macular edema leakage. In some cases, a central defect in the membrane (i.e., pseudohole) resembles a full-thickness macular hole. In most cases the visual acuity and fundus appearance remain stable after the epiretinal membrane contracts.

Macular pucker with pseudohole may resemble a full-thickness or a lamellar macular hole. In contrast to a full-thickness macular hole, the vision may be only slightly reduced, there is no cuff of subretinal fluid, and there are no drusen-like central deposits.

Management. In patients with a visual acuity of about 20/50 or less and symptoms of distortion or blur, vitrectomy with peeling of the membrane can be offered. Although some patients recover 20/20 vision, the median postoperative visual acuity improvement is approximately 2 to 3 Snellen lines. Vision outcomes are probably better with macular pucker of relatively recent (<1 year) onset.

TRAUMATIC MACULOPATHIES

Commotio Retinae

Commotio retinae is caused by the contrecoup mechanism. Shock waves caused by the impact traverse the fluid-filled eye and strike the retina. When commotio retinae is located in the macula, it is called Berlin's edema.

Clinical Features. The opacification of the outer retinal layers (Fig. 4.28) is caused by disruption of the outer segments of the photoreceptors and not by edema. In mild cases,

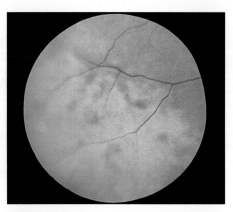

FIGURE 4.28. Peripheral commotio retinae.

fluorescein angiography shows no leakage (Fig. 4.29), indicating minimal damage to the pigment epithelium and an excellent prognosis for full return of vision. However, if there is subretinal hemorrhage or leakage on fluorescein angiography, the RPE is badly damaged, and the visual prognosis is poor.

Management. There is no treatment for commotio retinae.

Choroidal Rupture

As blunt trauma compresses the eye on its anteroposterior axis and expands it on its horizontal axis, it may cause a

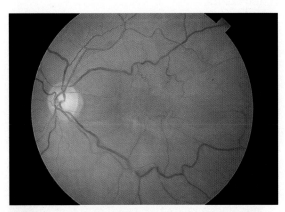

FIGURE 4.27. Severe macular pucker. Note the gray-appearing central epiretinal membrane and tortuosity of the perifoveal vessels.

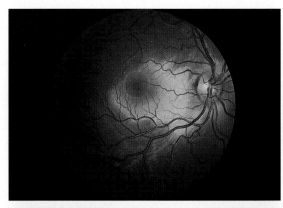

A

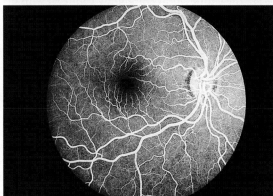

B

FIGURE 4.29. A: Berlin's edema. **B:** Normal fluorescein angiography in a case of Berlin's edema.

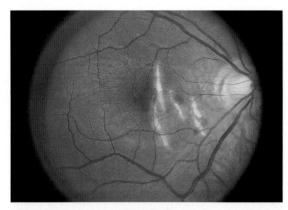

FIGURE 4.30. Multiple choroidal ruptures with subretinal hemorrhages temporal to the disc.

choroidal rupture, because Bruch's membrane is relatively rigid and breaks more easily. With it, the RPE and choriocapillaris break as well.

Clinical Features. Choroidal ruptures are usually temporal to and concentric to the optic disc (Fig. 4.30). They are usually accompanied by a subretinal hemorrhage, which may initially completely or partially mask the rupture. Because the overlying retina is usually intact, no nerve fiber bundle visual field defects are seen. A late but uncommon complication is CNV.

Management. There is no treatment for acute choroidal rupture. Nonsubfoveal CNV responds well to laser photocoagulation.

Avulsed Optic Nerve

Rarely, direct trauma to the eye or a blow to the back of the head tears the lamina cribrosa, resulting in avulsion of the optic nerve (Fig. 4.31).

Clinical Features. A gap is seen where the neural tissue of the optic nerve retracts back into the optic nerve sheath. Retinal and vitreous hemorrhages are detected.

Management. There is no treatment for avulsed optic nerve.

Purtscher's Retinopathy

Severe compression injury to the head or chest can result in complement-activated coagulation of leukocytes and other forms of microemboli which can occlude the retinal capillaries.

Clinical Features. Purtscher's retinopathy usually is bilateral. Fundus examination reveals multiple cotton-wool spots in the distribution of the radial peripapillary capillaries (Fig. 4.32). Multiple, superficial hemorrhages may also be present. The visual prognosis is guarded. Optic atrophy often develops to varying degrees. Poor vision results from macular infarction and/or optic nerve dysfunction.

Similar findings can be seen in patients with collagen-vascular disease, pancreatitis in chronic alcoholics, patients on renal dialysis, and any systemic disease state that results in widespread microemboli.

Management. There is no treatment for Purtscher's retinopathy.

Solar Retinopathy

Solar retinopathy is retinal damage caused by excessive exposure to light. Unlike laser burns which are thermal, solar retinopathy is a phototoxic lesion. In a phototoxic injury, the release of free radicals and lysosomal enzymes damages photoreceptor membranes. Blue and near-ultraviolet light have been found to be the most harmful wavelengths.

Clinical Features. Solar retinopathy is usually bilateral, but it can occur asymmetrically because the patient squints one eye. Initially, the fundus is normal. Later, there is a deep yellowish discoloration of the retina. In mild cases, the results of fluorescein angiography are normal, the photoreceptors and pigment epithelium regenerate, and the visual acuity and fundus return to normal. In moderate cases, there is a permanent depigmentation of the central pigment epithelium, and the visual acuity may be mildly reduced (Fig. 4.33). In severe cases, there is marked pigment clumping and only partial recovery of visual acuity.

Mild cases of solar retinopathy resemble adult foveomac-

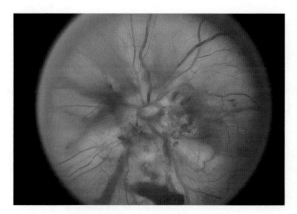

FIGURE 4.31. Avulsed optic nerve.

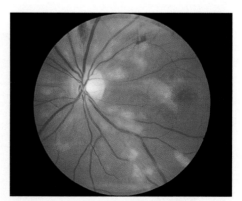

FIGURE 4.32. Multiple superficial nerve fiber layer infarctions (cotton-wool spots) along with some intraretinal hemorrhages in a patient with Purtscher's retinopathy.

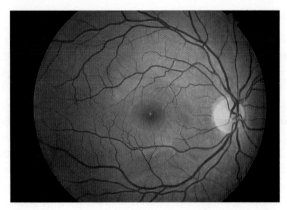

FIGURE 4.33. Small area of pigment epithelial atrophy in a patient who, as part of a religious cult, routinely looked directly at the sun.

ular dystrophy, and the patient's history is important in differentiating them. Solar retinopathy is usually seen in younger patients.

Management. There is no treatment for solar retinopathy.

Valsalva Maculopathy

Valsalva retinopathy is a condition in which an acute rise in intrathoracic or intraabdominal pressure against a closed glottis (i.e., Valsalva's maneuver) causes a marked increase in retinal venous pressure, which ruptures superficial capillaries, resulting in one or more superficial retinal hemorrhages.

Clinical Features. The typical patient complains of a sudden decrease in vision after coughing, sneezing, straining at stool, or heavy lifting. The hemorrhages are typically round and small (Fig. 4.34A) but may be as large as 1 to 3 disc areas. Fluorescein angiography shows no leakage (Fig. 4.34B).

A solitary subinternal membrane hemorrhage may also accompany posterior vitreous detachment. The ophthalmologist must carefully examine the peripheral retina to rule out tears.

Management. No treatment is necessary. The hemorrhages clear spontaneously, with no residual loss of vision.

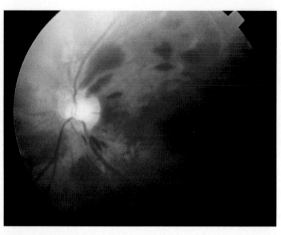

FIGURE 4.35. Terson's syndrome. Multiple superficial retinal hemorrhages are present in the posterior pole. (From Regillo CD. Posterior segment manifestations of systemic trauma. In: Regillo CD, Brown GC, Flynn HW. Vitreoretinal disease: The essentials. New York: Thieme; 1999:537, with permission.)

Terson's Syndrome

Terson's syndrome is a condition in which intraocular hemorrhage occurs as a result of either spontaneous or trauma-induced acute intracranial bleeding.

Clinical Features. The most common intraocular finding is multiple intraretinal hemorrhages. They are almost always bilateral, superficial, and concentrated in the posterior pole (Fig. 4.35). Significant vitreous hemorrhage can also occur. Visual acuity loss is often proportional to the extent of retinal and/or vitreous hemorrhage and, in many cases, the degree of intraocular hemorrhage is directly related to the severity of the intracranial hemorrhage. Late-appearing ocular sequelae include macular pucker and traction retinal detachments.

Some degree of intraocular hemorrhage is seen in 20% to 40% of patients with acute intracranial hemorrhages. The most common type of intracranial bleed associated with Terson's syndrome is a subarachnoid hemorrhage, the source of which is most often a spontaneous rupture of an anterior communicating aneurysm.

Management. No treatment is necessary. The retinal

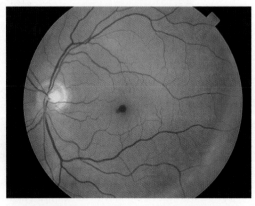 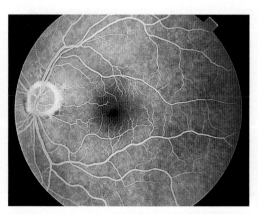

A B

FIGURE 4.34. A: Small, central, superficial hemorrhage in a patient who noticed decreased vision after heavy lifting. **B:** The fluorescein angiogram shows a blockage of background fluorescence.

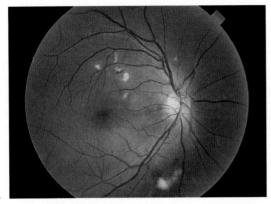
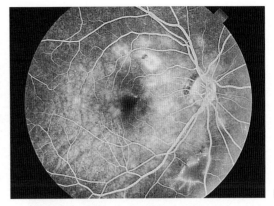

FIGURE 4.36. A: Multiple cotton-wool spots in a patient with radiation retinopathy. **B:** The late phase of the fluorescein angiogram shows leakage around the cotton-wool spots and from abnormal capillaries.

hemorrhages clear spontaneously and vision recovery is often good. Vitrectomy is sometimes employed for nonclearing vitreous hemorrhage or the relatively rare late sequelae.

Radiation Retinopathy

Radiation retinopathy is an ischemic injury to the retina caused by excessive radiation-induced damage to the retinal capillaries. A typical dose is 3,000 to 3,500 cGy, but as little as 1,500 cGy may suffice.

Clinical Features. The retinal signs are usually first noticed 6 months to 3 years after exposure. Initially, the patients are asymptomatic or have mildly decreased vision. Microaneurysms, hard exudates, soft exudates, superficial retinal hemorrhages, macular edema, neovascularization, and optic neuropathy may occur (Fig. 4.36A). Fluorescein angiography may reveal widespread capillary nonperfusion (Fig. 4.36B).

The retinal findings may closely resemble those of diabetic retinopathy. The key to the correct diagnosis is the history of radiation exposure, even if the radiation oncologist insists that the eyes were adequately shielded. In radiation retinopathy, when extensive capillary nonperfusion is found on fluorescein angiography, there are many fewer microaneurysms than would be expected in diabetic retinopathy.

Management. No treatment is known to prevent radiation retinopathy development or progression, although neovascularization may be treated with panretinal laser photocoagulation. The benefit of focal laser treatment is unproven.

PERIPHERAL RETINAL LESIONS

Paving Stone Degeneration

Paving stones are small, discrete areas of ischemic atrophy of the outer retina. Histopathologic analysis shows attenuation or absence of the choriocapillaris, absence of the RPE, absence of the outer retinal layers, and an adhesion between the remaining inner layers and Bruch's membrane.

Clinical Features. Paving stones are white and are often surrounded by a rim of hyperplastic RPE (Fig. 4.37). They occur singly or in groups and are sometimes confluent. The paving stones usually are anterior to the equator and are most commonly found in the inferior retina.

Management. Paving stones do not require treatment because they are not a predisposing factor to retinal breaks. They limit the spread of retinal detachment.

Lattice Degeneration

Lattice degeneration is focal atrophy of the inner retina with discontinuity of the internal limiting membrane and liquefaction of the overlying vitreous. There are strong vitreous adhesions at the edges of the lesion. Lattice degeneration increases in frequency with increasing axial length of the globe. It is found in 5% to 10% of the general population.

Clinical Features. The lesions are usually anterior to the equator and are elliptical, with the long axis circumferentially oriented (Fig. 4.38). Less commonly, the lesions accompany retinal blood vessels and have a radial (i.e., meridional) orientation. Blood vessels within the lattice often appear white or hyalinized. Sometimes, the underlying pigment epithelium is hyperplastic (i.e., pigmented lattice pattern). Between 20% and 40% of retinal detachments are complications of lattice degeneration. The causative breaks are atrophic holes

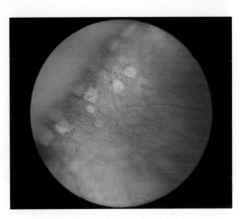

FIGURE 4.37. Peripheral paving stones.

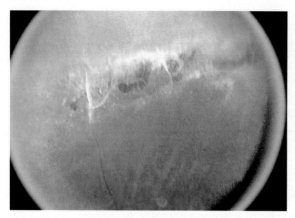

FIGURE 4.38. Patch of lattice degeneration with sclerosed-appearing vessels and hyperpigmentation.

within the lattice lesions or, more commonly, traction tears posterior to or at the ends of the lattice.

Management. Long-term follow-up studies have conclusively demonstrated that prophylactic treatment of asymptomatic lattice degeneration with and without atrophic holes is unnecessary. However, if a patient presents with a retinal detachment in one eye, many retinal surgeons treat lattice degeneration in the fellow eye.

Vitreoretinal Tufts

Vitreoretinal tufts are small foci of vitreous or zonular traction.

Clinical Features. Vitreoretinal tufts are slightly elevated (Fig. 4.39) and may have a cystic appearance. They can be surrounded by hyperplastic pigment epithelium. When posterior vitreous detachment occurs, vitreoretinal tufts may be the focus of a retinal tear.

Because they are elevated, vitreoretinal tufts may be difficult to differentiate from flap tears. Examination with indirect ophthalmoscopy and scleral depression or a Goldmann three-mirror lens is helpful.

Management. Asymptomatic vitreoretinal tufts do not require treatment.

RETINAL DETACHMENT

Posterior Vitreous Detachment

Posterior vitreous detachment (PVD) is the separation of the vitreous from the posterior portion of the retina (Fig. 4.40).

Clinical Features. The symptoms of posterior vitreous detachment are brief flashes of light or "floaters," which are vitreous collagen fibers, hemorrhage, or epipapillary glial tissue torn from the optic disc (Weiss ring) (Fig. 4.41). Posterior vitreous detachment occasionally causes peripapillary hemorrhage. At least one retinal tear is found in 15% of patients with acute posterior vitreous detachment. A tear is found in two thirds of patients with vitreous hemorrhage. In patients without vitreous hemorrhage, a break is found in only 2% to 4%.

When the vitreous is firmly attached to the retina, as at a vitreoretinal tuft, a meridional fold, or lattice degeneration, posterior vitreous detachment may tear the retina (Fig. 4.40). When a piece of retina is torn free from the adjacent retina, the tear is called operculated (Fig. 4.42). When the torn retina remains adherent to the adjacent retina, the tear is called a flap or horseshoe tear (Fig. 4.43). Flap tears are more likely to progress to retinal detachment than are operculated tears, because continuing vitreous traction helps to separate the retina from the underlying pigment epithelium.

Other causes of photopsias, such as migraine, and of vitreous hemorrhage must be ruled out.

Management. The fundus must be carefully inspected to rule out retinal tears. In the setting of a recent PVD, retinal tears are treated with transscleral cryotherapy or laser photocoagulation.

Acute Rhegmatogenous Retinal Detachment

In acute rhegmatogenous retinal detachment, liquefied vitreous gains access to the subretinal space through a retinal break (Greek: rhegma) and separates the sensory retina from the pigment epithelium (Fig. 4.44).

Clinical Features. In 97% of patients with rhegmatoge-

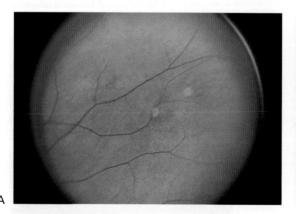
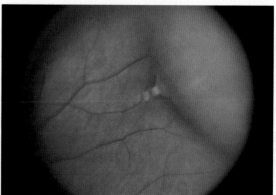

FIGURE 4.39. A: Two vitreoretinal tufts in the periphery. **B:** On scleral depression, the vitreous traction can be seen tenting the retina.

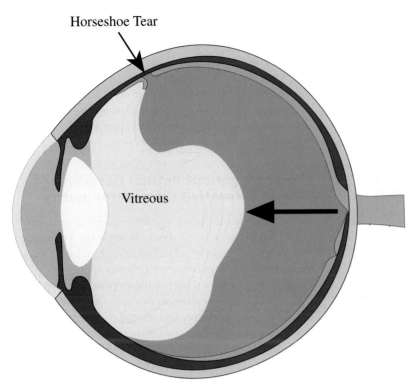

Horseshoe Tear

Vitreous

FIGURE 4.40. Posterior vitreous detachment. As the vitreous collapses, traction on areas of vitreoretinal adhesion may pull a strip of retina anteriorly, causing a flap or "horseshoe" tear.

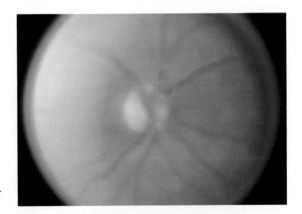

FIGURE 4.41. Weiss ring in a patient with posterior vitreous detachment.

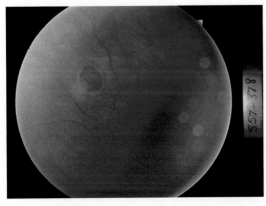

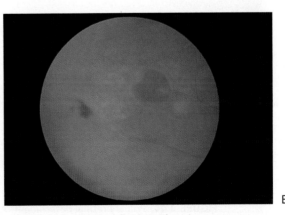

A

B

FIGURE 4.42. **A:** Acute operculated hole with a small rim of subretinal fluid. **B:** Chronic operculated hole with a pigmented demarcation line.

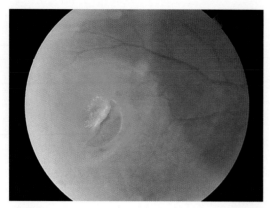

FIGURE 4.43. Flap ("horseshoe") retinal tear surrounded by sub-retinal fluid.

nous retinal detachment, a retinal break is found (Fig. 4.45). In the other 3%, it is presumed to be present. Vitreous hemorrhage is common in cases caused by a flap tear. In cases of recent onset, the detached retina is opaque and corrugated (Fig. 4.46). If the macula is detached, it frequently develops cystoid macular edema that is sometimes difficult to differentiate from a full-thickness macular hole. The subretinal fluid is usually nonshifting, but will undulate with eye movements. The intraocular pressure is often decreased in proportion to the area of detached retina, but may be increased with chronic retinal detachments.

Nonrhegmatogenous retinal detachment, retinoschisis, and choroidal detachment must be ruled out.

Management. For uncomplicated, primary rhegmatogenous retinal detachments, treatment approaches include scleral buckling (the gold standard), pneumatic retinopexy, and sometimes vitrectomy. Those complicated by vitreous hemorrhage, giant tears (Fig. 4.47), or significant proliferative vitreoretinopathy (see below) typically require vitrectomy, with or without scleral buckling.

Rhegmatogenous Retinal Detachment With Proliferative Vitreoretinopathy

When the retina detaches, pigment epithelial cells separate from Bruch's membrane, float through the vitreous, and proliferate on the inner retinal surface, the outer surface, or both. They also proliferate on vitreous strands. Glial cells also may proliferate on both retinal surfaces. The RPE and glial cells can form membranes that contract. In proliferative vitreoretinopathy, the proliferation and contraction are sufficient to cause clinically apparent signs.

Clinical Features. Signs of proliferative vitreoretinopathy include increased vitreous cells, posterior rolling of the edge of retinal breaks (Fig. 4.48), fixed folds (Fig. 4.49), equatorial vitreous traction, and subretinal bands.

Management. Rhegmatogenous retinal detachments with very early or limited proliferative vitreoretinopathy of-

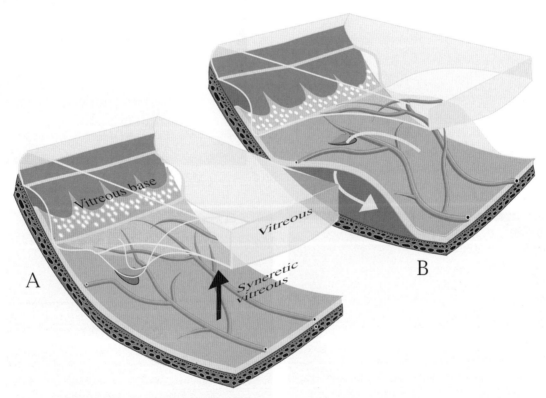

FIGURE 4.44. Primary retinal detachment. **A:** A posterior vitreous detachment produces traction on the peripheral retina, sometimes causing tears or holes. **B:** Fluid passes through the tear, dissecting through the subretinal space and creating a retinal detachment.

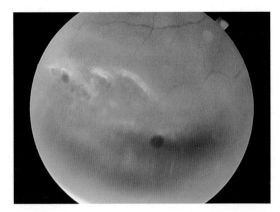

FIGURE 4.45. Retinal detachment caused by atrophic holes in lattice degeneration.

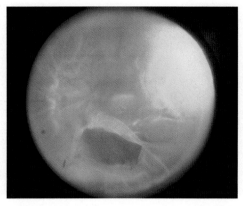

FIGURE 4.48. Equator-plus photograph of a patient with a total retinal detachment with proliferative vitreoretinopathy. There is a large inferior tear with a posteriorly rolled edge. The preequatorial area appears thin, because equatorial vitreous traction is pulling the peripheral retina centrally.

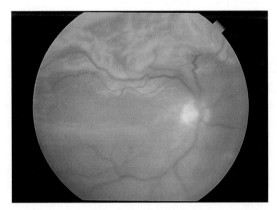

FIGURE 4.46. Corrugated, opaque appearance of the detached retina in a patient with rhegmatogenous retinal detachment.

ten can be repaired with a scleral buckling procedure alone. Most cases, however, require vitrectomy techniques. Long-acting gases or silicone oil are commonly needed. Perfluorocarbon liquids are useful intraoperative adjuncts to facilitate retinal reattachment. Relaxing retinotomies are sometimes required to get the retina to reattach.

Longstanding Retinal Detachment Without Proliferative Vitreoretinopathy

In rhegmatogenous retinal detachment caused by small breaks or by a dialysis, the detachment may remain localized indefinitely or progress slowly.

Clinical Features. The retina atrophies and becomes more transparent (Fig. 4.50). Demarcation lines may develop (Fig. 4.51). The underlying RPE becomes depigmented. RPE cells float through the vitreous cavity and proliferate on the outer surface of the retina (i.e., subretinal precipitates) or on vitreous strands (i.e., "tobacco dust") without progressing to proliferative vitreoretinopathy. In a

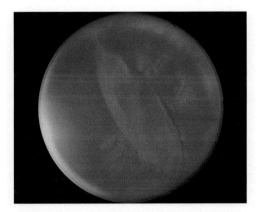

FIGURE 4.47. Equator-plus photograph showing a 6 clock-hour giant retinal tear with a rolled-over retina covering the optic disc.

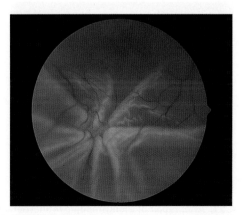

FIGURE 4.49. Fixed fold in a patient with a rhegmatogenous retinal detachment and proliferative vitreoretinopathy.

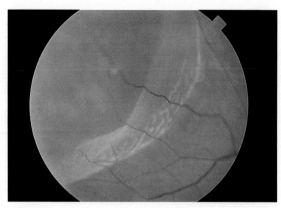

FIGURE 4.50. Rhegmatogenous retinal detachment caused by a small break along a retinal vein. Peripherally, the retina is thin where the detachment was localized for a long time. Posteriorly, the retina was more recently detached and is more opaque and corrugated than the peripheral area.

few cases, large pockets of fluid, called macrocysts, form in the retina. The intraocular pressure is often elevated.

Longstanding retinal detachment may be difficult to differentiate from senile retinoschisis, and long-term retinal detachment is part of the differential diagnosis of unilateral glaucoma.

Management. Cases with thick demarcation lines can usually be followed by observation alone. However, detachments with no or only a thin demarcation line usually require treatment. For very limited detachments, laser demarcation can be a useful alternative to surgical reattachment

Exudative Retinal Detachment

Exudative retinal detachments are caused by excessive leakage of fluid from the choroid or the retina. Common causes are neoplasms, inflammatory conditions (e.g., Harada's disease, posterior scleritis), nanophthalmos, uveal effusion syndrome, sympathetic ophthalmia, bullous CSCR, malignant hypertension, and Coats' disease.

Clinical Features. In cases caused by tumors, the subretinal fluid initially overlies or surrounds the lesion. Later, the subretinal fluid gravitates (i.e., "shifting fluid") to the most dependent part of the eye, usually forming two bullae inferiorly (Fig. 4.52). No retinal breaks occur.

Rhegmatogenous retinal detachment must be ruled out. If the retina can be seen immediately behind the lens, the detachment usually is exudative. Other findings depend on the cause of the detachment. Unlike rhegmatogenous detachments, one would not expect to find vitreous hemorrhage, vitreous pigment cells ("tobacco dust"), or, of course, a retinal break.

Management. Treatment is directed at the underlying condition (e.g., corticosteroids for inflammatory etiologies, radiation therapy for choroidal tumors, etc.). Visual prognosis is variable and depends on factors related to both the retinal detachment (e.g., extent and chronicity) and the inciting condition (e.g., location and curability).

Traction Retinal Detachment

In traction retinal detachment, the retina is pulled into the vitreous cavity by transvitreal (anteroposterior) traction. The most common causes are proliferative retinopathies, such as diabetic retinopathy and old penetrating injuries.

Clinical Features. Clinically, no breaks are found. The detached retina is smooth, immobile, and concave toward the pupil (Fig. 4.53), and it does not extend to the ora serrata. The examiner must remember that patients with proliferative retinopathy can also have combined traction and rhegmatogenous retinal detachment in which there may be corrugations and in which the retina is convex toward the pupil (Fig. 4.54).

Management. The traction must be released by vitrectomy in which various membrane peeling techniques are employed. Localized, extramacular detachments do not necessarily progress and, therefore, may be observed. Traction detachments that threaten to detach or already extend into the macula require surgery.

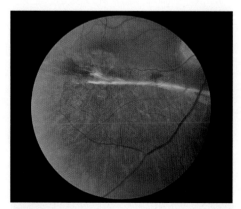

FIGURE 4.51. After repair of a longstanding retinal detachment, atrophic pigment epithelium and a thick demarcation line can be seen inferiorly.

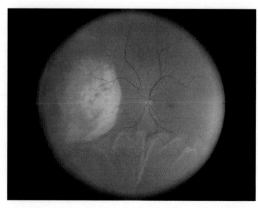

FIGURE 4.52. Large amelanotic malignant melanoma nasally with an inferior exudative retinal detachment.

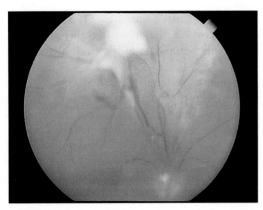

FIGURE 4.53. Superior traction retinal detachment in a patient with proliferative diabetic retinopathy.

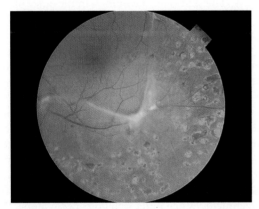

FIGURE 4.54. Combined early traction and rhegmatogenous retinal detachment. A small hole exists just inferior to the fibrovascular proliferation.

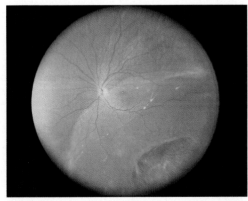

FIGURE 4.55. Equator-plus photograph showing a longstanding inferotemporal retinal detachment with a retinal dialysis from blunt eye trauma.

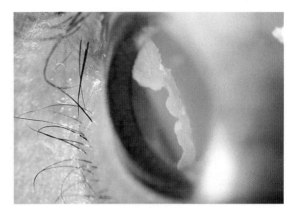

FIGURE 4.56. Avulsed vitreous base after blunt ocular trauma.

Traumatic Retinal Detachment

Clinical Features. There are five mechanisms by which blunt trauma can cause retinal breaks. The first type of traumatic break is caused by compression of the eye along its anteroposterior axis, with resultant horizontal expansion. This can result in true dialysis, which is a separation of the retina from the nonpigmented epithelium of the pars plana at the ora serrata (Fig. 4.55), or in linear tears along the anterior border of the vitreous base, the posterior border of the vitreous base, or both. Such tears are most common superonasally and inferotemporally and may be accompanied by an avulsed vitreous base (Fig. 4.56), which is pathognomonic of blunt trauma. The second type, posterior stretch tears (Fig. 4.57), are caused by the same mechanism. The third type of traumatic break is caused by traction on a distant focus of vitreoretinal traction, such as lattice degeneration or a vitreoretinal traction tuft. The fourth type is caused by focal retinal necrosis, in which a foreign object strikes the sclera directly under the retina (Fig. 4.58). These breaks are characterized by ragged edges. The fifth type, a macular hole, may follow severe Berlin's edema or be related to late vitreous contracture. Because traumatic retinal breaks usually occur in young patients with little liquid vitreous, the retinal detachments they cause typically progress slowly,

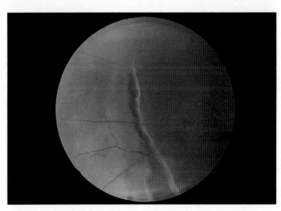

FIGURE 4.57. Traumatic stretch tear.

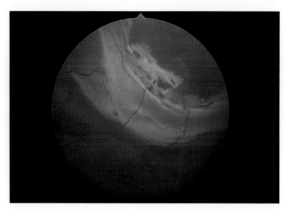

FIGURE 4.58. Necrotic tear caused by a direct blow to the eye.

with many of the features of longstanding retinal detachment (Fig. 4.55).

Management. Traumatic retinal breaks and detachments are treated like other retinal breaks and detachments.

CHOROIDAL DETACHMENT

Accumulation of fluid or blood in the suprachoroidal space elevates the choroid, pigment epithelium, and retina, creating what is called a choroidal detachment. The most common cause is hypotony during or after intraocular surgery. Serous choroidal detachments often are found in eyes with longstanding retinal detachment. Severe, often hemorrhagic, choroidal detachments that form during or after eye surgery are most common in elderly patients with myopia and glaucoma.

Clinical Features. Choroidal detachments have the same color as adjacent normal pigment epithelium. They may have a slightly corrugated appearance (Fig. 4.59). The pars plana may be seen without scleral depression.

Choroidal detachments can be mistaken for rhegmatogenous retinal detachment and choroidal melanoma. In

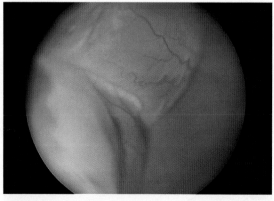

FIGURE 4.59. Superotemporal choroidal detachments after cataract surgery. The pars plana can be seen easily without scleral depression.

choroidal detachments, no breaks are found, and choroidal detachments have a denser, more solid appearance than retinal detachments. Serous choroidal detachments transilluminate.

Management. When hypotony is the cause of the choroidal detachment, the underlying cause, such as a cleft or a wound leak, must be identified and treated. Choroidal detachments, even large ones, often resolve spontaneously. In some cases, there can be a very shallow or flat anterior chamber, secondary intraocular pressure elevation, or severe pain, especially when there is suprachoroidal blood. These associated problems often represent indications for surgical drainage.

RETINOSCHISIS
Senile Retinoschisis

Senile retinoschisis is a peripheral splitting of the retina into two layers. The split is most common in the outer plexiform layer (Fig. 4.60). The cavity contains hyaluronic acid.

Clinical Features. Retinoschisis is usually seen in hyperopic eyes and is most commonly located inferotemporally and superotemporally. Prominent cystoid degeneration occurs at the ora serrata. The inner wall has a smooth surface and is dome shaped (Fig. 4.61). It may have sheathed retinal vessels and white opacities called snowflakes, which are the footplates of Müller's cell columns. Inner wall holes may be found. The outer wall has a pocked appearance and may have round holes (Fig. 4.62), with or without a pigmented demarcation line. The complications of senile retinoschisis are loss of peripheral visual field and rhegmatogenous retinal detachment. When outer wall holes occur alone, the detachments typically advance slowly, and demarcation lines around the holes are common. If inner and outer wall holes are present, the two layers of the schisis may collapse together, and the detachment may look like a typical rhegmatogenous retinal detachment and progress rapidly.

Factors that help to differentiate retinoschisis from a longstanding retinal detachment without proliferative vitreoretinopathy are the absence of a demarcation line, absence of underlying RPE degeneration, absence of tobacco dust, and an absolute scotoma on visual field testing.

Management. Because outer wall breaks rarely cause clinical retinal detachment, the only indication for treatment of retinoschisis is symptomatic, progressive retinal detachment.

Congenital or X-Linked Retinoschisis

Congenital retinoschisis is an X-linked recessively inherited condition in which the basic abnormality is splitting of the nerve fiber layer.

Clinical Features. The hallmark of congenital retinoschisis is the stellate or "spoke-wheel" macula (Fig. 4.63), which superficially resembles cystoid macular edema but does not

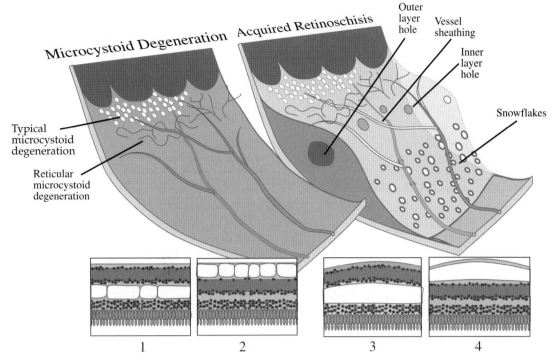

FIGURE 4.60. In typical microcystoid degeneration, pockets of hyaluronic acid form in the outer plexiform layer *(1)*. Reticular microcystoid degeneration is characterized by a cystic degeneration of the nerve fiber layer *(2)*. In typical retinoschisis, a continuous split in the outer plexiform layer is thought to be caused by a consolidation of the hyaluronic pockets of typical microcystoid degeneration *(3)*. Reticular microcystoid degeneration may lead to reticular retinoschisis when a continuous separation in the nerve fiber layer forms *(4)*. Round holes in the inner and outer retinal layers can occasionally lead to a rhegmatogenous retinal detachment.

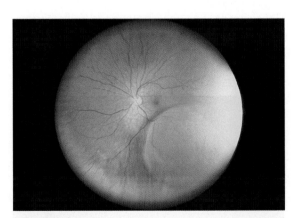

FIGURE 4.61. Equator-plus photograph showing a dome-shaped area of elevation of the inner retinal layer in a patient with senile retinoschisis.

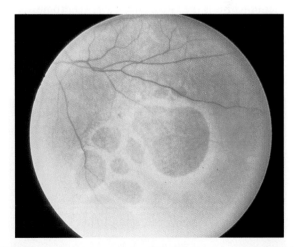

FIGURE 4.62. Large outer wall holes in an eye with senile retinoschisis.

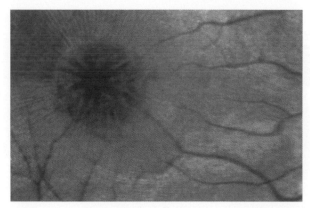

FIGURE 4.63. Spoke-wheel "cystoid" macular changes in a patient with juvenile retinoschisis.

show leakage on fluorescein angiography. Half of the patients have peripheral retinoschisis (inferotemporal, 90%; inferonasal, 58%) in which large inner wall holes (Fig. 4.64) with unsupported blood vessels are common. The ERG reflects the widespread inner retinal damage. Characteristically, the a wave is normal, and the b wave is decreased. The ERG is abnormal whether or not there are appreciable peripheral schisis cavities.

The most common reasons for the initial presentation are decreased vision (45%), strabismus (18%), vitreous hemorrhage (15%), and a positive family history (15%). Retinal detachment and vitreous hemorrhage is rare. The visual acuity is only moderately decreased, usually to the 20/70 level. After 20 years of age, the vision usually remains stable.

The only condition in which the macula resembles juvenile retinoschisis is the Goldmann-Favre syndrome.

Management. Because prophylactic photocoagulation to limit the spread of the area of schisis or to prevent retinal detachment is more likely to aggravate the condition than to

stabilize it, this approach is not indicated. Surgery is indicated for the rare, secondary complications of retinal detachment or nonclearing vitreous hemorrhage.

TOXIC RETINOPATHIES

Chloroquine Retinopathy

Excessive ingestion of chloroquine causes diffuse retinal deterioration. Traditionally, the damage was thought to be caused by progressive binding of chloroquine by melanin in the RPE cells, but later evidence indicated that the ganglion cells are also directly damaged. The cumulative dose of drug is the most important predictor of retinopathy. Less than 100 g causes no toxicity. When it is greater than 300 g, 70% of patients manifest some signs of toxicity. Plaquenil (hydroxychloroquine) retinopathy is similar to chloroquine retinopathy, but Plaquenil is much less toxic. Plaquenil toxicity is rarely seen with a total dose of less than 700 g or an average daily dose of 400 mg or less.

Clinical Features. The earliest signs of retinopathy are small scotomata on visual field testing, a supranormal EOG, an abnormal photostress test result, and decreased color vision. Because visual acuity is typically affected later, it cannot be relied on to detect early toxicity. Similarly, in an eye with early toxic reactions, the fundus may be normal. The earliest fundus abnormalities are small areas of depigmentation of the RPE (Fig. 4.65). By the time the classic bull's-eye maculopathy is evident (Fig. 4.66), considerable damage has been done.

The end-stage fundus appearance of chloroquine retinopathy resembles a bull's-eye pattern. The most common causes of a bull's-eye are Stargardt's disease, cone dystrophy, and AMD.

Management. The only treatment is to discontinue the drug. Although many patients have some recovery of vision, a few have damage that continues to progress.

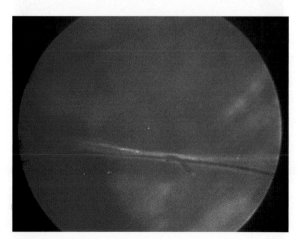

FIGURE 4.64. Large inner wall defect in a patient with juvenile retinoschisis. An unsupported retinal vessel bridges the gap.

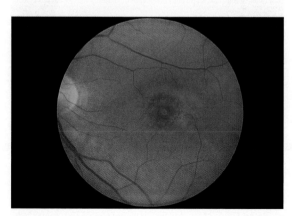

FIGURE 4.65. Early chloroquine retinopathy with a small bull's-eye lesion.

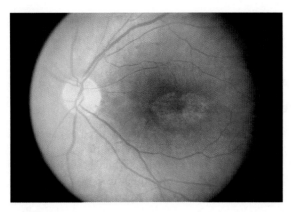

FIGURE 4.66. Fully developed bull's-eye lesion in a patient with chloroquine retinopathy.

Thioridazine Toxicity

There are two types of thioridazine (Mellaril) toxicity. In the acute form, large doses (e.g., 2,000 mg/day or more) are administered to psychotic patients, who experience an acute decrease in central vision. In the chronic form, patients who take thioridazine for long periods at lower doses (800 to 1,000 mg/day) have peripheral visual field loss, but they usually retain good central vision.

Clinical Features. The acute type of thioridazine toxicity

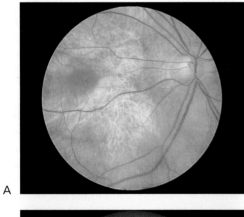

A

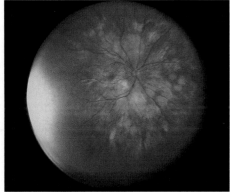

B

FIGURE 4.67. A: Posterior pole pigment epithelial atrophy in a patient with Mellaril (thioridazine hydrochloride) retinopathy. **B:** An equator-plus photograph shows multiple large areas of pigment epithelial atrophy.

is characterized by widespread stippling of the RPE, which includes the macula (Fig. 4.67A). In the chronic type, there are circumscribed areas of RPE loss (Fig. 4.67B).

In the acute type, the diagnosis is usually easy because of the history of ingestion of massive doses of thioridazine. The chronic type may resemble gyrate atrophy. The main difference is that the areas of atrophy in thioridazine toxicity are not as pronounced as those in gyrate atrophy.

Management. The drug must be discontinued with any signs of retinal toxicity.

Talc Retinopathy

In chronic intravenous drug abusers, talc particles gradually occlude pulmonary capillaries. Pulmonary shunts develop, allowing particles to gain access to the systemic circulation and to the eye, where they occlude retinal capillaries.

Clinical Features. In most cases, the refractile particles can be seen in the macula (Fig. 4.68). Macular capillary occlusions cause hypoxia and edema with decreased vision. Widespread areas of capillary nonperfusion in the periphery can lead to peripheral and optic disc neovascularization and to vitreous hemorrhage.

Proliferative talc retinopathy must be differentiated from other causes of peripheral neovascularization, such as diabetes, sarcoidosis, and Eales disease. Talc maculopathy can resemble radiation and diabetic retinopathies. The patient's history and recognition of the talc particles are important. The differential diagnosis of crystalline retinopathy in general includes canthaxanthine, tamoxifen, nitrofurantoin, primary and secondary oxalosis, cystinosis, and Bietti's disease.

Management. Patients with neovascularization and vitreous hemorrhage should be treated with photocoagulation.

Tamoxifen Retinopathy

Tamoxifen retinopathy is a rare form of crystalline retinopathy occasionally seen in patients taking the drug for extended periods of time.

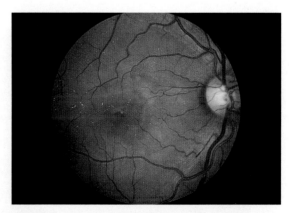

FIGURE 4.68. Multiple talc particles are present in the macula of a patient who was a longstanding intravenous drug abuser.

Clinical Features. Examination reveals subtle, yellow-white dots in the central macula with or without vision loss or other evidence of visual dysfunction. Corneal opacities and optic neuropathy have also been reported.

Management. The drug should be discontinued at the first signs of any visual dysfunction.

ALBINISM

Albinism can be divided into two somewhat overlapping types: oculocutaneous and ocular. In oculocutaneous albinism, which is inherited autosomal recessively, there is decreased melanin pigment in each melanosome. It can be subdivided into a tyrosinase-positive subtype, in which the skin, hair, and eyes have some pigment, and a tyrosinase-negative subtype, in which there is no pigment. In ocular albinism, the cutaneous findings are minimal. The total number of melanosomes is decreased, although each melanosome may be fully pigmented, and macromelanosomes are present. The disorder may have an X-linked recessive pattern of inheritance.

Clinical Features. The *sine qua non* of albinism is foveal hypoplasia (Fig. 4.69), which is the absence of the foveal reflex, absence of the yellow macula lutea pigment, absence of the normal hyperpigmentation of the foveal pigment epithelium, and failure of the retinal vasculature to create a foveal avascular zone. Other findings include congenitally subnormal vision, nystagmus, photophobia, iris transillumination, and a hypopigmented fundus. The visual acuity is usually markedly decreased, and the patients have searching nystagmus. Supranormal amplitudes are found on the ERG and EOG.

Women who are carriers of the X-linked variety often show partial iris transillumination. They may also have peripheral RPE mosaicism or a salt and pepper fundus. The visual functions of carriers are normal.

In some patients with lightly pigmented skin, the RPE may also be hypopigmented (i.e., "blond" fundus), but visual function and the fovea are normal.

Management. Periodic examination, genetic counseling, and low vision support constitute management.

TAPETORETINAL DISEASES

Retinitis Pigmentosa

Retinitis pigmentosa (RP) is characterized by progressive degeneration of the rods and cones. In most cases, there is associated migration of pigment epithelial cells into the retina. The disorder can have autosomal recessive, X-linked recessive, and autosomal dominant patterns of inheritance. The autosomal recessive and X-linked forms have the earliest onset (i.e., early childhood) and the worst prognosis. Patients with the autosomal dominant form may be symptom free until middle age. Genetic analysis has shown that the primary defect in most affected individuals is in the gene that codes for rhodopsin. There are two variants of RP: type I, in which the rods are affected earlier than the cones, and type II, in which the cones are affected earlier than the rods.

Clinical Features. In type I RP, the first symptoms are decreased scotopic vision and decreased peripheral vision. Central visual acuity is initially normal and may remain so, but it can be decreased because of macular atrophy (Fig. 4.70), cystoid macular edema, or the typical posterior subcapsular cataract.

Fundus findings include vitreous cells and opacities, narrowed arteries, diffuse depigmentation of the RPE, and comma-shaped intraretinal proliferation of pigmented cells (i.e., "bone spicules") that may be sparse or densely packed (Figs. 4.71 and 4.72). The waxy pallor of the optic disc is a late sign.

The diagnosis of type I RP is usually made by clinical examination alone. A careful family history can be helpful, as can examination of family members to detect the carrier state. The examiner looks for isolated patches of bone spicules, splotchy pigmentation of the RPE (i.e., salt and pepper pattern), or a bronze sheen in the macula. The diagnosis can be confirmed by an ERG. In the earliest stages of

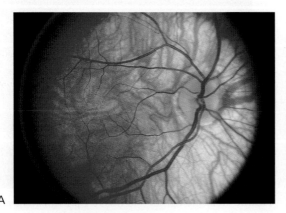
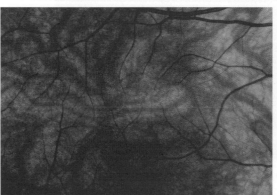

FIGURE 4.69. A: Depigmentation of the fundus occurs in albinism. **B:** Macular hypoplasia is present in the same patient.

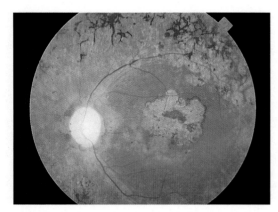

FIGURE 4.70. Narrowed arteries, pale optic disc, bone spicules, and atrophic macula can be seen in a patient with retinitis pigmentosa.

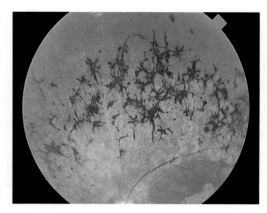

FIGURE 4.72. Densely packed bone spicules.

the disease, the scotopic ERG is more affected than the photopic. In late stages, the ERG is usually nonrecordable.

In type II RP, patients are usually not night blind until the visual field has contracted to less than 10°. Half of the patients have no intraretinal pigment deposition (i.e., retinitis pigmentosa *sine pigmento*). Nevertheless, they have cells in the vitreous, and the pigment epithelium has a paler appearance than normal. In early cases, the photopic ERG is more severely affected than is the scotopic.

Other causes of night blindness, such as vitamin A deficiency, congenital stationary night blindness, and the RP systemic syndromes, must be ruled out. Certain entities such as congenital syphilis and rubella have a salt and pepper appearance that may be confused with RP, but there is no migration of pigment cells into the sensory retina, and the ERG is usually normal or near normal. The "unilateral RP" probably does not exist, although there may be pigment migration into the sensory retina. Most cases are caused by blunt trauma, uveitis, and regressed, longstanding retinal detachment.

Management. If a significant cataract is present, cataract extraction with placement of a posterior chamber lens often provides a significant improvement in visual function.

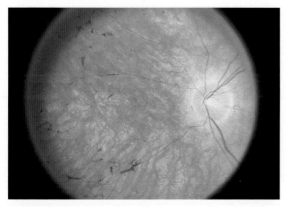

FIGURE 4.71. Narrowed arteries, pale or "washed-out" retinal pigment epithelium, and a few bone spicules.

Cystoid macular edema may respond to acetazolamide (500 mg/day) with some degree of improved visual acuity. Unfortunately, the beneficial effect is temporary for some patients. A prospective randomized trial showed that daily administration of 15,000 IU of vitamin A slowed the rate of deterioration detected by ERG, but there was no demonstrable benefit for visual acuity or the visual fields.

Sector Retinitis Pigmentosa

In sector retinitis pigmentosa, one area of the fundus has the prominent bone spicule and vascular changes of classic RP. The inferior retina is most commonly affected, and the changes are bilateral and symmetric. The remaining retina looks normal or almost normal, but careful electrophysiologic testing shows some impairment. Sector RP is inherited autosomal dominantly.

Retinitis Pigmentosa Syndromes

Laurence-Moon-Bardet-Biedl Syndrome

Laurence-Moon-Bardet-Biedl syndrome is an inherited condition that is characterized by an atypical pigmentary retinopathy. Affected individuals may also have mental retardation, hypogenitalism, short stature, polydactyly, obesity, and spastic paraplegia.

Refsum's Syndrome

Refsum's syndrome is caused by an inborn error of metabolism. In rhodopsin metabolism, vitamin A is esterified to palmitic acid, which is metabolized to phytanic acid. Because phytanic acid α-hydroxylase is deficient, phytanic acid accumulates in RPE cells, causing the sensory retina to deteriorate and resulting in an atypical type of RP (Fig. 4.73). Systemic findings include cerebellar ataxia, peripheral neuropathy, nerve deafness, and anosmia. There is also increased cerebrospinal fluid protein without pleocytosis. Patients may benefit from a diet low in phytanic acid.

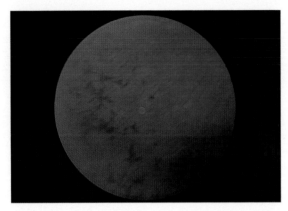

FIGURE 4.73. Irregular bone spicule-type pigmentation in the periphery of a patient with Refsum's syndrome.

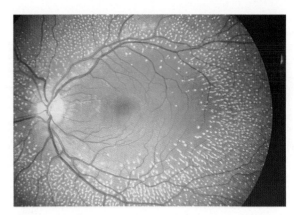

FIGURE 4.74. Multiple dot-like lesions at the level of the pigment epithelium in a patient with fundus albipunctatus.

Bassen-Kornzweig Syndrome

Bassen-Kornzweig syndrome is caused by failure to produce β-lipoprotein, with resultant malabsorption and vitamin A deficiency. The vitamin A deficiency causes night blindness with retinal degeneration. Bone spicules are usually not seen. Systemic findings include steatorrhea, acanthocytosis, ataxic neuropathy, and growth retardation. It must be stressed that the abnormalities caused by this condition can be reversed with vitamin A therapy if the diagnosis is made before significant retinal degeneration has occurred.

Spielmeyer-Vogt-Batten-Mayou Syndrome

Spielmeyer-Vogt-Batten-Mayou syndrome is characterized by seizures, progressive dementia, ataxia, and an RP-like syndrome with a bull's-eye macula. The diagnosis can be confirmed by the finding of vacuolation of peripheral lymphocytes and by metachromasia of skin fibroblasts in cell culture.

Progressive External Ophthalmoplegia

Progressive external ophthalmoplegia is a mitochondrially inherited disease characterized by gradual paresis of the extraocular muscles and eyelids. There is ophthalmoplegia (without diplopia) and ptosis. The severity of retinal involvement varies. The most common variant is benign, with salt and pepper RPE changes and normal visual function. The less common variant progresses to findings similar to those of RP. Systemic findings include facial weakness, dysphagia, small stature, limb girdle myopathy, and cardiac conduction defects. Affected patients may have complete heart block (Kearns-Sayre syndrome.)

Other Retinitis Pigmentosa–Related Syndromes

There are many syndromes in which the typical RP is associated with systemic abnormalities. The most common is Usher's syndrome, in which RP is associated with deafness.

Fundus Albipunctatus

Fundus albipunctatus is a descriptive term used to describe eyes that have myriad, small, white subretinal dots (Fig. 4.74). There are two variants. The first, retinitis punctata albescens, progresses to produce findings similar to those of retinitis pigmentosa. The second, albipunctate dystrophy, is a form of congenital stationary night blindness.

In patients with albipunctate dystrophy, the number of white dots may increase or decrease. The amplitude of the scotopic ERG is usually subnormal, but if the patient's eyes are patched and allowed to dark adapt for 3 hours, the amplitude typically recovers to normal. The same is true for dark adaptation, which may take hours to reach the final rod threshold. The visual acuity is usually normal, but there may be late macular atrophy.

Choroideremia

Choroideremia is an X-linked recessive tapetoretinal degeneration that becomes symptomatic in patients between 4

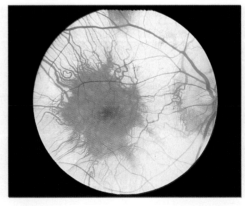

FIGURE 4.75. Central remaining island of pigment epithelium and choriocapillaris in a patient with advanced choroideremia.

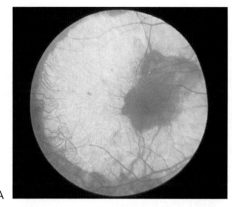
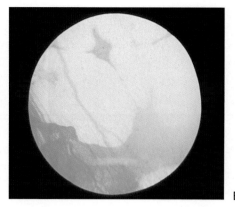

FIGURE 4.76. A Scalloped areas of pigment epithelium and choriocapillaris dropout in a patient with gyrate atrophy. **B:** Peripheral scalloped areas of choriocapillaris and pigment epithelial dropout in the same patient.

and 20 years of age. The primary defect is probably in the RPE. The symptoms are similar to those of RP. The fundus, unlike that seen in RP, has no pigment clumping. In its early stages, choroideremia is characterized by patchy atrophy of the peripheral RPE and choriocapillaris. Later, the RPE and choriocapillaris are completely absent, except in the macula (Fig. 4.75). The diagnosis is made by fundus examination, family history, and examination of carrier women who typically have a salt and pepper fundus.

Gyrate Atrophy

Gyrate atrophy is an autosomal recessive disease caused by an error in metabolism that results in hyperornithinemia. The age of onset is between 10 and 40 years. Its symptoms are similar to RP. The fundus has well-defined scalloped areas of absent choriocapillaris and RPE with an abrupt transition between normal and atrophic areas (Fig. 4.76). Patients and carriers can be diagnosed by measurement of ornithine ketoacid transaminase in cultures of skin fibroblasts. Lowering of serum ornithine with oral pyridoxine (vitamin B_6) therapy has been shown to slow the rate of retinal degeneration.

Stickler's Syndrome

Stickler's syndrome is an autosomal dominant condition whose hallmark is an optically empty vitreous, except for a thin layer of cortical vitreous behind the lens and bands of collagen that traverse the vitreous cavity and adhere to the retina (Fig. 4.77). Systematic abnormalities include orofacial abnormalities, such as midfacial flattening and cleft palate, and joint abnormalities, such as hyperextensibility, enlargement, and arthritis. Retinal detachment is common. Repair is frequently difficult, because the retinal breaks are at multiple levels in areas of circumferential and radial lattice degeneration (Fig. 4.78) and because there is a strong tendency for proliferative vitreoretinopathy. Other ocular abnormalities include retinoschisis, pigmentary retinal degeneration with a depressed ERG, cataract, glaucoma, optic atrophy, and high myopia.

Leber's Congenital Amaurosis

Leber's congenital amaurosis is a severe retinal dystrophy manifested at birth or early in infancy. The ERG pattern is nonrecordable. The fundus examination initially may be

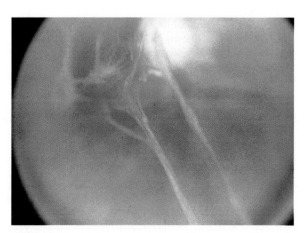

FIGURE 4.77. Vitreous bands in a patient with Stickler's syndrome.

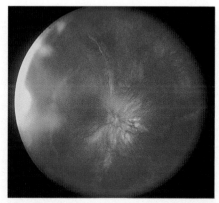

FIGURE 4.78. Equator-plus photograph showing multiple areas of radial and circumferential lattice in a patient with Stickler's syndrome.

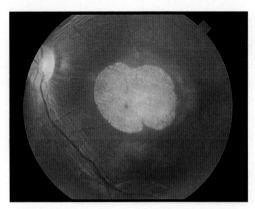

FIGURE 4.79. Macular atrophy and narrowed retinal arteries are seen in a patient with Leber's congenital amaurosis.

normal, or there may be a central area of atrophic RPE sometimes referred to as a macular coloboma (Fig. 4.79). Later, there is some degree of nonspecific, diffuse RPE mottling and sometimes intraretinal pigment deposits giving a retinitis pigmentosa–like picture. Affected patients usually are hyperopic and have pendular nystagmus. Keratoconus is also common. Mental retardation is sometimes present.

METABOLIC DISEASES

The *sphingolipidoses* are a group of diseases caused by a deficiency of the lysosomal enzymes necessary for the degeneration of gangliosides, cerebrosides, and sphingomyelin, which are collectively called sphingolipids. They are important components of cell membranes, especially in nervous tissue.

Patients with *Tay-Sachs disease* have mental retardation and experience early death. The sphingolipids accumulate in the ganglion cells of the retina, rendering them opaque. Because ganglion cells are more numerous in the perifoveolar retina than elsewhere and are absent in the foveola, the typical fundus finding is a cherry red spot (Fig. 4.80).

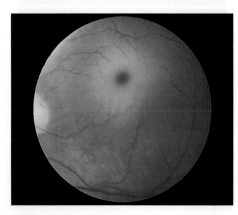

FIGURE 4.80. Cherry red spot in the macula of a patient with Tay-Sachs disease.

Niemann-Pick disease type B is also called the sea-blue histiocyte syndrome or chronic Niemann-Pick disease. It is the mildest form of the several varieties of Niemann-Pick and is commonly not diagnosed until the late teens or early adult years. Systemic findings include massive hepatosplenomegaly, infiltration of the lungs, and foam cells in the bone marrow. Unlike many of the other sphingolipidoses, there is no mental retardation and no functional involvement of the central nervous system. The typical ocular finding is a macular halo.

BIBLIOGRAPHY

American Academy of Ophthalmology. Retina and vitreous: Basic and clinical science course, section 12. San Francisco: Foundation of the AAO; 2000.

Armstrong JD, Meyer D, Xu S, et al. Long-term follow-up of Stargardt's disease and fundus favimaculatus. *Ophthalmology* 1998;105:448.

Benson WE, Shakin J, Sarin LK. Blunt trauma. In: Tasman W, Jaeger EA. Duane's clinical ophthalmology, vol 3. Philadelphia: JB Lippincott; 1992:1.

Berson EL, Rosner B, Sandberg MA, et al. A randomized trial of vitamin A and vitamin E supplementation for retinitis pigmentosa. *Arch Ophthalmol* 1993;111:761.

Bird AC, Bressler NM, Bressler SB, et al. An international classification and grading system for age-related maculopathy and age-related macular degeneration. *Surv Ophthalmol* 1995;39:367.

Bird AC. Retinal photoreceptor dystrophies. LI Edward Jackson memorial lecture. *Am J Ophthalmol* 1995;119:543.

Bird AC. Inherited outer retinal dystrophies. In: Tasman WS. Clinical decisions in medical retinal disease. St. Louis: Mosby; 1994:29.

Bressler NM, Bressler SB, Fine SL. Age-related macular degeneration. *Surv Ophthalmol* 1988;32:375.

Brown GC. Congenital fundus abnormalities. In: Regillo CD, Brown GC, Flynn HW. Vitreoretinal disease: The essentials. New York: Thieme; 1999:581.

Brown GC. Radiation retinopathy. In: Tasman W, Jaeger EA. Duane's clinical ophthalmology, vol 3. Philadelphia: JB Lippincott; 1992:1.

Byer NE. Long-term natural history of lattice degeneration of the retina. *Ophthalmology* 1989;96:1396.

Byer NE. Lattice degeneration of the retina. *Surv Ophthalmol* 1979;22:41.

Byer NE. Long-term natural history study of senile retinoschisis with implications for management. *Ophthalmology* 1986;93:1127.

Byer NE. The natural history of asymptomatic retinal breaks. *Ophthalmology* 1982;89:1033.

Carr RE. The generalized heredoretinal disorders. In: Regillo CD, Brown GC, Flynn HW. Vitreoretinal disease: The essentials. New York: Thieme; 1999:307.

Chu TG, Cano MR, Green RL, Liggett PE, Lean JS. Massive suprachoroidal hemorrhage with central retinal apposition: a clinical and echographic study. *Arch Ophthalmol* 1991;109:1575.

Clarkson JF, Altman RD. Angioid streaks. *Surv Ophthalmol* 1982;26:235.

Condon GP, Brownstein S, Wang NS, et al. Congenital hereditary (juvenile X-linked) retinoschisis. Histopathologic and ultrastructural findings in three eyes. *Arch Ophthalmol* 1986;104:576.

Cruess AF, Schachat AP, Nicholl J, et al. Chloroquine retinopathy: is fluorescein angiography necessary? *Ophthalmology* 1985;92:127.

Dabbs TR, Skjodt K. Prevalence of angioid streaks and other ocular complications of Paget's disease of bone. *Br J Ophthalmol* 1990;74:579.

Davis MD. Natural history of retinal breaks without detachment. *Arch Ophthalmol* 1974;92:183.

Deutman AF. Electro-oculography in families with vitelliform dystrophy of the fovea: detection of the carrier state. *Arch Ophthalmol* 1969;81:305.

Eagle RC, Lucier AC, Bernardino VB, et al. Retinal pigment epithelial abnormalities in fundus flavimaculatus. *Ophthalmology* 1980;87:1189.

Easterbrook M. Dose relationships in patients with early chloroquine retinopathy. *J Rheumatol* 1987;14:472.

Ficker L, Vafidis G, While A, Leaver P. Long-term follow-up of a prospective trial of argon laser photocoagulation in the treatment of central serous retinopathy. *Br J Ophthalmol* 1988;72:829.

Fishman GA, Baca W, Alexander KR, et al. Visual acuity in patients with Best vitelliform macular dystrophy. *Ophthalmology* 1993;100:1665.

Fishman GA, Farber M, et al. Visual acuity loss in patients with Stargardt's macular dystrophy. *Ophthalmology* 1987;94:809.

Fishman GA, Glenn AM, Gilbert LD. Rebound of macular edema with continued use of methazolamide in patients with retinitis pigmentosa. *Arch Ophthalmol* 1993;111:1640.

Flannery JG, Bird AC, Farber DB, Weleber RG, Bok D. A histopathologic study of a choroideremia carrier. *Invest Ophthalmol Vis Sci* 1990;31:229.

Folk JC, Arrindell EL, Klugman MR. The fellow eye of patients with phakic lattice retinal detachment. *Ophthalmology* 1989;96:72.

Gass JDM, Joondeph BC. Observations concerning patients with suspected impending macular holes. *Am J Ophthalmol* 1990;109:638.

Gass JDM. Diseases causing choroidal exudation and hemorrhagic localized detachment of the retina and retinal pigment epithelium. In: Gass JDM. Stereoscopic atlas of macular diseases. Diagnosis and treatment. 4th ed. St. Louis: Mosby; 1997:49.

Gass JDM. Macular dysfunction caused by vitreous and vitreoretinal interface abnormalities. In: Gass JDM. Stereoscopic atlas of macular diseases. Diagnosis and treatment. 4th ed. St. Louis: Mosby; 1997:903.

Gass JDM. Reappraisal of biomicroscopic classification of stages of development of a macular hole. *Am J Ophthalmol* 1995;119:752.

Gladstone GJ, Tasman W. Solar retinitis after minimal exposure. *Arch Ophthalmol* 1978;96:1368.

Greaves AH, Sarks JP, Sarks SH. Adult vitelliform macular degeneration: a clinical spectrum. *Aust N Z J Ophthalmol* 1990;18:171.

Green WR, Enger C. Age-related macular degeneration histopathologic studies. The 1992 Lorenz E. Zimmerman lecture. *Ophthalmology* 1993;100:1519.

Greven CM, Moreno RJ, Tasman W. Unusual manifestations of X-linked retinoschisis. *Trans Am Ophthalmol Soc* 1990;88:211.

Grossniklaus HE, Green WR. Pathologic findings in pathologic myopia. *Retina* 1992;12:127.

Guerry RK, Ham WT, Mueller HA. Light toxicity in the posterior segment. In: Tasman W, Jaeger EA. Duane's clinical ophthalmology, vol 3. Philadelphia: JB Lippincott; 1992:1.

Ham WT Jr, Mueller HA, Ruffolo JJ Jr, et al. Basic mechanisms underlying the production of photochemical lesions in the mammalian retina. *Curr Eye Res* 1984;3:165.

Hassan AS, Johnson MW, Schneiderman TE, et al. Management of submacular hemorrhages with intravitreal tPA injection and pneumatic displacement. *Ophthalmology* 1999;106:1900.

Hampton GR, Kohen D, Bird AC. Visual prognosis of disciform degeneration in myopia. *Ophthalmology* 1983;90:923.

Heckenlively JR, Arden GB. Principles and practice of clinical electrophysiology of vision. St. Louis: Mosby-Year Book; 1991.

Heckenlively JR. Retinitis pigmentosa. Philadelphia: JB Lippincott; 1988.

Hilton GF. Late serosanguineous detachment of the macula after traumatic choroidal rupture. *Am J Ophthalmol* 1975;799:997.

Ho AC. Miscellaneous macular degenerations. In: Regillo CD, Brown GC, Flynn HW. Vitreoretinal disease: The essentials. New York: Thieme; 1999:241.

Jalkh AE, Weiter JJ, Trempe CL, et al. Choroidal neovascularization in degenerative myopia: role of laser photocoagulation. *Ophthalmic Surg* 1987;18:721.

Jampol LM, Setogawa T, Rednam KRV, Tso MOM. Talc retinopathy in primates: a model of ischemic retinopathy. I. Clinical studies. *Arch Ophthalmol* 1981;99:1273.

Kaiser-Kupfer MI, Caruso RC, Valle D. Gyrate atrophy of the choroid and retina. Long-term reduction of ornithine slows retinal degeneration. *Arch Ophthalmol* 1991;109:1539.

Klein R, Klein BEK, Jensen SE, et al. The five-year incidence and progression of age-related maculopathy. The Beaver Dam study. *Ophthalmology* 1997;104:7.

Kozart DM. Anatomic correlates of the retina. In: Tasman W, Jaeger EA. Duane's clinical ophthalmology, vol 3. Philadelphia: JB Lippincott; 1994:1.

Krill AE, Deutman AF, Fishman M. The cone degenerations. *Doc Ophthalmol* 1973;35:1.

Kriss A, Russell-Eggitt I, Harris CM, Lloyd IC, Taylor D. Aspects of albinism. *Ophthalmic Paediatr Genet* 1992;13:89.

Leonard RE 2nd, Smiddy WE, Flynn HW Jr, et al. Long-term visual outcomes in patients with successful macular hole surgery. *Ophthalmology* 1997;104:1648.

Levine R, Brucker AJ, Robinson F. Long-term follow-up of idiopathic central serous chorioretinopathy by fluorescein angiography. *Ophthalmology* 1989;96:854.

Lim JI, Enger C, Fine SL. Foveomacular dystrophy. *Am J Ophthalmol* 1994;117:1.

Macular Photocoagulation Study Group. Argon laser photocoagulation for neovascular maculopathy. Five-year results from randomized clinical trials. *Arch Ophthalmol* 1991;109:1109.

Macular Photocoagulation Study Group. Five-year follow-up of fellow eyes of patients with age-related macular degeneration and unilateral extrafoveal choroidal neovascularization. *Arch Ophthalmol* 1993;111:1189.

Macular Photocoagulation Study Group. Persistent and recurrent neovascularization after krypton laser photocoagulation for neovascular lesions of age-related macular degeneration. *Arch Ophthalmol* 1990;108:825.

Macular Photocoagulation Study Group. Pretreatment fundus characteristics as predictors of recurrent choroidal neovascularization. *Arch Ophthalmol* 1991;109:1193.

Macular Photocoagulation Study Group. Risk factors for choroidal neovascularization in the second eye of patients with juxtafoveal or subfoveal choroidal neovascularization secondary to age-related macular degeneration. *Arch Ophthalmol* 1997;115:741.

Macular Photocoagulation Study Group. Persistent and recurrent neovascularization after krypton laser photocoagulation for neovascular lesions of ocular histoplasmosis. *Arch Ophthalmol* 1989;107:344.

Mansour AM. Systemic associations of angioid streaks. *J Intern Ophthalmol Clin* 1991;31:61.

Margherio RR, Cox MS Jr, Trese MT, et al. Removal of epimacular membranes. *Ophthalmology* 1985;92:1075.

McCulloch C, Arshinoff S. Choroideremia and gyrate atrophy. In: Tasman W, Jaeger EA. Duane's clinical ophthalmology, vol 3. Philadelphia: JB Lippincott; 1992:1.

McDonald HR, Schatz H, Johnson RN, Madeira D. Acquired macular disease. In: Tasman W, Jaeger EA. Duane's clinical ophthalmology, vol 3. Rev ed. Philadelphia: JB Lippincott; 1994: chap 23.

Mittra RA, Mieler WF. Drug and light ocular toxicity. In: Regillo CD, Brown GC, Flynn HW. Vitreoretinal disease: The essentials. New York: Thieme; 1999:545.

Murphy SB, Jackson WB, Pare JAP. Talc retinopathy. *Can J Ophthalmol* 1978;13:152.

O'Connell SR, Bressler NM. Age-related macular degeneration. In: Regillo CD, Brown GC, Flynn HW. Vitreoretinal disease: The essentials. New York: Thieme; 1999:213.

O'Donnell FE Jr, Green WR. The eye in albinism. In: Tasman W, Jaeger EA. Duane's clinical ophthalmology, vol 4. Philadelphia: JB Lippincott; 1992:1.

Ogden TE. Topography of the retina. In: Ryan SJ, Ogden TE. Retina. 2nd ed. St. Louis: CV Mosby; 1994:32.

Park SS, Sigelman J, Gragoudas ES. Retina. In: Tasman W, Jaeger EA. Foundations of clinical ophthalmology. Philadelphia: JB Lippincott; 1994:1.

Pece A, Avanza P, Galli L, Brancato R. Laser photocoagulation of choroidal neovascularization in angioid streaks. *Retina* 1997;17:12.

Petrukhin K, Koisti MJ, Bakall B, et al. Identification of the gene responsible for Best macular dystrophy. *Nat Genet* 1998;19:241.

Regillo CD, Blade KA, Custis PH, O'Connell SR. Evaluating persistent and recurrent choroidal neovascularization: the role of indocyanine green angiography. *Ophthalmology* 1998;105:1821.

Regillo CD, Benson WE. Retinal detachment: Diagnosis and management. 3rd ed. Philadelphia: Lippincott-Raven; 1998.

Regillo CD, Benson WE, Maguire JI, Annesley WH. Indocyanine green angiography and occult choroidal neovascularization. *Ophthalmology* 1994;101:280.

Regillo CD. Update on photodynamic therapy. *Curr Opin Ophthalmol* 2000;11:166.

Regillo CD. The present role of indocyanine green angiography in ophthalmology. *Curr Opin Ophthalmol* 1999;10:189.

Regillo CD, Custis PH. Surgical management of retinoschisis. *Curr Opin Ophthalmol* 1997;8:80.

Regillo CD, Tasman WS, Brown GC. Surgical management of complications associated with X-linked retinoschisis. *Arch Ophthalmol* 1993;111:1080.

Regillo CD. Posterior segment manifestations of systemic trauma. In: Regillo CD, Brown GC, Flynn HW. Vitreoretinal disease: The essentials. New York: Thieme; 1999:537.

Robertson DM, Ilstrup D. Direct, indirect, and sham laser photocoagulation in the management of central serous chorioretinopathy. *Am J Ophthalmol* 1983;95:457.

Ryan EH, Gilbert HD. Results of surgical treatment of recent-onset full-thickness macular holes. *Arch Ophthalmol* 1994;1112:1545.

Sanborn EG, Gonder R, Goldberg RE, Benson WE, Kessler S. Evulsion of the optic nerve: a clinicopathological study. *Can J Ophthalmol* 1984;19:10.

Sarks SH. Drusen and their relationship to senile macular degeneration. *Aust J Ophthalmol* 1980;8:117.

Schatz H, Yannuzzi LA, Gitter ER. Subretinal neovascularization following argon laser photocoagulation treatment for central serous chorioretinopathy. Complication or misdiagnosis? *Trans Am Acad Ophthalmol Otolaryngol* 1977;88:893.

Schubert HD. Ocular embryology. In: Regillo CD, Brown GC, Flynn HW. Vitreoretinal disease: The essentials. New York: Thieme; 1999:3.

Schultz PN, Sobol WM. Angioid streaks and pseudoxanthoma elasticum. *JAMA* 1991;265:45.

Silicone Study Group. Vitrectomy with silicone oil or perfluoropropane gas in eyes with severe proliferative vitreoretinopathy: results of a randomized clinical trial: Silicone Study report 2. *Arch Ophthalmol* 1992;110:780.

Sipperley JO, Quigley HA, Gass JDM. Traumatic retinopathy in primates: the explanation of commotio retinae. *Arch Ophthalmol* 1978;96:2267.

Smiddy WE, Flynn HW Jr, Nicholson DH, et al. Results and complications in treated retinal breaks. *Am J Ophthalmol* 1991;112:623.

Smiddy WE, Michels RG, Green WR. Morphology, pathology, and surgery of idiopathic vitreoretinal macular disorders. A review. *Retina* 1990;10:288.

Smith RE, Kelley JS, Harbin TS. Late macular complications of choroidal ruptures. *Am J Ophthalmol* 1974;77:650.

Song MK, Small KW. Macular dystrophies. In: Regillo CD, Brown GC, Flynn HW. Vitreoretinal disease: The essentials. New York: Thieme; 1999:293.

Steinmetz RL, Garner A, Maguire JI, Bird AC. Histopathology of incipient fundus flavimaculatus. *Ophthalmology* 1991;98:953.

Stickler GB, Belau PG, Farrell FJ, et al. Hereditary progressive arthro-ophthalmopathy. *Mayo Clin Proc* 1965;40:433.

Straatsma BR, Foos RY, Feman SS. Degenerative diseases of the peripheral retina. In: Tasman W, Jaeger EA. Duane's Clinical Ophthalmology, vol 3. Philadelphia: JB Lippincott; 1992:1.

Tasman W. Hyaloideoretinopathies. In: Regillo CD, Brown GC, Flynn HW. Vitreoretinal disease: The essentials. New York: Thieme; 1999:365.

Thomas MS, Grand MG, Williams DF, et al. Surgical management of subfoveal choroidal neovascularization. *Ophthalmology* 1992;99:952.

Thompson JT, Sjaarda RN, Lansing MB. The results of vitreous surgery for chronic macular hole. *Retina* 1997;17:493.

Tornambe PE, Hilton GF, and the Retinal Detachment Study Group. Pneumatic retinopexy: a multicenter randomized controlled clinical trial comparing pneumatic retinopexy with scleral buckling. *Ophthalmology* 1989;96:772.

Treatment of Age-related Macular Degeneration With Photodynamic Therapy (TAP) Study Group. Photodynamic therapy of subfoveal choroidal neovascularization in age-related macular degeneration with verteporfin. One-year results of 2 randomized clinical trials—TAP report 1. *Arch Ophthalmol* 1999;117:1329.

Tse DT, Ober RR. Talc retinopathy. *Am J Ophthalmol* 1980;90:624.

Vander JF, Duker JS, Jaeger EA. Miscellaneous diseases of the fundus. In: Tasman W, Jaeger EA. Duane's clinical ophthalmology, vol 3. Philadelphia: JB Lippincott; 1992:1.

Vander JF. Choroidal neovascularization associated with myopic macular degeneration. In: Tasman WS. Clinical decisions in medical retinal disease. St. Louis: Mosby; 1994.

Vine AK, Shatz H. Adult-onset foveomacular pigment epithelial dystrophy. *Am J Ophthalmol* 1980;89:680.

Welch JC, Spaeth G, Benson WE. Massive suprachoroidal hemorrhage. Follow-up and outcome of 30 cases. *Ophthalmology* 1988;95:1202.

Wendel RT, Patel AC, Kelly NE, Salzano TC, Wells JW, Novack GD. Vitreous surgery for macular holes. *Ophthalmology* 1993;100:1671.

Wray S, Boustany R-MN. Ophthalmic manifestations of defects in metabolism. In: Tasman W, Jaeger EA. Duane's clinical ophthalmology, vol 3. Philadelphia: JB Lippincott; 1992:1.

Yannuzzi LA, Slakter JS, Sorenson JA, Guyer DR, Orlock DA. Digital indocyanine green videoangiography and choroidal neovascularization. *Retina* 1992;12:191.

CHAPTER 5

Retinal Vascular Disease

Gary C. Brown
William Tasman

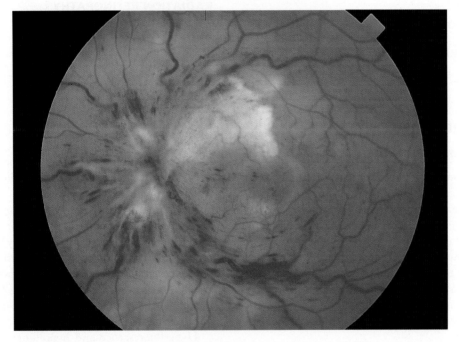

Central retinal vein obstruction associated with occlusion of a cilioretinal artery.

FUNDUS ANGIOGRAPHY

Fluorescein Angiography

Since its description by Novotny and Alvis in 1961, intravenous fluorescein angiography has become one of the most extensively used diagnostic modalities in ophthalmology. Sodium fluorescein is a hydrocarbon that is 80% bound to serum proteins when injected into the bloodstream. The 20% that is unbound can be excited by a blue light with a wavelength of 465 to 490 nm and caused to fluoresce a yellow-green color at a wavelength of 520 to 530 nm. The dye is 90% eliminated in the urine within 24 hours. It imparts an orange appearance to the skin and a yellow-orange appearance to the urine.

The complications of intravenous sodium fluorescein injection include nausea in 5% to 10% of patients and vomiting in 1% to 2%. These effects usually occur within 1 to 2 minutes after injection. Less frequently observed adverse effects include vasovagal reactions and true allergies, characterized by hives and pruritus. The incidence of true anaphylaxis is extremely low. Extravasation into extravascular spaces can lead to local tissue necrosis.

The vessels of the ciliary body and the choriocapillaris are permeable to sodium fluorescein. Ocular neovascularization is also permeable. The normal retinal vessels and the larger choroidal vessels are impermeable.

There are four phases to a normal fluorescein angiogram, although the first two may overlap (Fig. 5.1): the choroidal filling phase; the retinal arterial filling phase; the venous filling phase; and the recirculation phase.

Fluorescein dye usually enters the choroid about 10 to 15 seconds after intravenous injection, depending on the site of injection, the rapidity of injection, and the status of the systemic circulation. Filling the choroid is also referred to as the choroidal flush, because filling of the individual choriocapillaries cannot be seen. The choroid should be completely filled within 5 seconds after the first appearance of dye within it. Dye appears within a cilioretinal artery concomitantly with filling of the choroid.

The retinal arteries begin to fill approximately 1 to 2 seconds after the appearance of dye within the retinal arteries. Usually, the retinal veins are completely filled within 10 seconds after dye is first seen within the retinal arteries. During the recirculation phase, which usually begins a minute or so after the injection, there is decreasing fluorescence within the retinal vessels as the bolus of dye is distributed throughout the systemic vasculature.

Hyperfluorescence and hypofluorescence are the terms used when describing fluorescein angiographic patterns. *Hyperfluorescence* occurs when there is an abnormal accumulation of dye (Fig. 5.2) or a retinal pigment epithelial "window defect" (i.e., transmission defect), the absence or relative absence of the retinal pigment epithelium (Fig. 5.3). *Hypofluorescence* occurs when there is an absence of dye (Fig. 5.4) or blockage of fluorescence by blood (Fig. 5.5), melanin pigment, or some other substance.

Retinal capillary nonperfusion (Fig. 5.6) is a pattern that is important to recognize with fluorescein angiography. It is characterized by a homogenous gray appearance of fluorescence that comes predominantly from the underlying choroid. The larger remaining retinal vessels stand out in relief to the surrounding relative hypofluorescence and, in the later phases of the study, there is minimal leakage of dye into the retina in nonperfused areas.

Ocular neovascularization in the choroid, retina, or iris or on the optic disc routinely demonstrates leakage of fluorescein dye (Fig. 5.6). Fluorescence from new vessels is most often maximal during the early phases of the study. During

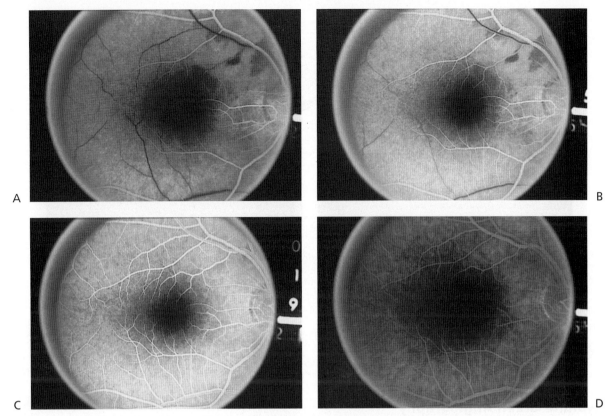

FIGURE 5.1. Normal intravenous fluorescein angiogram. **A:** Within 14 seconds after injection, the study is in the retinal arterial filling phase. A diffuse choroidal flush results from filling of the choriocapillaris, and several small choroidal filling defects are evident along the supertemporal retinal vascular arcade. The normal hypofluorescence in the foveal region occurs because of blockage of the choroidal fluorescence pattern in this region by taller retinal pigment epithelial cells and xanthophyll pigment in the outer retinal layers. **B:** Within 15 seconds after injection, the study is in the laminar venous filling phase. **C:** By 19 seconds after injection, the venous filling is nearly complete. **D:** Several minutes after injection, during the recirculation phase, the fluorescence of the choroid and the retinal vessels is less pronounced.

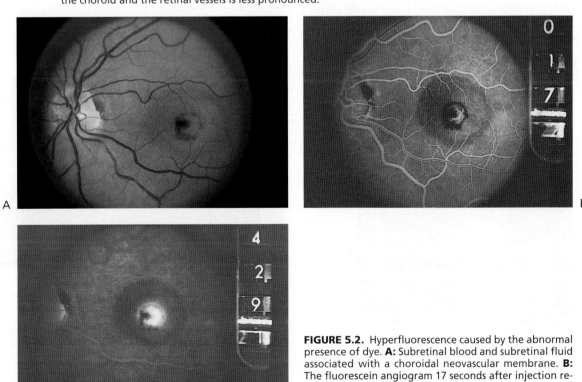

FIGURE 5.2. Hyperfluorescence caused by the abnormal presence of dye. **A:** Subretinal blood and subretinal fluid associated with a choroidal neovascular membrane. **B:** The fluorescein angiogram 17 seconds after injection reveals lacy hyperfluorescence of the membrane. **C:** At 429 seconds after injection, the hyperfluorescence of the membrane has increased and become more diffuse.

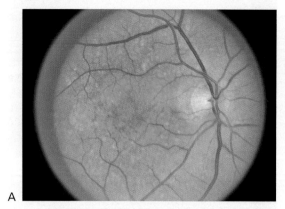
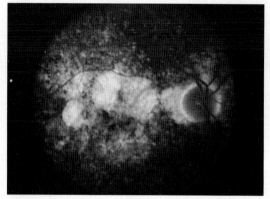

A   B

FIGURE 5.3. Hyperfluorescence from transmission defects. **A:** Retinal pigment epithelial (RPE) loss in the macula in an eye with atrophic, age-related macular degeneration. **B:** A fluorescein angiogram corresponding to **(A)** more than 13 minutes after injection reveals hyperfluorescence corresponding to the areas of RPE absence.

the later phases, minutes after injection, it becomes more diffuse.

Indocyanine Green Angiography

Indocyanine green (ICG) is a tricarbocyanine dye that absorbs at 790 to 805 nm and has a peak emission at 835 nm. These spectral properties allow ICG to be visualized through the ocular pigments, blood, and serous fluids better than fluorescein. ICG is almost 98% protein bound, and fluorescein is about 80% protein bound. This high degree of protein binding results in the tendency of ICG to remain intravascular, which facilitates visualization of the choroidal vessels and, in certain cases, choroidal pathologic processes. It is excreted unchanged by the liver via the biliary system.

The dye does not produce the nausea caused by sodium fluorescein after intravenous injection, but it can cause vasovagal reactions. Because it contains approximately 5% iodine by weight, it should not be given to patients with a history of iodine allergy.

ICG angiography usually demonstrates the choroidal vasculature better than fluorescein angiography (Fig. 5.7). Indications for the test are still being developed, but it appears most useful in exudative macular degeneration when fluorescein angiography fails to delineate the choroidal neovascularization. In some of these instances, ICG angiography can help to reveal the location and extent of choroidal neovascularization. It may also be of value in identifying the recurrence or persistence of choroidal neovascularization after laser therapy.

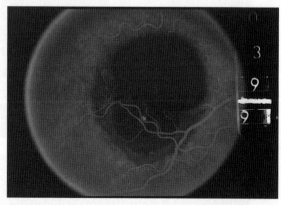

FIGURE 5.5. Hypofluorescence results from blockage by blood from a bleeding retinal arterial macroaneurysm, which can be seen as a focus of hyperfluorescence along the course of an inferotemporal retinal artery in this right eye. The preretinal blood superiorly blocks the fluorescence of the retinal and choroidal vasculature, but the subretinal blood inferiorly blocks the choroidal fluorescence and permits visualization of the retinal vessels.

FIGURE 5.4. Hypofluorescence caused by an absence of dye in an eye with choroidal hypoperfusion as a result of a severe ipsilateral carotid artery obstruction.

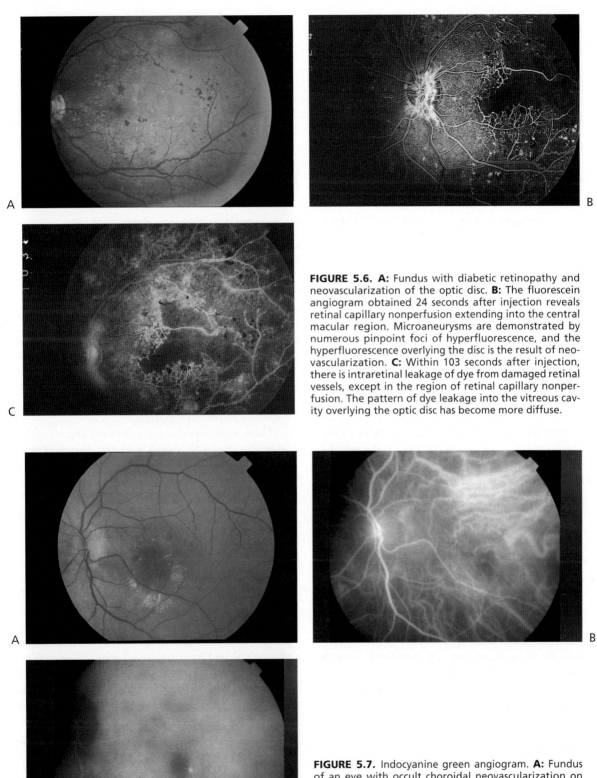

FIGURE 5.6. A: Fundus with diabetic retinopathy and neovascularization of the optic disc. **B:** The fluorescein angiogram obtained 24 seconds after injection reveals retinal capillary nonperfusion extending into the central macular region. Microaneurysms are demonstrated by numerous pinpoint foci of hyperfluorescence, and the hyperfluorescence overlying the disc is the result of neovascularization. **C:** Within 103 seconds after injection, there is intraretinal leakage of dye from damaged retinal vessels, except in the region of retinal capillary nonperfusion. The pattern of dye leakage into the vitreous cavity overlying the optic disc has become more diffuse.

FIGURE 5.7. Indocyanine green angiogram. **A:** Fundus of an eye with occult choroidal neovascularization on fluorescein angiography. **B:** In the early phases of the study, the large choroidal vessels are well visualized. **C:** Several minutes after injection, a focus of relative hyperfluorescence can be seen, which presumably represents staining or leakage of the dye from the neovascular complex.

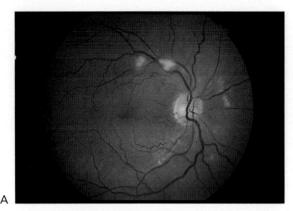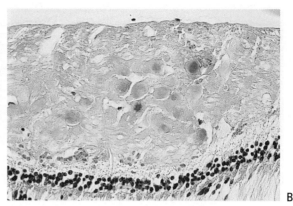

FIGURE 5.8. A: Cotton-wool spots located superotemporal to the optic nerve head. **B:** Histopathologic examination reveals a nerve fiber layer that is thickened by blockage of axoplasmic flow. Several cytoid bodies in a cotton-wool spot contain intensely eosinophilic nucleoids composed of dammed organelles. (Hematoxylin and eosin stain; original magnification ×100; courtesy of Ralph C. Eagle Jr, M.D.)

COTTON-WOOL SPOTS

A cotton-wool spot is a small focus of superficial retinal opacification that develops after focal retinal ischemia with secondary axoplasmic damming.

Clinical Features. Cotton-wool spots are usually white or yellow-white lesions that are less than 0.25 disc diameter (Fig. 5.8). They are located in the nerve fiber layer of the retina in the posterior pole, but are not seen in the periphery. With fluorescein angiography, they demonstrate relative hypofluorescence. In general, they resolve within 5 to 7 weeks, although those seen in patients with diabetic retinopathy can be more persistent.

Diabetic retinopathy is the most common cause of cotton-wool spots. Cotton-wool spots have been associated with numerous other abnormalities, such as systemic arterial hypertension, collagen vascular diseases, cardiac valvular disease, carotid artery obstructive disease, coagulopathies, metastatic carcinoma, trauma, and human immunodeficiency virus infection.

Management. Cotton-wool spots require no therapy. If no underlying disease is readily apparent, a systemic workup should be undertaken, possibly including a glucose tolerance test to rule out diabetes mellitus. An underlying cause or association can be found in about 95% of cases.

HARD EXUDATES

Hard exudates in the posterior segment represent the deposition of lipid from chronic leakage of plasma from incompetent vessels of the retina, choroid, or optic disc.

Clinical Features. Hard exudates appear as discrete, bright yellow lesions that are most frequently seen in the posterior pole. They can be globular or have a linear appearance (Fig. 5.9A). These exudates are typically located in the outer plexiform layer of the retina (i.e., Henle's layer; Fig. 5.9B), but in instances of severe exudation, such as Coats' disease, they can dissect into the subretinal space. In marked cases, the hard exudates can become confluent and extend into the central macula, usually causing severe visual loss (Fig. 5.9C). Hard exudates are usually undetectable with fluorescein angiography.

These lipid deposits are constantly changing. If leakage from the abnormal vessels worsens, the exudates can increase. If the leakage lessens or stops, the exudates eventually regress because of phagocytosis of the lipid by macrophages (i.e., gitter cells).

Hard exudates are associated with numerous retinal vascular diseases, including diabetic retinopathy, hypertensive retinopathy, retinal venous obstruction, retinal arterial macroaneurysm, radiation retinopathy, Coats' disease, and capillary hemangioma of the retina (i.e., von Hippel's lesion). The exudates are frequently associated with choroidal neovascularization in exudative macular degeneration and also with optic neuropathies. A unique variant is the macular star, which occurs most frequently with hypertensive retinopathy and optic neuropathies.

Management. Hard exudation in the central macular can lead to severe visual loss. Treatment of the underlying, leaking vascular abnormalities can be accomplished with laser photocoagulation in many instances, depending on the underlying disease.

VENOUS OBSTRUCTIVE DISEASE

Central Retinal Vein Obstruction

Michel is usually given credit for categorizing central retinal vein obstruction as a distinct clinical entity in 1878. Green and associates histopathologically studied 29 eyes with central retinal vein obstruction and found a thrombus within

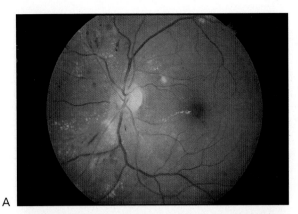

A

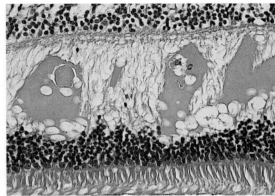

B

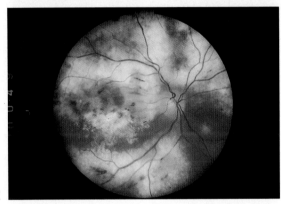

C

FIGURE 5.9. A: Multiple, discrete, yellow, hard exudates in the posterior pole of an eye with background diabetic retinopathy. **B:** Hard exudates are pools of proteinaceous fluid. Most are located in the outer plexiform layer, which is the watershed zone between the two circulations of the retina. (Hematoxylin and eosin stain; original magnification ×100; courtesy of Ralph C. Eagle Jr, M.D.) **C:** Severe, confluent hard exudation in an eye with marked background diabetic retinopathy of a patient with a serum triglyceride level approximately 10 times the normal level. The condition eventually progressed to proliferative diabetic retinopathy.

the lumen of the central retinal vein at or near the lamina cribrosa in each case. It has been suggested that the central retinal artery compresses the central retinal vein in the vicinity of the lamina cribrosa, leading to turbulence, endothelial damage, and subsequent thrombus formation in many cases.

Clinical Features. Central retinal vein obstruction usually develops in persons with a mean age of 65 years. Men appear to be affected at a higher rate than women, and in approximately 10% of cases, there is a history of a central or branch retinal vein obstruction in the contralateral eye.

Fundus examination typically shows dilated and tortuous retinal veins and a swollen optic disc (Fig. 5.10). Retinal

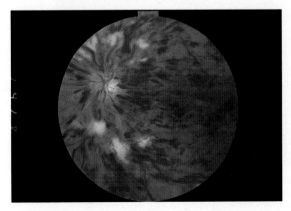

FIGURE 5.10. Central retinal vein obstruction.

hemorrhages are usually present in the posterior pole and the periphery. Macular edema is common. Neovascularization of the optic disc or retina may develop, although neovascularization of the iris is much more common.

Several nomenclature systems have been developed to describe central retinal vein obstruction. The obstructions can probably be best classified as nonischemic (i.e., perfused; Fig. 5.11) and ischemic (i.e., nonperfused) variants. A vein obstruction is considered to be nonperfused (Fig. 5.12) if retinal capillary dropout of at least 10 disc areas is evident on fluorescein angiography in a posterior pole view that also extends for a radius of 4 to 5 disc areas more peripheral to the macula. Electroretinography is also useful in classifying central retinal vein obstruction into these two basic categories. Clinically, the ischemic variants tend to have prominent relative afferent pupillary defects, poor visual acuity, numerous cotton-wool spots, and extensive intraretinal hemorrhages. Approximately one fourth to one third of all central retinal vein obstructions are ischemic in nature, and about 10% to 20% of the nonischemic cases progress to significant ischemia.

Overall, approximately 20% of eyes with central retinal vein obstruction develop iris neovascularization. Within the ischemic group, the rate rises to 50% of affected eyes. Iris neovascularization usually becomes evident between 2 weeks and 2 years after the obstructive event occurs, with a mean of 4 to 5 months.

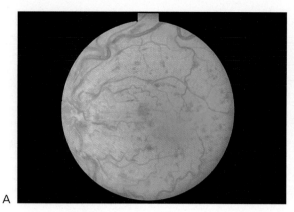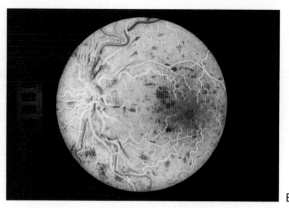

FIGURE 5.11. A: Nonischemic (i.e., perfused) central retinal vein obstruction in an eye with a visual acuity of 20/100. **B:** In the fluorescein angiogram obtained 30 seconds after injection, the retinal capillary bed is well perfused.

Whether or not posterior or anterior segment neovascularization occurs, the retinal hemorrhages from the obstruction slowly resolve over several months. Chronic cystoid macular edema and retinal pigment epithelial disruption in the macula are frequent sequelae that typically limit visual recovery. Frank macular ischemia also can contribute to permanently decreased vision. Optociliary collateral vessels often form on the optic disc after several months, as the hemorrhages resolve.

Systemic abnormalities associated with central retinal vein obstruction include systemic arterial hypertension, diabetes mellitus, and hyperviscosity states. Increased intraocular pressure also appears to be associated. Increased intraocular pressure can bow the lamina cribrosa posteriorly, theoretically contributing to compression of the central retinal vein, turbulence, and subsequent thrombus formation.

Management. No treatment has been consistently effective in stabilizing or improving the visual acuity of eyes with central retinal vein obstruction. Correction of associated systemic abnormalities, such as polycythemia, may benefit some patients.

Panretinal laser photocoagulation can cause regression of iris neovascularization when it develops in the setting of central retinal vein obstruction. For ischemic central retinal vein obstructions, panretinal laser photocoagulation before the development of iris neovascularization (Fig. 5.13) appears to reduce the risk of forming these new vessels and progression to neovascular glaucoma.

Branch Retinal Vein Obstruction

Branch retinal vein obstruction (i.e., occlusion) is a retinal vascular disease that usually affects persons in their sixties. Men and women appear to be affected equally. The disorder is more common in those with a history of systemic arterial hypertension. Approximately 10% of people with a branch retinal vein obstruction in one eye eventually develop a venous obstruction in the second eye.

Clinical Features. The obstruction usually occurs at an arteriovenous crossing, where the two vessels are bound by a common adventitial sheath. The retinal artery, which is typically located anterior to the vein, most likely compresses the

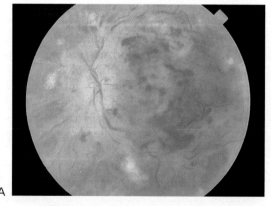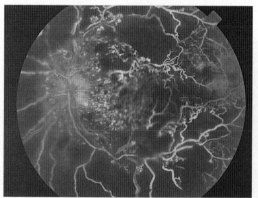

FIGURE 5.12. A: Examination of an ischemic (i.e., nonperfused) central retinal vein obstruction in an eye with visual acuity limited to hand motions shows marked intraretinal hemorrhage and numerous cotton-wool spots. **B:** The fluorescein angiogram corresponding to **(A)**, obtained 48 seconds after injection, reveals widespread retinal capillary nonperfusion.

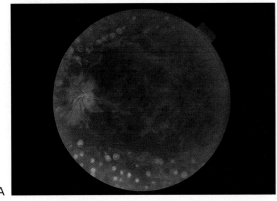
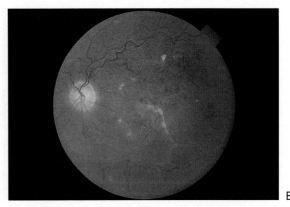

A

B

FIGURE 5.13. A: Panretinal laser photocoagulation in an eye with a nonperfused central retinal vein obstruction and vision limited to hand motions. **B:** One year later, the intraretinal blood has been reabsorbed, and changes in the retinal pigment epithelium are evident in the central macula. Such pigmentary changes are commonly seen after severe central or branch retinal vein obstructions.

vein, leading to turbulence, endothelial damage, and thrombus formation. If the blockage does not occur at an arteriovenous crossing, an inflammatory cause, such as sarcoidosis, is more likely.

Intraretinal hemorrhage and edema are seen in the distribution of the blocked vessel (Fig. 5.14). Cotton-wool spots may also be present. If the obstruction occurs within one of the vessels on the optic disc, the disc may be swollen. In longstanding cases, optociliary collaterals can develop on the optic disc, as can pigmentary changes in the central macula.

The visual acuity can range from 20/20 to counting fingers. The most common reason for decreased vision is macular edema, but retinal capillary nonperfusion and vitreous hemorrhage occurring secondary to posterior segment neovascularization are other causes. Traction and/or rhegmatogenous retinal detachment can occur in some cases. The rhegmatogenous component can develop when a retinal tear occurs adjacent to a tuft of retinal neovascularization under traction from the overlying vitreous gel.

Intravenous fluorescein angiography most often reveals a delay in retinal venous filling of the involved vessels; there

may also be delayed retinal arterial filling. Areas of retinal capillary nonperfusion can be seen, and in the late phases, there is often intraretinal leakage of dye, particularly in areas where the retinal capillary bed is intact (Fig. 5.15).

Retinal neovascularization or neovascularization of the optic disc can develop in eyes with vein obstructions that are ischemic, which is defined as significant retinal capillary nonperfusion ($\geq$5 disc diameters) on fluorescein angiography. Approximately 50% of the cases of branch retinal vein obstruction involving at least a quadrant of the fundus have significant ischemia. About 40% of such eyes eventually develop posterior segment neovascularization (Fig. 5.16).

Abnormalities that can be confused with branch retinal vein obstruction include retinal arterial macroaneurysm and certain cases of cavernous hemangioma of the retina. Exudative macular degeneration can mimic branch retinal vein obstructions that primarily involve the macula.

Management. Medical therapy has not benefitted eyes with branch retinal vein obstruction. Nevertheless, control of systemic arterial hypertension could theoretically be of benefit in preventing additional venous obstructive events.

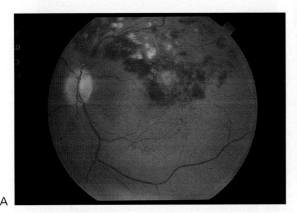
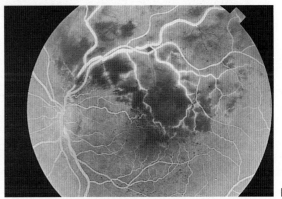

A

B

FIGURE 5.14. A: Superotemporal branch retinal vein obstruction. **B:** Fluorescein angiogram demonstrates retinal capillary nonperfusion in the distribution of the obstructed vessel.

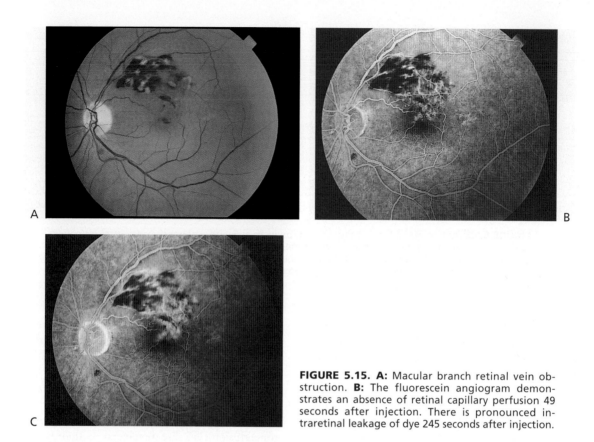

FIGURE 5.15. A: Macular branch retinal vein obstruction. **B:** The fluorescein angiogram demonstrates an absence of retinal capillary perfusion 49 seconds after injection. There is pronounced intraretinal leakage of dye 245 seconds after injection.

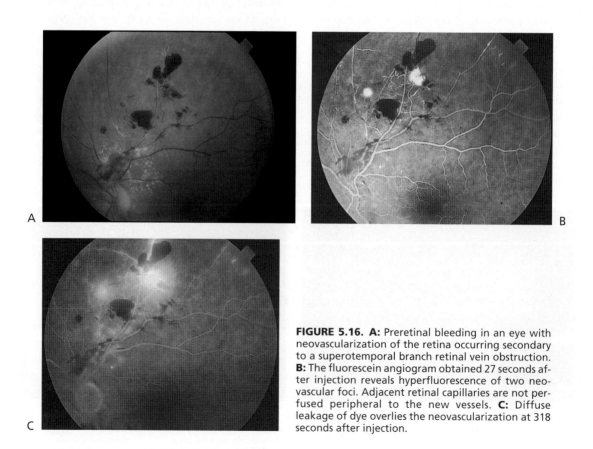

FIGURE 5.16. A: Preretinal bleeding in an eye with neovascularization of the retina occurring secondary to a superotemporal branch retinal vein obstruction. **B:** The fluorescein angiogram obtained 27 seconds after injection reveals hyperfluorescence of two neovascular foci. Adjacent retinal capillaries are not perfused peripheral to the new vessels. **C:** Diffuse leakage of dye overlies the neovascularization at 318 seconds after injection.

The Branch Vein Occlusion Study was a clinical trial that evaluated the efficacy of laser photocoagulation in eyes with branch retinal vein for improving visual acuity and for preventing posterior segment neovascular sequelae.

In affected eyes with 20/40 or worse vision (primarily caused by macular edema), an obstruction present 3 to 18 months, and absence of foveolar blood, the mean visual acuity in eyes treated with macular grid laser therapy was 20/40 to 20/50 at 3 years, but untreated eyes had a mean visual acuity of 20/70. When confluent intraretinal hemorrhage was present in the macula, treatment was delayed until the blood cleared sufficiently to assess macular capillary perfusion with fluorescein angiography and deliver laser treatment if indicated.

Treatment consisted of argon laser photocoagulation using 100-μm yellow-white burns in a grid fashion (Fig. 5.17). The treatment extended from the edge of the foveal avascular zone to the temporal macular vascular arcade. If macular edema was still present at 4 months after treatment and the vision remained decreased, treatment was repeated if fluorescein angiography still demonstrated retinal leakage.

Eyes with significant retinal capillary nonperfusion (i.e., >5 disc diameters wide on fluorescein angiography) were also randomized to receive sector scatter laser photocoagulation, delivering 200- to 500-μm, yellow-white burns to the

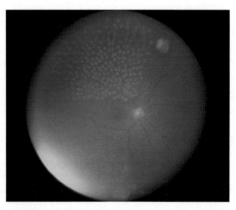

FIGURE 5.18. An equator-plus photograph demonstrates a sector panretinal photocoagulation with a full-scatter pattern in an eye with posterior segment neovascularization secondary to a branch retinal vein obstruction.

area affected by the obstruction (Fig. 5.18). This type of treatment was not administered closer than 2 disc diameters to the center of the fovea. If posterior segment neovascularization was diagnosed at the time of entrance into the study, the treatment reduced the incidence of vitreous hemorrhage from approximately 60% to 30% at 3-year follow-up. In eyes without posterior segment neovascularization initially,

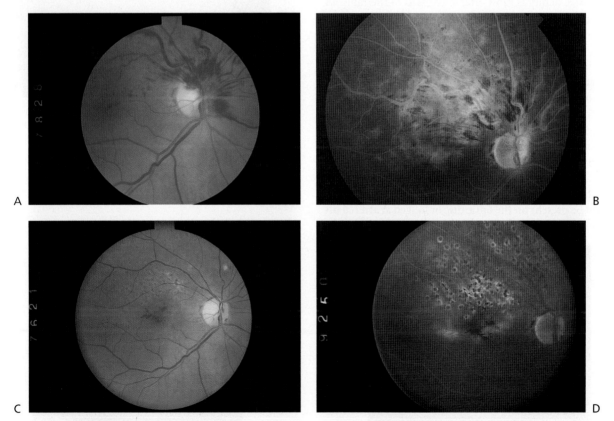

FIGURE 5.17. **A:** Superotemporal branch retinal vein obstruction. **B:** The fluorescein angiogram several minutes after injection reveals intraretinal leakage of dye and absence of retinal capillary nonperfusion. **C:** Several months after focal laser therapy, the macular edema has lessened. **D:** The fluorescein angiogram discloses decreased intraretinal leakage of dye after the laser therapy.

the chance of developing neovascularization was reduced from 31% to 19% with treatment. Overall, the Branch Vein Occlusion Study report recommended following these cases, with particularly close attention to the ischemic variants, and treating with sector scatter laser therapy after neovascularization develops.

ARTERIAL OBSTRUCTIVE DISEASE

Central Retinal Artery Obstruction

Central retinal artery obstruction is seen in about 1 of 10,000 outpatient ophthalmic visits. It is typically unilateral, and although it can be seen in all ages, the mean age of affected patients is about 65 years. The causes include emboli, hemorrhage under an atherosclerotic plaque, thrombosis, inflammation, spasm, systemic hypotension, hypertensive arterial necrosis, and dissecting carotid artery aneurysm.

Clinical Features. Patients with acute central retinal artery obstruction typically present with a history of sudden, painless visual loss. The fundus appearance is characterized by superficial retinal whitening that is most pronounced in the posterior pole (Fig. 5.19). A cherry red spot can be seen in the foveola, where the retina is thinnest.

The visual acuity is most often decreased to the range of counting fingers or hand motions. In approximately 10% of cases; however, a patent cilioretinal artery supplies the foveola (Fig. 5.20), and the vision may not significantly decrease or even improve to 20/20 to 20/50 within a few weeks after the onset of the obstruction.

Emboli are seen in the retinal arterial system in 20% of eyes with acute central retinal artery obstruction. Cholesterol emboli (i.e., Hollenhorst plaques; Fig. 5.21) appear as small, glistening crystals and are thought to originate predominantly from the carotid arteries. Calcific emboli (Fig. 5.22), usually originating from the cardiac valves, tend to be whiter and larger than the cholesterol variant. Both types can be present on the optic disc or lodged at arterial bifurcations.

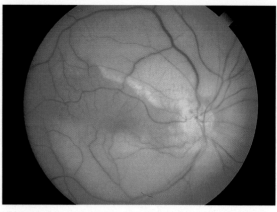

FIGURE 5.20. Central retinal artery obstruction with cilioretinal sparing between the disc and the fovea.

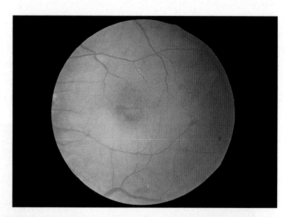

FIGURE 5.21. Hollenhorst plaque within a retinal arteriole in the fundus in an eye without a clinically evident retinal arterial obstruction.

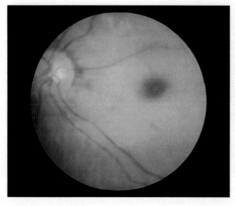

FIGURE 5.19. Acute central retinal artery obstruction with superficial retinal whitening and a cherry red spot in the foveola.

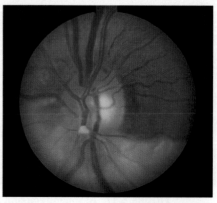

FIGURE 5.22. Inferior branch retinal artery obstruction secondary to a white calcific plaque. (Courtesy of Larry Magargal, M.D., Philadelphia, PA.)

Approximately 18% of eyes with a central retinal artery obstruction develop iris neovascularization, usually by 4 to 6 weeks after the obstruction. If iris neovascularization is already present when the central retinal artery obstruction occurs, the possibility of concurrent ocular ischemic syndrome should be considered.

Acute ophthalmic artery obstruction and combined central retinal artery and central retinal vein obstruction can be confused with acute central retinal artery obstruction. With an acute ophthalmic artery obstruction, the visual acuity is generally worse (often no light perception), the posterior pole whitening is more severe, and a cherry red spot is often absent (Fig. 5.23).

Eyes with a combined central retinal artery and central retinal vein obstruction have clinical features suggestive of both these entities (Fig. 5.24): superficial retinal whitening, a cherry red spot, dilated and tortuous retinal veins, and retinal hemorrhages. Retrobulbar injection and inadvertent penetration of the optic nerve is a common cause of this relatively rare combination. Approximately 80% of affected eyes progress to iris neovascularization with a median time of 6 weeks.

Management. The visual prognosis for eyes with acute central retinal artery obstruction and no cilioretinal foveolar sparing is grim, with most remaining legally blind. Globe massage, anterior chamber paracentesis, oxygen–carbon dioxide combination inhalation therapy, oral vasodilator treatments, and the use of systemic anticoagulants have all been advocated, but no consistent or significant improvement in vision has been demonstrated. If iris neovascularization develops, panretinal laser photocoagulation can be successful in promoting regression in as many as 65% of cases.

A thorough workup should be considered to ascertain underlying causes. More common underlying abnormalities include carotid artery obstructive disease, cardiac valvular disease, and collagen vascular diseases. In younger patients, the possibility of migraine and coagulopathies should also

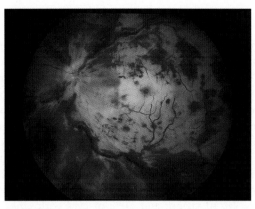

FIGURE 5.24. Combined central retinal artery and central retinal vein obstruction in a 20-year-old woman with systemic lupus erythematosus.

be entertained. Giant cell arteritis is seen in about 1% to 2% of cases and should be ruled out in any retinal arterial obstructive event in patients older than 55 years. Giant cell arteritis should be included in the differential diagnosis if the arterial obstruction is bilateral.

Branch Retinal Artery Obstruction

Branch retinal artery obstruction can occur as two variants: true branch retinal artery obstruction and cilioretinal artery obstruction.

Clinical Features. Patients with branch retinal artery obstructions usually present with a history of sudden, painless visual loss in part of the visual field of the affected eye. Superficial retinal whitening is seen in the distribution of the fundus supplied by the vessel (Fig. 5.25). The visual acuity generally returns to 20/40 or better. Although the visual defect may decrease in size, some residual field loss usually remains.

The causes of true branch retinal artery obstruction are similar to those of central retinal artery obstruction. Uncommonly, entities not associated with central retinal artery obstruction, such as toxoplasmosis retinochoroiditis

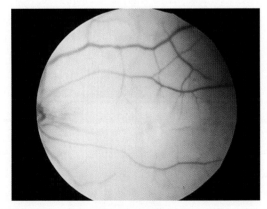

FIGURE 5.23. Acute ophthalmic artery obstruction. The inner and outer portions of the retina are severely opacified, and a cherry red spot is absent. Visual testing revealed no light perception.

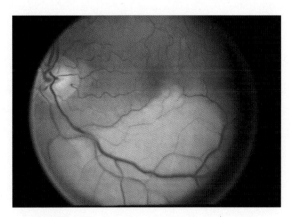

FIGURE 5.25. Branch retinal artery obstruction.

and thrombosis within a retinal arterial macroaneurysm, can cause branch retinal artery obstruction.

Cilioretinal arteries are direct or indirect (through the choroid) branches of the posterior ciliary arteries. They typically emerge from the temporal aspect of the optic disc separately from the central retinal artery. Three types of cilioretinal artery obstructions have been described: isolated cilioretinal artery obstruction (Fig. 5.26); cilioretinal artery obstruction associated with central retinal vein obstruction; and cilioretinal artery obstruction associated with anterior ischemic optic neuropathy (Fig. 5.27). Ninety percent of eyes with isolated cilioretinal artery obstruction eventually achieve 20/40 vision, and 70% of eyes with cilioretinal artery obstruction and associated central retinal vein obstruction reach 20/40 vision. Eyes with cilioretinal artery obstruction associated with anterior ischemic optic neuropathy usually remain legally blind.

The fundus appearance for a true branch retinal artery or cilioretinal artery obstruction is fairly characteristic. Viral retinitides, toxoplasmic retinochoroiditis, and fungal retinitides may rarely cause confusion.

Management. Ocular treatment is generally not given for branch retinal artery obstruction because it is not particularly effective and because the visual prognosis is relatively good.

The medical workup for branch retinal artery obstruction is similar to that for central retinal artery obstruction. The possibility of coexistent giant cell arteritis ranks high in the differential diagnosis in cases of cilioretinal artery obstruction associated with anterior ischemic optic neuropathy.

Ocular Ischemic Syndrome

In 1963, Kearns and Hollenhorst described the ocular symptoms and signs attributable to chronic, severe carotid artery obstruction, and they called the entity *venous stasis retinopathy*. The same term has been used to describe mild central retinal vein obstruction, a distinctly different entity. To avoid confusion, the term *ocular ischemic syndrome* is

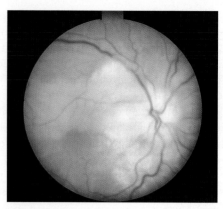

FIGURE 5.27. Cilioretinal artery obstruction associated with anterior ischemic optic neuropathy in a patient with giant cell arteritis.

preferable to designate the ocular findings found in conjunction with severe carotid artery obstruction.

The disease affects twice as many men as women, and the mean age at the time of diagnosis is 65 years. A carotid artery stenosis of at least 90% is necessary to cause the ocular ischemic syndrome (Fig. 5.28), although approximately 50% of patients have a 100% stenosis. Chronic ophthalmic artery insufficiency can also cause the ocular ischemic syndrome. Bilaterality is seen in 20% of cases.

Noninvasive vascular testing (e.g., duplex carotid ultrasonography) is about 90% successful in detecting a carotid artery stenosis of 50% or greater.

Atherosclerosis is the most common cause. Giant cell arteritis, inflammatory conditions of the large vessels, and Eisenmenger's syndrome are other known causes.

Clinical Features. Approximately 90% of patients with the ocular ischemic syndrome relate a history of visual loss

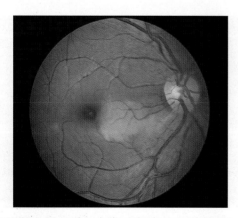

FIGURE 5.26. Isolated cilioretinal artery obstruction.

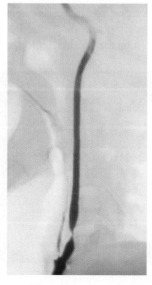

FIGURE 5.28. A carotid arteriogram reveals marked stenosis of the ipsilateral internal carotid artery in a patient with the ocular ischemic syndrome.

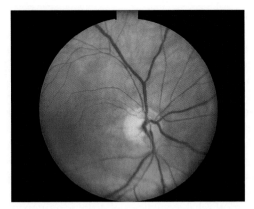

FIGURE 5.29. Examination of the fundus of a patient with the ocular ischemic syndrome reveals dilated, but not tortuous, retinal veins.

in the affected eye, usually occurring over a period of weeks to months. Forty percent relate a history of aching pain in the orbital region. The recovery time may be increased after exposure to bright light.

Rubeosis iridis affects two thirds of eyes at the time of diagnosis. Nevertheless, the intraocular pressure is elevated in only about half of the eyes with rubeosis, probably because of decreased aqueous production due to poor ciliary body perfusion. A mild anterior chamber cell and flare response is observed in about 20% of eyes.

Posterior segment signs (Fig. 5.29) include narrowed retinal arteries and dilated, but not tortuous, retinal veins in most eyes, with retinal hemorrhages in 80% (Fig. 5.30), and neovascularization of the disc or retina in about 35%. The retinal hemorrhages are generally dot and blot types, with a predilection for the midperipheral fundus. Less common signs include microaneurysms, a cherry red spot, cotton-wool spots, spontaneous pulsations of the retinal arteries, macular edema, and anterior ischemic optic neuropathy.

Fluorescein angiography reveals delayed choroidal filling in 60% of eyes (Fig. 5.31), a delayed retinal arteriove-

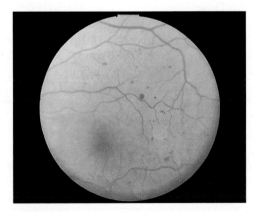

FIGURE 5.30. Retinal hemorrhages in a case of ocular ischemic syndrome.

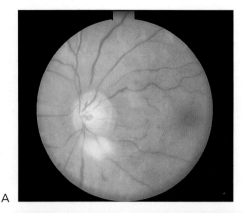

A

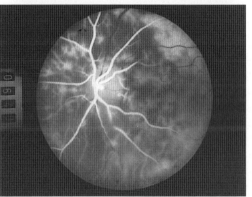

B

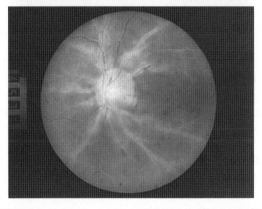

C

FIGURE 5.31. **A:** Fundus of the left eye in a patient with the ocular ischemic syndrome. The retinal arteries are narrowed, and myelinated nerve fibers are present at the inferior border of the optic disc. **B:** The fluorescein angiogram of the same eye discloses delayed choroidal filling approximately 1 minute after injection. **C:** At approximately 7.5 minutes after injection, there is marked staining of the large retinal vessels, particularly the arteries. (Courtesy of Larry Magargal, M.D.)

nous transit time in 95%, and late staining of the retinal vessels, especially the arteries, in 85%. Electroretinography shows diminution of the a and b waves (Fig. 5.32), indicating ischemia of the inner and outer retinal layers.

The 5-year mortality rate is about 40%, with death usually caused by cardiovascular disease. Systemic arterial hypertension is encountered in almost three fourths of pa-

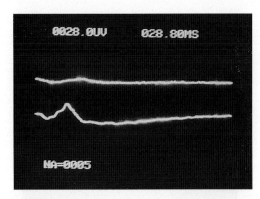

FIGURE 5.32. Electroretinogram of a normal left eye *(lower tracing)* and a right eye *(upper tracing)* with the ocular ischemic syndrome. There is diminution of the a and b waves in the ocular ischemic syndrome eye.

tients, diabetes in about half, previous cerebrovascular accident in one fourth, and peripheral vascular disease severe enough to require a bypass in about one fifth.

The disorder most likely to be confused with the ocular ischemic syndrome is mild central retinal vein obstruction. Helpful differentiating features include disc swelling seen with central retinal vein obstruction (i.e., the optic disc usually appears normal with the ocular ischemic syndrome), venous tortuosity with vein obstruction, and more retinal hemorrhages with venous disease. Light digital pressure on the lid can often induce retinal arterial pulsations with the ocular ischemic syndrome, although not in eyes with central retinal vein obstruction.

Diabetic retinopathy can mimic the ocular ischemic syndrome and can coexist with it. Eyes with the ocular ischemic syndrome alone do not usually have hard exudates. In markedly asymmetric cases of diabetic retinopathy, the ocular syndrome can exacerbate the proliferative retinopathy changes.

Management. The natural course of the ocular ischemic syndrome is uncertain. Nevertheless, after rubeosis iridis develops, more than 90% of eyes are legally blind within 1 year of diagnosis.

Panretinal photocoagulation causes regression of iris neovascularization in about 35% of cases, but it appears to be a temporizing procedure.

When a carotid obstruction is 100%, endarterectomy is generally unsuccessful. Extracranial to intracranial bypass has been advocated. Unfortunately, with long-term follow-up, this procedure does not favorably affect visual outcome or reduce the incidence of stroke compared with a group treated medically with antiplatelet agents.

Carotid endarterectomy can help to preserve or restore the vision in some cases. Moreover, in symptomatic patients with a 70% to 99% stenosis, it has reduced the incidence of severe stroke over a 2-year period from 26% to 9% compared with treatment using antiplatelet agents alone.

DIABETIC RETINOPATHY

Diabetic retinopathy is a leading cause of blindness in the industrial countries. It accounts for approximately 10% of cases of legal blindness (visual acuity ≤20/200) in the United States, and in patients between 45 and 74 years of ages, it causes 20% of the cases of new blindness. Blindness from diabetic retinopathy appears to be more common in women than men and in persons of African descent, particularly women, than Caucasians. Since 60% of diabetic patients are women, women comprise a majority of patients with diabetic retinopathy.

The most reliable predictor of diabetic retinopathy is duration of the disease. Among insulin-dependent diabetics, there is virtually no clinically apparent retinopathy within 4 to 5 years after the diagnosis is made. After 5 to 10 years, 25% to 50% of patients have retinopathy, and after 10 to 15 years, it can be detected in 75% to 95% of patients. Proliferative diabetic retinopathy is rare before 10 years of diabetes' duration, but after 20 to 25 years, it can be seen in 18% to 40% of patients.

It is uncertain exactly why diabetic retinopathy develops. Increased platelet adhesiveness and aggregation, decreased deformability of red and white blood cells, increased basement membrane formation in the retinal capillaries, and loss of autoregulation in the retinal vessels are all associated abnormalities that may lead to the damage seen in the retinal blood vessels.

Strict control of the serum glucose levels in type I (insulin-dependent) diabetics has reduced the onset of diabetic retinopathy and slowed the progression of mild disease. It has also slowed the onset and progression of nephropathy and neuropathy. It is uncertain whether the same data hold for type II (non–insulin-dependent) cases, although, theoretically, this should also be the case.

Clinical Features. Diabetic retinopathy can be subdivided into two basic forms: nonproliferative (i.e., background) and proliferative.

In *nonproliferative diabetic retinopathy,* the first fundus sign of background diabetic retinopathy is often a microaneurysm. These outpouchings from the retinal capillaries can be found in the superficial and deep retinal capillary beds (Fig. 5.33). They are 12 to 100 μm in diameter, although only those greater than 30 μm across are visible ophthalmoscopically. It is uncertain why they occur, but it has been suggested that a loss of intramural pericytes in diabetic retinal capillaries leads to weakening of the walls of the vessels. Microaneurysms can be differentiated from retinal hemorrhages, because they are generally hyperfluorescent, unlike hypofluorescent hemorrhages.

Retinal hemorrhages can be the splinter variants that occur in the nerve fiber layer, but more commonly, they are the dot and blot type and occur predominantly in the outer plexiform layer (Fig. 5.34). They are caused by leakage from microaneurysms and damaged retinal capillaries and

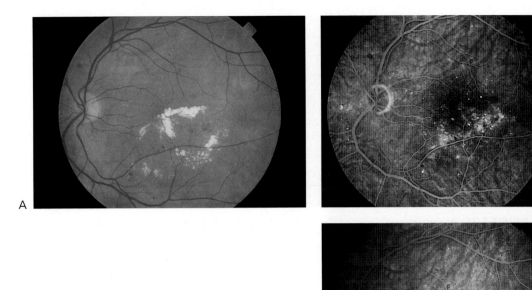

A

B

C

FIGURE 5.33. A: Fundus of an eye with background diabetic retinopathy. **B:** The fluorescein angiogram at approximately 1 minute after injection reveals multiple foci of pinpoint hyperfluorescence occurring secondary to the filling of microaneurysms with dye. **C:** At more than 8 minutes after injection, there is diffuse intraretinal leakage of dye from the microaneurysms.

venules. Hard exudates and retinal edema also occur primarily in the outer plexiform layer (Fig. 5.35). The hard exudates are constantly changing because of phagocytosis by macrophages. Cotton-wool spots in the nerve fiber layer can also be seen in many cases (Fig. 5.36). Intraretinal microvascular abnormalities are telangiectatic capillary and small vessel changes seen in severe nonproliferative disease (Fig. 5.37).

Retinal edema in the macula is commonly referred to as macular edema. When cystoid changes are visible, it is called cystoid macular edema. The Early Treatment Diabetic Retinopathy Study (ETDRS) emphasized an important term: *clinically significant macular edema* (Figs. 5.38 and 5.39). Eyes with clinically significant macular edema benefit from focal laser therapy. Clinically significant macular edema is determined ophthalmoscopically (not by fluorescein angiography) and is defined as:

Retinal thickening within 500 μm of the center of the fovea (Fig. 5.39A) or

Hard exudation within 500 μm of the center of the fovea if associated with retinal thickening (Fig. 5.39B) or

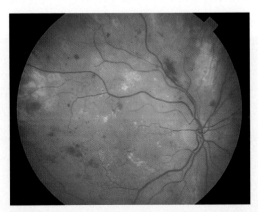

FIGURE 5.34. Retinal hemorrhages with background diabetic retinopathy. Most intraretinal hemorrhages are dot and blot types, although a streak hemorrhage in the nerve fiber layer can be seen superotemporal to the optic disc. Multiple foci of yellow, hard exudate are also evident.

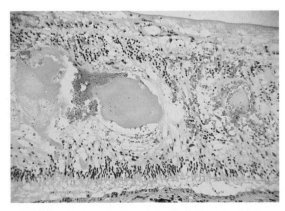

FIGURE 5.35. Hard exudates seen in diabetic retinopathy are located primarily in the outer plexiform layer of the retina. (Hematoxylin and eosin stain; original magnification ×40.)

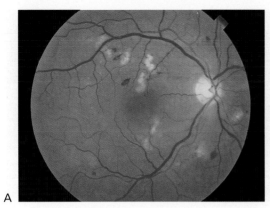 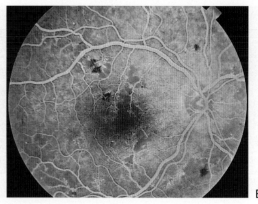

FIGURE 5.36. A: Cotton-wool spots in the nerve fiber layer of the retina in an eye with background diabetic retinopathy. **B:** Within 47 seconds after injection, the fluorescein angiogram of the eye in **(A)** reveals multiple foci of relative hypofluorescence corresponding to areas of retinal capillary nonperfusion in the regions of the cotton-wool spots.

Retinal thickening ≥1 disc area, any part of which is located within 1 disc diameter (1,500 μm) from the center of the fovea (Fig. 5.39C).

The term *preproliferative* (i.e., advanced or severe nonproliferative) *diabetic retinopathy* has been used to describe eyes that are at high risk of developing posterior segment neovascularization. Among the important signs of preproliferative retinopathy are numerous retinal hemorrhages in all four quadrants, venous abnormalities such as beading (Fig. 5.37) in two or more quadrants or loops (Fig. 5.40), and intraretinal microvascular abnormalities in one or more quadrants. The ETDRS found that the presence of one or more of these signs indicated a 50% or higher risk of developing proliferative retinopathy within 1 year.

In *proliferative diabetic retinopathy*, the eyes demonstrate, singularly or in combination, neovascularization of the disc (NVD), neovascularization of the retina (neovascularization elsewhere [NVE]), or neovascularization of the iris (NVI).

NVD arises from the optic disc or from the retina within

1 disc diameter of the optic disc (Fig. 5.41). It can grow along the posterior hyaloid face or anteriorly within Cloquet's canal. NVE arises from the retinal capillaries and veins and, less commonly, from the arteries. It grows through the internal limiting membrane of the retina to attach to the posterior hyaloid face (Fig. 5.42). Ninety percent of the posterior segment neovascularization seen with proliferative diabetic retinopathy is found within 6 disc diameters of the optic disc. As is the case with other proliferative retinopathies, the new vessels appear to stimulate contracture of the overlying vitreous, which subsequently places traction on the vessels and results in preretinal or vitreous hemorrhage (Fig. 5.43).

The Diabetic Retinopathy Study (DRS) identified certain posterior segment neovascular features that portended a particularly high risk of developing severe visual acuity loss (<5/200). These high-risk characteristics were as follows:

NVD greater than or equal to one fourth to one third of a disc area (one fourth of a disc area in eyes with large optic

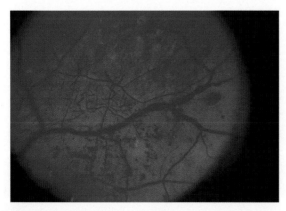

FIGURE 5.37. Telangiectatic vascular abnormalities (i.e., intraretinal microvascular abnormalities) in an eye with diabetic retinopathy. Venous beading is prominent.

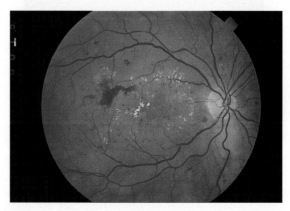

FIGURE 5.38. Diabetic fundus with clinically significant macular edema. The central, hard exudate is associated with retinal thickening.

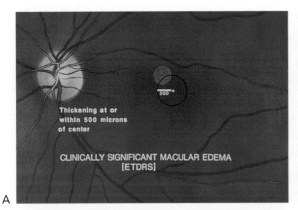

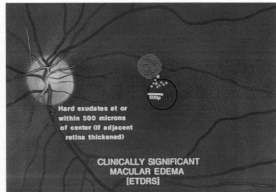

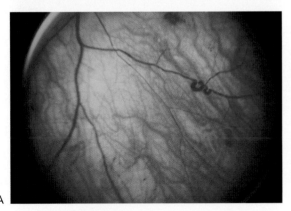

FIGURE 5.39. Clinically significant macular edema. **A:** Retinal thickening within 500 μm of the center of the fovea. **B:** Hard exudates, associated with retinal thickening, are located within 500 μm of the center of the fovea. **C:** Retinal thickening greater than 1 disc area, part of which is located within 1 disc diameter from the center of the fovea. (Courtesy of the Early Treatment Diabetic Retinopathy Study Group.)

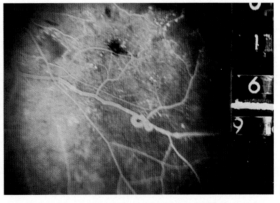

FIGURE 5.40. A: Venous loop in an eye with severe, nonproliferative diabetic retinopathy. **B:** In the fluorescein angiogram corresponding to **(A)**, obtained almost 17 seconds after injection, retinal capillary nonperfusion is evident adjacent to the loop.

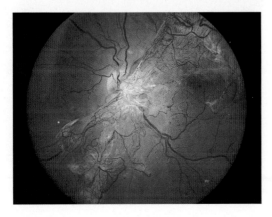

FIGURE 5.41. Pronounced neovascularization of the disc in an eye with proliferative diabetic retinopathy.

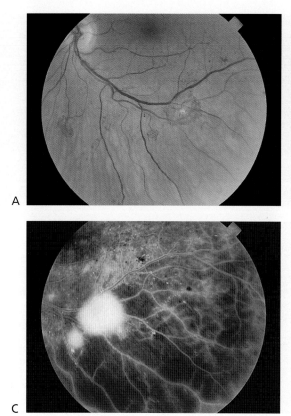

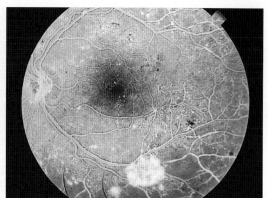

FIGURE 5.42. **A:** Neovascularization of the retina along the inferotemporal arcade in the fundus of an eye with proliferative diabetic retinopathy. **B:** The fluorescein angiogram obtained 24 seconds after injection reveals hyperfluorescence of the new vessels and retinal capillary nonperfusion adjacent and peripheral to the new vessels. **C:** Within 109 seconds after injection, the fluorescence of the neovascularization becomes more intense, and widespread retinal capillary nonperfusion is evident.

discs and one third of a disc area in eyes with small optic discs; Fig. 5.44) or

NVD of any size associated with preretinal or vitreous bleeding (Fig. 5.45) or

NVE at least 0.5 disc area and associated with preretinal or vitreous bleeding (Fig. 5.46).

Entities that can mimic diabetic retinopathy include radiation retinopathy, central retinal vein obstruction, the ocular ischemic syndrome, hypertensive retinopathy, and retinopathy of anemia. Sarcoidosis, Eales disease, and talc

retinopathy can cause changes similar to those seen with proliferative diabetic retinopathy.

Management. Strict glucose control can help to prevent the onset and progression of diabetic retinopathy. With a mean follow-up time of 6.5 years, the Diabetes Control and Complications Research Group demonstrated that strict glucose control in type I diabetics can reduce the chance of development of retinopathy by 76% and slow the progression in those who already have retinopathy by 54%. It also reduced the manifestations of nephropathy by approximately 50% and neuropathy by 60%.

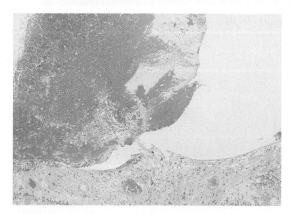

FIGURE 5.43. Traction on optic disc neovascularization by the vitreous gel in an eye with proliferative retinopathy. Intravitreal blood is also seen. (Hematoxylin and eosin stain; original magnification ×40).

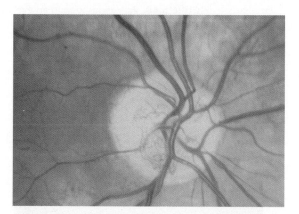

FIGURE 5.44. High-risk neovascularization of the optic disc is neovascularization greater than 25% to 33% of the disc area. (Courtesy of the Diabetic Retinopathy Study Group.)

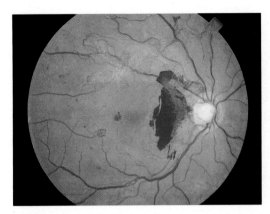

FIGURE 5.45. Neovascularization of the disc associated with pre-retinal bleeding.

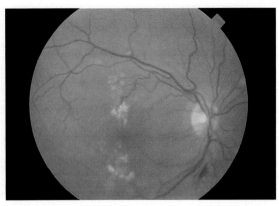

FIGURE 5.47. Focal treatment for the microaneurysmal abnormalities in an eye with background diabetic retinopathy and clinically significant macular edema.

For eyes with clinically significant macular edema or high-risk proliferative diabetic retinopathy, the mainstay of therapy is laser photocoagulation. The ETDRS demonstrated that eyes with clinically significant macular edema benefit from focal laser photocoagulation therapy. Microaneurysms within the temporal vascular arcade are treated directly with 50- to 100-μm spot burns, and 100-μm burns in the form of a grid pattern (burns spaced 0.5 burn width apart) are applied to areas of diffuse leakage or nonperfusion (Figs. 5.47 and 5.48). Nonperfused areas involving the fovea are not treated.

The ETDRS demonstrated that, at the end of 3 years, the progression of visual loss is halved with laser therapy in eyes with clinically significant macular edema. Overall, 12% of treated eyes had a doubling of the visual angle (e.g., 20/20 to 20/40, 20/40 to 20/80) during this period, whereas the corresponding rate for untreated eyes was 24%.

The DRS showed that eyes with high-risk characteristics benefited from full-scatter (i.e., panretinal) laser photocoagulation. In general, 1,500 to 2,000 burns, each approximately 500 μm in diameter, are applied to the peripheral retina, outside the macula (Fig. 5.49). Clinically significant macular edema should be treated concomitantly or, if possible, before starting panretinal treatment. Panretinal photocoagulation can also promote regression of iris neovascularization and therefore has the potential to stabilize or prevent neovascular glaucoma.

Among eyes with high-risk characteristics that were treated with panretinal photocoagulation, the incidence of severe visual loss (acuity $\leq$20/800) over a 5-year period was halved compared with the control eyes, which did not receive laser treatment. The percentage of eyes with severe visual loss at last follow-up was reduced from 30% to 15% with treatment. The complications of panretinal photocoagulation include decreased dark adaptation, peripheral visual field loss (i.e., construction of visual field), and decreased central vision (i.e., loss of visual acuity), primarily resulting from exacerbation of preexisting macular edema.

Pars plana vitrectomy can benefit eyes with proliferative diabetic retinopathy if there is significant nonclearing vitreous hemorrhage or macular retinal detachment, or if traction retinal detachment is threatening to occur (Fig. 5.50). Vitrectomy also is used if there is rubeosis iridis with an open anterior chamber angle and media opacification (e.g., vitreous hemorrhage) that would preclude delivery of panretinal photocoagulation. The Diabetic Retinopathy Vitrectomy Study (DRVS) demonstrated that, when the visual acuity is 20/800 or less secondary to vitreous hemorrhage, type I diabetic patients benefit more from early vitrectomy (1 to 2 months) than from waiting 6 months or longer for the hemorrhage to clear. Type II diabetic patients with dense vitreous hemorrhage can probably wait several months to allow spontaneous clearing unless there is underlying macular-threatening traction retinal detachment or some other condition, such as iris neovascularization, that necessitates earlier surgery. Overall, approximately 80% of eyes that undergo vitrectomy for nonclearing vitreous hemorrhage experience at least a two-line improvement in vision. The corresponding figure for traction retinal detachment is approximately 60%. Eyes with severe proliferative disease appear to have a better chance of retaining good vi-

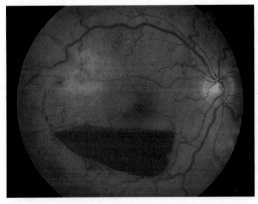

FIGURE 5.46. Neovascularization of the retina associated with preretinal bleeding into the subhyaloid space.

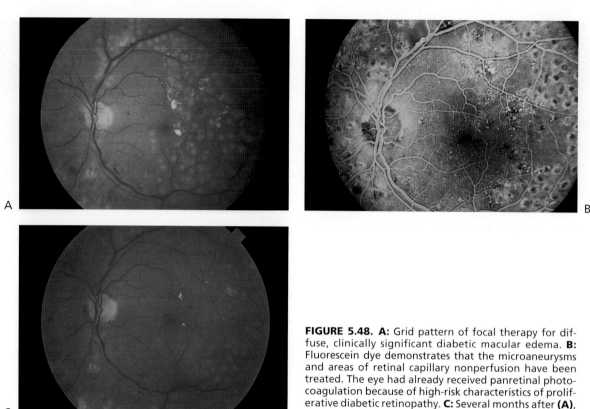

FIGURE 5.48. **A:** Grid pattern of focal therapy for diffuse, clinically significant diabetic macular edema. **B:** Fluorescein dye demonstrates that the microaneurysms and areas of retinal capillary nonperfusion have been treated. The eye had already received panretinal photocoagulation because of high-risk characteristics of proliferative diabetic retinopathy. **C:** Several months after **(A)**, the hard exudate has been absorbed by macrophages.

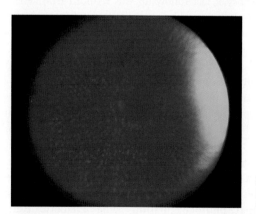

FIGURE 5.49. Argon laser, full-scatter, panretinal photocoagulation in an eye with proliferative diabetic retinopathy. The burns are located approximately one half of a burn width apart.

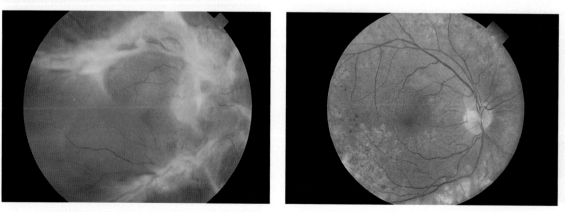

FIGURE 5.50. **A:** Proliferative diabetic retinopathy with traction retinal detachment in the macula. **B:** After vitrectomy, the retina is flat.

sion with early vitrectomy (i.e., 44% had ≥20/40 vision 4 years after surgery) versus delayed vitrectomy (i.e., 28% had ≥20/40 vision), but the possibility of total visual loss as a result of the surgical procedure must be considered.

HYPERTENSIVE RETINOPATHY

Many researchers have attempted to classify the changes seen with hypertensive retinopathy. One popular system is that described by Keith, Wagener, and Barker in 1939.

Clinical Features. Keith, Wagener, and Barker stratified the hypertensive changes into four groups (Figs. 5.51 through 5.54):

Group I: minimal narrowing of the retinal arteries

Group II: narrowing of the retinal arteries in conjunction with regions of focal narrowing and arteriovenous nicking

Group III: abnormalities seen in groups I and II, as well as retinal hemorrhages, hard exudation, and cotton-wool spots

Group IV (i.e., malignant hypertension): abnormalities encountered in groups I through III, as well as swelling of the optic nerve head

The changes seen in groups I and II are typically chronic, and those encountered in groups III and IV are seen with more acute rises in blood pressure. In an adult, diastolic blood pressure ≥110 mm Hg is usually necessary to induce the fundus changes seen in group III, and diastolic pressure ≥130 mm Hg usually correlates with the changes in group IV. The changes of groups III and IV can be seen in younger individuals at lower blood pressures.

Keith, Wagener, and Barker evaluated patients with hypertensive retinopathy before the use of effective antihypertensive regimens. In essentially untreated groups, they found the 3-year survival rates to be 70% for group I, 62% for group II, 22% for group III, and 6% for group IV. With the development and use of modern antihypertensive medications, survival rates have improved in all groups.

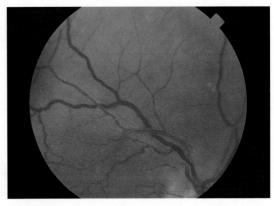

FIGURE 5.52. In grade II hypertensive retinopathy, the retinal arteries are narrowed, and arteriovenous nicking is evident.

Hypertensive choroidopathy frequently accompanies hypertensive retinopathy when the changes of group IV, and sometimes those of group III, are present. In the acute phase, yellow spots are visible at the level of the retinal pigment epithelium (Fig. 5.55). They are hyperfluorescent on fluorescein angiography and appear to occur secondary to fibrinoid necrosis within the choriocapillaris, leading to damage to the overlying retinal pigment epithelium. In severe cases, the intense leakage of plasma from these foci contributes to serous retinal detachment (Fig. 5.55). Over a period of weeks, these spots become pigmented or depigmented (Fig. 5.56). When the spots occur in a linear fashion, they are referred to as Siegrist's streaks.

Management. Treatment includes control of the blood pressure. With adequate systemic treatment, the fundus changes seen in groups III and IV resolve over a period of weeks to months. If visual acuity is affected in the short term, some improvement may be expected with resolution of the fundus changes such as the serous retinal detachments. However, visual recovery may be limited by retinal pigment epithelial disruption in the macula or optic nerve damage. Local ocular treatment has not been beneficial.

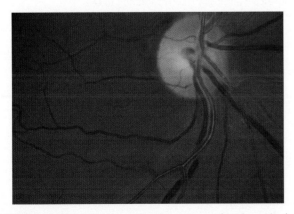

FIGURE 5.51. In grade I hypertensive retinopathy, the retinal arteries and arterioles have become narrowed.

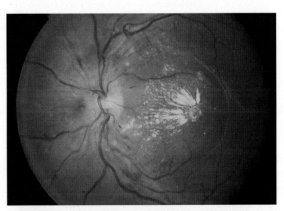

FIGURE 5.53. Grade III hypertensive retinopathy. The eye has retinal hemorrhages and hard exudates in the form of a hemimacular star.

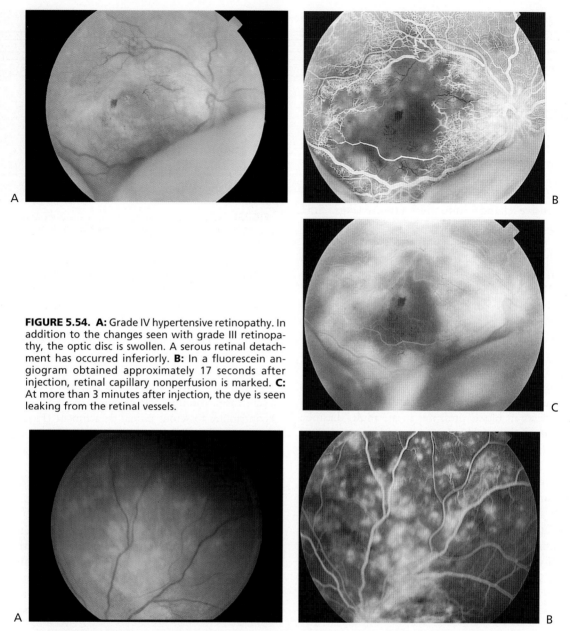

FIGURE 5.54. A: Grade IV hypertensive retinopathy. In addition to the changes seen with grade III retinopathy, the optic disc is swollen. A serous retinal detachment has occurred inferiorly. **B:** In a fluorescein angiogram obtained approximately 17 seconds after injection, retinal capillary nonperfusion is marked. **C:** At more than 3 minutes after injection, the dye is seen leaking from the retinal vessels.

FIGURE 5.55. A Acute hypertensive choroidopathy. Yellow, "acute" Elschnig's spots can be seen at the level of the retinal pigment epithelium. **B:** The fluorescein angiogram corresponding to **(A)** reveals leakage of dye corresponding to the yellow spots.

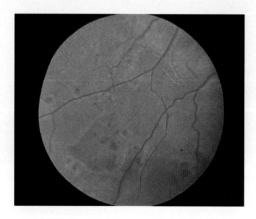

FIGURE 5.56. Chronic Elschnig's spots, characterized by pigmentary changes at the level of the retinal pigment epithelium.

PERIPHERAL PROLIFERATIVE RETINOPATHIES

Peripheral proliferative retinopathies are characterized by retinal neovascularization peripheral to the temporal vascular arcades. Although the predisposing factors are similar to those causing neovascularization of the optic disc and iris, the presence of concomitant optic disc neovascularization precludes the diagnosis. Sickle cell disease is the most common case of peripheral proliferative retinopathy.

Clinical Features. Peripheral proliferative retinopathy is seen in conjunction with a variety of systemic or ocular vascular conditions that have in common the potential to shut down the retinal vascular bed. This includes inflammatory conditions, such as sarcoidosis and pars planitis, that can lead to retinal vascular compromise.

In about 90% of cases, an underlying cause can be found. In the series of Brown and associates, sickle cell disease accounted for 49% of cases of peripheral retinal neovascularization. Other associated disorders included branch retinal vein obstruction (20%), diabetic retinopathy (9%), sarcoidosis (4%), intravenous drug abuse (4%; Fig. 5.57), ocular ischemic syndrome (1%), pars planitis (1%), Coats' disease (1%), and retinitis pigmentosa (1%). A list of disorders associated with peripheral retinal neovascularization is shown in Table 5.1.

Proliferative sickle retinopathy deserves special mention. Peripheral retinal neovascularization is seen most commonly in patients with hemoglobin SC disease, followed in order by hemoglobin SThal and hemoglobin SS disease. Approximately 29% of patients older than 50 years of age with sickle cell hemoglobinopathy have peripheral proliferative disease (Fig. 5.58). Signs of nonproliferative sickle retinopathy may accompany the proliferative changes and include "salmon patches" (Fig. 5.59), acute retinal hemorrhages that occur secondary to ruptured retinal vessels. When the hemorrhages are in the superficial retina, they can lead to iridescent spots, which are fine crystalline deposits

TABLE 5.1. CONDITIONS ASSOCIATED WITH PERIPHERAL RETINAL NEOVASCULARIZATION

Sickle cell hemoglobinopathies
   Hemoglobin SC
   Hemoglobin S thalassemia
   Hemoglobin SS
   Hemoglobin AS
   Hemoglobin AC
   Hemoglobin CB thalassemia
Diabetes mellitus
Venous obstructive disease
Inflammatory diseases
   Sarcoidosis
   Pars planitis
   Bird-shot chorioretinopathy
   Behçet's disease
   Acute retinal necrosis
Collagen vascular disease
   Systemic lupus erythematosus
   Scleroderma
Embolic disease
   Intravenous drug abuse
   Rheumatic fever
Arterial obstructive disease
   Ocular ischemic syndrome–large-vessel obstructive disease
     (e.g., aortic arch, carotid artery, ophthalmic artery)
   Branch retinal artery obstruction
Miscellaneous
   Retinopathy of prematurity
   Familial exudative vitreoretinopathy
   Eales disease
   Incontinentia pigmenti
   Chronic retinal detachment
   Retinitis pigmentosa
   Leukemia
   Radiation-induced retinopathy

under the internal limiting membrane of the retina that become evident as the blood resorbs. When the bleeding dissects to the level of the retinal pigment epithelium, a "black sunburst" (Fig. 5.60) or focal pigment epithelial hypertrophy may develop after the subretinal hemorrhage resolves.

The stages of proliferative sickle retinopathy have been classified by Goldberg:

Stage I: retinal capillary nonperfusion and other background changes

Stage II: arteriolar-venular anastomoses at the juncture of perfused and nonperfused retina

Stage III: peripheral retinal neovascularization

Stage IV: vitreous hemorrhage

Stage V: traction or rhegmatogenous retinal detachment

Eyes with peripheral proliferative retinopathy can have reduced vision secondary to vitreous hemorrhage, retinal detachment, macular edema, or retinal capillary nonperfusion involving the macula.

Management. A workup to determine the underlying cause should be undertaken for patients with peripheral proliferative retinopathy. The history alone often reveals the associated systemic disease, but a laboratory workup may be

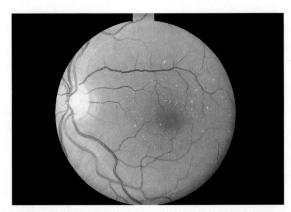

FIGURE 5.57. Talc particles are evident in the small retinal vessels of an eye of a chronic intravenous drug abuser with peripheral retinal neovascularization.

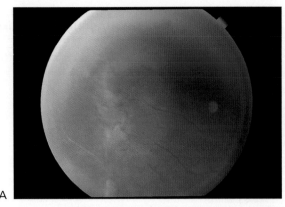 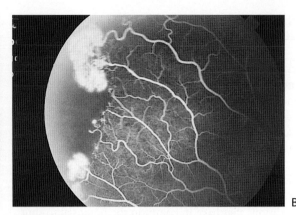

FIGURE 5.58. A: Peripheral retinal neovascularization in the eye of a patient with hemoglobin SC disease. **B:** The fluorescein angiogram corresponding to **(A)**, obtained 29 seconds after injection, reveals hyperfluorescence of the seafan-shaped neovascularization and peripheral retinal capillary nonperfusion that extends posteriorly to the posterior border of the seafan. Arteries that supply seafans are typically more tortuous (i.e., superior vessel) than the draining veins (i.e., inferior vessel).

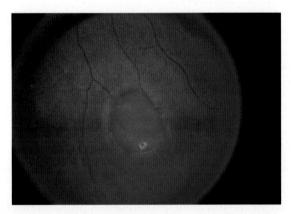

FIGURE 5.59. Retinal hemorrhage, also referred to as a salmon patch, in the eye of a patient with sickle hemoglobinopathy.

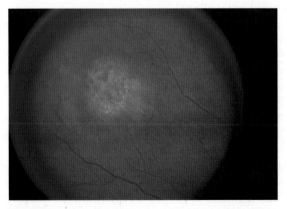

FIGURE 5.60. A "black sunburst" occurs as a sequela of a salmon patch.

necessary, including but not be limited to a complete blood count, fasting blood glucose level, hemoglobin electrophoresis, chest x-ray film, and angiotensin-converting enzyme level.

Scatter laser photocoagulation in the areas of retinal capillary nonperfusion has decreased the incidence of vitreous hemorrhage in eyes with proliferative sickle retinopathy. The same result has been demonstrated when the neovascularization occurs secondary to branch retinal vein obstruction. Eyes with diabetes-related retinal neovascularization and preretinal bleeding also benefit from scatter laser therapy.

Prospective clinical trials have not been performed to demonstrate the efficacy of preventing visual loss in eyes with peripheral retinal neovascularization from many of the causes listed in Table 5.1, although many clinicians believe that the data from studies with diabetic retinopathy, sickling hemoglobinopathy, and branch retinal vein obstruction can be extrapolated to these other conditions.

As with proliferative diabetic retinopathy, vitrectomy may be beneficial in instances of nonclearing vitreous hemorrhage or retinal detachment associated with the other causes of peripheral proliferative retinopathy.

RETINAL VASCULITIS

Vasculitis refers to inflammation of the blood vessels. The site of involvement may occur predominantly on the arterial side of the retinal circulation, the venous side, or both. In some instances, the vasculitis appears to affect the retinal vasculature alone, but in others, the ocular changes are a manifestation of a widespread systemic vasculitis that affects multiple organs.

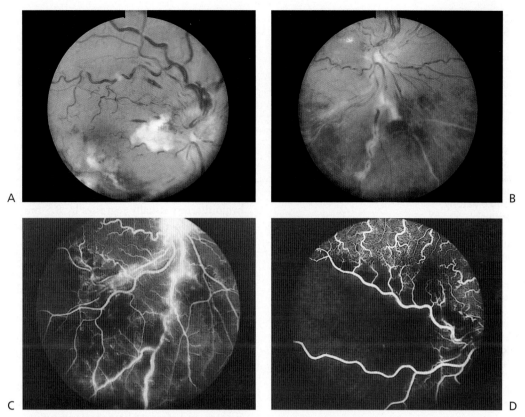

FIGURE 5.61. **A:** Macula of a patient with retinal arteritis and phlebitis as a result of Crohn's disease. Retinal whitening secondary to obstruction of a retinal arteriole is seen in the papillomacular bundle. **B:** Same fundus as in **(A)**, 2 months later. Sheathing of the retinal vessels, particularly the veins, is conspicuous. **C:** In the fluorescein angiogram corresponding to **(B)**, prominent staining of the sheathed retinal veins can be seen. **D:** A more peripheral fluorescein angiographic view demonstrates an area of confluent retinal capillary nonperfusion.

Clinical Features. There is an overlap between the arterial and venous changes seen with retinal vasculitis, although certain signs are seen more frequently with one type than another. The signs of retinal arteritis include arterial sheathing, arterial attenuation, cotton-wool spots, and superficial retinal opacification secondary to obstruction of larger arterioles

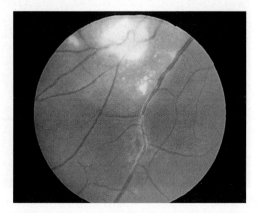

FIGURE 5.62. Sarcoidosis-related retinal phlebitis with perivascular exudates known as "candle-wax drippings."

and arteries. The signs of retinal phlebitis include retinal hemorrhages, retinal edema, telangiectases, microaneurysms, venous sheathing, venous dilations, and venous attenuation. Commonly, some combination of arterial and venous changes are seen (Fig. 5.61). Conditions that mainly affect the retinal veins include sarcoidosis (Fig. 5.62), multiple sclerosis, pars planitis, Eales disease, acute frosted retinal periphlebitis, and Crohn's disease. Conditions that result primarily in the signs of retinal arteritis include systemic lupus erythematosus, polyarteritis nodosa, and Behçet's syndrome.

Other signs of retinal vasculitis are anterior uveitis, cells in the vitreous cavity, and retinal or optic disc neovascularization. The neovascularization usually is associated with significant or widespread shutdown of the retinal vascular bed. Disorders causing vasculitis are shown in Table 5.2. The workup includes a careful history, physical examination, and appropriate laboratory evaluation.

Management. Regardless of whether there is active disease elsewhere, significant posterior segment vasculitis changes that affect or threaten vision may warrant the use of systemic corticosteroids. Although periocular steroids may be sufficient to control some cases, topical agents alone usu-

TABLE 5.2. CONDITIONS ASSOCIATED WITH RETINAL VASCULITIS

Infectious associations
    Herpes zoster virus
    Herpes simplex virus
    Cytomegalovirus
    Acquired immunodeficiency syndrome
    Syphilis
    Tuberculosis
    Toxoplasmosis
Collagen vascular diseases
    Systemic lupus erythematosus
    Polyarteritis nodosa
    Wegener's granulomatosis
    Giant cell arteritis
    Scleroderma
Other systemic diseases
    Diabetes mellitus
    Sarcoidosis
    Behçet's disease
    Multiple sclerosis
    Malignancy
    Ocular ischemic syndrome
    Crohn's disease
    Ankylosing spondylitis
    Goodpasture's syndrome
    Churg-Strauss syndrome
    Löffler's syndrome
    Whipple's disease
Miscellaneous
    Acute frosted retinal periphlebitis
    Eales disease
    Pars planitis
    Idiopathic conditions

Adapted from Brown GC. Retinal vasculitis. In: Margo CE. Diagnostic problems in clinical ophthalmology. Philadelphia: WB Saunders, 1994, with permission.

ally do not make a significant impact on posterior segment changes. In more advanced stages, when there is retinal capillary nonperfusion and retinal or optic disc neovascularization, full-scatter laser photocoagulation applied to the areas of retinal capillary nonperfusion may help to stabilize or cause regression of the neovascularization.

CONGENITAL MALFORMATIONS

Persistent Hyaloid Artery

During embryogenesis, the hyaloid artery gives rise to the vasa hyaloidea propria, which nourishes the primary vitreous, and the tunica vasculosa lentis, the series of vessels nourishing the lens. These two sets of vessels later regress, followed by regression of the hyaloid artery itself; the hyaloid artery usually regresses by 8.5 months of gestation. In approximately 3% of full-term neonates, the hyaloid artery still contains blood.

Clinical Features. A persistent hyaloid artery appears clinically as a sinuous single vessel extending from the optic disc, through Cloquet's canal, to insert on the posterior capsule of the lens. Its point of insertion on the capsule is called a Mittendorf's dot. In the adult, the vessel is usually bloodless (Fig. 5.63). Occasionally, it is blood-filled. Vitreous hemorrhage has been reported in adults with a blood-filled persistent hyaloid artery.

Persistent hyaloid arteries can be confused with larger, congenital precapillary arterial loops. Loops, however, have afferent and efferent branches and typically do not extend more than 5 mm into Cloquet's canal. Neovascularization of the optic disc occasionally also manifests with large vessels growing into Cloquet's canal. These are associated with proliferative disorders such as diabetic retinopathy, retinal vein obstruction, and the ocular ischemic syndrome from carotid artery obstruction.

Management. For most cases, no treatment is required for a persistent hyaloid artery. If a severe vitreous hemorrhage develops, pars plana vitrectomy may be necessary to facilitate clearing of the hemorrhage and restoration of visual acuity.

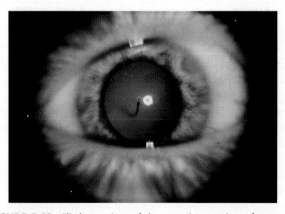

FIGURE 5.63. Slit lamp view of the anterior portion of a persistent hyaloid artery in an adult eye. Despite its appearance, the vessel was not filled with blood.

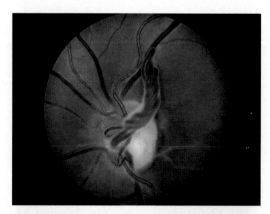

FIGURE 5.64. Prepapillary arterial loop surrounded by a fibroglial sheath that is probably a remnant of Bergmeister's papilla. The optic disc is pale, and the cilioretinal artery is sheathed secondary to the effects of toxemia of pregnancy 15 years earlier.

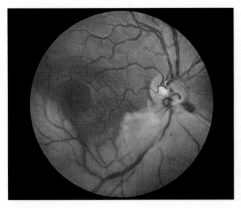

FIGURE 5.65. The prepapillary arterial loop is associated with a branch retinal arterial obstruction in the quadrant of the retina supplied by the loop.

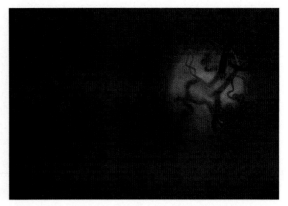

FIGURE 5.67. Multiple optociliary collateral veins are seen on a pale optic disc in the eye of a patient with a central nervous system meningioma. Macular retinal pigment epithelial changes resulted from a retinal venous obstruction.

Prepapillary Vascular Loops

Prepapillary vascular loops can be arterial or venous. The venous variant can be congenital or acquired. Acquired venous prepapillary vascular loops usually are multiple and referred to as optociliary collateral vessels.

Clinical Features. Congenital prepapillary loops are usually unilateral and single, and have an afferent and efferent limb that extend into Cloquet's canal. They vary in height from 0.5 to 5.0 mm (Fig. 5.64). Approximately one third are pulsatile, and about half are enclosed in a glial-appearing sheath that is probably a remnant of Bergmeister's papilla. Although some have a venous appearance, 95% are arterial. Seventy-five percent of affected eyes also have at least one cilioretinal artery.

The major complication associated with prepapillary arterial loops is retinal arterial obstruction in the sector of the retina supplied by the loop (Fig. 5.65). Approximately 10% of cases of loops reported have been associated with arterial obstruction. Amaurosis fugax has been described, as has vit-

reous hemorrhage, particularly in association with posterior vitreous detachment.

When multiple prepapillary loops are seen on the disc, they are almost always venous and acquired (Fig. 5.66). These optociliary collaterals arise secondary to retinal venous obstructive disease. They have been demonstrated to drain into the peripapillary choroidal circulation. Underlying causes include central retinal vein obstruction, branch retinal vein obstruction, optic nerve meningioma and glioma, glaucoma, and increased intracranial pressure. Optociliary collaterals associated with progressive visual loss and optic nerve pallor should increase the physician's index of suspicion concerning a possible optic nerve meningioma (Fig. 5.67).

A persistent hyaloid artery should not be confused with a prepapillary loop. The hyaloid artery is a single vessel that extends anteriorly to the posterior lens capsule.

Neovascularization of the optic disc can occasionally mimic a prepapillary loop when it extends into Cloquet's canal. Neovascularization is typically associated with abnormalities such as diabetic retinopathy, retinal venous

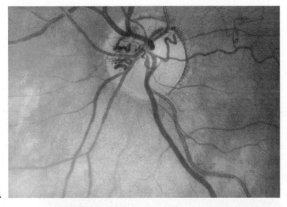
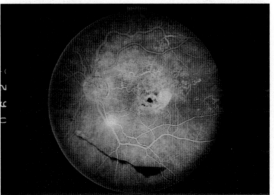

A   B

FIGURE 5.66. A: Multiple optociliary collateral veins on the optic disc developed after a branch retinal vein obstruction. **B:** The fluorescein angiogram reveals telangiectatic abnormalities in the superior macula. A hyperfluorescent area of retinal neovascularization is present along the vascular arcade inferotemporal to the optic disc.

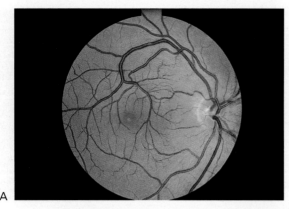
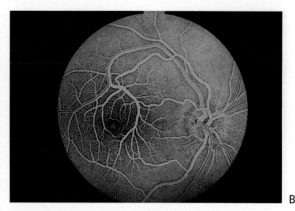

FIGURE 5.68. A: Grade I arteriovenous communication of the retina (retinal macrovessel). An enlarged retinal vein traverses the horizontal raphe, and a small foveolar cyst is present. **B:** Fluorescein angiogram reveals the small arteriovenous communication bordering the superior foveal avascular zone. A small focus of hyperfluorescence corresponds to the foveolar cyst.

obstruction and the ocular ischemic syndrome resulting from carotid artery obstruction. Neovascularization of the disc leaks on fluorescein angiography, but prepapillary loops do not leak fluorescein.

Management. No specific ocular treatment is indicated for prepapillary loops. With multiple venous loops associated with progressive visual loss and optic nerve pallor, imaging should be considered to rule out the possibility of an optic nerve tumor. Chronic papilledema from increased intracranial pressure should also be entertained as a possible cause for venous loops in this setting.

Congenital Retinal Arteriovenous Communications

A congenital retinal arteriovenous communication is an enlarged retinal vessel that acts as a shunt between the retinal arterial and venous circulations. The disorder typically occurs unilaterally.

Clinical Features. Archer and associates classified congenital arteriovenous communications of the retina into three groups.

Group 1 arteriovenous communications are the mildest variant and, clinically, can be very subtle. They are most readily recognized by their association with congenital retinal macrovessels, large retinal vessels (usually veins) that cross the horizontal raphe (Fig. 5.68). Foveolar cysts, which may be transient, have been seen with this abnormality and usually only mildly reduce the visual acuity.

Group 2 arteriovenous communications (Fig. 5.69) are larger than those of group 1. Each communication appears as a large vessel that leaves the optic disc, traverses the retina, and then returns to the disc, and there can be multiple arteriovenous communications. The visual acuity is usually normal.

Group 3 arteriovenous communications (Fig. 5.70) are conglomerations of large vessels that can be so pronounced that they replace optic nerve tissue. The abnormality can change its configuration with time. The visual acuity can vary from normal to severe visual loss.

Ocular complications that have been observed with larger arteriovenous communications include central retinal vein obstruction, neovascular glaucoma, macular hole,

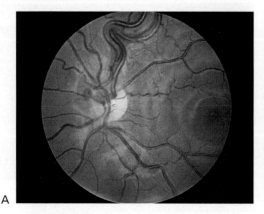
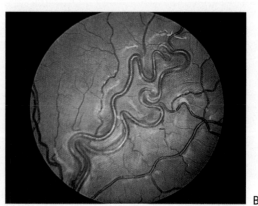

FIGURE 5.69. A: Grade II arteriovenous communication of the retina. **B:** The large communication extends to the midperipheral retina.

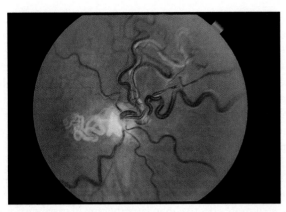

FIGURE 5.70. Grade III arteriovenous communication of the retina. Most of the optic nerve has been replaced by the enlarged vessels. Visual acuity testing revealed no light perception, and the patient also had an arteriovenous communication in the jaw. (Courtesy of Jerry Shields, M.D.)

macroaneurysmal abnormalities, retinal hemorrhage, and vitreous hemorrhage. The arteriovenous communications do not demonstrate leakage of dye during fluorescein angiography.

The larger and more pronounced the communication, the greater the chance it is associated with an arteriovenous communication in the central nervous system, face, or skin. Wyburn-Mason's syndrome has been used to describe the retinal arteriovenous communication when it is associated with other systemic arteriovenous communications. Theron and associates observed that, among the 80 cases reported by 1974, 25 (30%) were seen in conjunction with central nervous system arteriovenous communications. They typically occur ipsilateral to the ocular lesion or in the midline, often following the visual pathway. Subarachnoid hemorrhage can result.

Facial arteriovenous communications have occurred in about 40% of patients with retinal and central nervous system arteriovenous communications. They can occur in the maxilla, mandible, buccal mucosa, palate, or nasopharynx. Recurrent epistaxis and bleeding can occur with dental extraction. Skin lesions have been detected in approximately 25% of patients with retinal and central nervous system arteriovenous communications.

Acquired retinal arteriovenous communications can occur with retinal arterial obstructive diseases, including sickle cell retinopathies, retinal venous obstructive disease, diabetic retinopathy, and the ocular ischemic syndrome resulting from carotid artery obstructive disease. Enlarged retinal vessels on the optic disc can be seen with retinal capillary hemangioma (i.e., von Hippel lesion), retinoblastoma, and choroidal melanoma.

Management. The ocular lesions themselves are usually observed. If macroaneurysmal abnormalities occur and there is retinal edema or hard exudation into the fovea, laser therapy applied to the aneurysms can be considered.

Unfortunately, the central nervous system lesions are most often located deeply, making surgical excision difficult.

Dental extraction should be approached cautiously because of the possibility of severe hemorrhaging from an arteriovenous communication located in the maxilla or mandible.

COATS' DISEASE

Coats' disease is usually diagnosed between 2 and 16 years of age. In most cases, the diagnosis is made as a result of failing an eye test in school or, in infants, the appearance of a yellowish rather than red reflex. The disease occurs most often in boys, although girls may be affected. Unilaterality is the rule, but bilateral involvement does occur in about 8% of patients.

Clinical Features. Coats' disease is characterized by vascular abnormalities that appear as small, red "light bulbs" in the retinal periphery and by associated intraretinal and subretinal hard exudation (Fig. 5.71). The vascular changes include aneurysmal alterations, and on fluorescein angiography, capillary nonperfusion in the affected area of the retina is evident (Fig. 5.72). The exudate tends to accumulate in the posterior pole and the area of peripheral vascular abnormalities (Fig. 5.73).

The disease in children younger than 4 years of age may be expressed differently than in older children. Children younger than 4 years of age often present with leukocoria or strabismus and must be examined to rule out retinoblastoma. If the exudate is in the macular area, there is generally poor fixation in the affected eye. Although many eyes do not have an associated serous retinal detachment, some patients may present with a total retinal detachment, with the retina ballooned just behind the lens. In advanced cases for which there is no resolution of the disease after treatment, neovascularization of the iris may lead to neovascular glaucoma.

The most important disorder that must be differentiated from Coats' disease is the malignant intraocular tumor of infancy and childhood, retinoblastoma. The most difficult diagnostic scenario is when the retinoblastoma grows in an exophytic fashion, with the tumor primarily located beneath and detaching the retina.

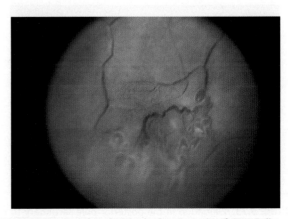

FIGURE 5.71. Peripheral retinal telangiectasia of Coats' disease.

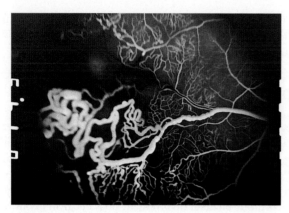

FIGURE 5.72. The fluorescein angiogram demonstrates nonperfusion in the area of a retinal vascular abnormality.

Haik suggests that computed tomography scanning is the single most valuable test for deciding this diagnostic dilemma, because it can help establish the diagnosis of retinoblastoma by identifying calcified subretinal densities, vascularities within the subretinal space (with contrast enhancement), and any associated orbital or intracranial abnormalities. Magnetic resonance imaging can also be helpful in providing insights into the structure and composition of tissues, but it is limited in its ability to detect calcium.

Another condition that must be differentiated from Coats' disease is angiomatosis retinae or retinal capillary hemangioma. This vascular anomaly can produce significant exudation like that seen in Coats' disease. Multiple retinal angiomas presenting in young patients are likely to be part of the angiophakomatosis, von Hippel–Lindau disease. This autosomal dominantly inherited condition is associated with visceral and central nervous system hemangioblastomas, with the latter occurring in about 18% of patients. Visceral cysts and tumors such as renal cell carcinoma and pheochromocytoma can also be part of this potentially life-threatening syndrome.

Cavernous hemangioma of the retina occurs in both sexes equally, is usually localized, has no associated exuda-

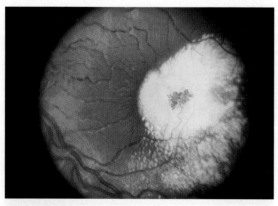

FIGURE 5.73. Exudation in the posterior pole secondary to the abnormal vasculature seen in Figure 5.72.

tion, and on fluorescein angiography, the lesion is demonstrated by dye within saccular vascular channels that do not exhibit any leakage.

Other conditions to be differentiated from Coats' disease include *Toxocara* endophthalmitis, persistent primary hyperplastic vitreous, familial exudative retinopathy, and retinopathy of prematurity (ROP). The diagnosis of these latter conditions can usually be made on the basis of the patient's history, clinical examination, and family history.

Management. Cryotherapy and laser photocoagulation applied to the areas of retinal telangiectasia have been used to reduce associated leakage. In our experience, cryotherapy has been more effective than laser therapy in cases with a significant amount of exudation. In cases with associated and frank retinal detachment, our preference is to perform cryotherapy for the abnormal vessels, external drainage of subretinal fluid, and scleral buckling to bring the retina into apposition with the pigment epithelium. Vitrectomy with internal drainage of subretinal fluid followed by photocoagulation or cryotherapy is also an option. Visual recovery in cases of massive retinal detachment is usually very limited.

RETINAL ARTERIAL MACROANEURYSM

Retinal arterial macroaneurysm was first described as a distinct clinical entity in 1973 by Robertson.

Clinical Features. Acquired retinal arterial macroaneurysms appear as fusiform dilations of retinal arteries or larger arterioles. They usually are located in the posterior pole, and approximately 10% of cases are bilateral. Women comprise 70% to 80% of cases, and approximately two thirds of affected patients have systemic arterial hypertension. In approximately 20% of patients, there are multiple macroaneurysms in an eye. The disease most commonly occurs in the sixth decade and beyond.

Macroaneurysms can cause decreased vision through two mechanisms: hemorrhage and macular edema. About 50% of patients present initially with hemorrhage. Hemorrhaging usually occurs only once. Hemorrhage from a macroaneurysm can occur into the retina, the subretinal space, or the vitreous cavity. The location of the blood is likely to be determined by the site of rupture of the aneurysm and/or the amount of bleeding that occurs. A pattern seen in about 40% of eyes with hemorrhage is the hourglass hemorrhage, with blood at two or more levels in the posterior pole (Fig. 5.74). Approximately 50% of eyes with hemorrhage from a microaneurysm eventually achieve 20/40 vision, but about 25% remain at a level of counting fingers or worse. Bleeding into the subretinal spaces carries a worse visual prognosis than bleeding at other levels.

Retinal edema can extend into the central fovea and adversely affect the vision. Hard exudates can also accumulate from chronic leakage of plasma from the abnormality (Fig. 5.75A). Depending on the series, approximately 30% to

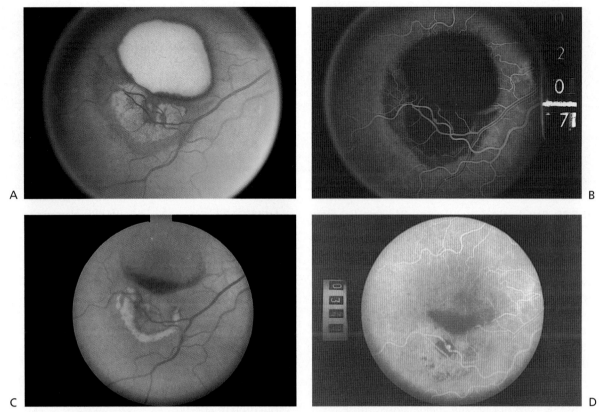

FIGURE 5.74. A: Subretinal and preretinal hemorrhage secondary to a ruptured retinal arterial macroaneurysm. The visual acuity was counting fingers. **B:** The fluorescein angiogram obtained 20 seconds after injection reveals prominent retinal vessels in the region of the subretinal blood, but the vessels are obscured in the area of preretinal blood. A small focus of hyperfluorescence along the course of a retinal artery corresponds to the macroaneurysm. **C:** Five weeks later, visual acuity had improved to 20/50 after reabsorption of much of the blood. **D:** The fluorescein angiogram of the eye in **(C)**, obtained 34 seconds after injection, demonstrates that the macroaneurysm remains hyperfluorescent.

60% of eyes have hard exudates at the time of diagnosis. If the central fovea is involved by edema, about 50% of eyes progress to 20/200 vision.

Fluorescein angiography typically reveals hyperfluorescence of the aneurysm that begins early and increases throughout the study (Fig. 5.75B). It can help to identify an aneurysm located along the course of a retinal artery when blood obscures the surrounding retina.

Most retinal arterial macroaneurysms are 100 to 300 μm in diameter, the size of some cerebral aneurysms. It is unknown whether people with retinal arterial macroaneurysms have a higher incidence of aneurysms elsewhere in the body.

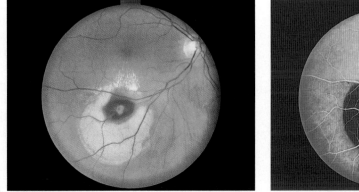
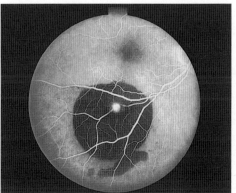

FIGURE 5.75. A: Retinal arterial macroaneurysm, with retinal edema and hard exudate involving the fovea. The visual acuity was 20/40. **B:** The fluorescein angiogram of the eye in **(A)**, obtained 90 seconds after injection, reveals hyperfluorescence of the aneurysm.

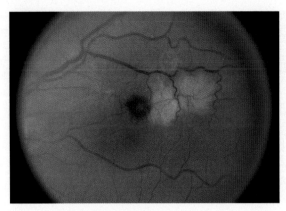

FIGURE 5.76. Branch retinal arterial obstruction distal to a spontaneously thrombosed retinal arterial macroaneurysm.

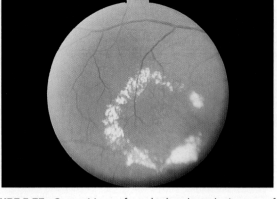

FIGURE 5.77. Group 1A parafoveal telangiectasis. An area of circinate exudate is present in the temporal macula.

Disorders that can mimic a retinal arterial microaneurysm include macular branch retinal vein obstruction, choroidal neovascularization, and causes of posterior segment neovascularization that could lead to preretinal hemorrhage, such as diabetic retinopathy.

Arterial and venous macroaneurysms can occur within the retinal vasculature in the distribution of a previous branch retinal vein obstruction. They can also be seen in cases of Coats' disease, Eales disease, and angiomatosis retinae.

Management. Treatment is generally not indicated for hemorrhages that occur secondary to retinal arterial macroaneurysms, particularly because bleeding is a one-time event and the aneurysm often autothromboses after the hemorrhage.

Although a large prospective study on the natural course of the disease when retinal edema involves the central fovea is lacking, most clinicians consider performing laser therapy in this setting to facilitate resolution of the edema. Light gray burns using 200- to 500-μm spots with the argon green laser can be applied to the aneurysm itself, although some prefer to surround the lesion. The major complication of treatment is obstruction of the retinal artery distal to the microaneurysm, which occurs in about one sixth of treated cases. However, retinal arterial obstruction can occur spontaneously (Fig. 5.76).

PARAFOVEAL TELANGIECTASIS

In 1956, Reese used the term *retinal telangiectasis* to describe a retinal vascular abnormality characterized by ectatic, incompetent retinal capillaries occurring in the macular or peripheral retina. In 1982, Gass and Oyakawa applied the term *idiopathic juxtafoveolar retinal telangiectasis* to the disorder, but it has since become more commonly referred to as *parafoveal telangiectasis*.

Clinical Features. It is thought that parafoveal telangiectasis can take two forms: congenital and acquired. Gass divided the condition into group 1 (A and B subgroups), group 2, and group 3.

Group 1A is congenital unilateral parafoveal telangiectasis. This form typically presents in middle-aged men, and it produces macular edema and hard exudates that can extend as far as 2 or 3 disc diameters from the central fovea (Fig. 5.77). The entity may be a variant of Coats' disease. The median vision at the time of presentation is 20/40, but this can drop to 20/200.

Group 1B is acquired unilateral parafoveal telangiectasis. This subtle form also affects middle-aged men, usually involving only a single clock hour of the perifoveolar retina. Visual loss is minimal.

Group 2 is the most common form of parafoveal telangiectasis. This variant affects both sexes and is seen primarily during the sixth and seventh decades of life. It is typically bilateral and tends to involve the temporal fovea in each eye (Fig. 5.78). The retinal capillaries can be subtly dilated, and the retina in the involved area appears slightly gray. Retinal pigment epithelial hyperplasia develops with time. Choroidal neovascularization is found in about 14% of eyes at the time of presentation and can develop later in others (Fig. 5.79). The median visual acuity in eyes without choroidal neovascularization is 20/40. Rarely, a familial variant can be seen.

Group 3 includes patients with bilateral telangiectasis and retinal capillary nonperfusion. Some cases may represent a variant of cerebroretinal vasculopathy, as described by Grand and associates.

Included in the differential diagnosis of parafoveal telangiectasis are diabetic retinopathy, radiation retinopathy, Coats' disease, and age-related macular degeneration if retinal pigment hyperplasia or choroidal neovascularization is present.

The association of parafoveal telangiectasis and diabetes mellitus deserves special mention. Among parafoveal telangiectasis patients with normal fasting blood glucose levels, Millay and colleagues found that the glucose tolerance test was abnormal in 35% of those with unilateral disease and in

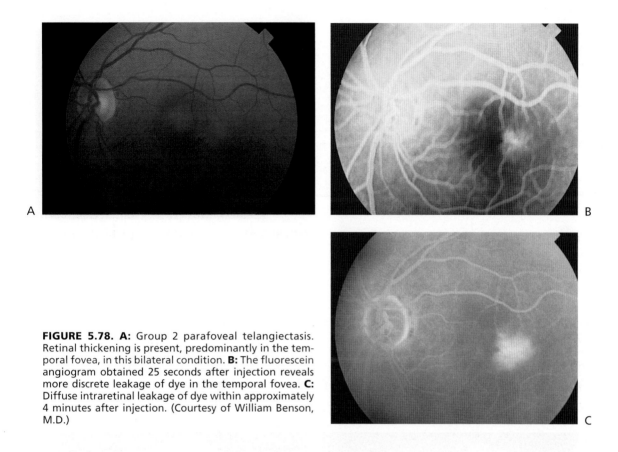

FIGURE 5.78. A: Group 2 parafoveal telangiectasis. Retinal thickening is present, predominantly in the temporal fovea, in this bilateral condition. **B:** The fluorescein angiogram obtained 25 seconds after injection reveals more discrete leakage of dye in the temporal fovea. **C:** Diffuse intraretinal leakage of dye within approximately 4 minutes after injection. (Courtesy of William Benson, M.D.)

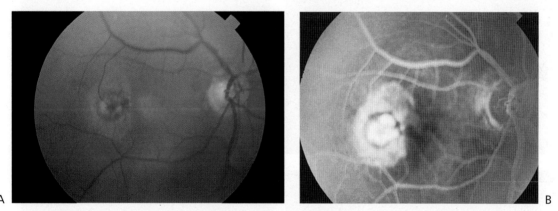

FIGURE 5.79. A: Gray-black pigmentation in an area of choroidal neovascularization in an eye with parafoveal telangiectasis. **B:** The fluorescein angiogram obtained 45 seconds after injection reveals marked hyperfluorescence centrally, corresponding to the choroidal neovascularization, and less intense hyperfluorescence surrounding the neovascular membrane, reflecting a disturbance in the retinal pigment epithelium. (Courtesy of William Benson, M.D.)

more than 60% of those affected bilaterally. Green and associates demonstrated histopathologic accumulations of basement membrane in the retinal capillary walls, similar to the findings seen in eyes with diabetic retinopathy.

Management. Laser therapy may benefit group 1A cases that are likely a variant of Coats' disease. It is probably of minimal benefit for the other variants. Treatment of associated choroidal neovascularization may also be necessary in selected cases. The relation between diabetes mellitus and parafoveal telangiectasis should not be forgotten, because some of these patients may eventually develop frank diabetes.

RADIATION RETINOPATHY

Radiation retinopathy appears to occur primarily as a result of retinal vascular damage. Radiation optic neuropathy is a variant that can also be seen with radiation retinopathy, and choroidopathy can occur as well. The abnormality can occur secondary to external beam irradiation (i.e., teletherapy) or localized plaque therapy (i.e., brachytherapy).

Although many clinicians are familiar with the term *rad* to quantify radiation doses, the term *centigray* (cGy) has supplanted it; 1 rad equals 1 cGy.

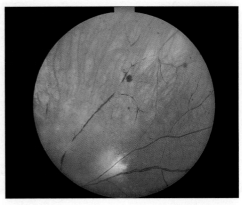

FIGURE 5.81. Hard exudation, retinal sheathing, retinal hemorrhages, and telangiectases occurred in an eye with radiation retinopathy.

Clinical Features. The posterior segment signs seen with radiation retinopathy include cotton-wool spots, retinal hemorrhages, hard exudates, microaneurysms, retinal vascular telangiectasias, vascular sheathing, macular edema, and neovascularization of the optic disc or retina (Fig. 5.80). Hard exudation appears to be more pronounced after brachytherapy than teletherapy (Figs. 5.81 and 5.82).

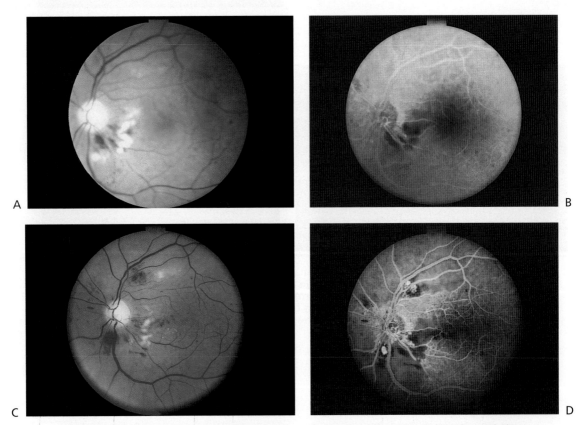

FIGURE 5.80. A: Radiation retinopathy occurring after external beam irradiation (i.e., teletherapy) is manifested by peripapillary cotton-wool spots and retinal hemorrhages. **B:** The fluorescein angiogram reveals peripapillary retinal capillary nonperfusion. **C:** Same fundus as in A, several months later. **D:** A repeat fluorescein angiogram reveals extensive retinal capillary nonperfusion. The eye eventually developed iris neovascularization and neovascular glaucoma.

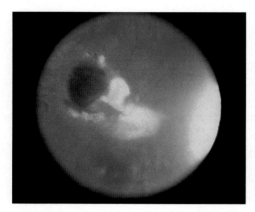

FIGURE 5.82. Equator-plus photograph of an eye with radiation retinopathy resulting from cobalt plaque irradiation (brachytherapy) for a choroidal melanoma. The hard exudation is extensive.

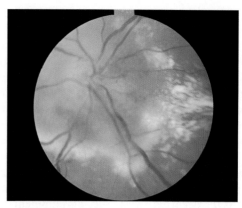

FIGURE 5.84. Acute radiation optic neuropathy is characterized by marked swelling of the optic disc and peripapillary hard exudate.

Retinal pigment epithelial changes are commonly seen, and central retinal artery obstruction and central retinal vein obstruction have rarely been reported.

Radiation retinopathy is related to the radiation dose and the fraction size. Tissue damage appears to increase with dose fractions greater than 250 cGy/day of extreme beam irradiation. Retinopathy has been reported after as little as 1,100 cGy of external beam irradiation, but 3,000 to 3,500 cGy usually are necessary to induce changes. The mean dose given in cases of radiation retinopathy occurring after teletherapy is about 5,000 cGy. After 7,000 to 8,000 cGy, 85% of patients demonstrate posterior segment changes within several months. The administration of chemotherapy may exacerbate radiation retinopathy, even when not given concomitantly with the irradiation. Patients with a preexisting microangiopathy, such as from diabetes mellitus, appear to be more prone to vascular damage from irradiation.

The latency period from the administration of external beam irradiation to the development of radiation changes is approximately 18 months, with a range of 6 to 36 months. For brachytherapy, the mean time is about 15 months, with a range of 4 to 32 months.

Fluorescein angiography may reveal areas of retinal capillary nonperfusion. In approximately 25% of eyes receiving external beam irradiation, the nonperfusion becomes so severe that iris neovascularization develops.

Radiation optic neuropathy can develop if the treatment is directed toward the anterior optic nerve (Fig. 5.83). Disc swelling can range from mild to severe, with striking peripapillary exudation in some cases (Fig. 5.84). The decrease in vision may be mild to severe, with approximately 20% of eyes demonstrating spontaneous improvement over several months.

The condition most likely to be confused with radiation retinopathy is diabetic retinopathy. Ophthalmoscopically, the two can be indistinguishable in some cases. Typically, there are more microaneurysms with diabetic retinopathy than with radiation retinopathy. Hypertensive retinopathy and central retinal vein obstruction can also present with a similar appearance.

The patient's history is essential for making the diagnosis of radiation retinopathy. Because of the latency, particularly when external beam irradiation is administered for neoplasms unassociated with the eye (e.g., oropharynx, brain), patients do not associate the radiotherapy with subsequent ocular changes.

Management. It has been suggested that focal grid laser therapy is of benefit in decreasing visual loss secondary to macular edema. Panretinal photocoagulation has been advocated when posterior segment neovascularization or iris neovascularization develops. Therapies such as hyperbaric oxygen and systemic corticosteroid treatment have not been shown to be consistently effective.

RETINOPATHY OF PREMATURITY

Our knowledge of ROP began in 1942 with the work of Terry, who referred to the condition as retrolental fibroplasia. In the early 1950s, Campbell's observations implicated the use of oxygen in the newborn nursery as playing a role in the

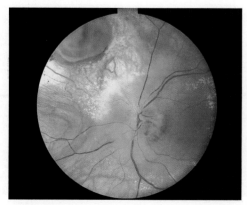

FIGURE 5.83. Radiation optic neuropathy in a left eye occurred after brachytherapy for a superotemporal choroidal melanoma.

pathogenesis of the disease; these concerns were delineated in the reports of the Cooperative Study of Retrolental Fibroplasia. Insights into this potentially blinding disease continued to be published. It seems clear that the two primary risk factors for the development of ROP are low birth weight and prematurity. Babies weighing less than 1,500 g at birth and born at approximately 26 to 28 weeks of gestation are most likely to manifest ROP. Some degree of ROP is seen in 25% to 30% of infants weighing less than 1,500 g and in 65% of infants weighing less than 1,250 g at birth. Those weighing less than 800 g run the greatest risk of needing treatment.

A major advance toward better understanding and managing ROP occurred with the development of the International Classification of ROP. This classification divided the retina into zones 1, 2, and 3, with the optic nerve as the central focal point for each of the concentric circles that define the three zones. The acute or active phases of the disease itself was divided into five stages. Stage 1 is defined as a thin structure within the plane of the retina that separates vascularized from avascular retina. Stage 2 represents an elevated ridge that has extended beyond the plane of the retina. In stage 3, there is extraretinal fibrovascular proliferation or neovascularization at the ridge. In stage 4, there is a partial traction-like retinal detachment; stage 4A indicates extramacular retinal detachment, and stage 4B indicates macular involvement. Stage 5 is defined as a total retinal detachment in an open or closed funnel configuration.

The term *plus disease* denotes significantly dilated and tortuous retinal vessels in the posterior pole. It indicates extensive vascular incompetence, and can be associated with vitreous haze, iris vessel engorgement, and poor pupillary dilation. Plus disease is a poor prognostic sign.

The classification scheme also specified the extent of disease in terms of clock hours. Overall, the farther posterior and the more quadrants involved with neovascularization, the worse the prognosis.

Clinical Features. Critical for the ophthalmologist examining premature infants is the ability to recognize *threshold dis-*

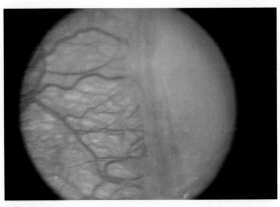

FIGURE 5.86. Stage 3 retinopathy of prematurity with extraretinal fibrovascular proliferation.

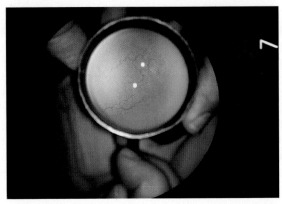

FIGURE 5.87. Clinical photograph of the neovascular "popcorn" posterior to the ridge in stage 2 retinopathy of prematurity.

ease, a term used to indicate the presence of plus disease (Fig. 5.85) with stage 3 changes greater than or equal to 5 contiguous or 8 cumulative clock hours (Fig. 5.86) in zone 1 or 2.

Prethreshold or regressing ROP can sometimes be confused with threshold disease when small neovascular lesions (i.e., popcorn) are seen posterior to the ridge (Figs. 5.87 and 5.88). The major complications during the active, proliferative

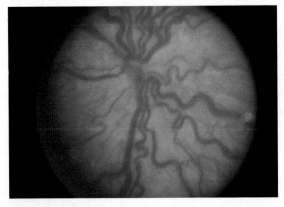

FIGURE 5.85. Dilated and tortuous arterioles and veins are in the posterior pole characteristic of "plus disease." Occasionally, iris engorgement may occur; this is an additional sign of significant plus disease.

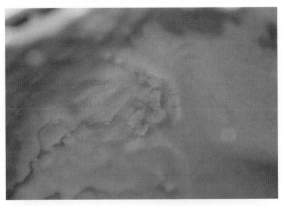

FIGURE 5.88. Gross histopathologic specimen of the neovascular popcorn seen in Figure 5.87.

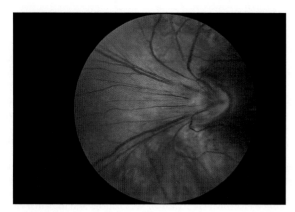

FIGURE 5.89. Temporal dragging of the retina in a 10-year-old boy with regressed retinopathy of prematurity.

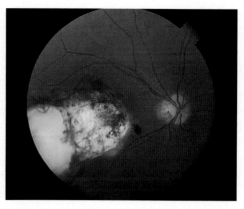

FIGURE 5.91. Chorioretinal scar in the posterior pole of a 36-year-old woman with retinopathy of prematurity. These scars have been confused with those secondary to toxoplasmosis.

phases of ROP include vitreous hemorrhage and traction retinal detachment.

In eyes with regressed ROP, one of the hallmark changes is dragging of the retina (Fig. 5.89). This usually occurs in the temporal retina and often causes some dragging or distortion in the macula. An accentuated form of dragging in regressed ROP is a falciform fold (Fig. 5.90). Such a fold through the macula, retinal detachment, and retrolental tissue were all considered unfavorable outcomes in the Cryotherapy for Retinopathy of Prematurity Cooperative Group study. Chorioretinal scarring may also occur in the fundus periphery or the posterior pole (Fig. 5.91). Another serious late occurrence in adult patients with ROP is exudative retinal detachment, which most likely results from vitreous traction (Fig. 5.92). The eyes affected by ROP tend to have high degrees of myopia and late rhegmatogenous retinal detachments.

The differential diagnosis for ROP includes dominant familial exudative vitreoretinopathy (FEVR), X-linked retinoschisis, incontinentia pigmenti, combined hamartoma of the retinal pigment epithelium, persistent posterior hyperplastic vitreous, Norrie's disease, and retinoblastoma. Of these, FEVR

is the most frequently seen. Retinal changes may simulate those seen in ROP (Fig. 5.93), but there is usually a history of normal birth weight and full-term gestation. Because of the usual dominant inheritance pattern, examination of family members helps to establish the diagnosis.

Management. Treatment of active ROP has included cryotherapy and laser photocoagulation. With either modality, treatment is applied to the entire peripheral avascular zone of retina. Cryotherapy creates large confluent scars, with a loss of retinal pigment epithelium and choroid (Fig. 5.94), but laser therapy produces more discrete scars (Fig. 5.95). Laser treatment, delivered with the indirect ophthalmoscope, is easier to deliver, and because of much less direct ocular manipulation, it appears less stressful to the infant. Comparable rates of regression have been reported for both types of treatment. Overall, the Cryotherapy for Retinopathy of Prematurity Cooperative Group study showed that unfavorable outcomes were reduced by almost half for eyes treated with threshold disease, as compared to those that were observed.

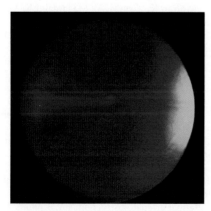

FIGURE 5.90. Temporal retinal fold. Vision is less than 20/200. This was considered an unfavorable outcome in the Cryotherapy for Retinopathy of Prematurity Cooperative Group study.

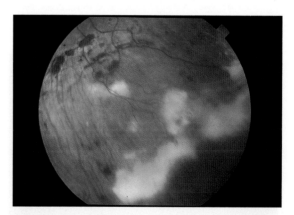

FIGURE 5.92. Exudative retinal detachment in a 23-year-old, one-eyed woman with retinopathy of prematurity. Because exudative detachments are probably caused by vitreous traction, a scleral buckle procedure was performed, which included cryotherapy to the abnormal peripheral vessels. This led to resolution of the exudative retinal detachment.

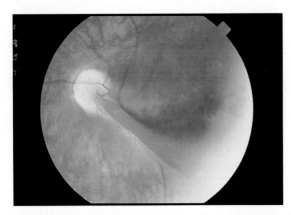

FIGURE 5.93. Temporal dragging of the retina in a patient with familial exudative vitreoretinopathy.

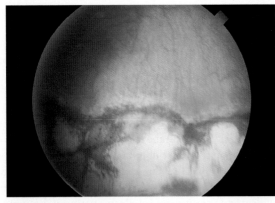

FIGURE 5.94. A large, confluent chorioretinal scar formed after cryotherapy. The retinal pigment epithelium and choroid have been destroyed.

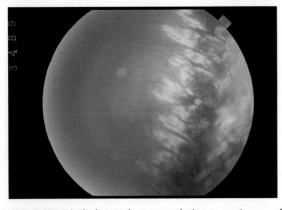

FIGURE 5.95. Diode laser photocoagulation scars 1 year after treatment.

BIBLIOGRAPHY

Abdel-Khalek MN, Richardson J. Retinal macroaneurysm. Natural history and guidelines for treatment. *Br J Ophthalmol* 1986;70:2.

Amoaku WM, Archer DB. Fluorescein angiographic features, natural course and treatment of radiation retinopathy. *Eye* 1990;4:657.

Archer DB, Amoaku WM, Gardiner TA. Radiation retinopathy. Clinical, histopathological, ultrastructural and experimental correlations. *Eye* 1991;5:239.

Archer DB, Deutman A, Ernest JR, Krill AE. Arteriovenous communications of the retina. *Am J Ophthalmol* 1973;75:224.

Benson WE, Brown GC, Tasman W, McNamara JA. Complications of vitrectomy for non-clearing vitreous hemorrhage in diabetic patients. *Ophthalmol Surg* 1988;19:862.

Benson WE, Brown GC, Tasman W. Diabetes and its ocular complications. Philadelphia: WB Saunders; 1988.

Branch Retinal Vein Occlusion Study Group. Argon laser scatter photocoagulation for prevention of neovascularization and vitreous hemorrhage in branch vein occlusion. *Arch Ophthalmol* 1986;104:34.

Branch Retinal Vein Occlusion Study Group. Argon laser photocoagulation for macular edema in branch vein occlusion. *Am J Ophthalmol* 1984;98:271.

Breckinridge A, Dollery CT, Parry EH. Prognosis of treated hypertension. Changes in life expectancy and causes of death between 1952–1967. *Q J Med* 1970;39:411.

British Multicentre Study Group. Photocoagulation for proliferative diabetic retinopathy. A randomized clinical trial using the xenon-arc. *Diabetologia* 1984;26:109.

Brown GC, Brown MM, Hiller T, Fischer DH, Benson WE, Magargal LE. Cotton-wool spots. *Retina* 1985;5:206.

Brown GC, Brown RH, Brown MM. Peripheral proliferative retinopathies. *Int Ophthalmol* 1987;11:41.

Brown GC, Donoso LA, Magargal LE, Goldberg RE, Sarin L. Congenital retinal macrovessels. *Arch Ophthalmol* 1982;100:430.

Brown GC, Duker J, Lehman R, Eagle R. Combined central retinal artery–central vein obstruction. *Int Ophthalmol* 1993;17:9.

Brown GC, Magargal LE. The ocular ischemic syndrome. Clinical, fluorescein angiographic and carotid angiographic features. *Int Ophthalmol* 1988;11:239.

Brown GC, Magargal LE, Sergott R. Acute obstruction of the retinal and choroidal circulations. *Ophthalmology* 1982;93:1371.

Brown GC, Magargal LE, Shields JA, Goldberg RE, Walsh PN. Retinal arterial obstruction in children and young adults. *Ophthalmology* 1981;88:18.

Brown GC, Magargal LE. Central retinal artery obstruction and visual acuity. *Ophthalmology* 1982;89:14.

Brown GC, Moffat K, Cruess A, Magargal LE, Goldberg RE. Cilioretinal artery obstruction. *Retina* 1983;3:182.

Brown GC, Ridley M, Haas D, Lucier AC, Sarin LK. Lipemic diabetic retinopathy. *Ophthalmology* 1984;91:1490.

Brown GC, Shields JA, Sanborn G, Augsburger JJ, Savino PJ, Schatz NJ. Radiation optic neuropathy. *Ophthalmology* 1982;89:1487.

Brown GC, Shields JA, Sanborn G, Augsburger JJ, Savino PJ, Schatz NJ. Radiation retinopathy. *Ophthalmology* 1982;89:1494.

Brown GC, Shields JA. Cilioretinal arteries and retinal arterial occlusion. *Arch Ophthalmol* 1979;97:84.

Brown GC, Tasman W. Congenital anomalies of the optic disc. New York: Grune & Stratton; 1983:12.

Brown GC. Central retinal vein obstruction. Diagnosis and management. In: Reinecke RD. Ophthalmology annual. Norwalk: Appleton-Century-Crofts; 1985:65.

Brown GC. Retinal arterial obstruction. Focal points 1994: clinical modules for ophthalmologists. *Am Acad Ophthalmol* 1994; 12(1):1.

Brown GC. Retinal arterial obstructive disease. In: Ryan SJ. Retina. Baltimore: CV Mosby; 1994;76:1361.

Brown GC. Retinal vasculitis. In: Margo CE. Diagnostic problems in clinical ophthalmology. Philadelphia: WB Saunders; 1994; 56:452.

Campbell K. Intensive oxygen therapy as a possible cause of retrolental fibroplasia: a clinical approach. *Med J Aust* 1951;2:48.

Central Vein Occlusion Study Group. Baseline and early natural history report. The central vein occlusion study. *Arch Ophthalmol* 1993;111:1087.

Chew EY, Murphy RP, Newsome DA, Fine SL. Parafoveal telangiectasis and diabetic retinopathy. *Arch Ophthalmol* 1986;104:71.

Cryotherapy for Retinopathy of Prematurity Cooperative Group. Multicenter trial of cryotherapy for retinopathy of prematurity: one year outcome: structure and function. *Arch Ophthalmol* 1990;108:1408.

Degenhart W, Brown GC, Augsburger JJ, Shields JA. Preretinal vascular loops. A clinical and fluorescein angiographic study. *Ophthalmology* 1981;88:1126.

Diabetes Control and Complications Trial Research Group. The effect of intensive treatment of diabetes on the development and progression of long-term complications in insulin-dependent diabetes mellitus. *N Engl J Med* 1993;329:977.

Diabetic Retinopathy Study Research Group. Four risk factors for severe visual loss in diabetic retinopathy. The third report from the Diabetic Retinopathy Study. *Arch Ophthalmol* 1979;97:654.

Diabetic Retinopathy Study Research Group. Photocoagulation treatment of proliferative diabetic retinopathy. Clinical application of Diabetic Retinopathy Study (DRS) findings. DRS report number 8. *Ophthalmology* 1981;88:583.

Diabetic Retinopathy Vitrectomy Study Group. Two-year course of visual acuity in severe proliferative diabetic retinopathy with conventional management. *Ophthalmology* 1985;92:492.

Diabetic Retinopathy Vitrectomy Study Research Group. Early vitrectomy for severe proliferative diabetic retinopathy in eyes with useful vision. *Ophthalmology* 1988;95:1307.

Diabetic Vitrectomy Study Research Group. Early vitrectomy for severe vitreous hemorrhage in diabetic retinopathy. Four-year results of a randomized trial: Diabetic Retinopathy Study report 5. *Arch Ophthalmol* 1990;108:958.

Early Treatment Diabetic Retinopathy Research Study Group. Photocoagulation for diabetic macular edema. Early Treatment Diabetic Retinopathy Study report number 1. *Arch Ophthalmol* 1985;103:1796.

EC/IC Bypass Study Group. Failure of extracranial-intracranial arterial bypass to reduce the risk of ischemic stroke. *N Engl J Med* 1985;313:1191.

European Carotid Surgery Trialists' Collaborative Group. MRC European carotid surgery trial: interim results for symptomatic patients with severe (70–99%) or with mild carotid stenosis. *Lancet* 1991;337:1235.

Farber MD, Jampol LM, Fox P, et al. A randomized clinical trail of scatter photocoagulation of proliferative sickle cell retinopathy. *Arch Ophthalmol* 1991;109:363.

Frangieh GT, Green WR, Barraguer-Somers E, Finkelstein D. Histopathologic study of nine branch retinal vein occlusions. *Arch Ophthalmol* 1982;100:1132.

Frisen L, Hoyt WF, Tengroth BM. Optociliary veins, disc pallor and visual loss: a triad of signs indicating spheno-orbital meningiomas. *Acta Ophthalmol* 1973;51:241.

Gass JD, Oyakawa R. Idiopathic juxtafoveolar retinal telangiectasis. *Arch Ophthalmol* 1982;100:769.

Gass JDM, Blodi BA. Idiopathic juxtafoveolar retinal telangiectasis. Update of classification and follow-up study. *Ophthalmology* 1993;100:1536.

Glaser DA, Shapiro MJ. Peripheral retinal neovascularization. In: Margo CE. Diagnostic problems in clinical ophthalmology. Philadelphia: WB Saunders; 1994:490.

Goldberg MF. Classification and pathogenesis of proliferative sickle retinopathy. *Am J Ophthalmol* 1971;71:649.

Graham EM, Stanford MR, Saunders MD, et al. A point prevalence study of 150 patients with retinal vasculitis. *Br J Ophthalmol* 1989;73:714.

Grand MG, Kaine J, Fulling K, et al. Cerebroretinal vasculopathy. A new hereditary syndrome. *Ophthalmology* 1986;95:649.

Green WR, Chan CC, Hutchins GM, Terry JM. Central retinal vein occlusion: a prospective histopathologic study of 29 eyes in 28 cases. *Retina* 1981;1:27.

Green WR, Quigley HA, de la Cruz Z, Cohen B. Parafoveal retinal telangiectasis. Light and electron microscopy studies. *Trans Ophthalmol UK* 1980;100:162.

Guyer DR, Yannuzzi LA, Slakter JS, et al. Diagnostic indocyanine green videoangiography. In: Ryan SJ. Retina, vol 2. Philadelphia: CV Mosby; 1994:985.

Haik BG. Advanced Coats' disease. *Trans Am Ophthalmol Soc* 1991;89:371.

International Committee for the Classification of the Late Stages of Retinopathy of Prematurity. An international classification of retinopathy of prematurity. II. The classification of retinal detachment. *Arch Ophthalmol* 1987;105:906.

Irvine AR, Wood IS. Radiation retinopathy as an experimental model for ischemic proliferative retinopathy and rubeosis iridis. *Am J Ophthalmol* 1987;103:790.

Jack RJ. Regression of the hyaloid vascular system. *Am J Ophthalmol* 1972;74:261.

Jampol LM, Goldbaum MH. Peripheral proliferative retinopathies. *Surv Ophthalmol* 1980;25:1.

Jones HE. Hyaloid remnants in the eyes of premature babies. *Br J Ophthalmol* 1963;47:39.

Karjalainen K. Occlusion of the central retinal artery and retinal branch arterioles. *Acta Ophthalmol* (suppl) 1971;109:5.

Kearns TP, Hollenhorst RW. Venous-stasis retinopathy of occlusive disease of the carotid artery. *Mayo Clin Proc* 1963;38:304.

Keith NM, Wagener HP, Barker NW. Some different types of essential hypertension: their cause and prognosis. *Am J Med Sci* 1939;197:332.

Kinsey VE. Retrolental fibroplasia: cooperative study of retrolental fibroplasia and the use of oxygen. *Trans Am Acad Ophthalmol Otolaryngol* 1955;59:15.

Kinyoun JL, Chittum ME, Wells CG. Photocoagulation of radiation retinopathy. *Am J Ophthalmol* 1988;105:470.

Kohner EM, Dollery CT, Bulpitt CJ. Cotton-wool spots in diabetic retinopathy. *Diabetes* 1969;18:691.

Lavin MJ, March RJ, Peart S, Rehman A. Retinal arterial macroaneurysms. A retrospective study of 40 patients. *Br J Ophthalmol* 1987;71:817.

Laser ROP Study Group. Laser therapy for retinopathy of prematurity. *Arch Ophthalmol* 1994;112:154.

Magargal LE, Brown GC, Augsburger JJ, Donoso LA. Efficacy of panretinal photocoagulation in preventing neovascular glaucoma following ischemic central retinal vein obstruction. *Ophthalmology* 1982;89:780.

Magargal LE, Donoso LA, Sanborn G. Retinal ischemia and risk of neovascularization following central retinal vein obstruction. *Ophthalmology* 1982;89:1241.

Mann I. The development of the human eye. 3rd ed. New York: Grune & Stratton; 1969.

Mansour AM, Walsh J, Henkind P. Arteriovenous anastomoses of the retina. *Ophthalmology* 1987;94:35.

Mansour AM, Wells CG, Jampol LM, Kalina RE. Ocular complications of arteriovenous communications of the retina. *Arch Ophthalmol* 1989;107:232.

Masuyama Y, Kodama Y, Matsura Y, Sawada A, Harada K. Clinical studies on the occurrence and the pathogenesis of opticociliary veins. *J Clin Neuro-ophthalmol* 1990;10:1.

McLeod D, Marshall J, Kohner EM, Bird AC. The role of axoplasmic transport in the pathogenesis of cotton-wool spots. *Br J Ophthalmol* 1977;61:177.

Michel J. Die spontane Thrombose der Vena centralis des Opticus. *Graefe's Arch Ophthalmol* 1878;24:37.

Millay RH, Klein ML, Handelman IL, Watzke RC. Abnormal glucose metabolism and parafoveal telangiectasia. *Am J Ophthalmol* 1986;102:363.

Nagpal KC, Goldberg MF, Rabb MF. Ocular manifestations of sickle hemoglobinopathies. *Surv Ophthalmol* 1977;21:391.

North American Symptomatic Carotid Endarterectomy Trial Collaborators. Beneficial effects of carotid endarterectomy in symptomatic patients with high-grade stenosis. *N Engl J Med* 1991;325:445.

Novotny HR, Alvis DL. A method of photographing fluorescence in circulating blood in the human retina. *Circulation* 1961;24:82.

Panton RW, Goldberg MF, Farber MD. Retinal arterial macroaneurysms. Risk factors and natural history. *Br J Ophthalmol* 1990;74:595.

Perry HD, Zimmerman LE, Benson WE. Hemorrhage from isolated aneurysm of a retinal artery. Report of two cases simulating malignant melanoma. *Arch Ophthalmol* 1977;95:281.

Reese AB. Telangiectasis of the retina and Coats' disease. *Am J Ophthalmol* 1956;42:1.

Ridley ME, Shields JA, Brown GC, Tasman W. Coats' disease. *Ophthalmology* 1982;89:1381.

Robertson DM. Microaneurysms of the retinal arteries. *Tr Am Acad Ophthalmol Otolaryngol* 1973;77:55.

Schatz H. Fluorescein angiography: basic principles and interpretation. In: Ryan SJ. Retina, vol 2. Philadelphia: CV Mosby; 1994:911.

Sivalingam A, Brown GC, Magargal LE, Menduke H. The ocular ischemic syndrome. II. Mortality and systemic morbidity. *Int Ophthalmol* 1989;13:187.

Sivalingam A, Brown GC, Magargal LE. The ocular ischemic syndrome. III. Visual prognosis and the effect of treatment. *Int Ophthalmol* 1991;15:15.

Tasman W. Coats' disease. In: Tasman W. Retinal diseases in children. New York: Harper & Row; 1971:59.

Theron J, Newton TH, Hoyt WF. Unilateral retinocephalic vascular malformations. *Neuroradiology* 1974;7:185.

Thompson JT, deBustros S, Michels RG, Rice TA. Results and prognostic factors in vitrectomy for diabetic vitreous hemorrhage. *Arch Ophthalmol* 1987;105:191.

Tso MOM, Jampol LM. Pathophysiology of hypertensive retinopathy. *Ophthalmology* 1982;89:1132.

Walsh JB. Hypertensive retinopathy: description, classification, and prognosis. *Ophthalmology* 1982;89:1127.

Wyburn-Mason R. Arteriovenous aneurysms of the mid-brain, retina, facial naevi and mental changes. *Brain* 1943;66:163.

CHAPTER 6

Tumors of the Uveal Tract

Jerry A. Shields
Carol L. Shields

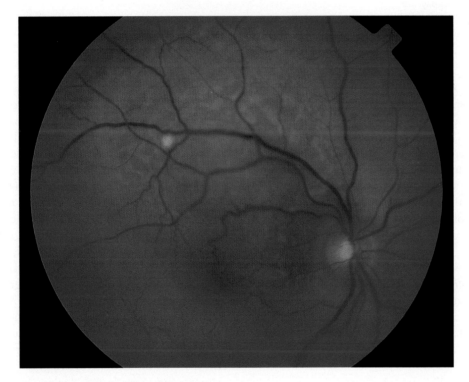

Fundus photograph of a choroidal melanoma adjacent to the optic disc, showing geographic orange pigment on the surface of the lesion.

IRIS TUMORS

Iris Nevus
Iris Melanoma
Adenoma of the Iris Pigment Epithelium

MELANOCYTIC TUMORS OF THE POSTERIOR UVEA

Choroidal Nevus
Ciliary Body Melanoma
Choroidal Melanoma

UVEAL METASTASIS

Anterior Uveal Metastasis
Choroidal Metastasis

CHOROIDAL HEMANGIOMA

Circumscribed Choroidal Hemangioma
Diffuse Choroidal Hemangioma

CHOROIDAL OSTEOMA

LYMPHOID TUMORS

LEUKEMIA

TUMORS OF THE NONPIGMENTED CILIARY EPITHELIUM

Medulloepithelioma
Acquired Adenoma and Adenocarcinoma

ACQUIRED TUMORS OF THE CILIARY AND RETINAL PIGMENT EPITHELIUM

Since publication of the first edition of *Atlas of Clinical Ophthalmology,* there have been several new developments related to intraocular tumors. As with the previous edition, space limitations do not permit a detailed account of all clinical variations, differential diagnoses, diagnostic techniques, pathology, management, and prognosis for all of the tumors that can develop in the iris, ciliary body, choroid, and pigment epithelium (PE). However, a comprehensive, extensively illustrated color atlas of intraocular tumors was recently published which covers details of virtually all intraocular tumors. The reader who wants more detailed information may consult the texts cited in the bibliography. Once again, less common uveal tumors such as leiomyoma, neurilemoma, neurofibroma, and several others are not discussed here. Some comments on tumors of the PE are included, since there have been recent developments regarding their natural course and clinical features.

IRIS TUMORS

Tumors of the iris can arise from the iris melanocytes, iris smooth muscle cells, and the iris PE. Systemic neoplasms such as lymphoma and metastatic tumors can also affect the iris. Nevus, malignant melanoma, and pigment epithelial tumors will be considered here.

Iris Nevus

Iris nevus is a benign tumor that arises in the melanocytes in the iris stroma. Although most iris nevi remain clinically stationary, they can occasionally give rise to malignant melanoma. Histopathologically, an iris nevus is usually composed of low-grade spindle-type cells. Occasionally, it is composed of deeply pigmented, round cells similar to those seen in the melanocytoma of the optic disc.

Clinical Features. An iris nevus classically appears as a variably-pigmented, well circumscribed lesion in the iris stroma (Fig. 6.1). It may involve any portion of the iris from the pupillary border to the iris root and may be flat or minimally elevated. Occasionally, an iris nevus may occupy an entire sector of the iris from the pupillary border to the anterior chamber angle. In some cases, an iris nevus may be clinically amelanotic (Fig. 6.2). An iris nevus can induce an irregular pupil (Fig. 6.2) or sector cortical cataract.

The differential diagnosis of iris nevus includes iris melanoma, adenoma of the iris PE, iris cyst, foreign body, iris granuloma, and other small circumscribed iris lesions.

Iris nevus is best diagnosed by recognition of the typical lesion with slit lamp biomicroscopy. Ancillary diagnostic studies, such as fluorescein angiography and ultrasonography, have little additional diagnostic value.

Management. An iris nevus is best managed by documentation with accurate drawings or photographs and examination on a yearly basis, looking for evidence of enlargement of the lesion. If growth is detected, malignant transformation into melanoma should be suspected.

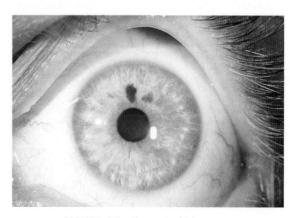

FIGURE 6.1. Pigmented iris nevus.

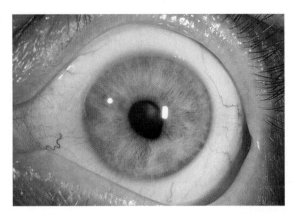

FIGURE 6.2. Minimally pigmented iris nevus with irregular pupil.

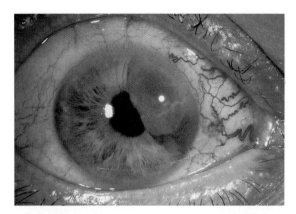

FIGURE 6.4. Minimally pigmented iris melanoma.

Iris Melanoma

An iris melanoma is a malignant melanocytic tumor that arises from the melanocytes of the iris stroma. Histopathologically, it is composed of spindle cells, epithelioid cells, or a combination of the two (mixed-cell type).

Clinical Features. An iris melanoma is characterized clinically as a variable pigmented, elevated, circumscribed or diffuse, melanocytic neoplasm that affects the iris stroma. It is typically larger than an iris nevus. The lesion most often is deeply pigmented and elevated (Fig. 6.3). In can be amelanotic, or it can be partially pigmented and partially nonpigmented (Fig. 6.4).

An important variant of iris melanoma is the diffuse iris melanoma. It grows as a flat, diffuse, often multifocal mass that covers a large area of the iris surface (Fig. 6.5). The patient with a diffuse iris melanoma typically presents with a clinical syndrome of progressive acquired hyperchromic heterochromia and ipsilateral secondary glaucoma.

Iris melanoma has the capacity to exhibit distant metastasis to the liver and other organs. Lesions that are diffuse and produce secondary glaucoma tend to have a greater tendency to spawn metastatic disease.

The differential diagnosis of iris melanoma is the same as mentioned previously for iris nevus. It is important to differentiate iris melanoma from similar conditions because of the malignant nature of this neoplasm. The diagnosis of iris melanoma is best made by recognition of the typical slit lamp features by an experienced observer. Although fluorescein angiography and ultrasonography have been employed, they add little useful diagnostic information. Fine needle aspiration biopsy can be employed to confirm the diagnosis of diffuse iris tumors when enucleation is being considered.

Management. Once the diagnosis of iris melanoma is clearly established, usually by documentation of progressive growth, the best management is surgical excision of the lesion. Lesions confined to the iris can be managed by removal by partial sector or peripheral iridectomy. Those that extend into the ciliary body require iridocyclectomy or iridogoniocyclectomy. The diffuse iris melanoma is often too large to resect locally and may require enucleation or plaque radiotherapy in selected cases.

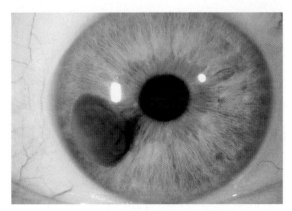

FIGURE 6.3. Pigmented iris melanoma.

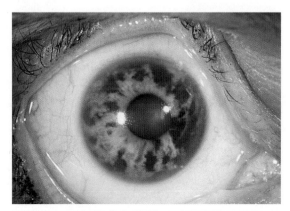

FIGURE 6.5. Diffuse iris melanoma.

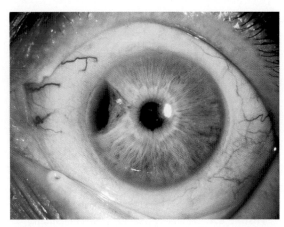

FIGURE 6.6. Round adenoma of the iris pigment epithelium.

Adenoma of the Iris Pigment Epithelium

An adenoma of the iris PE is a benign neoplasm that arises from the PE of the iris. Histopathologically, it is composed of columns or acini of pigmented epithelial cells.

Clinical Features. Clinically, an adenoma of the iris PE appears as a dark black lesion that can appear in the angle as a rounded mass (Fig. 6.6) or as an irregular, multinodular mass (Fig. 6.7). The lesion typically remains stable or progresses very slowly. Transformation into adenocarcinoma is exceedingly rare.

The differential diagnosis of adenoma of the iris pigment is the same as that for iris nevus and melanoma. The dark black color of the adenoma should suggest the diagnosis.

The diagnosis of adenoma of the iris PE is best made by recognition of its characteristic clinical features.

Management. Small asymptomatic tumors can be managed by simple observation. If the lesion shows progressive enlargement or early secondary glaucoma, removal by iridectomy or iridocyclectomy is warranted.

MELANOCYTIC TUMORS OF THE POSTERIOR UVEA

Choroidal Nevus

A choroidal nevus is a benign melanocytic tumor that arises in the choroid. Although most choroidal nevi remain clinically stationary for many years, they can occasionally give rise to malignant melanoma. Histopathologically, a choroidal nevus is usually composed of low-grade spindle-type cells. Occasionally it is composed of deeply pigmented, round cells similar to those seen in the melanocytoma of the optic disc. Such choroidal melanocytomas are very deeply pigmented.

Clinical Features. Ophthalmoscopically, a choroidal nevus is a variably pigmented, fairly well-circumscribed lesion that usually occurs in the more posterior portions of the choroid. It usually has a gray to black color and is often rather homogeneous (Fig. 6.8). Small drusen may be present on the surface of the lesion (Fig. 6.9). Occasionally, an iris nevus may be clinically amelanotic (Fig. 6.10). Choroidal nevi are usually less than 2 mm in thickness. Accumulation of a small amount of subretinal fluid can occasionally occur. The subretinal fluid may leak into the macular area, causing visual impairment.

The differential diagnosis of choroidal nevus includes small choroidal melanoma, hypertrophy of the retinal pigment epithelium (RPE), hyperplasia of the RPE, combined hamartoma of the retinal epithelium and RPE, subretinal hemorrhage, and other conditions. The amelanotic choroidal nevus must be differentiated from uveal metastasis, granuloma, and choroidal lymphoma. Choroidal nevus is best diagnosed by careful ophthalmoscopy by an experienced clinician who recognizes the typical clinical features. Fluorescein angiography may help to differentiate the lesion from subretinal hemorrhage or from lesions of the RPE.

Management. The best management of a choroidal nevus is periodic ophthalmoscopy, looking closely for enlargement of the lesion. Serial fundus photography is highly desirable in

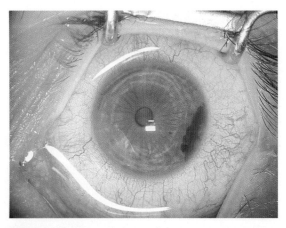

FIGURE 6.7. Irregular adenoma of the iris pigment epithelium.

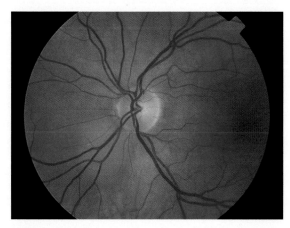

FIGURE 6.8. Homogeneous choroidal nevus in the macular area.

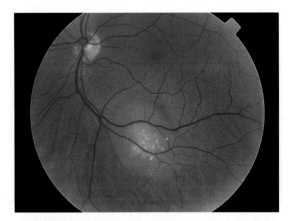

FIGURE 6.9. Choroidal nevus with surface drusen.

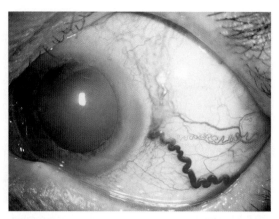

FIGURE 6.11. Episcleral dilated vessels over a ciliary body melanoma.

order to be certain of any growth. If growth is documented, the lesion should be managed as a small melanoma. When a nevus produces a secondary retinal detachment that causes visual impairment, laser photocoagulation to cause resolution of the subretinal fluid is often indicated.

Ciliary Body Melanoma

A ciliary body melanoma is a malignant neoplasm that arises from the melanocytes of the ciliary body. Like iris melanoma, it may contain spindle or epithelioid cells.

Clinical Features. Because of the hidden location behind the iris, ciliary body melanoma usually attains a relatively large size before it is detected clinically. However, external ocular signs such as dilated episcleral "sentinel" vessels (Fig. 6.11) or a focus of transscleral extension of the tumor (Fig. 6.12) can alert the clinician to a possible underlying neoplasm. Frequently, the tumor grows anteriorly through the iris root and appears in the anterior chamber angle (Fig. 6.13). More typically, however, it is confined to the ciliary body and can be detected only by slit lamp or fundus examination after wide dilation of the pupil (Fig. 6.14). Ciliary

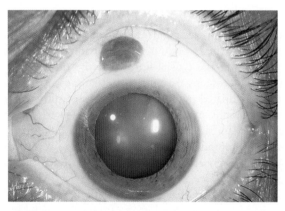

FIGURE 6.12. Extrascleral extension of a ciliary body melanoma.

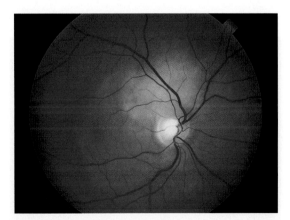

FIGURE 6.10. Amelanotic choroidal nevus superior to the optic disc.

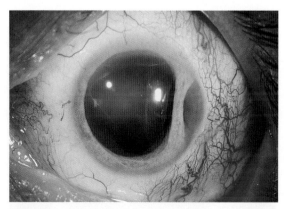

FIGURE 6.13. Ciliary body melanoma eroding through the iris into the anterior chamber.

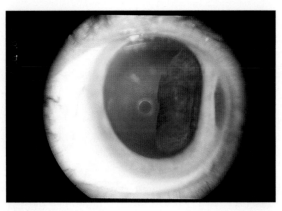

FIGURE 6.14. Large ciliary body melanoma seen through dilated pupil.

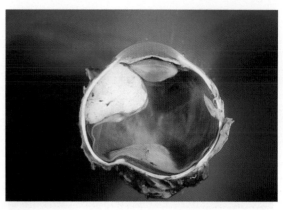

FIGURE 6.16. Gross pathology of a nonpigmented ciliary body melanoma.

body melanoma can be deeply pigmented (Fig. 6.15) or it can be amelanotic (Fig. 6.16).

The differential diagnosis of ciliary body melanoma includes iris pigment epithelial cyst and other less common ciliary body tumors such as melanocytoma, leiomyoma, and adenoma of the pigmented or nonpigmented ciliary epithelium. Ciliary body melanoma is best diagnosed by recognition of the typical features of the tumor with slit lamp biomicroscopy or indirect ophthalmoscopy through the widely dilated pupil. If the tumor is of sufficient size, ultrasonography may show the typical features of a uveal melanoma. In cases where the diagnosis is quite difficult, fine needle aspiration biopsy can be used. However, that is a difficult diagnostic technique that requires considerable experience.

Management. Ciliary body melanoma is most often managed by local removal of the tumor by partial lamellar iridocyclectomy or some variation thereof. The technique is described in the literature and is beyond the scope of this discussion. Tumors that are too large to resect locally may require treatment with a radioactive plaque or enucleation.

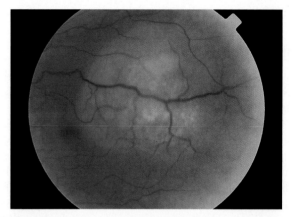

FIGURE 6.17. Small choroidal melanoma with surface orange pigment.

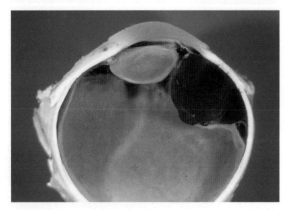

FIGURE 6.15. Gross pathology of a pigmented ciliary body melanoma.

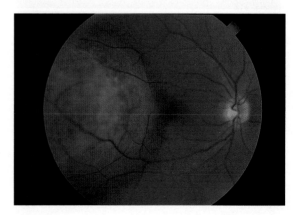

FIGURE 6.18. Dome-shaped pigmented choroidal melanoma in the macular area.

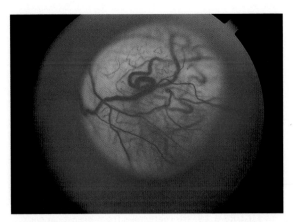

FIGURE 6.19. Mushroom-shaped nonpigmented choroidal melanoma. The prominent blood vessels in the tumor are highly typical of melanoma.

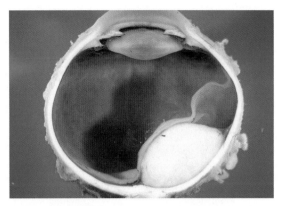

FIGURE 6.22. Gross pathology of a nonpigmented postequatorial choroidal melanoma.

Choroidal Melanoma

A choroidal melanoma is a malignant melanocytic tumor that arises from the melanocytes within the choroid. Like ciliary body melanoma, it contains spindle cells, epithelioid cells or a combination of the two (mixed-cell type).

Clinical Features. In its earliest stages, a malignant choroidal melanoma may be clinically indistinguishable from a large benign choroidal nevus. A small choroidal melanoma characteristically occurs as a black or gray choroidal mass with fairly well-defined borders. A typical early feature is the orange pigment on the surface of the tumor (Fig. 6.17). This correlates with clumps of macrophages at the level of the RPE that contain abundant lipofuscin pigment. A larger melanoma usually assumes a dome shape (Fig. 6.18). A melanoma that is clinically amelanotic is characterized by visible large blood vessels in the substance of the tumor. A choroidal melanoma can eventually break through Bruch's membrane, assuming a mushroom-shaped configuration (Figs. 6.19 and 6.20).

The growth patterns of choroidal melanoma can be best appreciated by examining gross sections of eyes enucleated for this disease. The tumors can be dome shaped and deeply pigmented (Fig. 6.21) or amelanotic (Fig. 6.22). The mushroom-shaped tumor typically produces a secondary nonrhegmatogenous retinal detachment (Figs. 6.23 and 6.24).

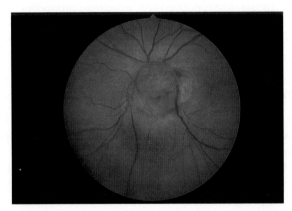

FIGURE 6.20. Juxtapapillary choroidal melanoma with a break through Bruch's membrane.

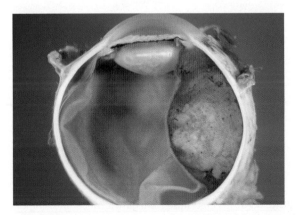

FIGURE 6.21. Gross pathology of a pigmented equatorial choroidal melanoma.

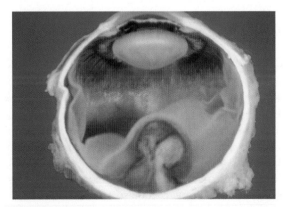

FIGURE 6.23. Gross pathology of a pigmented mushroom-shaped choroidal melanoma.

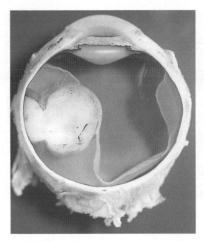

FIGURE 6.24. Gross pathology of a nonpigmented mushroom-shaped choroidal melanoma.

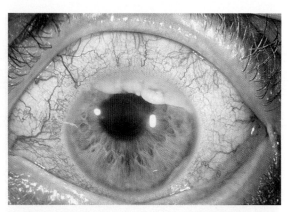

FIGURE 6.25. Iris metastasis from breast cancer.

The differential diagnosis of choroidal melanoma includes most elevated choroidal or subretinal lesions, such as choroidal nevus, choroidal metastasis, choroidal hemangioma, leiomyoma, neurilemoma, subretinal hemorrhage, the proliferative form of age-related macular degeneration, and tumors of the RPE. The most reliable way to make the diagnosis of choroidal melanoma is with the use of indirect ophthalmoscopy by an experienced observer. In cases that are atypical, ultrasonography, fluorescein angiography, indocyanine green angiography, the radioactive phosphorus uptake (^{32}P) test and fine needle aspiration biopsy may be helpful ancillary procedures.

Management. The management of choroidal melanoma is controversial. The details of this controversy are discussed in the literature and in the texts cited at the end of this chapter. Enucleation is generally recommended for large tumors with little hope of salvageable vision, and plaque radiotherapy is recommended for melanoma with a hope of salvageable vision. Smaller tumors that are not near the foveal area can be treated with heavy laser application. The treatment of uveal melanoma is variable and each case must be individualized.

UVEAL METASTASIS

Metastatic cancer to the uveal tract is the most common form of intraocular malignancy. However, many cases with small metastatic foci to the uveal tract have advanced systemic metastasis and few or no visual symptoms and, hence, do not come to medical attention. Therefore, in a clinical practice, uveal metastasis is not as common as primary uveal melanoma.

Most metastatic cancer to the intraocular structures resides in the uveal tract. Metastasis to the retina and optic disc are exceedingly uncommon. Metastatic tumors to the uvea most commonly reach the choroid, with metastasis to the iris and ciliary body being less common. All metastasis to the uvea comes through hematogenous routes, since there are no intraocular lymphatics. The primary malignancies that account for most uveal metastasis are breast cancer in women and lung cancer in men, although a number of other tumors can also spawn uveal metastasis. Since the clinical manifestations of anterior uveal metastasis often differ from those to the choroid, the two will be considered separately.

Anterior Uveal Metastasis

An anterior uveal metastasis is a malignant tumor that has spread from an extraocular primary site by hematogenous routes to the iris and/or ciliary body.

Clinical Features. Clinically, a metastasis to the anterior uvea can have several clinical variations. It can appear as a rather solitary fleshy mass or as a white, fluffy, loosely cohesive mass (Fig. 6.25). These friable tumors can seed tumor cells into the anterior chamber, producing a tumor-induced pseudohypopyon (Fig. 6.26). In other cases, an iris metastasis can bleed, causing a spontaneous hyphema (Fig. 6.27). Because of the friable nature of many anterior uveal metas-

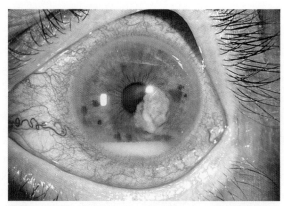

FIGURE 6.26. Iris metastasis from gastric cancer showing tumor-induced pseudohypopyon.

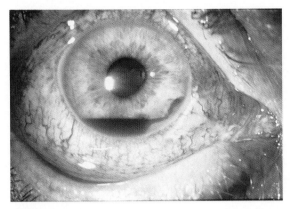

FIGURE 6.27. Iris metastasis from lung cancer showing spontaneous hyphema.

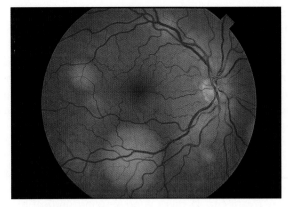

FIGURE 6.29. Multifocal choroidal metastasis.

tases, the neoplasm can simulate a granulomatous iridocyclitis or endophthalmitis.

The differential diagnosis of anterior uveal metastasis includes amelanotic uveal melanoma, granulomatous iridocyclitis, opportunistic infection, lymphoma, and other nonpigmented iris lesions.

The most important diagnostic step is recognizing the typical clinical features with slit lamp biomicroscopy. Since most patients with iridociliary metastasis have a history of systemic cancer, it is important to take a history to elicit previously treated neoplasm. In the occasional case where the iris metastasis is the first sign of a systemic malignancy, a fine needle aspiration biopsy can be performed to make the diagnosis and possibly to identify the primary site of the neoplasm.

Management. The management of an anterior uveal metastasis involves initiating a systemic evaluation to identify other sites of systemic metastasis. If chemotherapy is to be employed for the systemic disease, the anterior uveal metastasis can be cautiously observed for signs of regression. If systemic chemotherapy does not control the uveal metas-

tasis, ocular irradiation, giving approximately 3500 cGy over a 4- to 5-week period, is advisable.

Choroidal Metastasis

A choroidal metastasis is a malignant neoplasm that spreads to the choroid from a distant primary cancer.

Clinical Features. Clinically, a choroidal metastasis is usually different from a metastasis to the iris or ciliary body. It is confined by Bruch's membrane and does not exhibit the seeding that often characterizes anterior uveal metastasis. Hence, the choroidal metastasis is usually more circumscribed. It appears as a cream-yellow sessile or minimally elevated mass (Fig. 6.28). Unlike an amelanotic choroidal melanoma, it is often multifocal (Fig. 6.29) and bilateral. Choroidal metastasis located near the optic disc has a propensity to infiltrate the nerve and produce disc edema and superficial hemorrhage (Fig. 6.30).

The differential diagnosis of choroidal metastasis includes amelanotic choroidal melanoma, choroidal hemangioma, lymphoma, posterior scleritis, and granulomatous

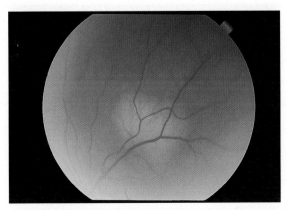

FIGURE 6.28. Solitary choroidal metastasis.

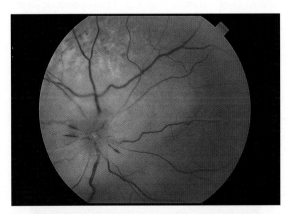

FIGURE 6.30. Peripapillary choroidal metastasis with optic nerve invasion.

inflammation. Choroidal metastasis is best diagnosed by ophthalmoscopic recognition of the typical fundus lesion. In cases where the lesion is atypical and the diagnosis is uncertain, fluorescein angiography and ultrasonography can provide diagnostic help. Transvitreal fine needle aspiration biopsy can be used to make a definitive diagnosis in cases where the diagnosis remains uncertain despite noninvasive diagnostic studies.

Management. The management of choroidal metastasis is similar to that described above for anterior uveal metastasis. If the patient is receiving chemotherapy for systemic disease, the choroidal metastasis can be followed without direct ocular treatment. If there is no systemic indication for chemotherapy, or if chemotherapy fails to control the choroidal metastasis, ocular radiotherapy should be employed. About half of the patients with choroidal metastasis require ocular irradiation and half can be successfully controlled with chemotherapy or hormone therapy.

CHOROIDAL HEMANGIOMA

Choroidal hemangioma is the most important vascular tumor of the uveal tract. It can occur as a circumscribed lesion that is unassociated with any extraocular manifestations or as a diffuse type that is usually associated with facial nevus flammeus or variations of the Sturge-Weber syndrome. Unlike uveal melanoma, uveal hemangioma occurs only in the choroid.

Circumscribed Choroidal Hemangioma

A circumscribed choroidal hemangioma is a localized benign vascular tumor that occurs in the posterior uveal tract.

Clinical Features. Circumscribed choroidal hemangioma usually appears as a sessile or minimally elevated, red-orange mass that has a similar color to the surrounding normal fundus. Smaller lesions (Fig. 6.31) are rather homogenous and do not usually produce a secondary retinal detachment. Larger lesions (Fig. 6.32) may produce overlying

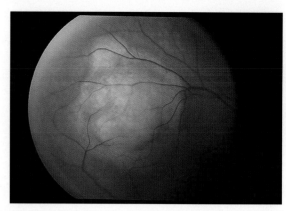

FIGURE 6.32. Circumscribed choroidal hemangioma with surface pigment changes.

proliferation or metaplasia of the RPE and secondary retinal detachment.

The differential diagnosis of choroidal hemangioma is the same as for choroidal melanoma and choroidal metastasis. The diagnosis of circumscribed choroidal hemangioma is best made by recognition of the typical red-orange color of the choroidal mass. Such a color is not usually seen with amelanotic choroidal melanoma, choroidal metastasis, or other choroidal masses.

Management. Since circumscribed choroidal hemangioma is a benign lesion that usually remains stationary or demonstrates only minimal enlargement, asymptomatic tumors generally require no treatment. If the tumor produces a secondary retinal detachment that causes visual impairment, laser photocoagulation to control the detachment is often warranted.

Diffuse Choroidal Hemangioma

The diffuse choroidal hemangioma occurs ipsilateral to a facial nevus flammeus, sometimes in association with the Sturge-Weber syndrome.

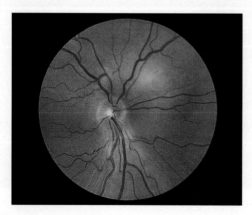

FIGURE 6.31. Circumscribed choroidal hemangioma adjacent to the optic disc.

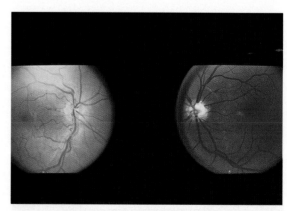

FIGURE 6.33. Diffuse choroidal hemangioma in the left eye showing the intense red color compared with the normal color of the right fundus (*left*).

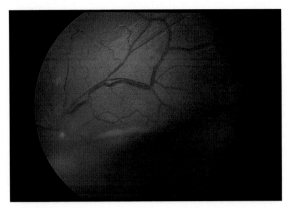

FIGURE 6.34. Diffuse choroidal hemangioma with secondary retinal detachment.

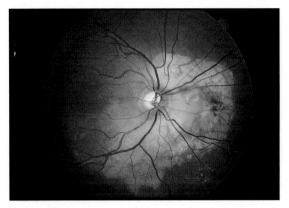

FIGURE 6.35. Juxtapapillary choroidal osteoma.

Clinical Features. Clinically, a diffuse choroidal hemangioma appears as a broad, red-orange thickening of the posterior choroid. The tumor appears redder than the background fundus, a finding sometimes called the "tomato catsup" fundus (Fig. 6.33). With time, the choroidal hemangioma produces cystic retinal degeneration and eventually an extensive secondary retinal detachment (Fig. 6.34).

The differential diagnosis of diffuse choroidal hemangioma includes other causes of choroidal thickening and secondary retinal detachment. Hence, it can be similar to a diffuse choroidal melanoma, choroidal metastasis, and possible posterior scleritis. The presence of an ipsilateral facial nevus flammeus in a patient with a nonrhegmatogenous retinal detachment should suggest the diagnosis. If there is any question regarding diagnosis, ultrasonography and fluorescein angiography can provide diagnostic assistance. Cranial computed tomography or magnetic resonance imaging to detect the meningeal calcification of the Sturge-Weber syndrome may also provide diagnostic help.

Management. The choroidal hemangioma of the Sturge-Weber syndrome can be difficult to manage. In its earliest stages, a refraction and treatment for hyperopic amblyopia is the best approach. Later, the secondary retinal detachment is best managed by laser photocoagulation or retinal detachment surgery, depending on the extent of the disease.

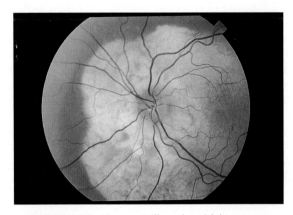

FIGURE 6.36. Circumpapillary choroidal osteoma.

CHOROIDAL OSTEOMA

Choroidal osteoma is a recently recognized osseous tumor of the choroid that has distinct clinical and histopathologic features. It is a benign choroidal tumor composed of mature bone that occupies a full-thickness area of the posterior choroid.

Clinical Features. Clinically, choroidal osteoma characteristically occurs as a well-delineated, sessile yellow-orange tumor in the posterior choroid, usually in a juxtapapillary (Fig. 6.35) or circumpapillary location (Fig. 6.36). Occasionally, a choroidal osteoma is located in the macular area and does not touch the optic disc (Fig. 6.37). The well-

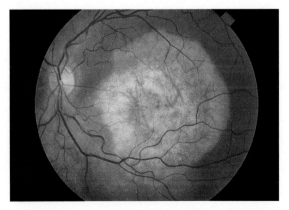

FIGURE 6.37. Choroidal osteoma in the macular area.

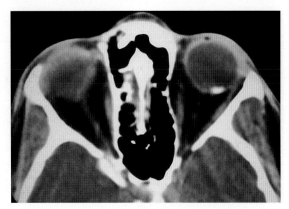

FIGURE 6.38. Computed tomogram showing choroidal osteoma.

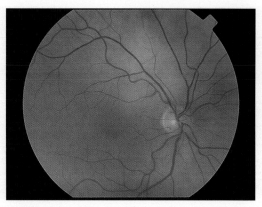

FIGURE 6.40. Choroidal lymphoma. Patient had systemic lymphoma and typical conjunctival infiltrate.

defined border is sometimes slightly irregular and occasionally has small pseudopodia-like projections. With time, a choroidal osteoma can cause subretinal neovascularization of choroidal origin and subretinal hemorrhage. The differential diagnosis of choroidal osteoma is the same as that already mentioned for amelanotic choroidal melanoma and choroidal metastasis. As with other lesions, the typical ophthalmoscopic features should be helpful in indicating the diagnosis of choroidal osteoma. Ultrasonography and computed tomography can be used to demonstrate a bony plaque at the level of the choroid, providing further support for the diagnosis (Fig. 6.38).

Management. There is no known treatment for a choroidal osteoma. When the tumor induces subretinal neovascularization or choroidal origin, laser treatment to the neovascular membrane may be warranted.

LYMPHOID TUMORS

Benign and malignant tumors of lymphoid origin can also affect the uveal tract. A uveal lymphoid lesion can occur with only ocular involvement, or it can be a part of a systemic lymphoma. It may be impossible clinically to distinguish a benign lymphoma (reactive lymphoid hyperplasia) from a malignant lymphoma on the basis of ocular examination. Lymphoma can occur as a retinovitreal infiltrate that can simulate intraocular inflammation, or it can occur as a uveal infiltration. Only the uveal variant will be considered here. A lymphoid tumor of the uvea is an infiltration of the uveal tract by benign or malignant tumor composed of a proliferation of abnormal lymphocytes.

Clinical Features. A lymphoid tumor of the iris appears as an amelanotic diffuse or circumscribed mass in the iris (Fig. 6.39). In the choroid, it appears as one or more yellow choroidal lesions that are indistinguishable from a choroidal metastasis (Fig. 6.40).

The differential diagnosis of uveal lymphoid tumor is the same as for uveal metastasis and amelanotic uveal melanoma. The diagnosis of a uveal lymphoma is best made by recognition of the uveal lesion with slit lamp biomicroscopy or indirect ophthalmoscopy. A general evaluation to detect a systemic lymphoma can be very helpful in establishing the diagnosis.

Management. The management of uveal lymphoma is the same as for uveal metastasis. Systemic chemotherapy should be employed for systemic disease, with the addition of ocular radiotherapy if tumor control is not achieved.

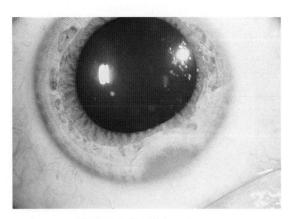

FIGURE 6.39. Iris lymphoma.

LEUKEMIA

Leukemia most often affects the ocular fundus by causing retinal hemorrhages secondary to the hematological alterations associated with the disease. However, direct infiltration of the uveal tract and the retina by leukemic cells occasionally occurs. Intraocular involvement by leukemia consists of infiltration of the uveal tract and retina by malignant leukocytes as part of the systemic disease.

Clinical Features. Leukemic infiltration of the iris usually appears as a diffuse friable mass in the inferior iris, often associated with a hyphema (Fig. 6.41). Early leukemic in-

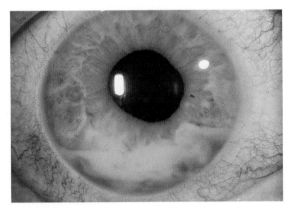

FIGURE 6.41. Iris involvement with leukemia.

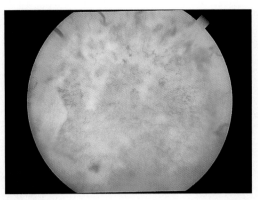

FIGURE 6.43. Massive retinal, choroidal, and optic nerve infiltration by leukemia.

volvement of the posterior segment appears as a gray thickening in the juxtapapillary area (Fig. 6.42). More advanced involvement appears as a massive yellow thickening of the optic nerve and adjacent retina and choroid (Fig. 6.43). The differential diagnosis of intraocular leukemia includes other diffuse amelanotic neoplasms such as lymphoma, metastatic carcinoma, and diffuse melanoma, as well as opportunistic infections, such as cytomegalovirus retinitis, that occur in immunosuppressed patients.

Most patients with intraocular involvement by leukemia have a long-term history of leukemia. The positive history and the clinical findings should suggest the diagnosis. In cases where differentiating between leukemic infiltration and opportunistic infection or other neoplasm is difficult, we have most commonly employed fine needle aspiration biopsy to help make the diagnosis.

Management. The management of leukemic infiltration of the intraocular structures is similar to the management of uveal metastasis. If chemotherapy that is employed for the systemic disease does not control the ocular disease, ocular irradiation should be initiated. In cases of infiltration of the optic nerve, irradiation should be promptly considered because of the poor visual prognosis.

TUMORS OF THE NONPIGMENTED CILIARY EPITHELIUM

Tumors that arise from the nonpigmented epithelium of the ciliary body can be divided into congenital and acquired types. The most important congenital tumor is the medulloepithelioma.

Medulloepithelioma

Intraocular medulloepithelioma most often occurs unilaterally in young children in the first decade of life. Intraocular medulloepithelioma is an embryonic neoplasm arising from the primitive medullary epithelium that is destined to form the nonpigmented ciliary epithelium in the adult. Cytologically, it can be benign or malignant, but it rarely exhibits distant metastasis. Both the benign and malignant variants can occur as a nonteratoid type or a teratoid type. The nonteratoid type consists of a proliferation of fairly well-differentiated cells of the nonpigmented ciliary epithelium. The teratoid type contains heterologous elements such as cartilage and skeletal muscle.

Clinical Features. In the early stages, medulloepithelioma appears as a gray-white tumor of the ciliary body (Fig. 6.44). As it slowly enlarges, it can cause a subluxation of the lens, secondary cataract, secondary glaucoma, retinal detachment, and a white pupillary reflex (leukokoria) (Fig. 6.45). A characteristic feature is the development of clear cysts that are visible near the surface of the lesion. These cysts frequently break away from the main lesion and float freely in the vitreous or aqueous cavity. The main lesion continues to slowly enlarge and can eventually fill the entire globe and, rarely, extend through the sclera into the orbit.

The differential diagnosis of intraocular medulloepithelioma includes retinoblastoma, persistent hyperplastic vitreous, ocular trauma, and other childhood conditions. The best method of diagnosis of medulloepithelioma is recognition of the clinical features described above, using slit lamp biomicroscopy and indirect ophthalmoscopy. If the diagno-

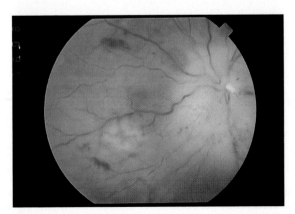

FIGURE 6.42. Juxtapapillary choroidal involvement with leukemia.

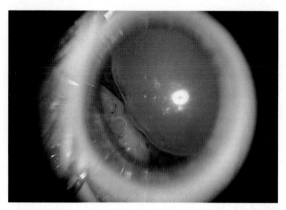

FIGURE 6.44. Circumscribed medulloepithelioma of the ciliary body.

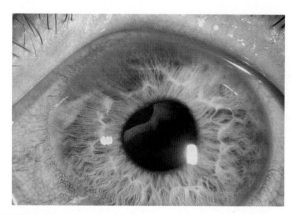

FIGURE 6.46. Adenoma of the nonpigmented ciliary epithelium with secondary cataract.

sis is uncertain, fine needle aspiration biopsy can be employed. In cases of larger tumors with opaque ocular media, B-scan ultrasonography can assist in recognition of the ciliary body mass.

Management. The management of intraocular medulloepithelioma is removal of the tumor by partial lamellar sclerouvectomy when the tumor involves less than 4 clock hours of the pars plicata. Although that procedure is often successful, there is a tendency for recurrence. Hence, many cases ultimately require enucleation. The systemic prognosis is generally quite favorable.

Acquired Adenoma and Adenocarcinoma

Acquired neoplasms can develop from the fully formed nonpigmented ciliary epithelium. Unlike the embryonic medulloepithelioma of childhood, these tumors do not contain teratoid elements. From a cytologic standpoint, they can be benign (adenoma) or malignant (adenocarcinoma). Even the malignant variant has little or no tendency to exhibit metastatic disease. An acquired adenoma or adenocarcinoma of the nonpigmented ciliary epithelium is a neoplasm

that develops from fully mature adult nonpigmented ciliary epithelium.

Clinical Features. Like the embryonic variant, the acquired tumor of the nonpigmented ciliary epithelium begins as an amelanotic mass of the pars plicata. It can have a smooth or irregular surface, and it occasionally contains clear cysts. It can produce a secondary cataract (Fig. 6.46). The differential diagnosis includes amelanotic melanoma of the ciliary body, metastatic carcinoma, leiomyoma, granuloma, and possibly other lesions. The experienced ocular oncologist can often make the diagnosis of this uncommon entity by slit lamp examination and indirect ophthalmoscopy. Fluorescein angiography and ultrasonography do not provide much diagnostic help in differentiating this lesion from the aforementioned conditions. Fine needle aspiration biopsy can be employed in difficult cases.

Management. The management of acquired tumor of the nonpigmented ciliary epithelium is removal of the mass by partial lamellar sclerouvectomy. Although this surgery is quite difficult, in many cases the tumor can be successfully removed (Fig. 6.47). Enucleation is necessary for larger or recurrent tumors.

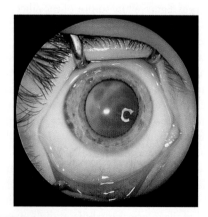

FIGURE 6.45. Larger medulloepithelioma causing a tumor cyclitic membrane and leukokoria.

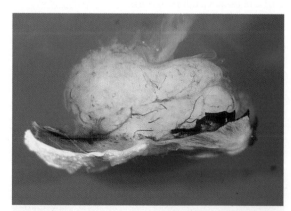

FIGURE 6.47. Appearance of the specimen shown in Figure 6.46 after removal by partial lamellar iridocyclectomy. The patient had a postoperative vision of 20/25 in the affected eye.

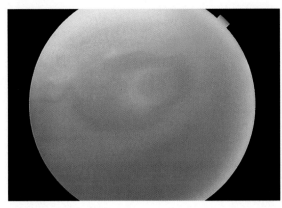

FIGURE 6.48. Adenoma of the retinal pigment epithelium. The photograph is hazy due to overlying vitreous cells, a common finding with this tumor.

ACQUIRED TUMORS OF THE CILIARY AND RETINAL PIGMENT EPITHELIUM

True tumors can develop in the PE of the ciliary body and retina. Both benign adenoma and malignant adenocarcinoma are locally aggressive tumors that lack potential to metastasize, but they can cause complications leading to visual loss. Since adenoma and adenocarcinoma are similar clinically and in their biologic behavior, they are discussed together.

Clinical Features. A neoplasm of the PE is usually, but not always, dark brown or black in color. When it develops in the ciliary body region, it can grow slowly and produce subluxation of the lens and invasion of the anterior chamber. When it arises in the retina, it appears as a relatively stable, abruptly elevated mass. It is known to occasionally develop in an eye that has experienced trauma or inflammation. It can also arise from an area of congenital hypertrophy of the RPE and from a small focus of hyperplasia of the PE. It is now recognized that a neoplasm of the PE can develop a feeding retinal artery and a draining retinal vein and can induce retinal exudation, exudative retinal detachment, and orbital extension.

The most important condition in the differential diagnosis is uveal melanoma. The typical features described may assist in suspecting the diagnosis. Fluorescein angiography and ultrasonography can also help in determining the diagnosis.

Management. If the diagnosis of acquired tumor of the PE is suspected and the lesion is asymptomatic, a period of observation is justified. Larger, more aggressive tumors can be managed by local resection if they are located in the ciliary body region. More posterior lesions may require irradiation of even enucleation.

BIBLIOGRAPHY

Shields JA, Shields CL. Intraocular tumors. A text and atlas. Philadelphia: WB Saunders; 1992.

Shields JA, Shields CL. Atlas of intraocular tumors. Philadelphia: Lippincott Williams & Wilkins; 1999.

(The above references are comprehensive and cite hundreds of additional references on the subject of intraocular tumors.)

Retinal Tumors

James J. Augsburger

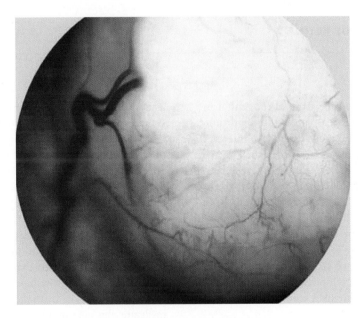

Macular retinoblastoma.

RETINOBLASTOMA

MEDULLOEPITHELIOMA

ASTROCYTOMA OF RETINA (ASTROCYTIC HAMARTOMA)

CAPILLARY HEMANGIOMA OF RETINA (VON HIPPEL TUMOR)

CAVERNOUS HEMANGIOMA OF RETINA

METASTATIC CARCINOMA TO RETINA

LEUKEMIC INFILTRATION OF RETINA

LYMPHOMATOUS INFILTRATION OF RETINA

HYPERTROPHY OF RETINAL PIGMENT EPITHELIUM

COMBINED HAMARTOMA OF RETINA

MASSIVE GLIOSIS OF RETINA

HYPERPLASIA OF RETINAL PIGMENT EPITHELIUM

ACQUIRED NONFAMILIAL RETINAL HEMANGIOMATOUS LESION

Retinal tumors comprise a broad spectrum of congenital and acquired, benign and malignant, isolated and syndromic, neoplastic and nonneoplastic intraocular lesions of interest to ophthalmologists. The clinical spectrum of retinal tumors includes retinoblastoma, lesions and conditions simulating retinoblastoma, and miscellaneous other tumors that arise from or involve the neurosensory retina, retinal pigment epithelium (RPE), and pigmented or nonpigmented ciliary epithelium. Several extremely rare tumors that are unlikely to be encountered by even the busiest practitioner (e.g., glioneuroma, adenocarcinoma of the RPE) are not covered. The reader is referred to an encyclopedic text on ophthalmic pathology for information about such lesions.

RETINOBLASTOMA

Retinoblastoma is a primary malignant intraocular neoplasm that arises from immature retinoblasts within the developing retina. It is the most common primary intraocular malignancy of childhood, occurring in about one in 15,000 individuals. Almost all cases occur in children under the age of 6 years. The neoplasm has strong tendencies to invade the brain via the optic nerve and to metastasize widely. Untreated children typically die of their disease within 2 to 4 years of onset of symptoms.

Clinical Features

Laterality and focality. Approximately 60% to 70% of retinoblastoma cases are unilateral, while the remaining 30% to 40% are bilateral. In unilateral cases, only a single tumor is usually present in the affected eye. In bilateral cases, multifocal tumors in both eyes are the rule.

Presenting signs and symptoms. The most common presenting symptom of retinoblastoma is leukokoria, a white pupil, in the tumor-containing eye or eyes (Fig. 7.1). Other common initial manifestations include strabismus (esotropia or exotropia; Fig. 7.2) and symptomatic or asymptomatic visual impairment. Less common presenting symptoms include an abnormal appearance of the eye (Fig. 7.2), such as a red eye, a cloudy cornea, or a change in color of iris, and pain in or around the eye.

Appearance of tumors. Very small retinoblastoma tumors typically appear as translucent, whitish-pink intraretinal patches (Fig. 7.3), while slightly larger intraretinal tumors appear as well-defined, white, nodular lesions with prominent feeder and drainer retinal blood vessels (Fig. 7.4). Larger tumors commonly produce a nonrhegmatogenous retinal detachment that frequently becomes total and bullous (exophytic growth pattern) (Fig. 7.5). In other cases, tumor cells flake off from the vitreal surface of the mass and infiltrate the gelatinous vitreous (endophytic growth pattern) (Figs. 7.5, 7.6). Many tumors exhibit elements of both endophytic and exophytic growth.

Some eyes with retinoblastoma develop implantation tumors on the iris and accumulation of tumor cells in the aqueous (Fig. 7.7). Most of these eyes have a form of

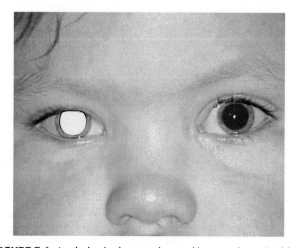

FIGURE 7.1. Leukokoria due to advanced intraocular retinoblastoma of right eye.

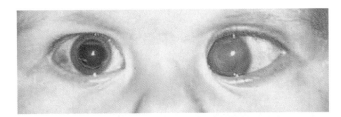

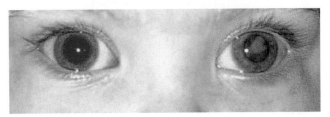

FIGURE 7.2. Strabismus as presenting manifestation of retinoblastoma. Left esotropia plus enlarged corneal diameter, corneal clouding, and loss of red reflex in left eye *(top)*. Left exotropia, plus slightly enlarged corneal diameter and loss of red reflex in left eye *(bottom)*.

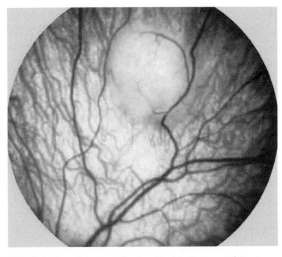

FIGURE 7.3. Small intraretinal retinoblastoma. White tumor is fed and drained by slightly dilated, mildly tortuous retinal blood vessels.

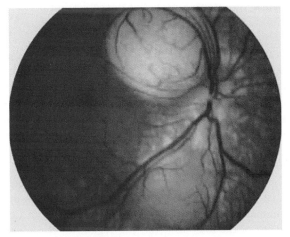

FIGURE 7.4. Slightly larger intraretinal retinoblastoma with prominent feeding and draining retinal blood vessels.

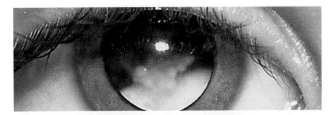

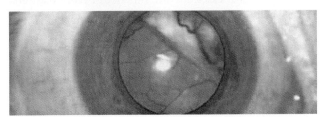

FIGURE 7.5. Endophytic and exophytic forms of retinoblastoma. Advanced endophytic retinoblastoma appears as avascular white mass inferiorly associated with prominent intravitreal tumor seeds *(top)*. Advanced exophytic retinoblastoma appears as ill-defined yellow-white vascularized fundus mass superiorly associated with total bullous retinal detachment *(bottom)*.

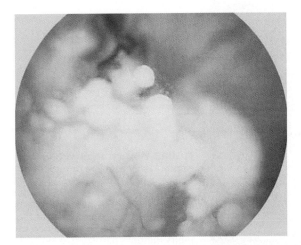

FIGURE 7.6. Prominent vitreous seeds of retinoblastoma overlying large intraretinal vascularized white retinal tumor.

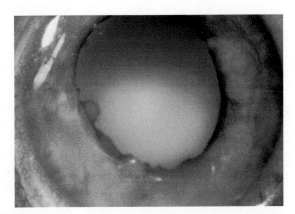

FIGURE 7.7. Eye with retinoblastoma showing implantation tumors on iris.

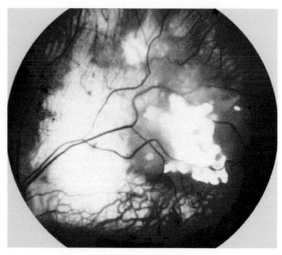

FIGURE 7.8. Retinoma. This spontaneously arrested retinoblastoma appears as a calcific tumor residue centrally surrounded by chorioretinal atrophy.

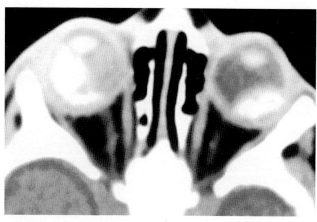

FIGURE 7.10. Computed tomography scan of bilateral retinoblastoma (without contrast enhancement). Intraocular tumors appear bright because of intralesional calcification.

retinoblastoma known as diffuse infiltrating retinoblastoma. Occasional retinoblastoma tumors stop growing spontaneously and either lose their malignant character or never acquire it. Such a tumor is called a retinoma. Tumors of this type (Fig. 7.8) tend to appear virtually identical to active retinoblastomas that have been treated successfully by irradiation. In other cases, massive intraocular retinoblastomas occasionally undergo spontaneous necrosis leading to phthisis bulbi.

Ancillary diagnostic studies. The three diagnostic studies most commonly used today in children with suspected retinoblastoma are ultrasonography, computed tomography (CT), and magnetic resonance imaging (MRI). B-scan ultrasonography generally reveals one or more soft tissue intraocular masses. In about 95% of cases, multifocal particu-

late intralesional calcification (characteristic of retinoblastoma) can be demonstrated (Fig. 7.9). CT demonstrates intraocular tumors and intralesional calcification better than ultrasonography (Fig. 7.10); however, not all retinoblastoma tumors become calcified. CT is also useful for evaluating the orbital optic nerve and for identifying extraocular tumor extension. MRI is the most useful and informative test currently available for evaluating sellar and parasellar regions of brain (to rule out ectopic intracranial retinoblastoma). At the same time, MRI appears to be less valuable than CT for assessing intraocular tumors because it does not show the intralesional calcification characteristic of this malignancy.

Genetics of retinoblastoma. Retinoblastoma appears to be due to loss or inactivation of both normal alleles of the "retinoblastoma gene," a DNA sequence localized to a small segment of the long arm (the 14q region) of chromosome

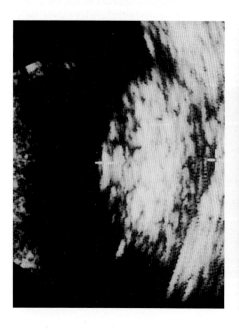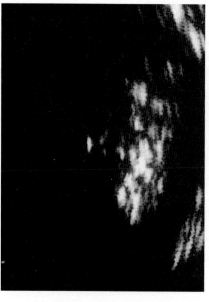

FIGURE 7.9. B-scan ultrasonography of retinoblastoma. Image of tumor obtained at typical gain setting (76 dB) for diagnostic examination of eye *(left)*. Tumor appears generally but nonuniformly bright (hyperreflective). Same tumor at reduced gain setting (60 dB) is ill defined but exhibits multiple persistent strong particulate intralesional echoes (foci of calcification) *(right)*.

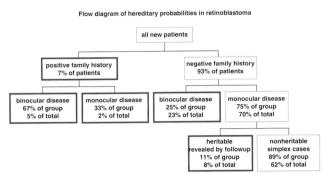

Flow diagram of hereditary probabilities in retinoblastoma

all new patients

positive family history
7% of patients

negative family history
93% of patients

binocular disease
67% of group
5% of total

monocular disease
33% of group
2% of total

binocular disease
25% of group
23% of total

monocular disease
75% of group
70% of total

heritable
revealed by followup
11% of group
8% of total

nonheritable
simplex cases
89% of group
62% of total

FIGURE 7.11. Flow diagram showing the hereditary probabilities in new cases of retinoblastoma. The boxes with red borders identify the heritable cases.

13. The timing of the loss or inactivation of the two normal alleles determines whether the disease is genetic (i.e., can be inherited by the offspring of an affected person) or somatic (i.e., cannot be inherited by the offspring of an affected person). In genetic retinoblastoma, at least one normal allele must be lost or inactivated prior to the first mitotic division of embryogenesis. This circumstance will arise if either the sperm or the egg contains defective DNA from an affected or carrier parent, or develops that defect by means of spontaneous mutation prior to fertilization. In somatic retinoblastoma, both alleles are present and active beyond the stage of the fertilized egg, but subsequent spontaneous mutation occurs to delete or inactivate both alleles in at least one immature retinal cell (retinoblast).

The majority of cases of retinoblastoma (about 62%) are sporadic (i.e., diagnosed in patients who have no family history of retinoblastoma and no affected family members on comprehensive familial ophthalmic examination). The hereditary probabilities in a newly diagnosed child with retinoblastoma are shown in Figure 7.11.

Natural history of retinoblastoma. Left untreated, retinoblastoma is usually relentlessly progressive, leading to death of the affected child from intracranial invasion along the optic nerve, widespread metastasis, or both within about 2 to 3 years of initial symptoms. In occasional cases, however, retinoblastoma undergoes either spontaneous regression, resulting in phthisis bulbi of the involved eye, or shows benign growth arrest, retinoma, which is self-limited and stable in most affected individuals.

Pathology. Retinoblastoma is characterized histopathologically by malignant neuroepithelial cells (retinoblasts) arising within the immature retina. The retinoblasts typically appear to have a large basophilic nucleus and scanty cytoplasm. Cellular necrosis and intralesional calcification (Fig. 7.12) are frequent associations, especially in larger tumors. In some cases, tissue differentiation occurs, often producing Flexner-Wintersteiner rosettes (Fig. 7.13, *left*) and occasionally resulting in Homer-Wright rosettes (Fig. 7.13, *center*). In occasional cases, photoreceptor differentiation of individual retinoblasts (fleurettes) can also be observed (Fig. 7.13, *right*). Retinoblastoma has a strong tendency to invade the optic nerve and choroid and to extend out of the globe via either the optic nerve or the scleral emissarial canals.

Syndromic associations. Some patients with retinoblastoma develop a primary nonretinoblastoma intracranial malignancy, which is usually categorized histopathologically as either a pineoblastoma or an ectopic intracranial retinoblastoma. Presenting features of this tumor include somnolence, headache, or other neurologic symptoms. Central nervous system (CNS) imaging studies show a solid tumor involving the suprasellar or parasellar regions of the brain. Ophthalmoscopy frequently reveals papilledema. Because

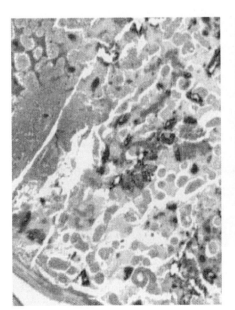
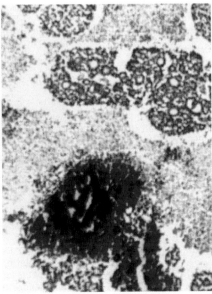

FIGURE 7.12. Histopathology of retinoblastoma. Low-power photomicrograph (*left*) and higher-power photomicrograph (*right*) showing cellular necrosis (pale, nonstaining areas) and intralesional calcification (intense reddish-purple foci) surrounding areas of viable retinoblastoma.

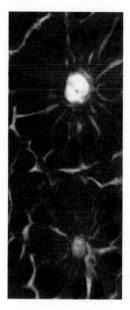
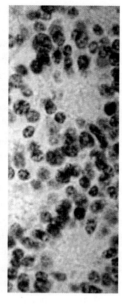
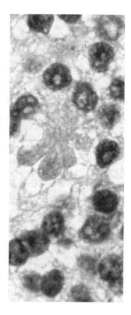

FIGURE 7.13. Tissue and cellular differentiation in retinoblastoma. **Left:** Flexner-Wintersteiner rosettes. **Center:** Homer-Wright rosettes. **Right:** Fleurette.

this type of tumor usually occurs in children with genetic retinoblastoma who have bilateral disease, this association is commonly referred to as trilateral retinoblastoma. The intracranial malignancy has a strong tendency to seed the cerebrospinal fluid (CSF) and thereby spawn implantation tumors all along the spinal cord. This malignancy is usually fatal.

Some children who develop retinoblastoma have a syndrome of multiple congenital anomalies attributed to a major deletion in the long arm of chromosome 13 (13q deletion syndrome). In children with this syndrome, the deletion is usually demonstrable by karyotype analysis. All infants with 13q deletion syndrome should be screened ophthalmoscopically for retinoblastoma.

Differential diagnosis. The principal differential diagnosis of retinoblastoma includes advanced Coats' disease (which tends to simulate advanced exophytic retinoblastoma), persistent hyperplastic primary vitreous, nematode endophthalmitis (which can simulate advanced endophytic retinoblastoma), retinopathy of prematurity with retrolental fibroplasia, retinal astrocytoma, intraocular medulloepithelioma, retinal capillary hemangioma (von Hippel tumor), and massive gliosis of the retina.

Management. Chemotherapy is the most commonly employed therapeutic option for children with advanced bilateral retinoblastoma in most parts of the world today. This type of therapy is also used in some children with advanced unilateral disease and in virtually all children with metastatic retinoblastoma. A cyclic, intravenous three-drug regimen consisting of carboplatin, etoposide, and vincristine (or some variation thereof) is currently the preferred combination in most centers. This treatment requires implantation of an indwelling venous port for repeated injection of the chemotherapeutic drugs. In some centers, the chemother-

apy is supplemented by cyclosporine A, a drug that is known to reduce resistance of tumor cells to chemotherapeutic agents. The child generally undergoes a chemotherapy cycle every 3 to 4 weeks, depending on his or her tolerance, for six to nine cycles. Because of the potential for drug-related immunosuppression and bone marrow toxicity, children undergoing such treatment require close systemic monitoring by their pediatricians and pediatric oncologists during the course of treatment.

In some children, chemotherapy alone induces complete clinical regression of all treated tumors (Fig. 7.14). More frequently, the chemotherapy shrinks the intraocular tumors, so that the residual lesions can be eradicated by local treatments such as laser therapy (Fig. 7.15), cryotherapy,

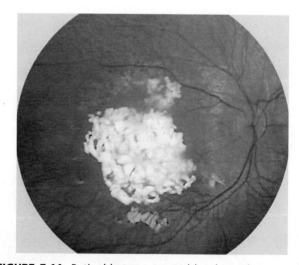

FIGURE 7.14. Retinoblastoma treated by chemotherapy only with carboplatin, etoposide, and vincristine. Regressed macular tumor appears as well-defined clump of calcific tissue surrounded by foci of chorioretinal atrophy.

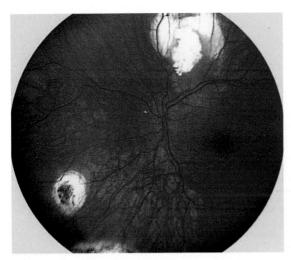

FIGURE 7.15. Retinoblastoma treated by chemotherapy plus laser therapy and cryotherapy. Superior tumor residue is completely calcific and partly surrounded by chorioretinal atrophy following laser therapy. The inferonasal lesion (also treated by laser) is completely atrophic, as is the inferior peripheral lesion (treated by cryotherapy).

and plaque radiotherapy (Fig. 7.16). This approach is referred to as chemoreduction followed by sequential aggressive local therapy. New tumors frequently arise in the peripheral fundus while the child is on chemotherapy, and residual lesions that regressed initially following the start of chemotherapy often relapse within 1 to 2 months after stopping chemotherapy. Vitreous seeds commonly regress markedly following chemotherapy but virtually always recur following discontinuation of the drug therapy. Because of these likely occurrences, children undergoing chemotherapy must be monitored closely during treatment and for an extended period of time following the completion of chemotherapy.

External beam radiation therapy (typically 4500 cGy delivered through precision lateral or oblique portals in a fractionated dose schedule over 4 to 5 weeks) was the primary treatment of choice for most children with advanced bilateral retinoblastoma until the advent of the chemotherapeutic regimen mentioned above. Although this method of treatment is frequently able to eradicate relatively large intraretinal tumors and multifocal intraretinal lesions (Fig. 7.17), it is often ineffective against vitreous seeding. It usually causes substantial orbital-facial bone growth arrest, induces development of posterior subcapsular radiation-induced cataracts, and causes other side effects. More importantly, long-term follow-up of retinoblastoma survivors who received external beam radiation therapy in childhood (especially prior to 6 months of age) has revealed a substantial increase in the expected frequency of malignant nonretinoblastoma neoplasms in the orbital-facial region (i.e., in the field of radiation). Most of this increased risk appears to be in children irradiated prior to 1 year of age. Because of this, most clinicians who deal with retinoblastoma regularly now try to avoid external beam radiation therapy. If such treatment must be used (e.g., in children who have failed chemotherapy with sequential aggressive local therapy), clinicians currently try to delay the radiotherapy until after the child is 1 year old.

Photocoagulation, the coagulation of tissues by means of intense light energy, is an effective local treatment for small- to medium-sized intraretinal retinoblastoma tumors. Therapeutic photocoagulation of retinal tissue can be produced with either a white light photocoagulator (e.g., xenon arc photocoagulator) or an ophthalmic laser (e.g., argon green laser). In retinal photocoagulation of retinoblastoma, the ophthalmologist creates an intense barrier of overlapping photocoagulator spots or a zone of confluent laser burns around the tumor in an attempt to obliterate its vas-

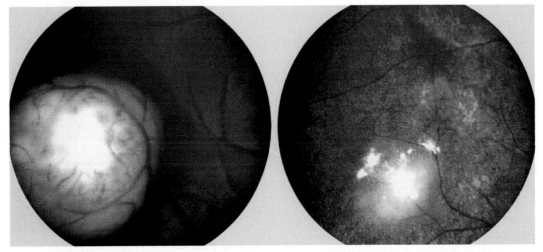

FIGURE 7.16. Retinoblastoma treated by plaque radiotherapy. **Left:** Tumor prior to treatment. **Right:** Regressed lesion 3 months following I-125 plaque radiotherapy. Lesion is markedly shrunken and exhibits foci of calcification.

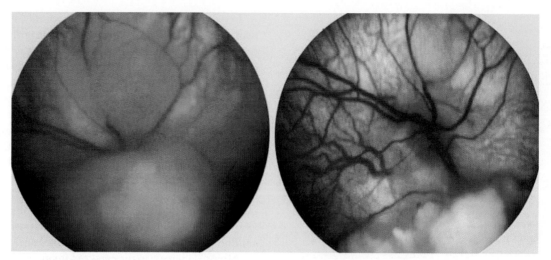

FIGURE 7.17. Retinoblastoma treated by external beam radiation therapy. **Left:** Multiple tumors prior to treatment. **Right:** Same tumors 6 months following irradiation (45 Gy over 5 weeks). Superior tumor has almost completely disappeared, and inferior tumor has regressed to a shrunken, calcific nodule.

cular supply. Multiple treatment sessions 1 to 3 weeks apart are frequently needed to ensure tumor destruction.

Noncoagulative laser therapy using a long wavelength (infrared) ophthalmic laser, relatively low power settings, long exposure times (typically 30 to 90 seconds per exposure), and a large spot size (typically 1 to 3 μm in diameter) has recently become popular as an alternative to conventional photocoagulation. This method of treatment has been widely promoted under the term *transpupillary thermotherapy* (TTT). In this treatment, the ophthalmologist attempts to heat the entire tumor for a prolonged duration without causing frank tissue coagulation. In the operating room, this therapy requires a commercially available adapter to an operating microscope or a specially adapted indirect ophthalmoscope. The end point of treatment is a uniform graying of the treated tissue after a total treatment duration of approximately 15 minutes. Just as with photocoagulation, this type of treatment must be repeated every 1 to 3 weeks until the tumor is totally eradicated (or until the treatment is judged to have failed).

Cryotherapy, the disruption of tissues by repeated freezing and thawing, is applicable to most eyes with one or multiple small tumors, provided that the tumors are peripherally located (i.e., not involving or near the central macula or optic disc) and there is no vitreous seeding. Tumors at and anterior to the ocular equator can usually be treated directly through the overlying conjunctiva, but those posterior to the equator generally require incision of the conjunctiva and dissection of subconjunctival connective tissues down to bare sclera for satisfactory placement of the cryoprobe tip. Cryotherapy can be used as a single treatment in some eyes with one or a few small- to medium-sized peripheral tumors, in conjunction with photocoagulation or noncoagulative laser therapy in eyes with multiple small- to medium-sized

anterior and posterior tumors, in conjunction with chemoreduction (as a locally destructive treatment in sequential aggressive local therapy), and as a subsequent treatment in some eyes with local tumor recurrences after plaque radiotherapy or external beam radiation therapy.

Plaque radiotherapy refers to delivery of ionizing radiation to a tumor by means of a temporary interstitial implant (the plaque) containing a radionuclide of specific known activity. The most commonly used radionuclides in eye plaques at this time are I-125 (a low-energy gamma emitter) and Ru-106 (a beta emitter). A plaque of appropriate diam-

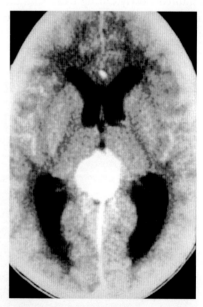

FIGURE 7.18. Ectopic intracranial retinoblastoma in child with bilateral retinoblastoma (trilateral retinoblastoma). Computed tomography scan of brain reveals prominent suprasellar mass that exhibits contrast enhancement.

eter (usually 2 to 4 mm larger than the estimated diameter of the tumor) is sutured to the sclera directly overlying the intraocular tumor. The plaque is left in place long enough to deliver a radiation dose of approximately 45 Gy to the tumor's apex (usually 2 to 4 days). The plaque is then removed at a second surgical procedure. This method of treatment frequently induces profound local regression of the treated tumor (Fig. 7.18).

Plaque radiotherapy is generally applicable to larger tumors than can be eradicated with cryotherapy, photocoagulation, or noncoagulative laser therapy. Larger tumors typically regress to well-defined calcific residues (type I regression), but medium-sized and smaller tumors frequently shrink down to residual soft tissue masses with a gray fleshy appearance (type II regression). Plaque radiotherapy can be used as a single treatment or as an element in sequential aggressive local therapy. Plaque therapy has the potential to cause delayed radiation retinopathy, radiation-induced optic papillopathy, and radiation-induced cataract but (because of the plaque's shielding) does not appear to increase the risk of second malignant neoplasms in the facial-orbital region the way that external beam radiation therapy does.

Observation without treatment is appropriate for children with a retinoma. However, because such tumors have occasionally been noted to become active later in life, all such children must be monitored on a regular basis throughout life.

Prognosis. Most children with retinoblastoma do not die of this malignancy, at least in developed countries in which affected children present at a relatively early stage of disease. Unfavorable prognostic factors for survival include metastatic disease, orbital extension, optic nerve invasion, and massive choroidal invasion. As long as the tumor is confined within the globe and does not massively involve the choroid, the size of the intraocular tumor and the degree of cellular or tissue differentiation are not important prognostic factors for survival.

Prognosis for survivors. Children with genetic retinoblastoma have a substantially heightened risk of developing an intracranial nonretinoblastoma malignancy within the first decade of life (see above) and of developing bony and soft tissue sarcomas in later years of life. These second malignancies are frequently fatal. All patients who survive their retinoblastoma must be monitored throughout their life for possible development of one or more nonretinoblastoma malignancies.

MEDULLOEPITHELIOMA

Intraocular medulloepithelioma is a rare primary intraocular tumor arising from the primitive ocular neuroectoderm. It is an uncommon tumor, but its precise frequency is unknown. It occurs in both benign and malignant varieties. It tends to be locally aggressive but rarely metastasizes. This tumor is usually congenital or infantile, but juvenile and even adult-onset cases have been reported. The average age of the affected individual at diagnosis is about 5 years. Medulloepithelioma affects all races and both sexes equally.

Clinical Features

Laterality and focality. Medulloepithelioma is almost always a unilateral, unifocal tumor. It usually arises in the ciliary body, but occasional lesions of this type have been found in the iris, retina, and optic nerve.

Presenting signs and symptoms. The usual presenting symptoms of medulloepithelioma are a red eye, a change in color of the iris (Fig. 7.19), a visible mass in the iris, and visual problems.

Appearance of tumors. The typical presenting findings are of a white, tan, or pink mass involving the ciliary body (Figs. 7.20, 7.21) and occasionally the root of iris (Figs.

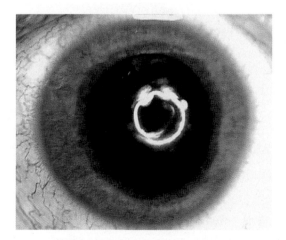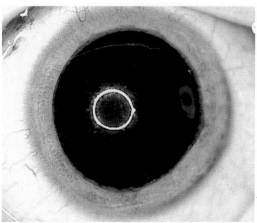

FIGURE 7.19. Heterochromia iridis as presenting manifestation of medulloepithelioma of ciliary body. Right iris *(left image)* appears substantially darker than the left iris *(right image)* due to florid iris neovascularization. The child's parents reported that this change of iris color developed abruptly less than 1 week prior to presentation.

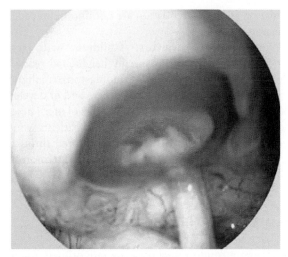

FIGURE 7.20. Medulloepithelioma of ciliary body. Anterior segment photograph taken during scleral depression in the pars plana region reveals pale ciliary body tumor with streaks of blood on its surface.

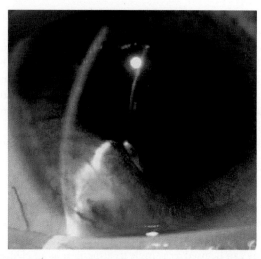

FIGURE 7.22. Medulloepithelioma of ciliary body with iris involvement presenting as fleshy, vascular peripheral iris tumor (slit lamp view).

7.22, 7.23), often in association with prominent surface cysts (Fig. 7.23). Neovascularization of iris is common in affected eyes. If the tumor was present congenitally, there may be an associated defect in the lens (coloboma; Figs. 7.23, 7.24) due to a deficiency of the zonule in the region of the ciliary body tumor.

Ancillary diagnostic studies. B-scan ultrasonography is frequently able to image a relatively large ciliary body tumor; however, conventional contact B-scan imaging is usually insufficient to demonstrate a small ciliary body mass. For such a lesion, either a water bath ultrasound or biomicroscopic ultrasonography is required for satisfactory imaging. CT scanning (Fig. 7.25) and MRI are generally capable of imaging ciliary body masses that cannot be demonstrated by conventional contact B-scan ultrasonography. They should be considered if medulloepithelioma of the ciliary

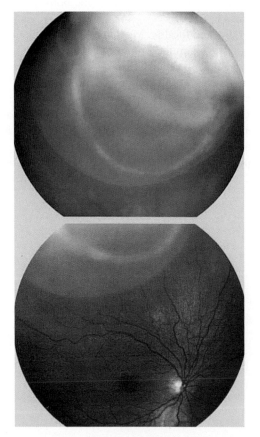

FIGURE 7.21. Cystic medulloepithelioma of ciliary body. **Top:** Solid portion of tumor appears opaque white while cystic portion appears gray with well-defined vitreal edge. **Bottom:** Cystic portion of mass is visible above normal optic disc and macula.

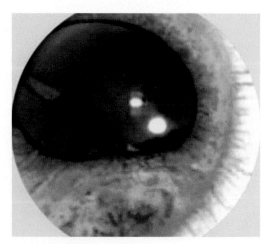

FIGURE 7.23. Fleshy vascularized iris mass and lens coloboma as presenting manifestations of congenital medulloepithelioma of ciliary body with iris involvement.

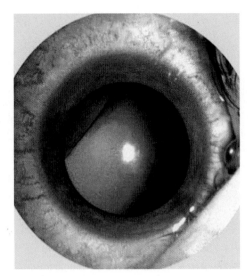

FIGURE 7.24. Sectorial notch in lens (lens coloboma) as sole presenting manifestation of ciliary body medulloepithelioma.

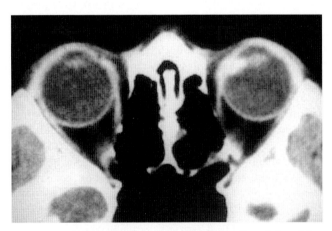

FIGURE 7.25. Computed tomography scan of medulloepithelioma of ciliary body nasally in left eye.

body is suspected and water bath ultrasonography and biomicroscopic ultrasonography are not available.

Natural history. The natural history of untreated medulloepitheliomas is essentially unknown. A few lesions of this type that have been observed for prolonged periods of time have remained relatively stable, but others have enlarged progressively over time. Because extraocular extension can occur in some advanced cases, surgical excision of the tumor or enucleation is usually performed shortly after the tumor is recognized.

Pathology. The characteristic histopathological feature of intraocular medulloepitheliomas is a structural arrangement of cells that closely resembles the neural medullary epithelium. The degree of cellular differentiation differs widely from case to case. Many well-differentiated medulloepitheliomas containing prominent rosettes and cystic spaces (Fig. 7.26, *left*) containing hyaluronic acid are common. Medulloepitheliomas that contain heterotopic elements such as hyaline cartilage (Fig. 7.26, *right*), striated muscle, or brain are referred to as teratoid medulloepitheliomas. Those that do not contain such elements are referred to as nonteratoid medulloepitheliomas. About two thirds of intraocular medulloepitheliomas are categorized as malignant pathologically, largely on the basis of invasiveness and extraocular extension of the tumor, especially if associated with a prominent degree of undifferentiation and numerous mitotic figures.

Differential diagnosis. The principal differential diagnosis of intraocular medulloepithelioma includes retinoblastoma, nematode granuloma, and juvenile xanthogranuloma.

Management. Enucleation is generally recommended if the eye is blind and painful, if the eye has advanced neovascular glaucoma due to tumor, if the tumor is very large, and if there is clinical evidence of extrascleral extension of tumor. **Microsurgical tumor excision** is sometimes performed if the intraocular tumor is relatively small, especially if the tumor involves only the peripheral iris and anterior ciliary body only and there is no evidence of neovascular glaucoma or extrascleral extension.

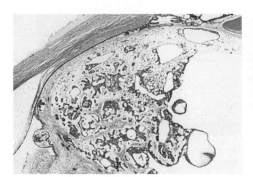

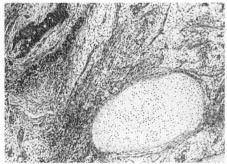

FIGURE 7.26. Histopathology of medulloepithelioma. **Left:** Low-power photomicrograph of nonteratoid medulloepithelioma showing cords and tubules of tumor cells and prominent associated cysts. **Right:** High-power photomicrograph of teratoid medulloepithelioma showing intralesional cartilage (oval area of pale tissue at lower right).

ASTROCYTOMA OF RETINA (ASTROCYTIC HAMARTOMA)

The retinal astrocytoma is a benign glioma arising from the astrocytes of the neurosensory retina. It tends to arise early in life, being detected in many affected persons during childhood or adolescence. It affects all races and both sexes equally. It is extremely rare, but its precise frequency has not been determined. This tumor is regarded by many ophthalmic pathologists as a hamartoma rather than a true neoplasm. In some patients, it occurs as a manifestation of the tuberous sclerosis syndrome.

Clinical Features

Laterality and focality. The retinal astrocytoma occurs in unilateral and bilateral forms. The bilateral form is usually characterized by multifocal tumors in both eyes, and most patients with such lesions have tuberous sclerosis. The unilateral form is usually characterized by a single tumor in the affected eye, and most patients with this form of the disease do not appear to have tuberous sclerosis.

Presenting signs and symptoms. Affected patients usually have no visual symptoms unless one or more tumors involve the macula. In rare instances, a retinal astrocytoma remote from the fovea causes a nonrhegmatogenous retinal detachment that involves the macular retina and abruptly blurs the vision in that eye.

Appearance of tumors. The typical ophthalmoscopic finding is that of one or more whitish superficial retinal tumors ranging from thin translucent patches through somewhat thicker opalescent lesions to well-defined opaque nodules (Figs. 7.27 to 7.30). The retinal vasculature tends to be somewhat irregular at the site of each lesion, but prominent tortuous feeder and drainer retinal blood vessels similar to those in retinoblastoma do not occur.

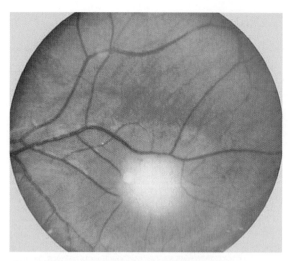

FIGURE 7.28. Astrocytoma (astrocytic hamartoma) of retina. Small, homogeneously white intraretinal tumor in fundus midzone. The tumor appears soft and noncalcified.

Ancillary diagnostic studies. Fluorescein angiography generally reveals a prominent network of superficial and deep intralesional blood vessels. B-scan ultrasonography shows a solid soft tissue mass that, in some cases, contains focal calcifications. CT scanning is sometimes able to image larger intraocular tumors, but it is more useful for showing associated paraventricular intracranial tumors in patients who have tuberous sclerosis (see below).

Syndromic associations. A substantial but currently unspecified proportion of individuals with one or more retinal astrocytomas is found to have other manifestations of tuberous sclerosis. This syndrome is characterized by cutaneous lesions (adenoma sebaceum of the face, subungual fibromas, ash leaf spots, shagreen patches), CNS lesions (benign par-

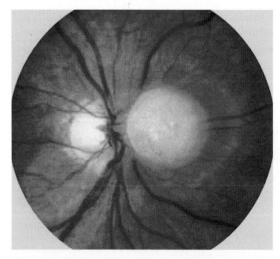

FIGURE 7.27. Astrocytoma (astrocytic hamartoma) of retina. Opaque white intraretinal tumor just nasal to optic disc. The tumor appears solid and has a faintly bumpy surface texture.

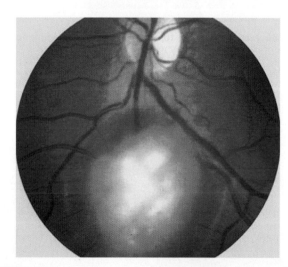

FIGURE 7.29. Astrocytoma (astrocytic hamartoma) of retina. Opaque yellow-white superficial retinal tumor is not associated with dilated, tortuous retinal blood vessels or surrounding subretinal or intraretinal exudates.

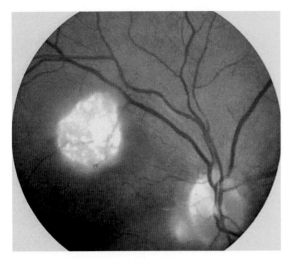

FIGURE 7.30. Multiple retinal astrocytomas (astrocytic hamartomas) in patient with tuberous sclerosis. Larger lesion is located just above center of macula, and small lesion is located just temporal to optic disc.

aventricular astrocytomas of the brain, retinal astrocytomas), and various visceral lesions (cysts in the lungs, liver, and other organs; benign tumors in the heart; rhabdomyomas), and a host of other abnormalities.

Genetics. Tuberous sclerosis is inherited as an autosomal-dominant disease with incomplete penetrance in some families. Several chromosomal loci have been linked with tuberous sclerosis, the most common of which is located on the long arm of chromosome 9 (locus 9q32-34).

Natural history. Retinal astrocytomas appear to have extremely limited malignant potential; however, some tumors of this type have been noted to grow to a rather large size and lead to bullous retinal detachment and blindness in the affected eye.

Pathology. The typical retinal astrocytoma consists of a mass of enlarged fibrous astrocytes containing small oval nuclei and interlacing cytoplasmic processes (Fig. 7.31). Larger lesions frequently contain foci of calcification.

Differential diagnosis. The principal differential diagnosis of retinal astrocytoma includes intraretinal retinoblastoma, nematode granuloma of the retina, and retinal capillary hemangioma.

Management. In most cases, no treatment is required. For patients whose tumor enlarges progressively and eventuates in a blind, painful eye, enucleation seems to be the only available treatment.

CAPILLARY HEMANGIOMA OF RETINA (VON HIPPEL TUMOR)

The retinal capillary hemangioma (hemangioblastoma) is a benign retinal vascular tumor that occurs in unifocal and multifocal, monocular and binocular, and hereditary and nonhereditary forms. It is rarely if ever congenital but tends to develop in most patients by the second to fourth decades of life. It affects both sexes equally and has no racial predilection. Its precise frequency is unknown. Untreated tumors commonly cause substantial visual impairment and sometimes lead to total blindness. Most patients with multifocal binocular disease have other features of the von Hippel–Lindau syndrome.

Clinical Features

Laterality and focality. The usual patient has a single lesion in one eye, but some patients have multifocal or bilateral tumors or both. The precise relative frequency of unilateral, unifocal lesions versus bilateral, multifocal retinal capillary hemangiomas is unknown.

Presenting signs and symptoms. Blurred vision in the affected eye or loss of visual field are the usual presenting symptoms. In some patients, the affected eye is blind by the time any problem is recognized. In advanced cases, the patient presents with a blind painful eye due to secondary glaucoma. In families known to have members with the von Hippel–Lindau syndrome, ophthalmic screening examinations frequently identify asymptomatic small tumors in one or both eyes.

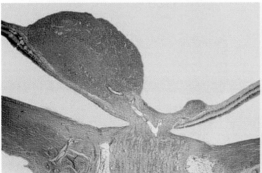
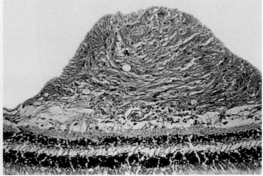

FIGURE 7.31. Histopathology of retinal astrocytomas. **Left:** Lower-power photomicrograph showing two retinal tumors arising from the inner portion of sensory retina near the optic disc. **Right:** Higher-power photomicrograph showing tumor composed of benign fibrous astrocytes.

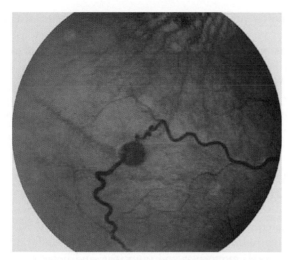

FIGURE 7.32. Capillary hemangioma of retina (von Hippel tumor). Fundus photograph shows small red intraretinal tumor fed and drained by prominent dilated tortuous retinal blood vessels. Superior to the lesion is an area of chorioretinal atrophy subsequent to prior cryotherapy of another retinal capillary hemangioma.

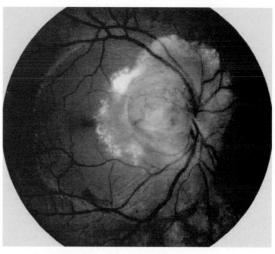

FIGURE 7.34. Capillary hemangioma (von Hippel tumor) involving optic disc. Reddish vascular tumor is surrounded by intraretinal and subretinal exudates. Dilated afferent and efferent retinal blood vessels are not usually observed with tumors at the disc.

Appearance of tumors. The classic retinal capillary hemangioma is a discrete reddish retinal vascular tumor connected to prominent, dilated, tortuous afferent and efferent retinal blood vessels (Figs. 7.32 to 7.35). Intraretinal and subretinal exudates (Figs. 7.33, 7.34) and nonrhegmatogenous retinal detachment with vitreoretinal traction (Fig. 7.35) are frequently associated with such tumors.

Ancillary diagnostic studies. Fluorescein angiography reveals rapid blood flow through the vascular tumor, shows fluorescein leakage through the walls of the vascular lesion, and distinguishes the feeder arteriole from the draining venule. CT scanning and MRI can be used to search for in-

tracranial vascular tumors and abdominal visceral tumors of the von Hippel–Lindau syndrome.

Genetics. The von Hippel–Lindau syndrome is an autosomal-dominant disease that has been linked to a defect in the short arm of chromosome 3 (locus 3p25-26). This syndrome is highly penetrant in affected families. Most individuals who have multifocal, bilateral retinal capillary hemangiomas have this syndrome, while most persons with a single tumor in one eye do not.

Natural history. Some untreated retinal capillary hemangiomas remain stable or enlarge minimally over long periods, but most tumors of this type enlarge progressively and lead to exudative, hemorrhagic, and fibrotic complications if followed without treatment.

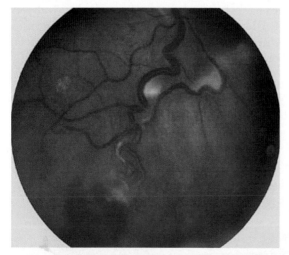

FIGURE 7.33. Capillary hemangioma of retina (von Hippel tumor). Typical globular red retinal lesion with dilated, tortuous afferent and efferent retinal blood vessels. A line of intraretinal exudates is present approximately halfway between the hemangioma and the optic disc.

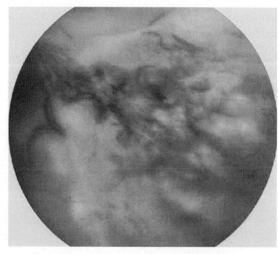

FIGURE 7.35. Large capillary hemangioma of peripheral retina (von Hippel tumor) with an associated exudative-tractional retinal detachment.

Pathology. The vascular tumor consists of small capillary-like blood vessels lined by endothelial cells and supported by a delicate tumor stroma that contains vacuolated fibrous astrocytes (Fig. 7.36).

Differential diagnosis:

- Idiopathic acquired nonfamilial retinal hemangiomatous lesion
- Hemangiomatous retinal neovascularization associated with:
    - Prior scleral buckling surgery for retinal detachment
    - Retinitis pigmentosa
    - Retinopathy of prematurity
    - Familial exudative vitreoretinopathy

Baseline assessment. CT scan or MRI of the CNS and abdomen are generally recommended as part of the patient's baseline systemic evaluation to rule out clinically important extraocular lesions of the von Hippel–Lindau syndrome in the CNS (hemangioblastomas) and abdominal viscera (renal cell carcinomas, pheochromocytomas); they are particularly important in patients with a personal or family history consistent with the von Hippel–Lindau syndrome and in those with multifocal and/or bilateral retinal hemangiomas.

Management. Photocoagulation is applicable to small tumors that do not involve the optic disc or central macula in eyes that do not have an exudative retinal detachment or vitreous clouding.

Cryotherapy is appropriate for small- to medium-sized tumors of the equatorial or oral zone of fundus and can be used even in the presence of localized exudative retinal detachment.

Diathermy can be used to treat some medium-to-large tumors. This treatment is generally performed as a penetrating treatment using a needle-like diathermy tip inserted into the hemangioma transsclerally via a lamellar scleral bed just external to the lesion. Scleral buckling is usually performed at the same time.

Scleral buckling and vitrectomy are sometimes performed in conjunction with endodiathermy, endophotocoagulation, and even **endoresection** of the tumor in eyes with bullous exudative retinal detachment or tractional retinal detachment.

Enucleation is usually reserved for patients with a blind painful eye due to tumor or for those with an unsightly phthisical eye.

Observation appears to be appropriate management for selected patients who have one or more small tumors not causing visual problems, especially if they are not producing any exudative or hemorrhagic problems.

CAVERNOUS HEMANGIOMA OF RETINA

The cavernous hemangioma of the retina is a benign retinal vascular tumor having characteristic clinical and pathological architecture. This lesion is very uncommon, but its precise frequency is unknown. It affects both sexes and occurs in all races. Most affected patients have a single lesion in one eye and no evidence of a multi-system syndrome.

Clinical Features

Laterality and focality. The typical patient has a single lesion in one eye; however, some patients have multifocal or bilateral tumors or both. The precise relative frequency of unilateral, unifocal lesions and bilateral, multifocal hemangiomas is unknown.

Presenting signs and symptoms. Most patients with a cavernous hemangioma of the retina are asymptomatic when their tumor is detected on ophthalmic examination. In some cases, vision is blurred due to the macular location of the lesion. In other cases, the patient reports floaters attributable to intravitreal bleeding from the hemangioma.

Appearance of tumors. Ophthalmic examination typically reveals a localized cluster of dark red vascular saccules

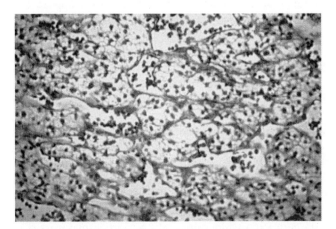

FIGURE 7.36. Histopathology of retinal capillary hemangioma. Tumor consists of small vascular channels lined by mature endothelial cells and a stroma of pale tumor cells.

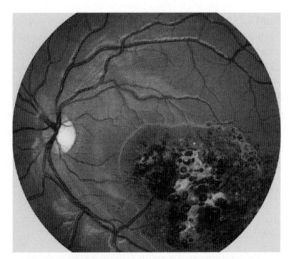

FIGURE 7.37. Cavernous hemangioma of retina. Macular retinal lesion appears as cluster of aneurysmal vascular saccules with some associated white superficial fibrosis (gliosis).

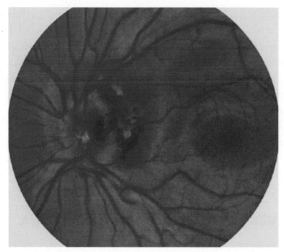

FIGURE 7.38. Cavernous hemangioma of retina involving optic disc. Tumor consists of a collection of small vascular saccules containing dark red blood.

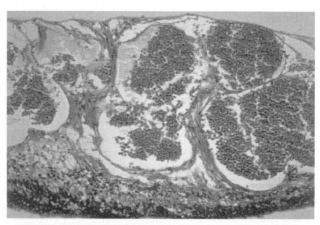

FIGURE 7.39. Histopathology of cavernous hemangioma of retina. Tumor consists of a cluster of large-caliber, thin-walled intraretinal vascular saccules lined by normal vascular endothelial cells.

(Figs. 7.37, 7.38) frequently in proximity to a central large-caliber retinal vein. There may be whitish fibrous tissue on the surface of the lesion, and this white tissue can be mistaken on casual viewing for intraretinal exudate. If the component vascular saccules are relatively large, plasma-erythrocyte separation can be seen in some of the saccules. In some affected eyes, one can find intraretinal and preretinal or intravitreal blood arising from the surface of the tumor.

Ancillary diagnostic studies. Fluorescein angiography reveals slow blood flow through the vascular lesion, accentuates the central vein of the lesion, and confirms plasma-erythrocyte separation in some of the larger vascular saccules.

Genetics. In most patients with retinal cavernous hemangioma, the fundus tumor is a sporadic, nonfamilial, nonsyndromic lesion. However, some patients appear to have an uncommon familial disorder characterized by other benign cavernous or telangiectatic vascular lesions of the skin and CNS.

Natural history. Most retinal cavernous hemangiomas that have been observed for prolonged periods have remained stable in size and clinical appearance. Occasional hemangiomas of this type bleed repeatedly into the vitreous over the course of many years.

Pathology. The retinal capillary hemangioma consists of a cluster of large-caliber, thin-walled intraretinal vascular saccules lined by normal vascular endothelial cells (Fig. 7.39). The tumor thickens and replaces the neurosensory retina at the affected site.

Differential diagnosis:

- Coats' disease (idiopathic retinal telangiectasis)
- Idiopathic perifoveal telangiectasia

Baseline patient assessment. CT scanning or MRI of the CNS is probably appropriate in patients with a personal or family history of retinal or CNS vascular lesions; however, such studies are probably not necessary in patients with a unifocal, unilateral lesion and no symptoms or neurologic signs suggesting an intracranial abnormality.

Management. Observation is recommended for most lesions of this type because of their benign nature and usual lack of progression.

Coagulation (**photocoagulation or cryotherapy**) is applicable to small- to medium-sized lesions that bleed repeatedly.

Excision of the lesion via posterior vitrectomy can be performed in eyes with massive or nonclearing intravitreal hemorrhage from the hemangioma.

METASTATIC CARCINOMA TO RETINA

Metastatic carcinoma to the retina is an extraocular primary malignancy that has metastasized via the bloodstream to the retina. Although metastatic tumors to the eye are relatively common, most such lesions involve the uveal tract. The retina is an uncommon site for a metastasis to appear. The great majority of retinal metastatic lesions are unifocal and unilateral.

Clinical Features

Laterality and focality. The great majority of retinal metastatic lesions are unilateral and unifocal; however, bilateral and multifocal retinal metastatic tumors have been reported.

Presenting signs and symptoms. Patients with a metastatic retinal tumor tend to have visual symptoms corresponding to the location of the tumor. In some patients, the tumors are detected on routine ophthalmic evaluation of asymptomatic eyes.

Appearance of tumors. The usual metastatic tumor to the retina is a white to tan, placoid intraretinal mass (Fig. 7.40). The most common exception to this appearance is the metastatic melanoma from the skin, which typically ap-

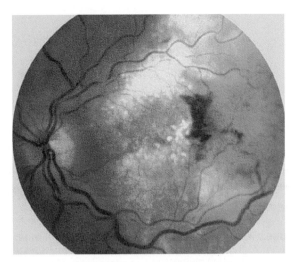

FIGURE 7.40. Metastatic cutaneous malignant melanoma to retina. Tumor is an ill-defined tan infiltration of the retina *(at right in photograph)* associated with extensive surrounding intraretinal exudates and some localized surface hemorrhage.

pears dark brown to almost black. If the tumor involves the optic disc, it appears as an infiltrative lesion, often with finely dispersed tumor cells in the overlying vitreous.

Ancillary diagnostic studies. On fluorescein angiography, a metastatic retinal lesion generally appears hypofluorescent early and somewhat hyperfluorescent late. Leakage of fluorescein from the retinal blood vessels damaged by the lesion is frequently apparent in the late frames.

Systemic implications. The patient who develops a metastatic lesion to the retina is likely to have other bodily sites of metastasis. Consequently, such a patient's prognosis for long-term survival is correspondingly poor.

Natural history. If untreated, most metastatic carcinomas to the retina progress, leading eventually to retinal detachment and marked visual loss.

Pathology. The pathology of metastatic carcinomas to the retina depends largely on the nature of the metastasizing cancer. The retina is thickened and replaced by metastatic tumor cells in the area of involvement.

Differential diagnosis:

- Microbial infiltrate (e.g., *Candida, Nocardia, Cryptococcus,* etc.)
- Nonmicrobial inflammatory granuloma (e.g., sarcoid granuloma)
- Leukemic or lymphomatous infiltrate

Baseline patient assessment. Comprehensive systemic history and physical examination is essential in patients suspected of having a metastatic retinal tumor for identifying other metastatic lesions and, if necessary, finding the primary malignancy. Chest x-ray, mammography, CT scanning, MRI and other studies of these types are needed to evaluate the patient for metastatic lesions in other bodily sites not detectable by physical examination.

Management. External beam radiation therapy is commonly used to treat visually significant metastatic retinal tumors in patients who are not in a terminal phase of their illness.

Chemotherapy hormone therapy, or **immunotherapy** is appropriate in patients with generalized metastatic disease, assuming that there is a reasonable chance of salvage.

Observation is probably appropriate in most terminal patients, especially in ones who have a healthy fellow eye.

Enucleation of the affected eye is occasionally required for pain relief in patients who develop a blind, painful eye due to their retinal tumor.

LEUKEMIC INFILTRATION OF RETINA

Leukemic infiltration of the retina is an extravascular proliferation of leukemic cells within the substance of the retina. Lesions of this type are uncommon, but their precise frequency is unknown. They occur in individuals of any age, but peaks of incidence mirror peaks of incidence of leukemia in general. Retinal involvement is much more common as a manifestation of leukemic relapse than as an initial site of disease. Hemorrhagic retinal lesions are much more common in leukemic patients than are true malignant infiltrates.

Clinical Features

Laterality and focality. Leukemic retinal infiltrates may be unifocal or multifocal and unilateral or bilateral.

Presenting signs and symptoms. The usual symptoms are blurred vision, dim vision, and floaters.

Appearance of tumors. The typical leukemic retinal infiltrate is a fuzzy, flat, white retinal lesion (Fig. 7.41) that is frequently associated with retinal hemorrhages and overlying intravitreal cells (Fig. 7.42).

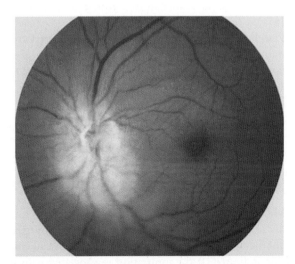

FIGURE 7.41. Leukemic infiltration of retina and optic disc in a patient with chronic myelogenous leukemia. Tumor appears as an ill-defined yellowish infiltration that partly obscures the retina and optic disc.

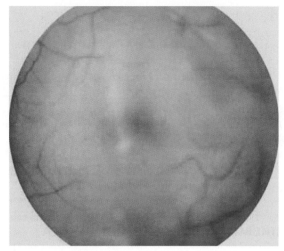

FIGURE 7.42. Leukemic cells in the vitreous of a boy with relapse of acute lymphoblastic leukemia.

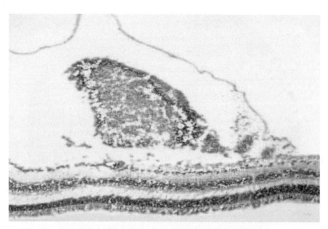

FIGURE 7.43. Histopathology of leukemic retinal infiltrate. This photomicrograph shows an accumulation of leukemic cells under the internal limiting membrane.

Ancillary diagnostic studies. All patients with suspected leukemic retinal infiltration should be evaluated thoroughly from a hematologic perspective (i.e., with complete blood count and differential count, bone marrow aspiration or biopsy, complete systemic staging evaluation, and probably lumbar puncture for CSF cytology). In addition, if there is still uncertainty about the ocular diagnosis, the ophthalmologist should consider pars plana vitrectomy or retinal biopsy to confirm the diagnosis.

Systemic implications. Concurrent CNS leukemia is common in patients who develop a retinal leukemic infiltrate. Consequently, CNS imaging and lumbar puncture are especially indicated in any patient suspected of having leukemic relapse in the eye. Not surprisingly, leukemic infiltration of the retina is an unfavorable prognostic factor for survival.

Natural history. Untreated leukemic infiltrates tend to progress at a variable rate and to eventuate in profound visual loss in the affected eye.

Pathology. The infiltrated retina and overlying vitreous contain leukemic cells in various quantities (Fig. 7.43). Leukemic cells are commonly observed in the lumina of retinal blood vessels.

Differential diagnosis:

- Microbial infiltrate (e.g., *Candida, Nocardia, Cryptococcus,* etc.)
- Nonmicrobial inflammatory granuloma (e.g. sarcoid granuloma)
- Lymphomatous infiltrate

Management. In terminal patients, no treatment for the ocular lesions is indicated. In patients who are salvageable, **chemotherapy** appropriate to the precise type of leukemia is usually indicated. If the infiltration is associated with profound visual loss because of macular or optic nerve involvement, **palliative external beam radiation therapy** should also be considered.

LYMPHOMATOUS INFILTRATION OF RETINA

Lymphomatous infiltration of the retina is a malignant intraretinal or subretinal collection of atypical lymphoid cells. Such tumors are uncommon, but their precise frequency is unknown. Lymphomatous retinal infiltrates usually occur as a feature of primary lymphoma of the CNS and retina, but they rarely occur as a metastatic tumor in patients with systemic non-Hodgkin's lymphoma. The disease generally affects older adults and occurs somewhat more commonly in women than in men.

Clinical Features

Laterality and focality. Retinal lymphomatous infiltrates can involve one or both eyes, but bilateral involvement is distinctly more common (about 80% of cases). However, asynchronous ocular involvement is often noted in affected patients who develop binocular disease.

Presenting signs and symptoms. The usual symptoms are blurred vision and floaters.

Appearance of tumors. The characteristic retinal lesions are geographic yellowish-white subretinal pigment epithelial lesions (Fig. 7.44) and fuzzy, ill-defined intraretinal patches (Fig. 7.45), both of which are frequently associated with overlying, finely dispersed white cells in the vitreous.

Ancillary diagnostic studies. Patients suspected of having primary retinal lymphoma should undergo CT scanning or MRI of the brain and lumbar puncture for CSF cytology. If primary CNS lymphoma is confirmed by such studies, pathologic confirmation of the intraocular diagnosis by biopsy may be judged unnecessary. However, diagnostic posterior vitrectomy with cytopathologic assessment of intravitreal cells or even transscleral retinal biopsy must be considered when the CNS evaluation is negative for lymphoma and when the intraocular lesions are not absolutely characteristic. The vitreous from eyes with suspected intraocular lymphoma can also be evaluated to determine lev-

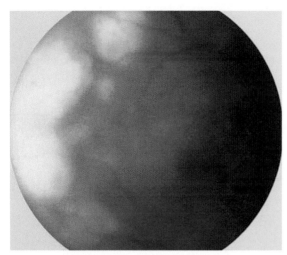

FIGURE 7.44. Lymphomatous infiltration of retina in a patient with primary lymphoma of the retina and central nervous system. Tumor appears as geographic, relatively flat, yellowish-white subretinal pigment epithelial infiltrates *(left in photograph)* surrounded by less distinct satellite lesions. The lesions appear a bit hazy because of associated diffuse fine intravitreal cells.

els of interleukins (IL) 10 and 6. Recent evidence suggests that an IL-10/IL-6 ratio greater than 1 is strongly suggestive of lymphoma.

Natural history. Untreated infiltrative lymphoid lesions of the retina tend to progress and result in progressive visual loss in the affected eye or eyes. However, some lesions have been noted to wax and wane without specific intervention.

Pathology. The infiltrative retinal and subretinal pigment epithelial lesions are composed of malignant lymphoid cells that typically have the cytologic features of large cell lymphoma (Fig. 7.46).

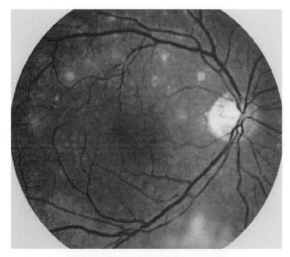

FIGURE 7.45. Primary lymphoma of retina (confirmed pathologically). Multiple small deep retinal or subretinal amelanotic foci are evident above macula, and an ill-defined area of lymphomatous inner retinal whitening is present inferiorly from optic disc.

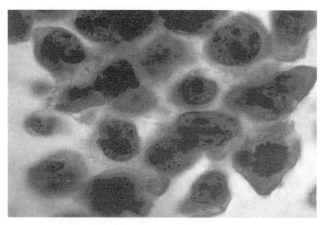

FIGURE 7.46. Cytopathology of subretinal lymphoid infiltrate. High-power photomicrograph showing malignant lymphoid cells, some exhibiting mitotic figures, obtained by fine needle aspiration biopsy.

Differential diagnosis:

- Microbial infiltrate (e.g., *Candida, Nocardia, Cryptococcus,* etc.)
- Nonmicrobial inflammatory granuloma (e.g., sarcoid granuloma)
- Leukemic infiltrate

Systemic implications. Patients who have primary CNS lymphoma or a visceral non-Hodgkin's lymphoma are at great risk for death due to complications of that disease.

Management. If only the eyes are involved, ocular irradiation by **external beam radiation therapy** (35 to 45 Gy in fractionated schedule) is generally recommended. If there is concurrent CNS lymphoma, aggressive **chemotherapy** and sometimes whole brain irradiation are usually recommended. The role of chemotherapy in primary intraocular lymphoma without evidence of CNS lymphoma or visceral lymphoma is controversial. Local intraocular relapses of lymphoma in previously irradiated eyes can sometimes be treated effectively by repeated intravitreal injections of methotrexate.

HYPERTROPHY OF RETINAL PIGMENT EPITHELIUM

Hypertrophy of the RPE is a benign congenital hamartoma of the RPE. The lesion occurs in typical and atypical forms and in unifocal and multifocal patterns. The prevalence of this lesion is unknown, but it appears to be relatively common. There is no apparent racial or gender predilection.

Clinical Features

Laterality and focality. There are three distinct clinical patterns of these lesions:

1. Unifocal unilateral—the typical solitary lesion referred to as *congenital hypertrophy of the RPE*

2. Multifocal unilateral—this clustering of lesions is commonly referred to as *grouped pigmentation of the retina* (or "bear tracks")
3. Multifocal bilateral or atypical—this clinical pattern is observed most commonly as a marker phenomenon for Gardner's syndrome and several other forms of familial adenomatous polyposis–carcinoma of the colon

Presenting signs and symptoms. These lesions are virtually always asymptomatic and detected on routine ophthalmic examination.

Appearance of tumors. The characteristic tumors are gray to black, flat fundus lesions at the retinal pigment epithelial level (Figs. 7.47 to 7.49). These lesions typically occur in the midzone to periphery of the fundus, but they occasionally occur in the macular and juxtapapillary regions of the fundus. Flatness of the lesion can usually be confirmed by slit lamp biomicroscopy of the fundus, binocular indirect ophthalmoscopy with scleral depression over the lesion, or, if necessary, B-scan ultrasonography.

Typical unilateral unifocal lesions appear as nummular or geographic lesions with well-defined, smooth margins (Fig. 7.47). These lesions may have one or more central lacunae of depigmentation. Typical unilateral multifocal lesions generally appear less dense in terms of the pigmentation of the individual lesions but are frequently densely clustered in a small area of the retina (Fig. 7.48). The atypical bilateral multifocal lesions tend to be more irregular and angulated in shape and less uniform in pigmentation than are the other two types of lesions (Fig. 7.49). These lesions tend to be scattered widely in the fundus and not localized to one area.

Ancillary diagnostic studies. No diagnostic studies are generally indicated for characterization of these retinal lesions.

Syndromic associations. As noted above, atypical multifocal, bilateral fundus lesions of congenital hypertrophy of

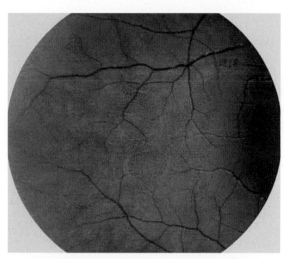

FIGURE 7.48. Hypertrophy of retinal pigment epithelium (RPE), multifocal type. The lesion appears as a cluster of gray to black, well-defined RPE lesions that have been likened to bear tracks on the retina.

the RPE tend to be identifying markers for Gardner's syndrome and some other autosomal-dominant colonic polyposis–carcinoma syndromes in affected kindred. Because of this, the ophthalmologist should always review the family history of any individual with multifocal, bilateral, atypical hypertrophy of the RPE and also recommend comprehensive colonic evaluation of all such patients.

Natural history. Most retinal lesions of this type change minimally if at all over extended periods of follow-up. In rare instances, malignant change (to adenocarcinoma of the RPE) has been documented in lesions of this type. Because of this, periodic life-long monitoring of such lesions is probably advisable.

Pathology. The lesions of hypertrophy of the RPE consist of well-defined foci of taller than normal retinal pigment

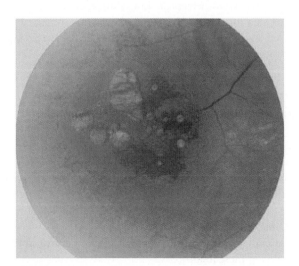

FIGURE 7.47. Hypertrophy of retinal pigment epithelium (RPE), unifocal type. Black lesion appears well circumscribed and nummular, and has several white lacunae of RPE depigmentation.

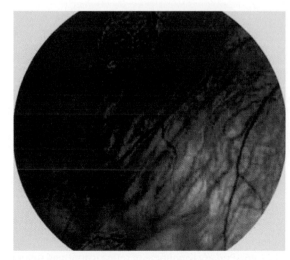

FIGURE 7.49. Hypertrophy of retinal pigment epithelium, atypical-multifocal-bilateral type, associated with colonic adenomatous polyposis–carcinoma.

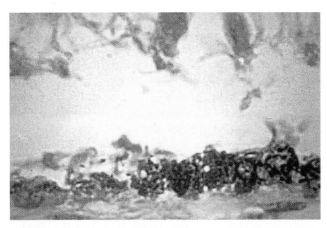

FIGURE 7.50. Histopathology of hypertrophy of retinal pigment epithelium (RPE). High-power photomicrograph showing abrupt transition between normal RPE *(on left)* and abnormally thickened RPE densely packed with melanin granules *(on right)*. The overlying retina is artifactitiously detached and degenerated.

epithelial cells containing an increased number of large oval melanin granules (Fig. 7.50).

Differential diagnosis:

- Hyperplasia of RPE
- Metastatic melanoma to retina
- Malignant melanoma of choroids

Management. No treatment is indicated for typical lesions of this type.

COMBINED HAMARTOMA OF RETINA

The combined hamartoma of the retina is a benign tumor comprised of retinal pigment epithelial cells, neurosensory retina, retinal vascular elements, and vitreous. This lesion is usually detected during infancy or early childhood and is probably congenital in a large proportion of affected individuals. Although it can cause profound visual impairment, it has no recognized malignant potential. It sometimes occurs in association with other features of neurofibromatosis type 2.

Clinical Features

Laterality and focality. The combined hamartoma of the retina is almost always unifocal and unilateral. With rare exceptions, it arises in a juxtapapillary or circumpapillary location.

Presenting signs and symptoms. The most common presenting feature is amblyopia in the involved eye due to macular involvement.

Appearance of lesion. The typical lesion is a geographic white "gliotic" retinal lesion with deep intrinsic gray-black pigmentation, especially at its margins, and marked tortuosity of the retinal blood vessels in the area of the lesion (Figs. 7.51, 7.52). The retinal vascular pattern and chorioretinal appearance peripheral to lesion are normal.

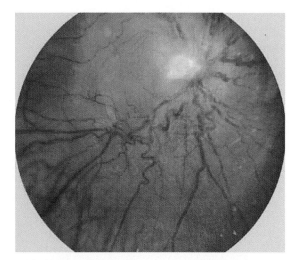

FIGURE 7.51. Combined hamartoma of retina. Typical lesion surrounds optic disc, appears gray in its deeper layers, and exhibits superficial whitish gliosis with pronounced tortuosity and angulation of involved retinal blood vessels.

Ancillary diagnostic studies. Fluorescein angiography accentuates the prominent tortuous intralesional retinal blood vessels but provides no important differential diagnostic information. B-scan ultrasonography can image thicker lesions but is also not particularly helpful in differential diagnosis. CT scanning and MRI can reveal bilateral acoustic neuromas (the characteristic feature of neurofibromatosis type 2) in patients who have that syndromic association.

Syndromic associations. Although most cases have been sporadic and nonsyndromic, a substantial number of cases have been associated with neurofibromatosis types 2 (central neurofibromatosis, bilateral acoustic neuromas), and an oc-

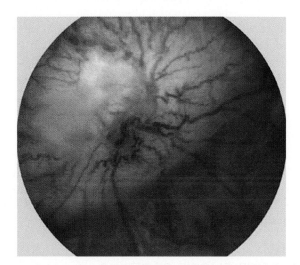

FIGURE 7.52. Combined hamartoma of retina. Lesion surrounds and completely obscures optic disc. Tumor in this case is approximately 3 mm thick and has well-defined margins. It is gray in its deeper layers and appears whitish on its surface due to superficial gliosis. The involved retinal blood vessels are markedly angulated and tortuous.

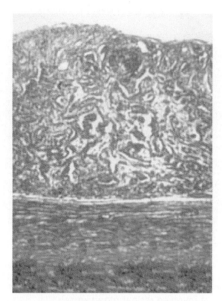

FIGURE 7.53. Histopathology of combined hamartoma of retina. High-power photomicrograph shows tumor to be composed of interlacing cords of retinal pigment epithelial cells and blood vessels within disorganized and thickened neurosensory retina.

casional case has been linked with neurofibromatosis type 1 (von Recklinghausen's disease). Consequently, neurofibromatosis should always be considered in youngsters found to have a combined hamartoma of the retina.

Natural history. Most such lesions are minimally progressive after detection. In those cases that change during follow-up, the apparent progression is usually due to contraction of the vitreoretinal surface of the lesion and not to cellular proliferation of the lesion per se.

Pathology. The few pathologic specimens that have been reviewed have been composed of interlacing cords of retinal pigment epithelial cells and blood vessels within disorganized and thickened neurosensory retina (Fig. 7.53) and a proliferation of benign fibrous cells on its vitreal surface.

Differential diagnosis:

■ Choroidal malignant melanoma (because of the dark intrinsic pigmentation)
■ Retinoblastoma (because of the whitish appearance of the surface gliosis in many lesions)

Management. No treatment is generally indicated. Posterior vitrectomy has been employed in a few cases to remove the vitreoretinal fibrosis, but such procedures have met with limited visual success.

MASSIVE GLIOSIS OF RETINA

Massive gliosis of the retina is a benign proliferation of retinal glial cells in response to some underlying injury or other local process. Recognized causes of such lesions include se-

vere ocular trauma, chronic intraocular inflammation, retinal vascular occlusive diseases, and even congenital malformations. In spite of its name, massive gliosis does not necessarily involve a large portion of fundus; this is because the word "massive" in the term refers to the "mass-like" nature of the lesion rather than its size. Massive gliosis is rare, but its precise frequency is unknown. It can arise at any age, but it is rarely identified in childhood.

Clinical Features

Laterality and focality. Massive gliosis of the retina is almost always a unilateral unifocal lesion.

Presenting signs and symptoms. If the lesion develops in childhood, amblyopia is possible. If the lesion develops later in life, profound visual loss usually occurs in the affected eye.

Appearance of tumors. The typical lesion (when it can be observed ophthalmoscopically) is a gray-white to black fundus tumor (Fig. 7.54), depending on the proportion of pigment-laden retinal pigment epithelial cells contained in the lesion. In many patients, no fundus view is possible because of dense cataract, vitreous opacification, or other media abnormalities. Most affected eyes have an extremely limited visual potential.

Ancillary diagnostic studies. B-scan ultrasonography reveals a soft tissue mass that can be difficult if not impossible to distinguish from a posterior uveal malignant melanoma. Fluorescein angiography has rarely been attempted because the optical media of the eye are usually hazy or opaque.

Natural history. Progression of lesions of this type has rarely been observed, in part because enucleation is commonly recommended if the mass is extremely large and in part because the ophthalmoscopic view of the lesion is typically poor to nil in most affected eyes.

Pathology. The tumor is composed of benign spindle-shaped fibrous astrocytes, an abundant fibrous extracellular

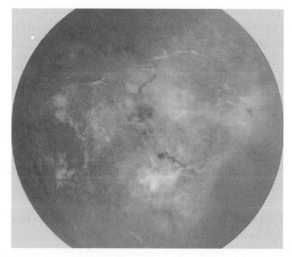

FIGURE 7.54. Localized form of massive gliosis of retina showing prominent superficial white glial proliferation, marked retinal pigment epithelial hyperplasia with intraretinal pigment migration, and abnormal intralesional blood vessels.

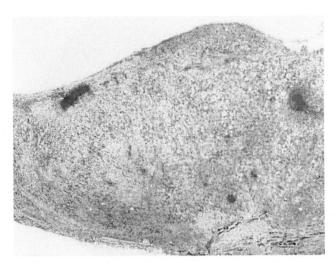

FIGURE 7.55. Histopathology of massive gliosis of retina. Tumor is composed of spindle-shaped fibrous astrocytes, abundant fibrous extracellular matrix, and numerous thick-walled intralesional blood vessels. Retinal pigment epithelial cells are present within basal aspect of mass.

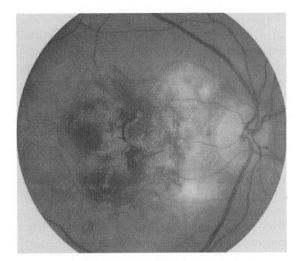

FIGURE 7.56. Hyperplasia of retinal pigment epithelium in macula.

matrix, and numerous dilated thick-walled blood vessels scattered throughout the lesion (Fig. 7.55).

Differential Diagnosis:

■ Choroidal malignant melanoma
■ Eccentric disciform lesion

Management. If the lesion is recognized for what it is, simple observation is all that is indicated. In many cases, however, the affected eye comes to enucleation because posterior uveal melanoma cannot be excluded.

HYPERPLASIA OF RETINAL PIGMENT EPITHELIUM

RPE hyperplasia is a benign reactive proliferation of RPE cells that develops in response to traumatic insult of some type, including focal infection and noninfectious inflammation. It is a rather common lesion, but its prevalence in the general population is unknown. It can develop at any age but is rarely congenital.

Clinical Features

Laterality and focality. The lesion is usually unifocal and unilateral.

Presenting signs and symptoms. These lesions are usually asymptomatic unless they involve the macula.

Appearance of lesions. The typical RPE hyperplasia is a focal irregular black retinal lesion, usually with some associated circummarginal chorioretinal atrophy and intraretinal pigment cell migration (Fig. 7.56). On high magnification fundus biomicroscopy, intraretinal migration of the black RPE pigment is usually evident.

Ancillary diagnostic studies. No diagnostic studies are generally indicated for lesions of this type.

Natural history. The lesions of RPE hyperplasia, once developed, usually remain dormant or change minimally during long-term follow-up. However, occasional lesions of this type have enlarged substantially during follow-up, suggesting either malignant change or erroneous initial clinical diagnosis.

Pathology. The lesion consists of an increased number of retinal pigment epithelial cells that are also larger than normal. The cells are densely packed with large spherical melanin granules. The overlying sensory retina is partially degenerated, and the retinal pigment epithelial cells extend into the sensory retina.

Differential diagnosis:

■ Choroidal malignant melanoma
■ Unifocal hypertrophy of RPE

Management. No treatment is generally indicated for typical lesions of this type. However, enucleation is usually performed when malignant change is suspected on the basis of substantial or rapid tumor progression during follow-up.

ACQUIRED NONFAMILIAL RETINAL HEMANGIOMATOUS LESION

The acquired nonfamilial retinal hemangiomatous lesion is a benign nodular retinal vascular tumor of the peripheral fundus that resembles a retinal capillary hemangioma. It typically occurs in older adults as a manifestation of peripheral chorioretinal degeneration with subretinal neovascularization, but similar lesions also occur in younger patients with certain underlying chorioretinal disorders.

Clinical Features

Laterality and focality. This lesion is almost exclusively unilateral and unifocal. It usually develops in the oral zone of the fundus adjacent to the ora serrata, most commonly in the inferotemporal quadrant.

Presenting signs and symptoms. The lesion is asymptomatic in most affected patients because of its peripheral location, but it can cause blurred vision if an exudative response extends to the macula or vitreous hemorrhage occurs.

Appearance of tumors. The typical lesion is a red to pink, globular oral zone mass associated with subretinal and intraretinal exudation (Fig. 7.57). Unlike the classic retinal capillary hemangioma, this lesion tends not to have any prominent dilated, tortuous retinal feeder and drainer blood vessels.

Ancillary diagnostic studies. Fluorescein angiography usually reveals slow filling of the retinal vascular network that ramifies on the surface of the tumor, but it also commonly suggests at least partial vascular supply from the underlying choroid. In the late frames, one usually observes profuse leakage of fluorescein into the overlying vitreous and surrounding subretinal fluid.

Natural history. The tumor characteristically changes minimally if at all in size during postdetection follow-up; however, the exudation associated with the vascular tumor can increase over time and result in exudative retinal detachment that threatens or involves the macula. In some cases, the lesion can also be the source of intermittent intravitreal bleeding.

Pathology. The few lesions of this type that have been examined histopathologically have consisted of hemangiomatous neovascular proliferations arising from the peripheral uvea via a defect in Bruch's membrane. They are composed of cavernous vascular channels lined by uveal-type endothelial cells, extravasated blood, and fibrous connective tissue.

Association with chorioretinal disorders. Although most lesions of this type occur in eyes with peripheral chorioretinal degeneration of aging, some lesions that appear virtually identical have been associated with various forms of retinitis pigmentosa (Fig. 7.58), familial exudative vitreoretinopathy, and cicatricial retinopathy of prematurity.

Differential diagnosis:

- Retinal capillary hemangioma
- Choroidal malignant melanoma with retinal invasion

Management. Most lesions of this type require no treatment. If progressive exudative retinal detachment or recurrent episodes of intravitreal bleeding develop, then transscleral **cryotherapy** may be advisable.

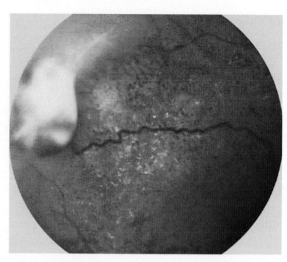

FIGURE 7.58. Acquired hemangiomatous lesion of peripheral retina in a young man with advanced retinitis pigmentosa.

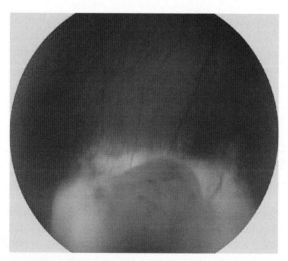

FIGURE 7.57. Typical acquired nonfamilial retinal hemangiomatous lesion in the inferior periphery with associated thick subretinal and intraretinal exudates.

BIBLIOGRAPHY

Alpek EK, Ahmed I, Hochberg FH, et al. Intraocular-central nervous system lymphoma: clinical features, diagnosis, and outcomes. *Ophthalmology* 1999;106:1805.

Arnold AC, Hepler RS, Yee RW, Maggiano J, Eng LF, Foos RY. Solitary retinal astrocytoma. *Surv Ophthalmol* 1985;30:173.

Baud O, Cormier-Daire V, Lyonnet S, et al. Dysmorphic phenotype and neurological impairment in 22 retinoblastoma patients with constitutional cytogenetic 13q deletion. *Clin Genet* 1999;55:478.

Bell D, Yang HK, O'Brien C. A case of bilateral cavernous hemangioma associated with intracerebral hemangioma. *Arch Ophthalmol* 1997;115:818.

Benz MS, Scott IU, Murray TG, et al. Complications of systemic chemotherapy as treatment of retinoblastoma. *Arch Ophthalmol* 2000;118:577.

Bhatnagar R, Vine AK. Diffuse infiltrating retinoblastoma. *Ophthalmology* 1991;98:1657.

Blach LE, McCormick B, Abramson DH. External beam radiation therapy and retinoblastoma: long-term results in the comparison of two techniques. *Int J Radiat Oncol Biol Phys* 1996;35:45.

Blodi CF, Russell SR, Pulido JS, Folk JC. Direct and feeder vessel photocoagulation of retinal angiomas with dye yellow laser. *Ophthalmology* 1990;97:791.

Blumenkranz MS, Ward T, Murphy S, et al. Applications and limitations of vitreoretinal biopsy techniques in intraocular large cell lymphoma. *Retina* 1992;12:S64.

Blumenthal EZ, Papamichael G, Merin S. Combined hamartoma of the retina and retinal pigment epithelium: a bilateral presentation. *Retina* 1998;18:557.

Bornfeld N, Schuler A, Bechrakis N, et al. Preliminary results of primary chemotherapy in retinoblastoma. *Klin Padiatr* 1997; 209:216.

Bouzas EA, Parry DM, Eldridge R, Kaiser-Kupfer MI. Familial occurrence of combined pigment epithelial and retinal hamartomas associated with neurofibromatosis 2. *Retina* 1992;12:103.

Campochiaro PA, Conway BP. Hemangiomalike masses of the retina. *Arch Ophthalmol* 1988;106:1409.

Canning CR, McCartney ACE, Hungerford J. Medulloepithelioma (diktyoma). *Br J Ophthalmol* 1988;72:764.

Cardoso RD, Brockhurst RJ. Perforating diathermy coagulation for retinal angiomas. *Arch Ophthalmol* 1976;94:1702.

Chamot L, Zografos L, Klainguti G. Fundus changes associated with congenital hypertrophy of the retinal pigment epithelium. *Am J Ophthalmol* 1993;115:154.

Chan CC, Vortmeyer AO, Chew EY, et al. VHL gene deletion and enhanced VEGF gene expression detected in the stromal cells of retinal angioma. *Arch Ophthalmol* 1999;117:625.

Chan HSL, DeBoer G, Thiessen JJ, et al. Combining cyclosporin with chemotherapy controls intraocular retinoblastoma without requiring radiation. *Clin Cancer Res* 1996;2:1499.

Chang JH, Spraul CW, Lynn ML, et al. The two-stage mutation model in retinal hemangioblastoma. *Ophthalmic Genetics* 1998;19:123.

Cohen SY, Quental G, Guiberteau B, Coscas GJ. Retinal vascular changes in congenital hypertrophy of the retinal pigment epithelium. *Ophthalmology* 1993;100:471.

Cole EL, Zakov ZN, Meisler DM, et al. Cutaneous malignant melanoma metastatic to the vitreous. *Arch Ophthalmol* 1986;104:98.

Colvard DM, Robertson DM, Trautman JC. Cavernous hemangioma of the retina. *Arch Ophthalmol* 1978;96:2042.

Crino PB, Henske EP. New developments in the neurobiology of the tuberous sclerosis complex. *Neurology* 1999;53:1384.

Dithmar S, Holz FG, Volcker HE. Massive reaktive Gliose der Netzhaut. *Klin Monatsbl Augenheilkd* 1997;211:338.

el-Asrar A, al-Momen AK, Kangave D, et al. Correlation of fundus lesions and hematologic findings in leukemic retinopathy. *Eur J Ophthalmol* 1996;6:167.

el-Asrar A, al-Momen AK, Kangave D, Harakati MS. Prognostic importance of retinopathy in acute leukemia. *Doc Ophthalmol* 1995-96;91:273.

Eng C, Li FP, Abramson DH, et al. Mortality from second tumors among long-term survivors of retinoblastoma. *J Natl Cancer Inst* 1993;85:1121.

Fishburne BC, Wilson DJ, Rosenbaum JT, Neuwelt EA. Intravitreal methotrexate as an adjunctive treatment of intraocular lymphoma. *Arch Ophthalmol* 1997;115:1152.

Friedrich CA. von Hippel–Lindau syndrome: a pleomorphic condition. *Cancer* 1999;86:2478.

Garcia-Arumi J, Sararols LH, Cavero L, et al. Therapeutic options for capillary papillary hemangiomas. *Ophthalmology* 2000;107:48.

Gass JDM. Focal congenital anomalies of the retinal pigment epithelium. *Eye* 1989;3:1.

Glenn GM, Linehan WM, Hosoe S, et al. Screening for von Hippel–Lindau disease by DNA polymorphism analysis. *JAMA* 1992;267:1226.

Gottlieb F, Fammartino JJ, Stratford TP, Brockhurst RJ. Retina angiomatous mass. A complication of retinal detachment surgery. *Retina* 1984;4:152.

Green WR. Vascular and circulatory conditions and diseases. In: Spencer WH. Ophthalmic pathology. An atlas and textbook. 3rd ed. Philadelphia: WB Saunders; 1985:1515.

Green WR. Peripheral retinal lesions, degenerations, and related conditions. In: Spencer WH. Ophthalmic pathology. An atlas and textbook. 3rd ed. Philadelphia: WB Saunders; 1985:837.

Griffiths PD, Martland TR. Tuberous sclerosis complex: the role of neuroradiology. *Neuropediatrics* 1997;28:244.

Grossniklaus HE, Thomas JW, Vigneswaren N, Jarrett WH. Retinal hemangioblastoma. A histologic, immunohistochemical, and ultrastructural evaluation. *Ophthalmology* 1992;99:140.

Guyer DR, Schachat AP, Vitale S, et al. Leukemic retinopathy. Relationship between fundus lesions and hematologic parameters at diagnosis. *Ophthalmology* 1989;96:860.

Hardwig P, Robertson DM. von Hippel–Lindau disease: a familial, often lethal, multi-system phakomatosis. *Ophthalmology* 1984; 91:263.

Haines JL, Short MP, Kwiatkowski DJ, et al. Localization of one gene for tuberous sclerosis within 9q32-9q34, and further evidence for heterogeneity. *Am J Human Genetics* 1991;49:764.

Haller JA, Knox DL. Vitrectomy for persistent vitreous hemorrhage from a cavernous hemangioma of the optic disk. *Am J Ophthalmol* 1993;116:106.

Hussain SE, Hussain N, Boniuk M, Font RL. Malignant nonteratoid medulloepithelioma of the ciliary body in an adult. *Ophthalmology* 1998;105:596.

Irvine F, O'Donnell N, Kemp E, Lee WR. Retinal vasoproliferative tumors. Surgical management and histological findings. *Arch Ophthalmol* 2000;118:563.

Jampel HD, Schachat AP, Conway B, et al. Retinal pigment epithelial hyperplasia assuming tumor-like proportions. Report of two cases. *Retina* 1986;6:105.

Kasner L, Traboulsi EI, Delacruz Z, Green WR. A histopathologic study of the pigmented fundus lesions in familial adenomatous polyposis. *Retina* 1992;12:35.

Kivela T, Tarkkanen A. Recurrent medulloepithelioma of the ciliary body. Immunohistochemical characteristics. *Ophthalmology* 1988;95:1565.

Kreusel KM, Bornfeld N, Lommatzsch A, et al. Ruthenium-106 brachytherapy for peripheral retinal capillary hemangioma. *Ophthalmology* 1998;105:1386.

Lafaut BA, Meire FM, Leys AM, et al. Vasoproliferative retinal tumors associated with peripheral chorioretinal scars in presumed congenital toxoplasmosis. *Graefes Arch Clin Exp Ophthalmol* 1999;237: 1033.

Landau K, Dossetor F, Hoyt WF, Muci-Mendoza R. Retinal hamartoma in neurofibromatosis 2. *Arch Ophthalmol* 1990;108:329.

Leonardy NJ, Rupani M, Dent G, Klintworth GK. Analysis of 135 autopsy eyes for ocular involvement in leukemia. *Am J Ophthalmol* 1990;109:436.

Leys AM, Van Eyck LM, Nuttin BJ, et al. Metastatic carcinoma to the retina: clinicopathologic findings in two cases. *Arch Ophthalmol* 1990;108:1448.

Lloyd WC, Eagle RC, Shields JA, et al. Congenital hypertrophy of the retinal pigment epithelium. Electron microscopic and morphometric observations. *Ophthalmology* 1990;97:1052.

Mack HG, Jakobiec FA. Isolated metastases to the retina or optic nerve. *Int Ophthalmol Clin* 1997;37:251.

Maher ER, Kaelin WG. von Hippel–Lindau disease. *Medicine* 1997;76:381.

Maher ER, Moore AT. von Hippel–Lindau disease. *Br J Ophthalmol* 1992;76:743.

McCabe CM, Mieler WF. Six-year follow-up of an idiopathic retinal vasoproliferative tumor. *Arch Ophthalmol* 1996;114:617.

McDonald HR, Schatz H, Johnson RN, et al. Vitrectomy in eyes with peripheral retinal angioma associated with traction macular detachment. *Ophthalmology* 1996;103:329.

Medlock RD, Shields JA, Shields CL, et al. Retinal hemangioma-like lesions in eyes with retinitis pigmentosa. *Retina* 1990;10:274.

Messmer EP, Heinrich T, Hoepping W, deSutter E, Havers W, Sauerweim W. Risk factors for metastases in patients with retinoblastoma. *Ophthalmology* 1991;98:136.

Messmer EP, Fritze J, Mohr C, et al. Long-term treatment effects in patients with bilateral retinoblastoma: ocular and mid-facial findings. *Graefes Arch Clin Exp Ophthalmol* 1991;229:309.

Meyers SM, Gutman FA, Kaye LD, Rothner AD. Retinal changes associated with neurofibromatosis 2. *Trans Am Ophthalmol Soc* 1995;93:245.

Moore AT, Maher ER, Rosen P, et al. Ophthalmological screening for von Hippel–Lindau disease. *Eye* 1991;5:723.

Mohney BG, Robertson DM. Ancillary testing for metastasis in patients with newly diagnosed retinoblastoma. *Am J Ophthalmol* 1994;118:707.

Mullaney PB, Jacquemin C, Abboud E, Karcioglu ZA. Tuberous sclerosis in infancy. *J Pediatr Ophthalmol Strabismus* 1997;34:372.

Murphree AL, Villablanca JG, Deegan WF, et al. Chemotherapy plus local treatment in the management of intraocular retinoblastoma. *Arch Ophthalmol* 1996;114:1348.

Niemela M, Lemeta S, Sainio M, et al. Hemangioblastomas of the retina: impact of von Hippel–Lindau disease. *Invest Ophthalmol Vis Sci* 2000;41:1909.

Nikaido H, Mishima H, Ono H, et al. Leukemic involvement of the optic nerve. *Am J Ophthalmol* 1988;105:294.

Nork M, Ghobrial MW, Peyman GA, Tso MOM. Massive retinal gliosis. A reactive proliferation of Müller cells. *Arch Ophthalmol* 1986;104:1383.

Nyboer JH, Robertson DM, Gomez MR. Retinal lesions in tuberous sclerosis. *Arch Ophthalmol* 1976;94:1277.

Ohkoski K, Tsiaras WG. Prognostic importance of ophthalmic manifestations in childhood leukemia. *Br J Ophthalmol* 1992;76:651.

O'Keefe M, Fulcher T, Kelly P, et al. Medulloepithelioma of the optic nerve head. *Arch Ophthalmol* 1997;115:1325.

Olsen TW, Frayer WC, Myers FL, et al. Idiopathic reactive hyperplasia of the retinal pigment epithelium. *Arch Ophthalmol* 1999;117:50.

Palmer JD, Gragoudas ES. Advances in treatment of retinal angiomas. *Int Ophthalmol Clin* 1997;37:159.

Paulino AC. Trilateral retinoblastoma: is the location of the intracranial tumor important? *Cancer* 1999;86:135.

Peterson K, Gordon KB, Heinemann MB, DeAngelis LM. The clinical spectrum of ocular lymphoma. *Cancer* 1993;72:843.

Peyman GA, Rednam KRV, Mottow-Lippa L, Flood T. Treatment of large von Hippel tumors by eye wall resection. *Ophthalmology* 1983;90:840.

Peterson K, Gordon KB, Heinemann MB, DeAngelis LM. The clinical spectrum of ocular lymphoma. *Cancer* 1993;72:843.

Pollack IF, Lunsford LD, Flickinger JC, Dameshek HL. Prognostic factors in the diagnosis and treatment of primary central nervous system lymphoma. *Cancer* 1989;63:939.

Reddy SC, Quah SH, Low HC, Jackson N. Prognostic significance of retinopathy at presentation in adult acute leukemia. *Ann Hematol* 1998;76:15.

Renardel de Lavalette VW, Cruysberg JRM, Deutman AF. Familial congenital grouped pigmentation of the retina. *Am J Ophthalmol* 1991;112:406.

Ridley ME, McDonald HR, Sternberg P, Blumenkranz MS, Zarbin MA, Schachat AP. Retinal manifestations of ocular lymphoma (reticulum cell sarcoma). *Ophthalmology* 1992;99:1153.

Ridley M, Green J, Johnson G. Retinal angiomatosis: the ocular manifestations of von Hippel–Lindau disease. *Can J Ophthalmol* 1986;21:276.

Ruhswurm I, Zehetmayer M, Till P, et al. Kavern ses H mangiom der Papille: klinische und echographische Befunde. *Klin Monatsbl Augenheilkd* 1996;209:380.

Sahel JA, Frederick AR, Pesavento R, Albert DM. Idiopathic retinal gliosis mimicking a choroidal melanoma. *Retina* 1988;8:282.

Saleh RA, Gross S, Cassano W, Gee A. Metastatic retinoblastoma successfully treated with immunomagnetic purged autologous bone marrow transplantation. *Cancer* 1988;62:2301.

Schachat AP, Shields JA, Fine SL, et al. Combined hamartomas of the retina and retinal pigment epithelium. *Ophthalmology* 1984;91:1609.

Schachat AP, Markowitz JA, Guyer DR, Burke PJ, Karp JE, Graham ML. Ophthalmic manifestations of leukemia. *Arch Ophthalmol* 1989;107:697.

Shields CL, Santos MCM, Diniz W, et al. Thermotherapy for retinoblastoma. *Arch Ophthalmol* 1999;117:885.

Shields CL, Shields JA, De Potter P, et al. Plaque radiotherapy in the management of retinoblastoma: use as a primary and secondary treatment. *Ophthalmology* 1993;100:216.

Shields JA, Shields CL, Singh AD. Metastatic neoplasms in the optic disc. *Arch Ophthalmol* 2000;118:217.

Shields JA, Shields CL, Singh AD. Acquired tumors arising from congenital hypertrophy of the retinal pigment epithelium. *Arch Ophthalmol* 2000:118:637.

Shields JA, Eagle RC, Shields CL, De Potter P. Congenital neoplasms of the nonpigmented ciliary epithelium (medulloepithelioma). *Ophthalmology* 1996;103:1998.

Shields JA, Decker WL, Sanborn GE, Augsburger JJ, Goldberg RE. Presumed acquired retinal hemangiomas. *Ophthalmology* 1983;90:1292.

Singh AD, Santos MCM, Shields CL, et al. Observations on 17 patients with retinocytoma. *Arch Ophthalmol* 2000;118:199.

Smith BJ, O'Brien JM. The genetics of retinoblastoma and current diagnostic testing. *J Pediatr Ophthalmol Strabismus* 1996;33:120.

Traboulsi EI, Krush AJ, Gardner EJ, et al. Prevalence and importance of pigmented ocular fundus lesions in Gardner's syndrome. *N Engl J Med* 1987;316:661.

Tsai P, O'Brien JM. Combined hamartoma of the retina and retinal pigment epithelium as the presenting sign of neurofibromatosis-1. *Ophthalmic Surg Lasers* 2000;31:145.

Vadmal M, Kahn E, Finger P, Teichberg S. Nonteratoid medulloepithelioma of the retina with electron microscopic and immunohistochemical characterization. *Pediatr Pathol Lab Med* 1996;16:663.

Watzke RC. Cryotherapy for retinal angiomatosis. A clinicopathologic report. *Arch Ophthalmol* 1974;92:399.

Webster AR, Maher ER, Moore AT. Clinical characterization of ocular angiomatosis in von Hippel–Lindau disease and correlation with germline mutation. *Arch Ophthalmol* 1999;117:371.

Whitcup SM, deSmet MD, Rubin BI, et al. Intraocular lymphoma. Clinical and histopathologic diagnosis. *Ophthalmology* 1993;100:1399.

Whitcup SM, Stark-Vancs V, Wittes RE, et al. Association of interleukin-10 in the vitreous and cerebrospinal fluid and primary central nervous system lymphoma. *Arch Ophthalmol* 1997;115:1157.

Wittebol-Post D, Hes FJ, Lips CJM. The eye in von Hippel–Lindau disease. Long-term follow-up of screening and treatment: recommendations. *J Intern Med* 1998;243:555.

Zimmer-Galler IE. Robertson DM. Long-term observation of retina lesions in tuberous sclerosis. *Am J Ophthalmol* 195;119:318.

CHAPTER 8

Intraocular Inflammation

Jonathan B. Belmont
David H. Fischer

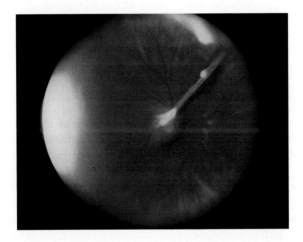

Wide-angle postvitrectomy photograph of a young patient with ocular toxocariasis. The characteristic falciform fold still is evident and the three yellowish areas along the fold and peripheral to it represent areas of residual scar from the release of traction attachments during vitrectomy. There is a serous detachment around the disc.

ANTERIOR UVEITIS

Acute Nongranulomatous Anterior Uveitis
Chronic Iridocyclitis in Juvenile Rheumatoid Arthritis

INTERMEDIATE UVEITIS

Pars Planitis
Fuchs' Heterochromic Cyclitis

POSTERIOR UVEITIS

Toxoplasmosis
Toxocariasis
Candida Retinitis
Cytomegalovirus Retinitis
Acute Multifocal Posterior Placoid Epitheliopathy
Acute Retinal Necrosis Syndrome
Bird-Shot Vitiliginous Chorioretinitis
Ocular Histoplasmosis Syndrome

DIFFUSE UVEITIS

Sarcoidosis

Sympathetic Ophthalmia
Vogt-Koyanagi-Harada Syndrome
Behçet's Disease
Lyme Disease
Syphilis
Tuberculosis
Acquired Immunodeficiency Syndrome

MASQUERADE SYNDROMES

Intraocular Foreign Body
Large Cell Lymphoma
Leukemia

POSTERIOR SCLERITIS

ENDOPHTHALMITIS

Endogenous Endophthalmitis
Exogenous Endophthalmitis

Uveitis is a general term denoting intraocular inflammation that either primarily or secondarily involves one (or more) components of the uveal tract. Although components of the uveal tract are comprised of the iris, ciliary body, and choroid, all layers of the eye may be involved by inflammation. Because the uveal tract is supplied by the systemic circulation, systemic diseases and local diseases that affect blood vessels can involve the uvea as well as contiguous ocular tissues and structures.

Classification of uveitis relates to the area or anatomic structure(s) involved, as well as to time course (i.e., acute, chronic, acute recurrent, and chronic recurrent), laterality (i.e., unilateral or bilateral), character of inflammation (i.e., nongranulomatous or granulomatous), and associated findings (e.g., glaucoma, cystoid macular edema, etc.). Uveitis may also be classified as either endogenous or exogenous in nature. Frequently, all of the above parameters are combined to provide a detailed and precise description of the ocular inflammation present in any given patient, a process called "naming." Naming of the inflammatory process is the first step in diagnosis and management in that it allows narrowing of the differential diagnosis by providing a specific and discrete set of clinical findings to "match" against the known clinical findings of various uveitic entities and syndromes. For example, a patient presenting with acute, unilateral, nongranulomatous iridocyclitis would be "matched" with those clinical entities known to present with a compatible clinical picture, narrowing the differential diagnosis, helping to direct a diagnostic workup, and assisting in formulation of initial therapy.

From the standpoint of uveitis classification, it is also frequently helpful to think of eye inflammation by compartmentalizing the eye. The anterior segment has a specific subset of diseases that are common to that area; acute iritis and iridocyclitis are the most common forms of *anterior uveitis.*

Most forms of anterior uveitis are characterized by episodes of pain, redness, and photophobia, and a tendency for synechiae formation. Iritis refers to inflammation of the iris. If the ciliary body is also involved, the condition is called iridocyclitis. Inflammation of the intermediate area or midzone of the eye is classified as *intermediate uveitis*; the pars planitis syndrome is an example. *Posterior uveitis* affects the deeper tissues, such as the retina and choroid; ocular toxoplasmosis and cytomegalovirus (CMV) retinitis are examples of posterior uveitis. Posterior uveitis syndromes characteristically occur without episodes of pain, redness, or photophobia, and floaters—with or without blurring of vision—frequently herald their onset. Choroiditis refers to inflammation primarily in the choroid. Because the choroid is contiguous with (and may involve) the retina, the condition may also be called chorioretinitis or, if the retina is the primary locus of inflammation, retinochoroiditis. *Diffuse uveitis* refers to intraocular inflammation that affects the front and back of the eye; conditions such as sarcoidosis can manifest in this manner. The clinical features of some diseases may fit more than one of these compartmental classifications.

The terms nongranulomatous and granulomatous are pathologic terms that denote Boyd's cellular response to an inciting agent. Lymphocytes, polymorphonuclear leukocytes, and plasma cells are found in nongranulomatous uveitis, and epithelioid and giant cells characterize granulomatous disease. A typical clinical picture is associated with each form. Nongranulomatous uveitis is usually anterior, has an acute onset, exhibits fine keratic precipitates (KPs), and often resolves with aggressive corticosteroid therapy or, sometimes, even spontaneously. The onset of granulomatous uveitis is often insidious, and the disorder frequently has a chronic course and is characterized by large "mutton-fat" KPs, Koeppe and Busacca nodules, and retinal vascular sheathing (Figs. 8.1, 8.2, 8.3). There is considerable overlap

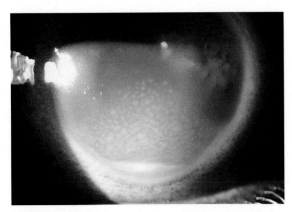

FIGURE 8.1 Anterior granulomatous uveitis in the left eye of a 26-year-old African-American man is indicated by a dependent accumulation of white cells (i.e., hypopyon), mutton-fat keratic precipitates, and a superotemporal Busacca nodule.

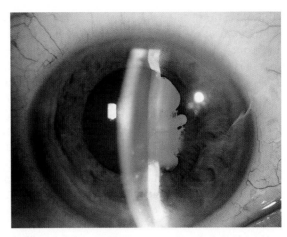

FIGURE 8.3. Slit lamp photograph demonstrating the characteristic anterior segment findings of granulomatous uveitis including keratic precipitates, posterior synechiae, and Koeppe nodules along the pupillary border. The presence of flare and cells is demonstrated by fluorescein in the anterior chamber.

in the clinical presentation of these types, but it is still valuable for the clinician to think in these terms. This method of classification suggests certain underlying causes, enabling a more focused diagnostic evaluation.

The causes of uveitis include infectious agents (e.g., bacteria, protozoa, viruses, and spirochetes) and immunologic conditions in which the immune response initiates and potentiates acute and/or chronic inflammation. Underlying conditions may be related to the intraocular inflammation. Systemic diseases such as sarcoidosis or rheumatoid arthritis and infectious conditions such as syphilis or CMV infection in patients with acquired immunodeficiency syndrome (AIDS) may manifest primarily in the eye. Clinical and laboratory workups may help to elucidate the underlying problem.

In many cases, prompt and accurate diagnosis and appropriate therapeutic intervention can control or resolve inflammation and prevent the inflammatory sequelae of intraocular scarring, which may otherwise lead to complications or visual loss. Primary immune-related processes

are usually treated with antiinflammatory agents. Corticosteroids are most commonly used for eye disease, and can be administered topically, in the form of periocular injections, or systemically through oral or intravenous routes. For some conditions, antiinfectious and antiinflammatory agents may be combined. The rationale is to treat the infectious and inflammatory components together to eradicate the disease promptly and reduce intraocular scarring. A biopsy of appropriate eye tissues may yield useful information in selected cases. Although uncommon, anterior chamber taps, vitreous taps, or partial-thickness eye wall biopsies may help to identify potentially irreversible, vision-threatening forms of disease.

ANTERIOR UVEITIS

Acute Nongranulomatous Anterior Uveitis

Acute nongranulomatous anterior uveitis, commonly referred to as iritis or iridocyclitis, affects the front part of the eye. This form is the most common of all uveitis syndromes. Acute nongranulomatous anterior uveitis often is associated with the histocompatibility antigen HLA-B27 and linked with a predisposition for developing ankylosing spondylitis. Ninety percent of the patients who have the two diseases concomitantly are also positive for the HLA-B27 marker. Other diseases associated with this form of acute ocular inflammation include ulcerative colitis, Crohn's disease, Reiter's syndrome, psoriatic arthritis, and gastroenteropathies secondary to *Yersinia* and *Klebsiella pneumoniae* infections. These disease associations should be looked for in any individual presenting with acute nongranulomatous anterior uveitis. The HLA-B27 genotype is often the link that binds them together.

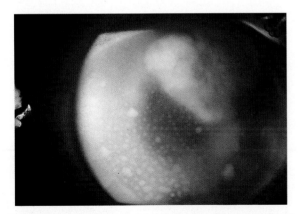

FIGURE 8.2. The right eye of the patient in Figure 8.1, showing typical granulomatous keratic precipitates on the posterior corneal surface inferiorly and a large iris granuloma (i.e., Busacca nodule) superiorly. Although cellular haze prevents sharp focus, synechiae formation around the pupil from Koeppe nodules completes the classic picture of granulomatous inflammation.

Clinical Features. The hallmark of acute nongranulomatous anterior uveitis is acute inflammation characterized by intense redness, pain, photophobia caused by ciliary spasm, and diminished vision, which usually prompts the individual to visit a physician. Symptoms generally evolve over hours to days. Findings include hyperemia of the conjunctival vessels, especially the ciliary zone; multiple fine clear keratic precipitates; intense cell and flare reaction in the anterior chamber; and in severe cases a dependent accumulation of cells, called hypopyon (see Fig. 8.1). If untreated, posterior synechiae form between the pupil margin and the lens, fixing the pupil in a moderately miotic position (Fig. 8.4). If the posterior synechiae encompass 360 degrees of the pupil, aqueous flow into the anterior chamber is blocked, resulting in the iris bowing forward, a condition called iris bombé (Fig. 8.5). The resulting closed anterior chamber angle causes an acute rise in intraocular pressure. In most cases of acute anterior uveitis, the intraocular pressure is diminished because of ciliary body dysfunction. Occasionally, intense inflammation can cause a rise in intraocular pressure despite an open angle because of acute trabeculitis. Acute inflammation of the iris vessels may cause their dilation and confuse the diagnosis with rubeosis iridis (Fig. 8.6). Prompt antiinflammatory therapy restores normal architecture.

The inflammatory cells and debris in the anterior segment can make fundus examination difficult. The posterior segment of the eye is generally normal, although cystoid macular edema may occur, especially in patients with severe anterior segment inflammation. If the inflammation is only partially treated or becomes subacute, spillover of inflammatory cells and debris into the vitreous may occur, and may contribute to blurring of vision. Most patients seek attention promptly because of the pain or an acute decrease in vision.

Management. The management of acute nongranulomatous anterior uveitis involves the intensive use of cyclo-

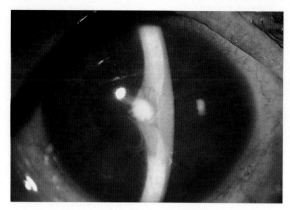

FIGURE 8.5. Iris bombé.

plegic and steroidal agents, and the secret to successful therapy is prompt aggressive treatment. Cycloplegics such as 1% Cyclogyl administered four times daily or, in severe cases, 1% Atropine administered four times daily help to dilate the pupil, relieve ciliary spasm, and reduce pain. However, a side effect of this therapy is blurred near-range vision, which may incapacitate younger individuals. Fortunately, these effects are dose dependent. Topical steroids are the primary antiinflammatory agents, with an initial treatment rate of one drop every hour while awake. If no improvement occurs within 24 to 48 hours, high-dose topical steroid therapy can be supplemented with subconjunctival injections of intermediate-acting steroids or occasionally supplemented with a short course of high-dose oral steroid therapy (60 to 100 mg/day in divided doses). If an infectious process is identified, appropriate antibiotic or antiviral therapy should be started.

The prognosis for the cessation of inflammation is uniformly good, but in severe or recalcitrant cases it may take weeks to months for the inflammatory cycle to resolve completely. Recurrences of inflammation, usually developing in

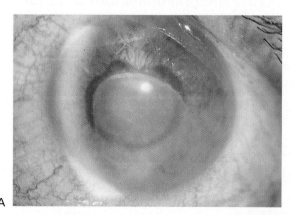

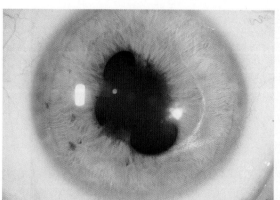

A

B

FIGURE 8.4. **A:** The rapid onset of pain, photophobia, redness, tearing, and diminished vision are classic features of acute iridocyclitis. The photograph shows the fibrin membrane generated by transudation from acutely inflamed tissues. Synechiae involve most of the lens but are partially broken superiorly. **B:** Inactive iridocyclitis. The eye is white and noninflamed, but telltale synechiae formation and pigment are seen on the lens capsule, producing a scalloped or irregular pupil that is characteristic of a prior acute uveitis process.

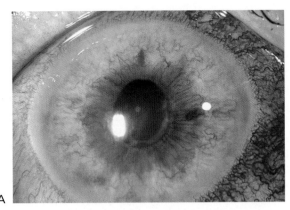 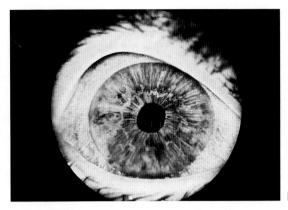

A   B

FIGURE 8.6. A: Acute iridocyclitis. Dilated iris vessels can often change the coloration of the iris. The conjunctiva, especially along the limbus, is intensely red. Iris details are slightly hazy because of anterior segment inflammation. Synechiae are seen with the fibrin membrane along the inferior aspects of the pupil. **B:** An iris fluorescein angiogram of the patient in **(A)** demonstrates the dilated vessels but normal anatomy of the iris. This is a common sequela of subacute iridocyclitis.

a stereotypical manner, are not uncommon, and the patient should be counseled to seek prompt attention if this occurs.

The disease process is usually seen in teenagers and young or middle-aged adults, and it has a tendency to become less intense in the later years. Sometimes, only one or two bouts occur during a lifetime, although a higher recurrence rate is more common.

Chronic Iridocyclitis of Juvenile Rheumatoid Arthritis

Chronic iridocyclitis associated with juvenile rheumatoid arthritis is an indolent, smoldering disease that usually begins between ages 3 and 15, occurring more often in girls than boys.

Clinical Features. Affected individuals are frequently unaware of the low-grade inflammation, because minimal red-

ness or pain occurs. A parent often notices an irregular pupil, or a school screening finds diminished vision, bringing the individual under medical supervision. The clinical findings are the direct antithesis of acute anterior nongranulomatous uveitis. Evaluation discloses a low-grade inflammatory process with small, white KPs, sometimes with a low-grade granulomatous response (Fig. 8.7). Examination often reveals synechiae, and the pupil can be small or irregular, with scalloped edges seen on dilation. Band keratopathy is frequently noted in patients with longstanding chronic inflammation.

This form of anterior uveitis is chronic and indolent in nature, often with minimal symptoms manifested over months to years. Cataract formation is not an unusual finding, and secondary glaucoma of an indolent nature is a feared complication (Fig. 8.8). The hallmark of this low-grade intraocular inflammation and systemic disease is the

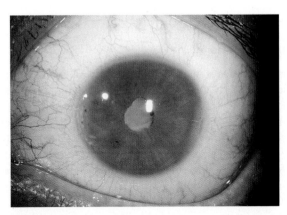

FIGURE 8.7. Chronic iridocyclitis secondary to juvenile rheumatoid arthritis. Patchy, irregular pupillary dilation with pigment along the lens capsule suggests breakage of old synechiae. The media are relatively clear, although band keratopathy is evident at the 3- and 9-o'clock positions on the peripheral cornea. The findings of a white eye and band keratopathy are characteristic of chronic iridocyclitis secondary to juvenile rheumatoid arthritis.

FIGURE 8.8. Secondary cataract as a result of chronic iridocyclitis in juvenile rheumatoid arthritis. The white, noninflamed eye has some subtle limbal calcium deposits at the 3- and 9-o'clock positions. Synechiae have formed, except for a pupillary area at the 12-o'clock position. The advanced cataract is characteristic of the late-stage sequelae of chronic inflammation related to juvenile rheumatoid arthritis.

pauciarticular form of rheumatoid arthritis seen in juveniles. Although the joint involvement usually precedes eye inflammation, it may occur years after the uveitis is diagnosed. Generally, the wrists, ankles, or knees are involved by mild inflammation. Two to five joints may be affected.

The diagnosis is based on the characteristic ocular and systemic clinical features and on serology testing. These individuals are generally rheumatoid factor negative and antinuclear antibody positive. Conditions that must be excluded include sarcoidosis and spirochetal diseases.

Management. The management of this form of chronic iridocyclitis involves the use of cycloplegics to prevent synechiae formation. Because this is a long-term disease process, the extended use of a cycloplegic, such as Atropine, may be indicated to keep the pupil from binding and producing secondary complications such as iris bombé. Typically, one to four drops daily of low-dose topical steroids are needed to reduce the potential for side effects of the inflammation. Long-term steroid use, however, is associated with the risks of cataract formation and glaucoma. Over many years of treatment, these are the two most feared complications. The former may be successfully treated with intraocular surgery. If topical antiglaucoma medications are ineffective, surgery may also correct the latter condition. In end-stage disease, often occurring in the patient's later years, ciliary dysfunction and hypotony are the more sinister problems. This expected course has prompted some ophthalmologists to treat the initial and long-term disease aggressively with oral nonsteroidal anti-inflammatory agents or even with cytotoxic or alkylating medications to attempt to resolve all traces of inflammation. The rationale of aggressive treatment is that intraocular integrity may be better maintained over the many years the disease is present, but the added risks of aggressive treatment make this approach controversial.

INTERMEDIATE UVEITIS

Pars Planitis

Pars planitis syndrome is a bilateral ocular inflammatory disease that usually affects otherwise healthy young people of grade-school through college age. The condition goes by many names, including intermediate uveitis, peripheral uveitis, and chronic cyclitis. The cause of pars planitis is usually idiopathic, although a small percentage of individuals have or may later develop associated demyelinating disease. Lyme disease has also been implicated in some patients.

Clinical Features. The main patient complaint concerns floaters, which are caused by a cellular reaction in the vitreous. There is usually minimal pain, redness, and photophobia. Slit lamp examination often reveals minimal aqueous cell and flare although moderate iritis may be present, especially during a flare-up of inflammation. Posterior synechiae

are uncommon, but may develop. Inflammatory cells are typically noted in the vitreous, posterior to the lens. The chronic, low-grade inflammation results in a buildup of cellular material at the vitreous base and over the pars plana (Fig. 8.9). This initially results in a whitish and congealed-appearing accumulation of cells in the inferior pars plana, a finding called "snowbanking" that is the distinctive feature of pars planitis (Fig. 8.10). Pars plana "snowbanking" is best visualized with indirect ophthalmoscopy and scleral depression or with a Goldman three-mirror lens. Retinal periphlebitis and edema of the disc and macula frequently exist in patients with active pars planitis.

Pars planitis generally pursues an indolent course, often punctuated with spontaneous exacerbations and remissions. For many individuals, the effects of the inflammation are annoying but do not significantly impair vision, although central vision may be severely compromised if macular edema occurs.

Management. Treatment usually consists of cautious observation in patients who do not have significant cystoid macular edema, severe or disabling floaters, or significant anterior segment inflammation. In those patients who do require treatment, use of intensive high-dose topical steroid therapy is often effective in gradually achieving control of the inflammation, and may be very useful in unmasking steroid responders for whom treatment with periocular injection with depot corticosteroid agents is contraindicated. Subtenons steroid injections and/or oral steroid therapy are often helpful in resolving or controlling inflammation that has not responded satisfactorily to high-dose topical steroid therapy. Treatment with stronger agents such as cyclosporine or alkylating agents is rarely indicated.

Complications include cataracts and a slightly higher incidence of retinal detachment, which can be treated surgically. The long-term prognosis is good, especially if the inflammation is mild. The disease may resolve, sometimes after many years' duration.

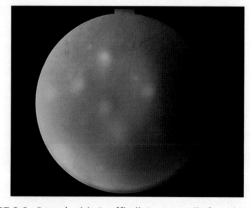

FIGURE 8.9. Pars planitis "puffballs" are usually found inferiorly and associated with peripheral periphlebitis. These fluffy exudates in the vitreous are commonly seen in patients with the pars planitis syndrome.

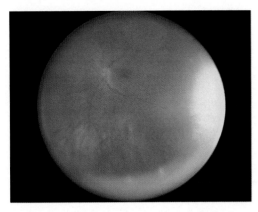

FIGURE 8.10. Pars planitis syndrome causes inferior "snowbanking" and precipitates along the inferior edge of the vitreous base, as seen in the wide-angle photograph with the transillumination light reflex at the periphery. Indirect ophthalmoscopy and scleral depression commonly are needed to evaluate this area.

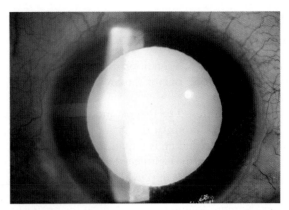

FIGURE 8.12. Fuchs' heterochromic cyclitis and cataract. This dense, mature cataract in a young individual is characteristic of one of the more common complications of Fuchs' heterochromic cyclitis.

Fuchs' Heterochromic Cyclitis

Fuchs' heterochromic cyclitis is a form of anterior and intermediate uveitis. The condition is usually unilateral and chronic in nature, and eventually results in iris heterochromia (a change in the color of the iris), as well as posterior subcapsular cataract in many patients. The cause of this disorder is unclear; it may be an immune-related process or a manifestation of a low-grade degenerative process.

Clinical Features. The classic presentation usually involves minimal symptoms and the findings of a low-grade aqueous cell and flare reaction; stellate, white, granulomatous KPs involving the entire endothelial surface; and over many years, a characteristic change in the surface contours and the coloration of the iris (Fig. 8.11). The age of onset is usually in the twenties to forties, with women slightly more

affected than men. Occasionally, floaters may be the presenting symptom. Loss of yellowish pigment within the iris stroma and subtle blunting of surface details of the iris stroma are seen early. With time, frank iris heterochromia develops, with generalized thinning and atrophy of the iris stroma. In blue-eyed individuals, this often results in the involved iris appearing darker than the noninvolved iris, since atrophy of the iris stroma allows the darkly pigmented underlying iris pigment epithelium to show through. In brown-eyed individuals, the involved iris often appears lighter in coloration than the iris in the noninvolved eye. The heterochromic iris is appreciated better in daylight. Although posterior synechiae are rare, glaucoma and cataract formation are long-term complications of the disease. Rare occurrences of occult-retained metallic intraocular foreign body may cause heterochromia from siderosis and may mimic iris heterochromia associated with Fuchs' heterochromic iridocyclitis; x-ray and computed axial tomography scan findings are generally useful in ruling out this entity.

Management. Fuchs' heterochromic cyclitis responds variably to topical steroids and cycloplegic or systemic steroids. The complications of long-term use of these drugs may at times outweigh their potential benefits. Many affected individuals can be followed routinely without treatment and reevaluated at 6-month intervals, although at times the iritis may be sufficiently active to warrant judicious treatment with topical steroids. The primary complications include cataract and secondary glaucoma (Fig. 8.12). Cataracts respond well to most forms of intraocular surgery, including the standard extracapsular procedures with intraocular lens implantation. Glaucoma control may be somewhat more problematic, with surgical options indicated for later forms of the disease. The long-term prognosis is good.

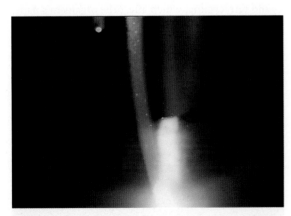

FIGURE 8.11. Stellate keratic precipitates from Fuchs' heterochromic cyclitis. Although difficult to photograph, these small, white, stellate keratic precipitates, with pseudopods along the edges, extend over the entire endothelial surface of the cornea. In conjunction with heterochromia, this is a classic feature of Fuchs' uveitis syndrome.

POSTERIOR UVEITIS

Toxoplasmosis

Ocular toxoplasmosis, a condition caused by an obligate intracellular parasite, is one of the more common forms of posterior uveitis.

Clinical Features. The toxoplasmosis organism, *Toxoplasma gondii*, is a protozoa that has a predilection for the retina. The classic finding is retinochoroiditis. The organism reaches the eye through hematogenous spread. Eating uncooked meats that are infected with *T. gondii* and ingesting the organism from aerosolized fecal material of infected cats are the more common ways in which the organism enters the human body. Usually, the immune system can bring the infection under control, and the infected individual may notice only flu-like symptoms. However, the organisms may enter the eye and cause localized disease.

The primary lesion is a localized zone of inflammation in the retina, manifested as a whitish-yellow area of retinal swelling with indistinct borders (Fig. 8.13). Cellular exudation into the overlying vitreous results in a hazy ophthalmoscopic view. The lesion may occur anywhere in the retina. In immunocompetent individuals, the infectious process usually heals spontaneously, with characteristic chorioretinal scarring and pigment proliferation (Fig. 8.14). Sometimes, months to years later, the edge of the scar may become reactivated. This clinical picture is the most common (Figs. 8.15 and 8.16).

The clinical findings are usually characteristic, but serologic testing may be helpful. In a primary infection, test results for immunoglobulin M (IgM) antibodies are usually positive for the first few months, followed by elevated immunoglobulin G (IgG) levels. However, over many years, because of the low level of systemic antibodies, the IgG level may be quite low, and a high index of suspicion based on the clinical findings may be more important than results of the serologic studies.

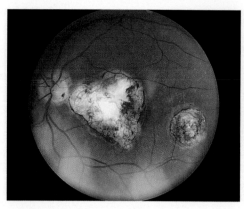

FIGURE 8.14. Full-thickness chorioretinal scars in a patient with recurrent ocular toxoplasmosis. The patient's vision has been reduced to the level of legal blindness. A peripheral scar is seen temporally in the macular area, but there is no active inflammation or infection.

In immunocompetent individuals, the body's own defense mechanisms are often capable of bringing the intraocular infection under control. However, the scars resulting from the infection may damage the eye. If the infection affects the macular area, irreversible visual loss may occur. If infection occurs near the optic nerve, secondary neuritis may develop and cause optic atrophy and sectoral visual field loss (Fig. 8.17). Lesions along blood vessels can obstruct arteries or veins, resulting in hemorrhage, macular, edema, and visual field loss (see opening figure). Peripheral lesions may heal without any apparent symptoms.

Management. Treatment is aimed at prompt resolution of the infectious process in vision-threatening areas. Classically, sulfadiazine and the folic acid antagonist pyrimethamine have been used. Folinic acid is administered to reduce the bone marrow toxicity of pyrimethamine. Antibiotics such as clindamycin, trimethoprim-sulfamethoxazole, and tetracycline, which affect the organism's pathways

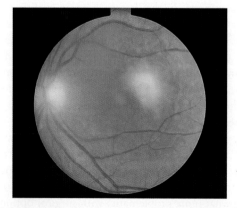

FIGURE 8.13. Acute toxoplasmosis retinochoroiditis in the macula of a 15-year-old Caucasian girl. Old toxoplasmosis scars were observed in the other eye. (Courtesy of Peter V. Palena, M.D., Philadelphia, PA.)

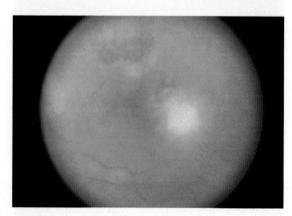

FIGURE 8.15. Acute, recurrent toxoplasmosis at the edge of a macular scar. The cellular reaction in the overlying vitreous results in hazy ophthalmoscopic views and gives the classic appearance of a "headlight in fog." (Courtesy of Peter V. Palena, M.D.)

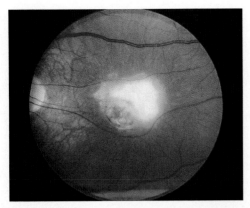

FIGURE 8.16. In this case of ocular toxoplasmosis with recurrent, active retinochoroiditis along the edge of an old macular scar in an early resolution stage, the overlying cellular exudation has cleared.

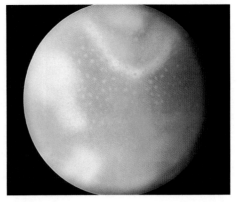

FIGURE 8.18. Chronic or recurrent ocular toxoplasmosis with endophthalmitic findings. The large geographic zones of retinochoroiditis shown superiorly are characteristic of chronic, low-grade endophthalmitic toxoplasmic choroiditis, which often occurs secondary to chronic steroid use. The small, white dots are granulomatous deposits of cells located along the back surface of the posterior hyaleid, analogous to the granulomatous keratic precipitates seen on the corneal endothelium.

of protein transcription, have been used. Corticosteroids have also been advocated for severe inflammation, although caution is indicated because high doses of these drugs, especially in the form of periocular injections, may be contraindicated because of their immunosuppressive action, which may potentiate the infectious process (Fig. 8.18).

The drugs used in the treatment of ocular toxoplasmosis may have significant side effects, and patients undergoing treatment must be closely monitored. Because the folic acid antagonists may cause bone marrow suppression, a platelet and complete blood count should be obtained at least weekly. With sulfadiazine, the rare but devastating complication of Stevens-Johnson syndrome must be watched for. Clindamycin may cause necrotizing enterocolitis, and tetracycline should not be prescribed for pregnant patients. Corticosteroids given topically or systemically are not without hazards. These treatment regimens, however, are often effective in reducing intraocular scarring and preserving visual function. For small, peripheral lesions or those that do not threaten vision, observation only may be a viable option.

Toxocariasis

Ocular toxocariasis is caused by the second stage larvae of *Toxocara canis* and *Toxocara cati*. *Toxocara canis* is a common intestinal parasite in dogs, and *Toxocara cati* is found in cats. Young individuals, from toddlers to teenagers, most frequently acquire the disease. Classically, the organism enters the body through the ingestion of dirt contaminated with *Toxocara* ova. The animal vector is usually an infected puppy.

Clinical Features. Unilateral blurring of vision is often the presenting symptom in ocular toxocariasis infection in children older than 2 years of age. In preverbal patients, leukokoria may be the only presenting symptom, and retinoblastoma must be excluded. A characteristic whitish dome-shaped granuloma is noted ophthalmoscopically (Fig. 8.19). Granuloma formation within the choroid results from hematogenous spread of *Toxocara* to the eye; anterior

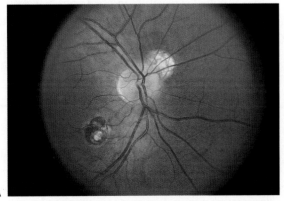

A

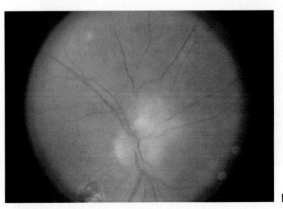

B

FIGURE 8.17. A: Juxtapapillary toxoplasmosis scar at the superonasal aspect of the right optic disc. **B:** Three years later, a lesion developed in the same area and involved the optic disc. (Courtesy of Peter V. Palena, M.D., Philadelphia, PA.)

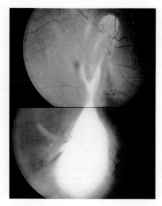

FIGURE 8.19. Traction retinal detachment with inferior peripheral granuloma secondary to ocular toxocariasis. A falciform fold has been created, dragging the optic nerve vessels inferiorly. The macular area is also dragged inferiorly, resulting in a secondary strabismus. (Courtesy of Jerry Shields, M.D., Philadelphia, PA.)

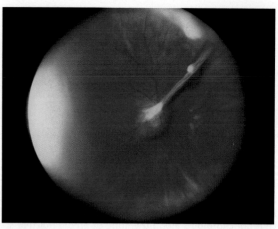

FIGURE 8.21. Wide-angle postvitrectomy photograph of a young patient with ocular toxocariasis. The characteristic falciform fold is still evident and the three yellowish areas along the fold and peripheral to it represent areas of residual scarring from the release of traction attachments during vitrectomy. There is a serous detachment around the disc.

uveitis and vitritis may be present or absent, but are generally severe in the endophthalmitis form of ocular toxocariasis. The granuloma may be peripheral or central (i.e., near or involving the macula; Fig. 8.20) or may involve the optic nerve head. Rarely, the organism may travel beneath the retina, creating "snail tracks." Most of the intraocular inflammation in ocular toxocariasis occurs after the death of the *Toxocara* larva and occurs as the eye reacts immunologically to antigens released from the dead or dying organism. Chronic inflammation leads to localized granuloma formation and may be associated with formation of retinal folds, vitreous traction bands, or generalized diffuse whitish inflammatory debris throughout the vitreous cavity (Fig. 8.21). In eyes with central lesions, destruction of the macular region or the optic nerve may cause a loss of vision.

Ocular toxocariasis is not associated with visceral larval migrans, a disease in which fever, hepatosplenomegaly, and

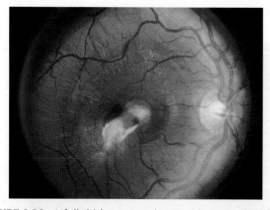

FIGURE 8.20. A full-thickness macular granuloma resulted from *Toxocara canis* infection and caused severe visual loss. All layers of the retina are involved by this condition. Secondary choroidal neovascularization may be a late sequela, as occurred in this case, producing the greenish appearance next to the old scar and mild degrees of subretinal blood.

systemic involvement occur. Ova and parasites are not present in stools, and the peripheral eosinophil count is characteristically normal. Intraocularly, eosinophilia may be found in the aqueous and vitreous if the eye fluids are sampled. The *Toxocara* antigen and antibody can also be detected in this manner. Unless secondary problems such as traction retinal detachment or opaque vitreous are encountered, intraocular biopsy for diagnostic and therapeutic reasons is usually unnecessary.

The outcome, depending on the intraocular location of the organism, can be quite good, and the disease is generally self-limited after the inflammatory process is quieted.

Management. Thiabendazole, the treatment of choice for visceral larval migrans, is not indicated for treatment of ocular toxocariasis because the organism has generally perished by the time that the eye changes are noted; secondary inflammation is responsible for the ocular symptoms and findings. Ocular inflammation may be self-limited in many cases, although active iritis and/or vitritis may require treatment with topical and/or periocular steroid injection. Vitrectomy may become a consideration in patients with chronic smoldering active inflammation, and removal of the antigen-laden vitreous in these patients often results in permanent quiescence of intraocular inflammation.

Candida Retinitis

Candida albicans retinitis is an uncommon disease seen in a specific clinical population that includes patients who are immunosuppressed as a result of disease or treatment of a disease that requires immunosuppressive therapy. Cancer patients receiving immunosuppressive agents, AIDS patients, patients with long-term indwelling catheters (e.g., hemodialysis, hyperalimentation), intravenous drug abusers, and debilitated patients are the most susceptible. The infection is usually indolent elsewhere in the body but spreads hematogenously to the eye.

Clinical Features. Multiple infectious foci initially develop within the choroid and secondarily involve the retina, appearing as multiple yellow-white spots. The infection subsequently spreads into the vitreous cavity. Intraocular inflammation evolves slowly, usually developing over a period of days to weeks, and the classic findings at diagnosis are small "puffballs" of localized fungal infection within the vitreous gel (Fig. 8.22). Symptoms may be minimal or nonexistent initially, although as the disease progresses, floaters become the most common complaint. If the organism affects the macular or parafoveal areas, diminished vision may also be a presenting symptom. Ocular candidal infection is often bilateral.

Management. The diagnosis is usually made by the characteristic clinical findings of puffballs in the vitreous, and is often confirmed by blood cultures or culture of a wound or catheter sample. If a diagnosis cannot be firmly established on the basis of blood, wound, or catheter cultures, diagnostic vitrectomy with staining and culture of the biopsy specimen usually demonstrates fungal organisms. Treatment involves administration of intravenous amphotericin B or oral fluconazole. Intravitreal injection of amphotericin B is often useful at the time of intraocular biopsy. The active infectious process generally responds promptly to antibiotic therapy. Depending on the intraocular location of the infection, scarring may be minimal, with complete return of vision. However, scars in the macular region may result in irreversible visual loss (Fig. 8.23). Because the affected individuals usually are quite ill from other causes, the ocular findings may not come to light until the systemic problems have been addressed. The ophthalmologist can be of great help in reducing visual problems by being alert to the characteristic pattern of the disease.

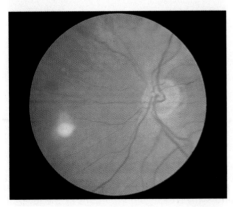

FIGURE 8.22. Candidal endophthalmitis. A candidal "puffball" is observed nasally in this immunocompromised patient on long-term intravenous therapy. The only complaint expressed by the patient was occasional floaters.

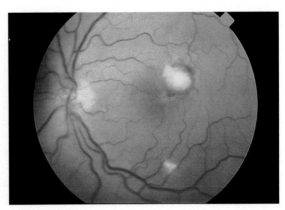

FIGURE 8.23. Candidal endophthalmitis with a macular lesion. Macular candidal infection causes gradual, progressive visual loss. Secondary scarring often prohibits good visual function. The small zone of blood at the superior edge suggested secondary choroidal neovascularization, which was confirmed angiographically.

Cytomegalovirus Retinitis

CMV infection of the retina and surrounding ocular structures is a condition usually found in immunosuppressed individuals. The immune system may be compromised by the disease itself or by the use of immunosuppressive agents. CMV retinitis is the most common cause of visual morbidity in persons with AIDS. In renal transplant patients, the most common infectious complication is systemic CMV infection, which may involve the retina and cause a necrotizing retinitis.

Clinical Features. The onset of CMV retinitis is frequently insidious in nature. Early symptoms may include low-grade floaters and/or painless worsening of vision in one or both eyes. Anterior segment reaction is usually absent. Ophthalmoscopic examination reveals patchy, bone-white or grayish-white areas of full-thickness retinitis. Hemorrhage is occasionally noted both within and along the margins of areas of retinitis. Retinitis may begin peripherally or posteriorly (Fig. 8.24A) and characteristically progresses by contiguous spread into adjacent areas of retina. As the infection spreads contiguously it leaves atrophic necrotic retina and retinal pigment epithelium in its wake, with retinal pigment epithelial hyperplasia and atrophy as well as retinal gliosis. Generally, the edges of the areas of infection are the areas of active infection and, given the observed pattern of progressive contiguous spread and advancement, are often referred to as a "brushfire border." Monitoring of the advancing edge of active infection is important in the management of CMV retinitis, since retinal function is effectively irretrievably lost in involved areas (Fig. 8.24B). Large areas of necrotic retina may result in retinal detachment. As in most cases of intraocular infection in immunocompromised patients, other opportunistic causes of infection should be excluded.

Management. Control of CMV retinitis depends on

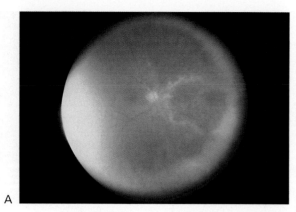 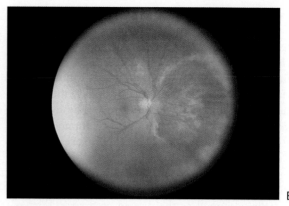

FIGURE 8.24. **A:** Cytomegalovirus (CMV) retinitis. Individuals who are immunocompromised because of disease or drug treatment are at risk of developing CMV retinitis. The wide-angle photograph demonstrates an area of retinitis nasal to the disc, with the active edge displaying a yellowish, patchy distribution. The central area of the lesion denotes destroyed retina, and the main ocular complaint was temporal visual loss, although central vision was 20/20. The transillumination light is evident at the periphery. **B:** CMV retinitis. The same individual, 2 months later, had progressive temporal visual loss and spreading of the active edge of the retinitis in a "brushfire" fashion.

prompt diagnosis. Indications for treatment are changing as new medications are discovered. Intravenous ganciclovir and foscarnet (Foscavir) remain the primary antiviral agents of choice. Oral ganciclovir has also been approved for use and in some patients can control advancing retinitis while avoiding both the inconvenience and the potential complications of intravenous drug delivery. Although they are virostatic, these agents are effective in controlling the progressive nature of the disease in many individuals. Remission usually occurs, but there may be exacerbations. The intraocular ganciclovir sustained-release implant (Vitrasert) can also be used to provide localized antiviral therapy for CMV retinitis, and intravitreal injections of ganciclovir are helpful if the implant is not available. Pars plana vitrectomy with silicone oil injection is often the initial surgical approach used for treating CMV-associated retinal detachments. Newer therapeutic agents are also under investigation.

The visual prognosis depends on the time of diagnosis and the amount of retina that has been damaged or destroyed. If the immune status can be returned to normal, CMV usually disappears through normal immune responses. In renal transplantation cases, reducing immunocompromising drugs can often halt the progression of CMV retinitis.

Acute Multifocal Posterior Placoid Epitheliopathy

Acute multifocal posterior placoid pigment epitheliopathy (AMPPE) is a descriptive term given to an unusual and relatively uncommon posterior segment inflammatory process. AMPPE generally occurs in adults, and often has its onset after a relatively mild nonspecific viral illness.

Clinical Features. The presenting symptoms are spots, floaters, and blurred vision in one or both eyes. Fundus examination reveals multiple yellowish to cream-colored areas that are approximately 1 disc diameter or smaller, scattered throughout the posterior pole, and occasionally seen in the periphery (Fig. 8.25). There may be associated low-grade vasculitis with a cellular reaction and vitritis. Occasionally, iridocyclitis is also seen. Symptoms may be severe if the plaques involve the central foveal zone. If the lesions are extrafoveal, the symptoms may be minimal. The disease is often bilateral.

Management. The disease is usually self-limited and resolves within 6 to 8 weeks, leaving subtle pigmentation in the areas of the cream-colored plaques. Treatment other than observation is controversial; corticosteroids may have a place in therapy if there are vision-threatening areas of in-

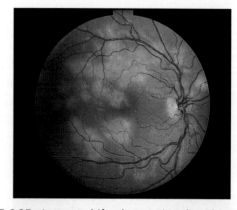

FIGURE 8.25. Acute, multifocal, posterior placoid epitheliopathy presents with cream-colored lesions at the level of the pigment epithelium and choriocapillaris, often after a viral illness. This individual's main complaint was fixed spots surrounding the central visual area. His acuity was 20/20 and remained so after the process healed.

volvement. Fluorescein angiography usually shows early blocked fluorescence and late hyperfluorescence and staining in the affected areas (Fig. 8.26). Rarely, cerebral vasculitis may be associated with the condition, and the clinician needs to be alert for this finding. The prognosis is good for the return of good functional vision, depending on the location of the initial lesions. In a small subgroup, the disease process may recur months to years later.

Acute Retinal Necrosis Syndrome

Acute retinal necrosis syndrome is a viral disease that affects immunocompetent individuals of any age. The condition is bilateral in one third of cases. The cause is unknown, although the varicella-zoster virus is considered the offending agent in most cases.

Clinical Features. Patients present with blurred vision and ocular pain in one or both eyes. The hallmark findings are small, opaque spots of grayish-white full-thickness retinitis in the retinal periphery and secondary vasculitis that is often obstructive (Fig. 8.27). Over a period of days, these spots increase in size and coalesce, resulting in a 360-degree involvement (Fig. 8.28) with subsequent extension into the posterior pole. In rare cases, the posterior pole can be affected earlier in the disease. Blindness can occur within weeks as the posterior pole becomes involved. Retinal detachment occurs in as many as one quarter of affected individuals (Fig. 8.29).

Management. Acyclovir, the agent of choice, is given intravenously for 7 to 10 days, and high-dose oral or parenteral steroid therapy is often employed. Concomitant aspirin therapy is recommended by many, and is felt to counter and minimize retinal ischemia due to associated retinal vasculitis. Prompt treatment with acyclovir is felt to minimize the chances for involvement of the fellow eye, and prolonged treatment with oral acyclovir for least several months is often recommended even after the acute phase of

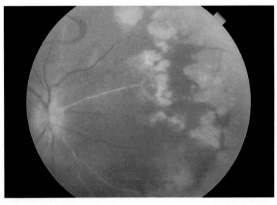

FIGURE 8.27. Acute retinal necrosis demonstrating the hallmark finding of grayish-white patches in the retinal periphery prior to becoming confluent. The arterioles are white due to immune reactants staining the arterial wall.

retinitis has responded to initial parenteral acyclovir therapy.

The visual prognosis can be good if the disease is discovered early. A high index of suspicion is critical, because a delayed diagnosis can result in visual loss. Small, peripheral retinal detachments can be walled off by photocoagulation. In severe cases, proliferative vitreoretinopathy may develop because of the large amount of tissue loss and pigment proliferation. Pars plana vitrectomy with silicone oil injection may be the only way to reattach the retina in this subgroup of patients.

Bird-Shot Vitiliginous Chorioretinitis

Bird-shot choroidopathy (sometimes referred to as vitiliginous choroidopathy) is an unusual and rare syndrome. Although its cause is unknown, this syndrome is frequently associated with positive test results for the HLA-29 antigen, and it usually affects middle-aged women.

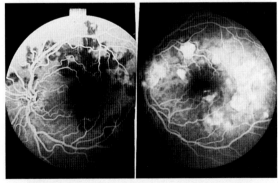

FIGURE 8.26. Fluorescein angiographic findings of acute, multifocal, posterior placoid epitheliopathy. The picture on the left shows the characteristic early-phase blockage of fluorescein caused by edema of the choriocapillaris, and the right photograph shows late staining of the inflamed areas. The person's visual acuity was 20/20.

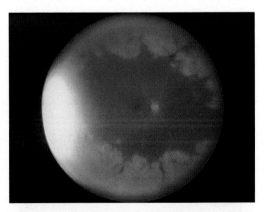

FIGURE 8.28. Acute retinal necrosis syndrome. This wide-angle photograph reveals the characteristic peripheral whitening of the retina from small spots of retinitis coalescing into broad areas. Vasculitis is also seen with whitening of the vessels and blood along the vessel borders.

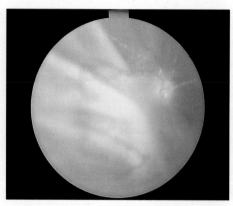

FIGURE 8.29. Acute retinal necrosis (ARN) syndrome and secondary retinal detachment. The classic findings of retinal detachment, seen in two thirds of individuals with ARN, are early fixed folds caused by a severe pigment epithelial response; white plaques in the arteries, thought to be immune reactants; and minimal compromise of the arterial circulation.

Clinical Features. The classic diagnostic feature of bird-shot vitiliginous chorioretinitis is cream-colored spots, often as large as 0.5 to 1 disc diameter, that are scattered throughout the fundus (Fig. 8.30). With time, these spots may coalesce. Associated with this is a low-level vasculitis and cystoid macular edema, with disc leakage demonstrated on fluorescein angiography. Iridocyclitis and a vitreous cellular reaction are other common features. The condition often lasts months to years and may be progressive. The complications of chronic ocular inflammation such as cystoid macular edema (CME) and cataract formation may adversely affect vision.

The diagnosis depends on the clinical picture. The HLA-29 genotype has been associated with bird-shot vitiliginous chorioretinitis in as many as 80% of affected persons. Other causes of chorioretinitis, such as spirochetal disease, sarcoidosis, and tuberculosis, must be excluded.

Management. Treatment consists of antiinflammatory drugs, including corticosteroids and, in recalcitrant cases, cyclosporine or other immunosuppressive agents. Although acyclovir has been suggested as concomitant therapy, controversy persists about adding this drug to the regimen. The poor prognosis reflects the chronicity of the disorder and frequent involvement of the macula. A thorough understanding of the cause of the condition is needed to design effective therapy.

Ocular Histoplasmosis Syndrome

The ocular histoplasmosis syndrome has been used to describe a primary choroidopathy thought to be caused by the fungus *Histoplasma capsulatum*. This organism is found most commonly in the Ohio River valley area but is also present in the Mid-Atlantic and Southeastern states. It is found in surface soil, particularly that which contains the droppings of certain birds. The organism is thought to be inhaled with the dust from a contaminated area.

Clinical Features. The classic findings are limited to the fundus and are manifested as the classic triad of small, whitish "punched-out" areas, peripapillary scarring, and choroidal neovascularization in the posterior segment (CNV; Fig. 8.31). The punched-out areas are less than 1 mm in diameter and can occur anywhere in the fundus. Vitreous inflammation is notably absent. The scarring adjacent to the disc is manifested by chorioretinal atrophy and a rim of pigment at the disc margin. Submacular choroidal neovascularization is manifested initially as a thickened, gray-green area deep to the retina. Fluorescein angiography is essential in delineating the location and extent of the choroidal neovascular membrane. Hemorrhage from the choroidal neovascular membrane and subsequent disciform scarring are vision-threatening complications (Fig. 8.32).

Patients are asymptomatic unless macular involvement develops, in which case central vision can be lost. There is no anterior segment reaction.

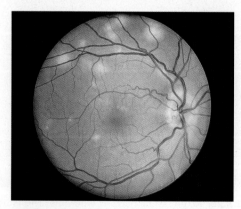

FIGURE 8.30. Bird-shot choroiditis. The classic finding is a creamy yellow, multifocal choroiditis. The central vision is excellent; the patient's main complaints were floaters and peripheral spots.

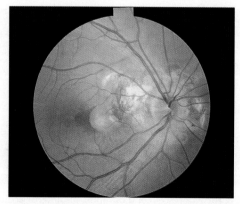

FIGURE 8.31. Presumed ocular histoplasmosis syndrome. The classic findings of juxtapapillary chorioretinal scars and macular scarring, with a greenish yellow area and blood along the edge, fulfill the clinical picture of choroidal neovascularization. Peripheral scars are often seen.

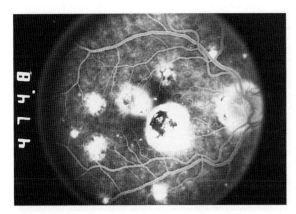

FIGURE 8.32. Fluorescein angiogram of an eye with presumed ocular histoplasmosis syndrome. Macular scars are present from old choroidal neovascularization, which has cicatrized but has destroyed central vision. Peripheral scars and juxtapapillary chorioretinal scars are also seen in this photograph.

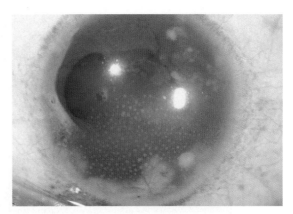

FIGURE 8.33. Anterior segment granulomatous involvement in a case of ocular sarcoidosis. White, mutton-fat, granulomatous keratic precipitates; nodules in the iris stroma (i.e., Busacca nodules); a low-grade cellular response; and adhesions of the pupil to the lens (i.e., synechiae formation secondary to Koeppe nodules) were found in this African-American patient with chronic sarcoid iridocyclitis.

Management. Careful and ongoing assessment of macular function using an Amsler grid and careful periodic inspection of the macula are necessary for patients suspected of having choroidal neovascular involvement and for those previously treated for choroidal neovascularization. Fluorescein angiography plays a crucial role in the diagnosis and follow-up of these patients.

Choroidal neovascularization in the ocular histoplasmosis syndrome is treated with laser photocoagulation, similar to that used in age-related macular degeneration. Vitrectomy with extraction of the choroidal neovascular membrane is often successful in restoring macular function in patients with subfoveal choroidal neovascularization that cannot be treated with conventional laser therapy. Photodynamic therapy may also be a useful treatment option in patients with subfoveal choroidal neovascularization. Systemic antifungal treatment has not proven to be helpful.

DIFFUSE UVEITIS

Sarcoidosis

Sarcoidosis is a multisystem systemic disease of unknown cause in which lymphoid tissue develops noncaseating, granulomatous inflammation. Usually, sarcoidosis is a disease that affects 20- to 40-year-old individuals, with persons of African descent and women more predisposed than other patient subgroups. The lungs are the most frequently involved organs, but the skin, liver, spleen, joints, and heart may also be involved. Ocular involvement occurs in 17% of cases of systemic involvement. Ocular sarcoidosis can take many forms, but it is often the presenting sign of the systemic disease.

Clinical Features. Acute iridocyclitis may be the earliest form of sarcoid uveitis. Patients complain of ocular pain, photophobia, and redness, and on slit lamp examination,

flare and cells are seen in the anterior chamber. The uveitis may be granulomatous or nongranulomatous. Fine, gray KPs initially may be seen on the posterior surface of the cornea. The condition often becomes chronic, and mutton-fat KPs develop as the disease process continues. The granulomatous nature of sarcoidosis is responsible for some of the ocular features, including conjunctival granulomas, mutton-fat KPs, Busacca nodules within the iris stroma, and Koeppe nodules along the pupil margin (Fig. 8.33).

Posterior segment findings in ocular sarcoidosis may include vitritis, pars plana snowbanking, cyclitis, choroiditis, optic neuritis, cystoid macular edema, retinal arteritis, retinal phlebitis, and optic nerve granulomas (Figs. 8.34; 8.35A, B). All or none of these may be found. White, fluffy opacities may be seen in the inferior vitreous, and yellow-white exudates, called candle-wax drippings, and sheathing of the peripheral retinal veins may be seen (Fig. 8.36).

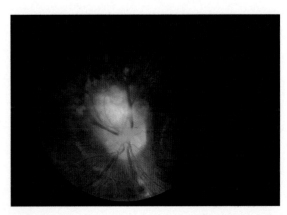

FIGURE 8.34. Optic nerve granuloma. Granulomatous disease can involve the optic nerve, producing a large blind spot and diminished visual function. A granuloma is seen off the superior border of the papilla.

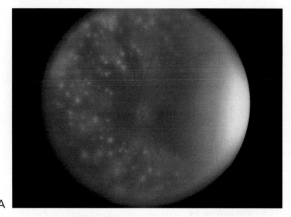
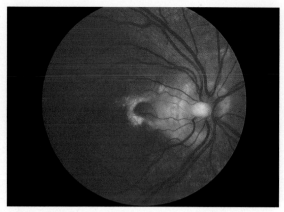

FIGURE 8.35. A: Scattered peripheral multifocal lesions characteristic of ocular sarcoidosis. **B:** The macula of the same patient demonstrating a choroidal neovascular membrane.

The characteristic granulomatous anterior, posterior, or diffuse uveitis should alert the clinician to search for systemic involvement. The workup should include a chest x-ray, serum angiotensin-converting enzyme assay, and if necessary, a gallium scan limited to the head, neck, and mediastinum. Biopsy of ocular tissues such as conjunctival granulomas (Fig. 8.37) or lacrimal gland granulomas may be helpful in confirming the diagnosis.

Management. The management of sarcoidosis is related to the level of eye inflammation and its structural damage. Topical, periocular, or systemic corticosteroids are the basic elements of treatment. Cycloplegic agents may also be helpful in reducing synechiae formation. The ophthalmologist should work with the internist to determine whether systemic therapy would benefit extraocular areas.

Oral steroid therapy may be needed initially in patients with severe inflammation, and chronic low-dose oral steroid therapy, such as 20 mg of prednisone daily, may be needed to control chronic inflammation or reduce exacerbations. If inflammation is not controlled, secondary scarring can occur. This can result in corneal scars, iris bombé from synechiae between the pupillary margin and the lens surface, cataract formation, chronic cystoid macular edema, optic nerve dysfunction, and vascular ischemic events caused by inflammatory obstructive phenomena.

Sympathetic Ophthalmia

Sympathetic ophthalmia is a rare condition seen after penetrating trauma to one eye (called the "inciting" eye) that results in an inflammatory reaction in the other eye (called the "sympathizing" eye). It occurs after approximately one of 500 cases of penetrating eye injury and after one of 10,000 cases of intraocular surgery.

The most common sequence involves a traumatic rupture of one eye followed by inflammation in the second eye usually beginning 2 weeks to 1 year later, although cases have occurred within 5 days to as long as many years later (Figs. 8.38 and 8.39). The injury to the "inciting eye" may be as minimal as an intraocular penetration occurring during anterior chamber paracentesis. The cause is unclear but may include microbial hypersensitivity and immune reacti-

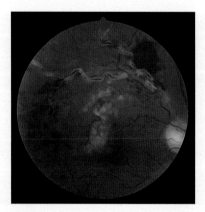

FIGURE 8.36. The classic findings of "candle-wax drippings" in ocular sarcoidosis are observed near the superior arcade. Because of the intense periphlebitis, capillary bleeding has occurred superiorly, and macular function is diminished because of edema.

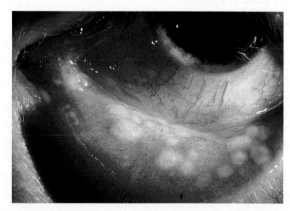

FIGURE 8.37. Conjunctival granulomas in ocular sarcoidosis. The classic yellowish follicular deposits are characteristic of ocular sarcoidosis and are easy to biopsy in an office setting.

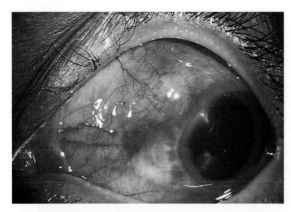

FIGURE 8.38. Sympathetic ophthalmia. This young person suffered trauma 3 weeks before evaluation. Examination of the traumatized eye revealed an occult scleral rupture superotemporally, low-grade inflammation, and irregular healing. The visit was prompted by acute uveitis in the sympathizing eye.

vation of intraocular antigens. Intraocular surgery is a form of controlled trauma that may result in sympathetic ophthalmia, although this is a rare event.

Clinical Features. The patient presents with symptoms of iritis, including ocular pain, photophobia, redness, and decreased vision in both eyes. Sympathetic ophthalmia produces a diffuse granulomatous uveitis in both eyes. The result of this process may be mutton-fat KPs, granulomatous nodules on the iris, and focal areas of inflammation at the level of the retinal pigment epithelium, called Dalen-Fuchs nodules. The choroid is markedly swollen from increasing cellular infiltration, and choroidal exudation may cause serous retinal detachment. Over time, the granulomatous inflammation can cause chorioretinal scarring and poor vision if not treated aggressively (Fig. 8.40A, B).

Management. The clinician must remain alert to the possibility of sympathetic ophthalmia after ocular trauma. Prompt treatment of ruptures with primary closure and meticulous attention to cleanliness of the wound, with all uveal tissues cleaned from wound edges, may reduce the risk

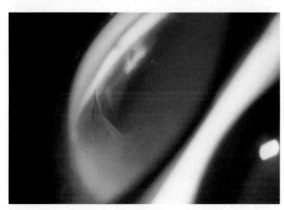

FIGURE 8.39. A superotemporal gonioscopic photograph of the eye in Figure 8.38 shows the internal scleral rupture that resulted in sympathetic ophthalmia.

of sympathetic ophthalmia. Rarely, enucleation of the "inciting" eye may be indicated, especially if the condition is caught within 2 weeks or less from the inciting event or if the inciting eye is blind or painful. Evidence suggests this may reduce inflammation in the sympathizing eye. However, observation is indicated if the inciting eye has good vision, because it may have better visual function at the end of the disease.

Treatment includes high-dose systemic corticosteroids along with periocular or topical medications and longer-acting immunosuppressive medications such as chlorambucil, methotrexate, or cyclosporine. Although treatment may require months to years, the final outcome can be good.

Vogt-Koyanagi-Harada Syndrome

Vogt-Koyanagi-Harada (VKH) syndrome is a rare and unusual form of diffuse granulomatous uveitis. This condition is usually more severe in more highly pigmented individuals. In the United States, the VKH syndrome is seen most commonly in individuals of Native American or Asian ancestry.

Clinical Features. Acute serous detachment of the retina is the hallmark of the VKH syndrome (Fig. 8.41) and may be accompanied by multiple areas of yellowish or yellowish-white edema of the retinal pigment epithelium, as well as by retinal vasculitis and by swelling of the optic disc. Associated anterior iritis may be severe and may be either granulomatous or nongranulomatous in appearance. Some patients will experience associated headache and stiffness of the neck or other neurologic symptoms such as tinnitus. With time, many patients will manifest associated dermatologic changes including poliosis (whitening of the lashes) and vitiligo (patchy depigmentation of the skin). Neither the vitiligo nor poliosis is generally present at the outset of the disease.

Management. Successful management of VKH requires a high index of suspicion for the disease based on the characteristic physical findings. A spinal tap may reveal leukocytosis, and other laboratory tests can exclude other granulomatous conditions. Affected individuals are often positive for the Dw-54 marker.

Treatment of this immunologic condition includes the use of systemic corticosteroids and sometimes includes immunosuppressive agents such as chlorambucil or methotrexate. Cyclosporine may also be used in the treatment of this condition. The final outcome depends on the control of inflammation and prevention of scar formation. Visual function may remain quite good, although the course may be long term and indolent (Fig. 8.42).

Behçet's Disease

Behçet's disease is a form of diffuse uveitis of unknown cause that is associated with significant dermatologic and vascular features. It is found in young adults, and although

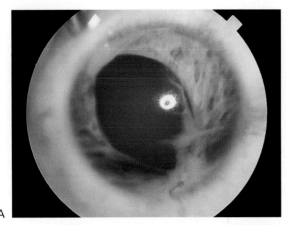
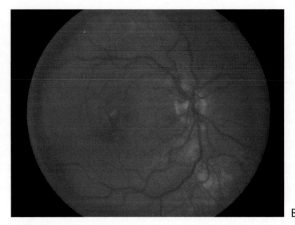

FIGURE 8.40. A: An injured eye in a 5-year-old that developed sympathetic ophthalmia. **B:** Dalen-Fuchs nodules in the macular region of the same patient that have gone on to choroidal neovascularization with leakage of fluid and bleeding.

rare in the United States, it is the most common form of uveitis in Japan. The ophthalmologist may be the first to recognize the condition because of the unusual presentation and clinical findings.

Clinical Features. The most common ocular findings are a posterior uveitis and occlusive vasculitis that may involve both arteries and veins (Fig. 8.43), although some patients may present initially with a hypopyon iridocyclitis without posterior segment findings. Clinically, the hypopyon may be seen in an eye that is otherwise relatively noninflamed. Behçet's disease can be severe, and irreversible damage can easily lead to blindness if the condition is not diagnosed or if it remains untreated.

The features of painful oral aphthous ulceration, genital ulceration, and uveitis fulfill the triad of physical findings characteristic of Behçet's disease. Other associated systemic findings may include phlebitis, polyarthritis, and cerebral vasculitis. Because of this systemic involvement, Behçet's disease may be life-threatening.

Management. Successful treatment requires prompt recognition and suppression of inflammation. Laboratory studies may be helpful, and patients commonly have the HLA-B5 marker. Therapeutic agents include systemic corticosteroids, cyclosporine, and immunosuppressive agents such as chlorambucil. The final outcome depends on the amount of damage caused by the initial vasculitis, which often results in arterial occlusion and retinal necrosis. The end result, however, may be satisfactory if the process is diagnosed and treated promptly. Localized treatment, such as laser therapy for the ischemic complications of vasculitis, is sometimes helpful, and the proper management of Behçet's disease should include consultation with a skilled internal medicine specialist.

Lyme Disease

Lyme disease is a spirochetal infection (*Borrelia burgdorferi*) that is transmitted through a deer tick vector. Lyme disease

FIGURE 8.41. The hallmark of Vogt-Koyanagi-Harada syndrome is an exudative retinal detachment, shown here with hazy vitreous, dilation of the vessels and optic nerve, and the retina separated, with subretinal fluid puddling inferiorly because of dependent positioning.

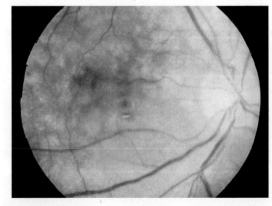

FIGURE 8.42. Resolution of an exudative retinal detachment in a patient with Vogt-Koyanagi-Harada syndrome is often associated with pigment dispersion, a condition called a sunset fundus. If the macular area has been maintained during treatment, the end result may be good vision.

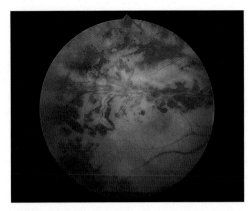

FIGURE 8.43. Acute retinal vasculitis in a patient with Behçet's syndrome. The central vision remained good, although an inferior visual field defect resulted from the vasculitis in the superior arcade.

may involve many organ systems, and although it rarely involves the eye, the ophthalmologist may be the first to diagnose the disease.

Clinical Features. The eye findings are protean and reflect low-grade inflammation, which may be granulomatous in nature. Ocular findings may include corneal disease in the form of a nummular keratitis, low-grade iridocyclitis, pars planitis syndrome (which may be one of the more common presentations), or low-grade optic neuritis and chorioretinitis (Fig. 8.44). Because of the wide array of ocular findings, some degree of suspicion is needed for the correct diagnosis. Serologic testing and DNA probes are improving Lyme disease diagnosis.

Management. The management of Lyme disease depends on the systemic and ocular findings. Systemic and ocular treatments include antibiotic use orally or intravenously. There is some controversy about the optimum duration of antibiotic treatment, which can range from weeks to months. Treatment of the ocular manifestations

also usually involves the use of corticosteroids given topically, periocularly, or systemically to reduce the inflammatory complications of the disease. The extent of steroid use depends on the severity and vision-threatening nature of the ocular findings. The outcome can be good if the condition is caught early and scarring is minimal.

Syphilis

Ocular syphilis may occur as both an acquired and a congenital form of disease, and can confuse the uveitis diagnosis. In acquired syphilis, eye involvement can occur in the secondary, latent, and tertiary phases of the disease. Untreated acquired syphilis and congenital syphilis are associated with multisystem abnormalities.

Clinical Features. The protean ocular findings of acquired syphilis may be acute or chronic in nature, and are often granulomatous in character. Any portion of the ocular system may be involved. Some characteristic findings of acute ocular infection are anterior uveitis, diffuse and focal chorioretinitis, retinal vasculitis, and optic neuritis (Fig. 8.45). Late findings include interstitial keratitis, chorioretinal scars, "salt-and-pepper" retinal pigment epithelial scarring, and optic atrophy. The Argyll-Robertson pupil, which fails to react to light but preserves accommodation, classically has been associated with syphilis. The systemic complications of tertiary syphilis include cardiovascular and meningovascular disease, generalized paresis, and tabes dorsalis.

Ocular findings associated with congenital syphilis may include anterior uveitis, chorioretinitis, interstitial keratitis, and optic atrophy. The interstitial keratitis develops in the first or second decade of life and is bilateral. There is cellular infiltration and vascularization of the corneal stroma. Eventually, the cornea becomes thin, with patchy opacification and residual ghost vessels in the stroma (Fig. 8.46). The

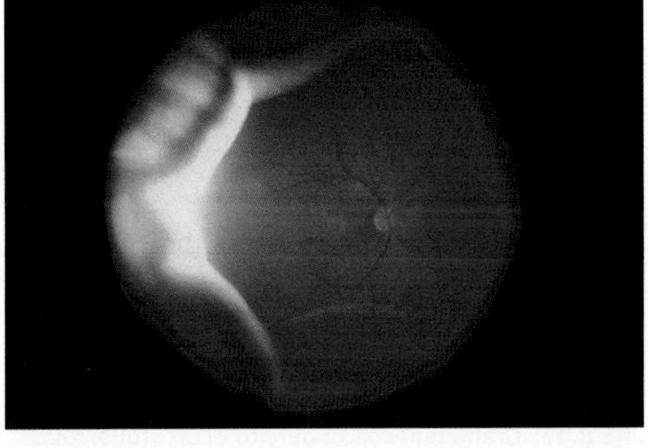

FIGURE 8.44. A wide-angle photograph of a peripheral choroidal detachment with puddled subretinal fluid and a secondary exudative retinal separation inferiorly in a patient with Lyme disease also shows a macular lesion. Prompt resolution occurred with corticosteroids and antibiotic treatment.

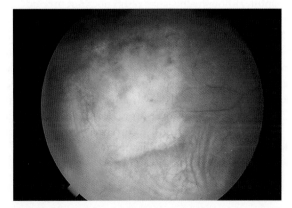

FIGURE 8.45. Resorbing retinitis secondary to ocular syphilis. This patchy retinitis with pigment along the superior border may be found in early, latent, or late ocular syphilis. The patient previously presented with an acute loss of vision secondary to severe vitritis. The patchy, focal retinitis was noticed after a course of intraocular antibiotics.

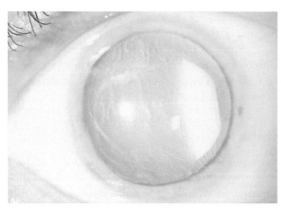

FIGURE 8.46. Interstitial keratitis in secondary syphilis. The interstitial keratitis, revealed in vessels by transillumination, extends into the corneal surface.

chorioretinitis results in pigment clumping interspersed with atrophic white areas, producing the classic salt-and-pepper fundus of ocular syphilis. The systemic features of congenital syphilis include Hutchinson's teeth (i.e., widely spaced, peg shaped), saddle nose, nerve deafness, arthropathy, and mental retardation.

The workup of patients suspected of having ocular syphilis begins with a careful history of sexual activity, including eliciting a history of chancre, which is a manifestation of the primary infection. Because history alone is frequently unproductive, serologic testing using the Venereal Disease Research Laboratory (VDRL) test and fluorescent treponemal antibody absorption (FTA-ABS) test is required. The VDRL test result is usually positive during the acute phase of the disease but can become negative over many years or if the condition is in remission. The FTA-ABS result, however, usually remains positive for life. Both tests should be ordered. Theoretically, a negative VDRL test result with a positive FTA-ABS result can be compatible with ocular syphilis. A VDRL assay of spinal fluid may also be helpful, although a negative result does not preclude central nervous system syphilis.

Management. Ocular syphilis is treated with oral, intramuscular, or intravenous antibiotics. A full systemic course is indicated for ocular and extraocular involvement. If macular scarring is minimized, good vision may be obtained. The VDRL test result falls slowly after treatment and is useful in following patients over time. Because the spirochetes are slow-growing organisms, recurrences are possible, and follow-up VDRL testing is indicated.

Tuberculosis

Tuberculosis is a chronic disease caused by *Mycobacterium tuberculosis*. Any organ system, including the eye, can be affected. Ocular tuberculosis is rare, although it is becoming more common with the advent of AIDS and the use of immunosuppressive agents in the treatment of other diseases.

Clinical Features. A posterior granulomatous choroiditis is the most common finding in ocular tuberculosis (Fig. 8.47). Retinal vasculitis in the form of sheathing of the veins and arteritis is common. Blurred vision is usually the presenting symptom and is generally related to vitritis. Chronic iridocyclitis may also occur, although it may be solely immunologic in nature, without active organisms. In overwhelming systemic infections, tuberculous endophthalmitis has been reported.

As with many of these rare conditions, a high index of suspicion is necessary for the initial diagnosis. Skin testing and a chest radiograph are indicated as part of the ophthalmologist's workup, but an internal medical consultation also is indicated before determining the diagnosis and treatment.

Management. Treatment is accomplished with antitubercular medications, which include isoniazid and rifampin. Because resistant strains commonly develop, single drug therapy should not be used. Topical corticosteroids and cycloplegics may be used to treat anterior uveitis. Posterior uveitis may be treated with the judicious use of systemic corticosteroids after consultation with the internist.

Acquired Immunodeficiency Syndrome

The human immunodeficiency virus (HIV) may affect the eye directly, but more frequently because of the underlying systemic immunodepression the eye becomes vulnerable to a number of opportunistic infections and neoplastic conditions, including CMV retinitis, *Candida* retinitis, herpes zoster infection, toxoplasmosis, *Pneumocystis carinii* infection, and Kaposi's sarcoma.

AIDS is a bloodborne and sexually transmitted disease. Groups at increased risk include homosexual or bisexual men, intravenous drug users, transfusion recipients, hemophiliacs, prostitutes, healthy sex partners of those with

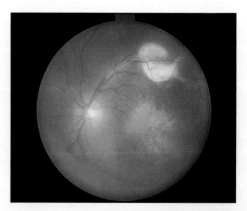

FIGURE 8.47. Granulomas secondary to ocular tuberculosis. The media are slightly hazy because of low-grade vitritis. Off the superior arcade is an old granuloma that has healed with glial scarring. In the macular region is an orange-brown macular granuloma, causing a drop in vision to 20/50. This patient had been treated 5 years previously for Pott's disease.

AIDS, and infants born to mothers with AIDS. The ophthalmologist may be the first to diagnose AIDS in a seemingly healthy individual.

Clinical Features. The cotton-wool spot (i.e., a retinal nerve fiber layer infarct) is the most common eye finding of ophthalmic examination (Fig. 8.48). These localized areas of ischemia are usually located in the posterior pole and may be related to circulating immune complexes. Cotton-wool spots may be found in as many as 100% of HIV-positive individuals over the course of the disease. In most cases, cotton-wool spots are asymptomatic. The diagnosis must exclude other causes of cotton-wool spots, such as diabetes, high blood pressure, collagen vascular disease, and retinal venous occlusion.

Management. Serologic testing is necessary to confirm the diagnosis of AIDS, and a physician skilled in the treatment of this patient population should be consulted. The cotton-wool patches usually are evanescent, and although there may be some mild associated microangiopathy, no treatment is indicated.

AIDS-Related Toxoplasmosis

Clinical Features. Toxoplasmosis may be seen in individuals with HIV infection. If the immunosuppression is moderate to severe, the toxoplasmic retinochoroiditis may be multifocal and endophthalmitic in nature with numerous foci of retinochoroiditis and with marked vitritis (Fig. 8.49). This is a different presentation than that seen in the immunocompetent patient.

Management. The management of ocular toxoplasmosis in patients with HIV-related conditions is somewhat more aggressive than in immunocompetent individuals. Sulfa compounds, clindamycin, and Daraprim have been advocated for the therapy of intraocular infections and are given in high doses to these patients.

The complications of the ocular disease are related to the amount and location of the resulting scars. The condition

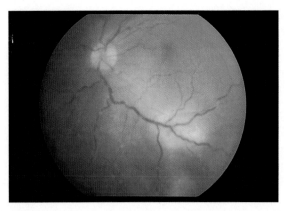

FIGURE 8.49. *Toxoplasma gondii* retinochoroiditis in a patient with acquired immunodeficiency syndrome (AIDS). The findings of precipitates along peripheral vessels, low-grade vasculitis, and deep retinochoroidal lesions scattered throughout the fundus are characteristic of the immunocompromising effects of AIDS in a patient with ocular toxoplasmosis. The immunocompromising events create multifocal lesions.

can become chronic because of the poor cell-mediated immunity in HIV-positive patients. Although central nervous system toxoplasmosis is a common complication of AIDS, intraocular infections are somewhat rare.

AIDS-Related Kaposi's Sarcoma

Clinical Features. Kaposi's sarcoma is one of the more common cancers associated with AIDS. Ocular manifestations consist of small, reddish lesions and tumorous areas on the conjunctiva or contiguous ocular adnexa (Fig. 8.50). These lesions may initially be misdiagnosed as subconjunctival hemorrhages, but the localized elevation of the area and the lack of spontaneous resolution differentiate the lesions. Biopsy is definitive, and antineoplastic agents are used for treatment.

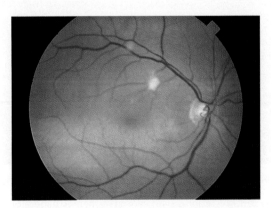

FIGURE 8.48. An asymptomatic young individual was found to have cotton-wool patches and subtle microangiopathy. Serologic testing revealed human immunodeficiency virus as the cause.

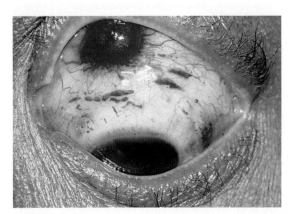

FIGURE 8.50. Kaposi's sarcoma. The conjunctival nodule was originally misdiagnosed as a subconjunctival hemorrhage. Biopsy revealed Kaposi's sarcoma. (Courtesy of Jerry Shields, M.D., Philadelphia, PA.)

AIDS-Related Progressive Outer Retinal Necrosis

Herpes zoster infection in the immunocompromised HIV-positive individual can result in a severe, progressive outer retinal necrosis (PORN). It is a severe, potentially blinding disease that can cause irreversible loss of vision within days to weeks if not diagnosed and treated aggressively.

Clinical Features. Patients present with blurred vision and occasionally with ocular pain in one or both eyes. The hallmark of the disease is seen ophthalmoscopically in the form of small, punctate, opaque foci representing inflammation in the outer retina, occurring initially in the periphery (Fig. 8.51). Within days, the small spots coalesce to form a sheet of retinal necrosis that often extends 360 degrees around the globe. Cells in the vitreous are common. If the condition affects the posterior pole, optic nerve, or macular area, the necrosis may cause severe and irreversible loss of vision. Sometimes, systemic herpes zoster infection is detected several weeks before the eye involvement. In most cases, intense systemic immunosuppression has occurred, associated with CD4 counts below 50.

Management. The management of progressive outer retinal necrosis is difficult. The use of foscarnet, ganciclovir, and acyclovir, alone or in combination, has been advocated. Prompt evaluation and treatment may preserve vision. Retinal detachments are common in this condition, and the injection of silicone oil to tamponade the retina may preserve sight.

AIDS-Related Cytomegalovirus Retinitis

CMV retinitis is the most common ocular infection with the greatest ocular morbidity in AIDS patients. CMV retinitis was discussed earlier in this chapter and is reemphasized here because of the frequency with which this opportunistic virus affects the AIDS patient.

Clinical Features. The presenting symptom is a painless decrease in vision in one or both eyes. No significant anterior segment reaction occurs, and ophthalmoscopic examination reveals patchy areas of whitish or grayish-white full-thickness necrotizing retinitis (Fig. 8.52). The necrotizing retinitis extends through contiguous spread into adjacent noninvolved retina, and progressive retinal destruction can lead to blindness. The more the immune system is compromised, the greater is the chance for rapid progression. CD4 counts in affected individuals are usually below 50.

Management. Treatment involves the use of anti-CMV drugs such as ganciclovir or foscarnet. Because these agents are not viricidal, treatment must be continued for the duration of the disease. In difficult cases, intravitreal injections have been used, as have ganciclovir intravitreal implants. If the immune system remains severely suppressed, recurrences may develop.

AIDS-Related *Pneumocystis carinii* Infection

Pneumocystis carinii is a ubiquitous protozoan organism that almost never causes disease in individuals with normal immune systems but becomes an opportunistic pathogen in immunosuppressed patients. *P. carinii* pneumonia is the most common form of systemic involvement, affecting 80% of patients with AIDS.

Clinical Features. Eye findings are rare, but choroiditis is the most common ocular manifestation (Fig. 8.53). This is seen ophthalmoscopically as multiple, yellow-white subretinal lesions that are 0.5 to 1 disc diameter. They are found more frequently in the posterior pole. There is no significant ocular inflammatory reaction, and patients are usually asymptomatic unless the macula is involved.

Management. These individuals are severely immunosuppressed, and their systemic status often overshadows the

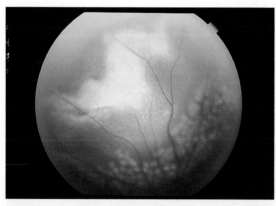

FIGURE 8.51. Progressive outer retinal necrosis (PORN). The PORN syndrome is associated with acute peripheral retinal necrosis, indicated here by the whitish areas located peripherally in the superior retina. Laser burns had been placed inferiorly to help wall off the area.

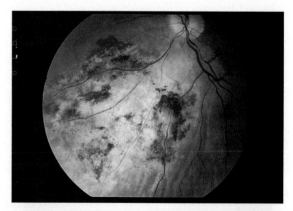

FIGURE 8.52. Cytomegalovirus (CMV) retinitis secondary to acquired immunodeficiency syndrome. The characteristic finding of yellowish CMV retinitis with secondary hemorrhage along the edges is seen off the inferior nasal areas of the human immunodeficiency virus–positive individual, who had a CD4 count below 50.

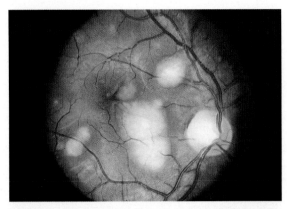

FIGURE 8.53. *Pneumocystis carinii* choroiditis in a patient with acquired immunodeficiency syndrome. Multifocal, whitish lesions are seen at the level of the choroid. Macular involvement often reduces vision, although the lesions are asymptomatic and clear promptly with appropriate antibiotic therapy. (Courtesy of Trent Wallace, M.D., Nashville, TN.)

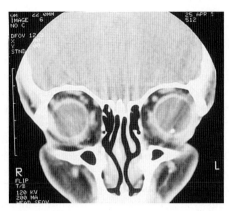

FIGURE 8.55. Intraocular foreign body. The computed tomography scan reveals a small pellet in the inferior pars plana of the left eye that was caused by an undiagnosed injury 6 months earlier. Courtesy of Trent Wallace, M.D., Nashville, TN.)

ocular portion of the disease. *P. carinii* infection, including the choroiditis, is treated with trimethoprim-sulfamethoxazole (Bactrim) and pentamidine given parenterally or orally. These drugs may have significant side effects and should be prescribed by a physician familiar with their use.

MASQUERADE SYNDROMES

Ophthalmologists use the term masquerade syndrome to describe eyes with uveitis (or simulated uveitis) in which the cause of inflammation is either neoplastic or nonuveitic in origin (Fig. 8.54). It is important to be aware of these conditions so that they do not escape clinical recognition and proper therapy. With a careful history and physical examination and a high index of suspicion, most masquerade syndromes can be discovered and treated correctly.

Intraocular Foreign Body

Clinical Features. A foreign body may penetrate the eye in such an unobtrusive manner that the seriousness of the event is not appreciated. A piece of metal from a lawn mower or a hammer may be tolerated in the eye for several months (Fig. 8.55). If iron is part of the metallic makeup, it can generate a condition called siderosis, which is manifested by low-grade inflammation around the site, cataractous changes, and chronic inflammation (Fig. 8.56).

Management. If a careful history reveals any possibility of an intraocular foreign body, a CT scan is needed to look for the metallic fragments. If siderosis has involved the retina, the electroretinogram may show a diminished b wave, and this may be helpful in making the diagnosis. Heterochromia of the iris can also be seen in chronic cases of siderosis. Surgical extraction of the foreign body is indicated and curative.

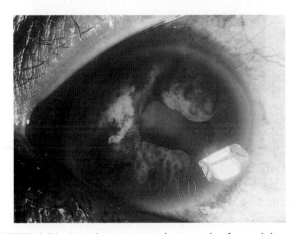

FIGURE 8.54. Anterior segment photograph of an adult male with what was believed to be uveal granulomas. Notice that there are no signs of active inflammation and the lesions turned out to be metastatic carcinoma.

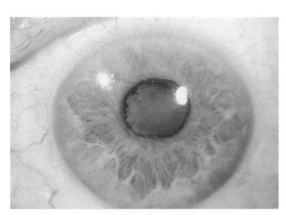

FIGURE 8.56. Siderosis secondary to an intraocular foreign body. Low-grade iridocyclitis, synechiae formation, cataract, and a change in iris coloration are characteristic of an occult intraocular metallic foreign body.

Large Cell Lymphoma

Clinical Features. Large cell lymphoma (e.g., reticulum cell sarcoma, non-Hodgkin's lymphoma) is the most common and feared nonmelanoma cancer of the eye among older persons. The characteristic symptoms are chronic, bilateral spots and floaters from infiltration of the vitreous cavity (Fig. 8.57). Other findings include yellow-white, patchy subretinal infiltrates of lymphoma cells (Fig. 8.58), occasional vasculitis, and rarely, anterior segment involvement. Neurologic symptoms can occur. Large cell lymphomas often arise primarily within the eye, without systemic or central nervous system involvement. Systemic lymphoma primarily infiltrates the choroid and manifests as a thickening of the choroidal tissues.

   Management. The diagnosis of intraocular large cell lymphoma depends on a high index of suspicion. Investigation includes CT scans, MRI, and a spinal tap, looking for central nervous system involvement. An intraocular vitreous biopsy may help in diagnosing large cell lymphoma (Fig. 8.59). The treatment of intraocular lymphoma is undergoing reevaluation, but it usually includes irradiation and aggressive chemotherapy.

Leukemia

Clinical Features. In younger individuals, leukemia may present as infiltrative lesions in the eye (Fig. 8.60). Ocular disease may present as hypopyon, vitreous infiltration, optic nerve infiltration, or secondary vasculitis. The ophthalmologist may be the first to diagnose the leukemia because of the ocular findings or to diagnose an acute leukemic exacerbation in a person previously in remission. The cells may masquerade as inflammatory cells, but because they are infiltrative, the condition is usually progressive.

   Management. An anterior chamber tap or vitrectomy can aid diagnosis. Consultation with an oncologist should be obtained for further diagnosis and treatment.

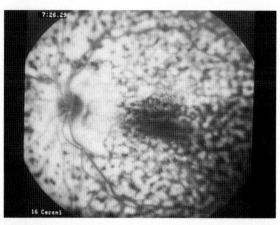

FIGURE 8.58. Fluorescein angiogram demonstrating the "leopard spots" pattern resulting from patchy subretinal infiltrates in a patient with reticulum cell sarcoma.

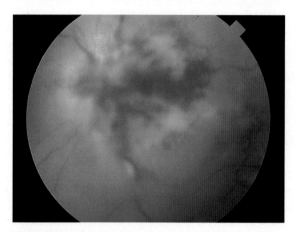

FIGURE 8.59. Disc area of a patient with acquired immunodeficiency syndrome demonstrating infiltration from intraocular lymphoma. A specimen was obtained by needle biopsy.

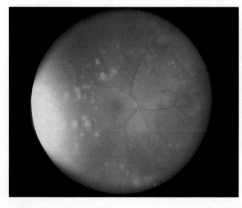

FIGURE 8.57. Reticulum cell sarcoma. A wide-angle photograph shows whitish, multifocal deposits at the level of the pigment epithelium, characteristic of reticulum cell sarcoma. A biopsy specimen revealed the characteristic histopathology.

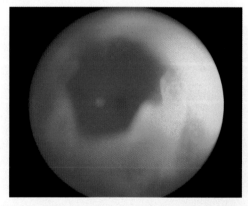

FIGURE 8.60. The wide-angle photograph shows a central core vitrectomy used to sample cells from a progressive opacification of the vitreous, which was thought to be cytomegalovirus retinitis in a leukemic individual in remission. The cells were positive for leukemia, and the patient died of fulminant systemic leukemia soon after the ocular diagnosis was made. (Courtesy of James J. Augsburger, M.D., Philadelphia, PA.)

POSTERIOR SCLERITIS

Posterior scleritis is a disorder in which intense inflammation and swelling primarily involve the posterior sclera. The primary disorder appears to be an immune reaction directed towards scleral collagen (similar to the immune reaction seen in joints of patients with rheumatoid arthritis), causing scleral swelling, dilation of blood vessels within the overlying choroid, and inflammation and other changes in adjacent ocular tissues.

Clinical Features. There is an acute onset of deep-seated and aching pain, usually in one eye only. Blurred vision and pain on eye movement may be present or absent. Fundus examination reveals subretinal edema or thickening that may resemble an ocular tumor, and serous elevation of the overlying retina may also be seen (Fig. 8.61). In less acute cases, choroidal folds may be noted. Depending on the area of involvement, visual acuity may be affected by optic nerve swelling or by elevation and distortion of the macula. Fluorescein angiography reveals a characteristic picture of initial pinpoint hyperfluorescence leading to pooling of fluorescein dye subretinally. The ultrasound scan shows fluid between the layers of the eye and orbital tissues (Fig. 8.62).

Posterior scleritis frequently occurs in the absence of any significant underlying systemic disease, although rheumatoid arthritis, Crohn's disease, and Wegener's granulomatosis have all been associated with posterior scleritis, and must be ruled out. Thorough medical evaluation and laboratory testing for collagen vascular disorders are indicated.

Management. Therapy is focused on controlling the inflammation. Short-term systemic corticosteroid therapy often brings prompt relief, although recurrences are possible. Nonsteroidal antiinflammatory agents are helpful. Posterior scleritis has a variable course, and if inflammatory damage is minimal, visual function can remain excellent.

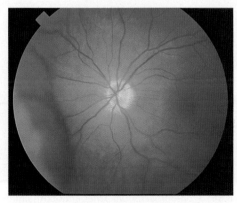

FIGURE 8.61. Posterior scleritis. The findings of acute pain and a mass, seen here in the fundus nasally, are characteristic of posterior scleritis.

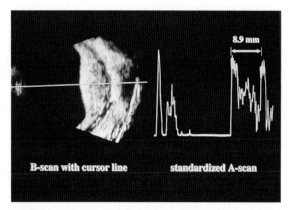

FIGURE 8.62. The A- and B-scan ultrasonograms of the area described in Figure 8.61 show the mass. The characteristic fluid line seen posteriorly is called the T sign. The scan denotes the size of the lesion. (Courtesy of James J. Augsburger, M.D., Philadelphia, PA.)

ENDOPHTHALMITIS

Endophthalmitis refers to severe infection involving all the coats of the eye. The infectious process, depending on the underlying cause, may present in different manners. If the infectious nidus is internal and has spread from another infected organ, it is called endogenous. If the infectious process follows intraocular surgery or penetrating ocular trauma, it is called exogenous. Both forms of endophthalmitis are true ophthalmic emergencies that can lead to blindness if not diagnosed and treated appropriately and aggressively.

Endogenous Endophthalmitis

Clinical Features. Endogenous endophthalmitis is usually associated with systemic infection. In immunocompromised individuals, such as those receiving long-term intravenous therapy or hyperalimentation or those debilitated from other causes, an infectious nidus of bacteria or fungi reaches the eye through the choroidal or retinal circulation.

The initial symptoms may be minimal, such as spots and floaters. Severe visual loss may result from opacification of the vitreous; full-thickness inflammation of the retina, choroid, and sclera; and opacification in the anterior segment. Initially, the findings may mimic acute nongranulomatous anterior uveitis, but the rapid progression and the nature of the clinical picture are usually characteristic of endogenous endophthalmitis (Fig. 8.63).

Management. Immediate vitrectomy surgery or vitreous biopsy is needed to identify the offending organism. Intravenous and intraocular broad-spectrum antibiotic treatment should be initiated promptly until the specific organism is isolated. If caught early, endogenous endophthalmitis has a good visual prognosis, but severe cases can lead to severe scarring, blindness, phthisis bulbi, or loss of the eye.

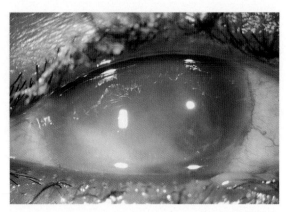

FIGURE 8.63. Subacute bacterial endocarditis (SBE) and endogenous endophthalmitis. Severe vitritis and an acute-onset fibrinoid and exudative reaction were detected in the anterior chamber of a patient with SBE. Culture-proven streptococci were recovered.

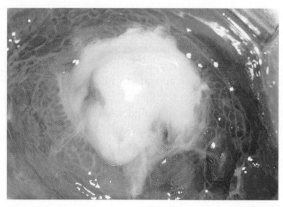

FIGURE 8.65. Severe postoperative endophthalmitis. Severe coagulative necrosis of the cornea from *Serratia* endophthalmitis is evident 3 days after routine cataract surgery. Despite aggressive therapy, vision in this eye was lost.

Exogenous Endophthalmitis

Clinical Features. Exogenous endophthalmitis refers to intraocular infection, usually bacterial, which occurs after intraocular surgery or penetrating ocular trauma. The offending agents can occur from many sources, although the usual source in postsurgical endophthalmitis is patient flora or contamination of instruments or fluids, yielding an infectious culture in the eye. Depending on the series reported, the incidence of endophthalmitis after cataract surgery is one in 500 to 10,000 surgical cases. The technique involved, the degree of intraocular manipulation, and the duration and complexity of surgery may influence the infection rate.

The clinical features include postoperative pain out of proportion to normal postoperative healing within 24 hours to 1 week after surgery, a steamy inflammation of the cornea with a fibrinoid anterior chamber reaction, and hypopyon (Fig. 8.64). The size of the hypopyon often reflects the bac-

terial load or aggressiveness of the offending organism. Gram-positive bacteria, such as *Staphylococcus epidermidis*, are some of the more common causes of postoperative endophthalmitis and generally produce milder disease. *Staphylococcus aureus, Streptococcus pneumoniae,* and Gram-negative organisms usually produce much more severe clinical findings. The onset of pain, redness, and hypopyon and, sometimes, complete opacification of the cornea with intraocular pus formation can occur within 8 hours (Fig. 8.65). Endophthalmitis after penetrating ocular trauma can be caused by multiple organisms, including *Bacillus cereus,* a particularly virulent organism, which can lead to rapid destruction of the eye.

Bleb-associated endophthalmitis is a special case of postsurgical endophthalmitis. Symptoms may develop months to years after the procedure. Unlike chronic endophthalmitis, the onset is sudden. *Haemophilus influenzae* and *S. pneumoniae* are common pathogens.

Chronic postoperative endophthalmitis can arise after extracapsular cataract surgery. Usually developing 2 weeks

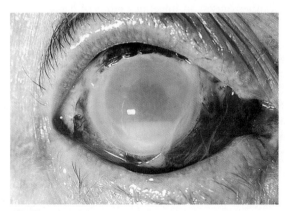

FIGURE 8.64. Acute postoperative endophthalmitis. One day after cataract surgery, the characteristic findings of redness, pain, discomfort, and hypopyon were exhibited by this elderly individual with β-hemolysin streptococcal endophthalmitis. Fluorescein staining shows severe superficial punctate keratopathy of the cornea.

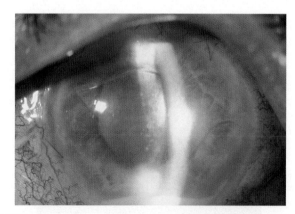

FIGURE 8.66. *Propionibacterium acnes* endophthalmitis is characteristically indolent, producing minimal pain and photophobia. Granulomatous keratic precipitates and a small hypopyon are seen.

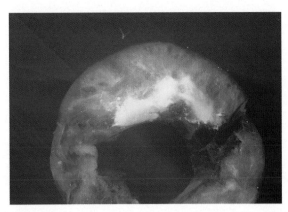

FIGURE 8.67. A biopsy specimen of a peripheral capsular bag shows the whitish lesions characteristic of *Propionibacterium acnes* infection. These can often be seen clinically and help to make the diagnosis.

to 2 months postoperatively, low-grade granulomatous inflammation causes mild discomfort, occasional hypopyon, vitritis, and blurred vision. Occult infection with *Propionibacterium acnes* often is the cause, although *S. aureus* can also result in an identical clinical picture. The infecting organism becomes sequestered in the capsular bag and causes low-grade inflammation.

Management. The secret to successful treatment is early recognition and appropriate therapy. Depending on the amount of scarring of important tissues, vision may be quite good, especially if the organism is not virulent and is caught early. Unfortunately, the loss of ciliary body function, corneal opacification, retinal obliteration due to toxins or severe uncontrolled inflammation, and loss of optic nerve function can cause blindness. In chronic endophthalmitis due to *P. acnes*, removal of the lens and capsular bag or intracameral antibiotics to eradicate the infection usually ensures the return of good vision (Figs. 8.66 and 8.67).

Endogenous or exogenous endophthalmitis can result in complete loss of vision or loss of the eye. The secret to preservation of ocular integrity and vision is prompt recognition and appropriate and aggressive treatment directed to the offending organism. Visual outcome can be good if the infection is caught early.

BIBLIOGRAPHY

Michaelson SB. Color atlas of uveitis diagnosis. 2nd ed. St. Louis: Mosby; 1992.

Nussenblatt RB, Whitcup SM, Palestine AG. Uveitis. Fundamentals in clinical practice. 2nd ed. St. Louis: Mosby; 1996.

Opremcak EM. Uveitis: A clinical manual for ocular inflammation. New York: Springer-Verlag; 1995.

Pepose JS, Holland GN, Wilhelmus KR. Ocular infection and immunity. St. Louis: Mosby; 1996.

Rao NA, Augsburger JJ, Forster DJ. The uvea: Uveitis and intraocular neoplasms. New York: Gower; 1992.

Roitt IM. Essential immunology. 3rd ed. Malden, MA: Blackwell Science; 1997.

Neuro-ophthalmology

Peter J. Savino
Helen V. Danesh-Meyer

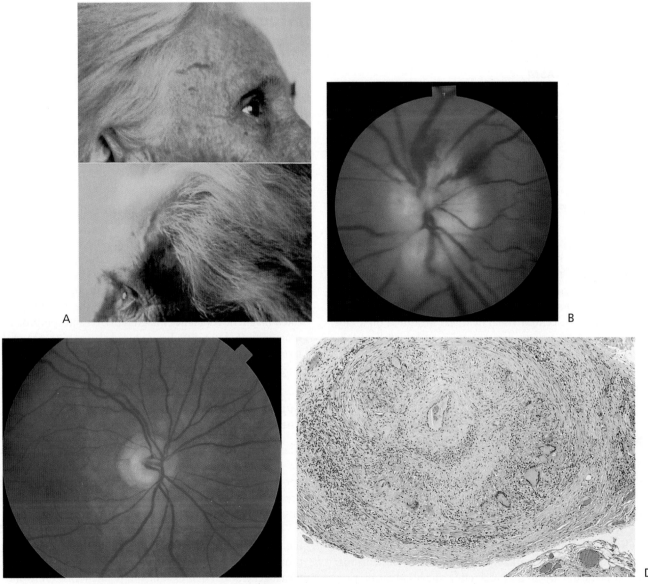

A: Patient with visual loss demonstrating large, indurated and nonpulsatile superficial temporal arteries (horizontal on her right temple and vertical on her left. **B:** Pale swollen optic disc with a characteristic chalk-white appearance. Nerve fiber layer hemorrhages are visible superiorly. The infarction extends into the retina inferiorly. **C:** Optic disc after resolution of an arteritic anterior ischemic optic neuropathy. The disc is pale but is also cupped, another typical feature of giant cell arteritis. **D:** Temporal artery biopsy specimen in which the lumen is almost obliterated. The vessel wall is thickened by an intense infiltrate of chronic inflammatory cells that includes multinucleated giant cells. An elastin stain (not shown) revealed segmental loss of the internal elastic lamina.

LESIONS OF THE VISUAL PATHWAY

The visual pathway begins with the neurosensory layer of the retina (i.e., rods and cones) and extends to the visual receptive area of the occipital cortex. A thorough knowledge of the neuroanatomy of the visual pathway is needed to understand the localizing value of the visual field test. For many years, the central visual field was measured on a tangent screen with various sizes of targets, and the full peripheral visual field was measured by the Goldmann perimeter. Modern visual field analysis usually is done by an automated method that measures a variable amount of the central field, depending on the program selected.

Normal Visual Field

The size of the "normal" monocular visual field depends on the size and color of the test target. However, it is considered to be 60 degrees nasally, 100 degrees temporally, 60 degrees superiorly, and 70 degrees inferiorly. The binocular field is an ovoid that is 200 degrees laterally and 130 degrees vertically. The normal blind spot, which represents the area of the optic disc, is remarkably constant in its dimensions. Because the disc lies in the nasal retina, the blind spot is projected into the temporal field. Measured at 1 m, its center is 15.5 degrees temporal to fixation and 1.5 degrees below the horizontal meridian. It is 5.5 degrees wide and 7.5 degrees high, and because there are no receptive cells in the disc the blind spot is an absolute scotoma. With both eyes open, the blind spot cannot be detected because of the overlapping binocular field.

The diagnosis of lesions involving the visual pathways is made by associated neuro-ophthalmic signs. Primary among these is the pattern of visual field loss. The pattern can be exquisitely localized, pointing to specific anatomic areas of the visual pathway (Fig. 9.1). Although the era of sophisticated magnetic resonance imaging (MRI) and computed tomography (CT) studies has reduced the importance of determining the visual field, it remains a valuable, inexpensive diagnostic procedure.

Types of Visual Field Defects and Terminology

The pattern of a visual field defect depends on the composition and configuration of the visual pathway fibers in the affected area. It is helpful to divide the visual pathway into prechiasmal (i.e., retina and optic nerve), chiasmal, and postchiasmal sections.

There are essentially five patterns of field defects resulting from visual pathway lesions: central or centrocecal scotoma; arcuate or altitudinal scotoma; temporal wedge scotoma; generalized depression; and hemianopia. Only one of these defects, the hemianopia, occurs with lesions between the optic chiasm to the occipital lobe. The other four defects are produced by lesions that may be at any location between the retina and the prechiasmal optic nerve.

Certain terms are used to describe visual field defects. A

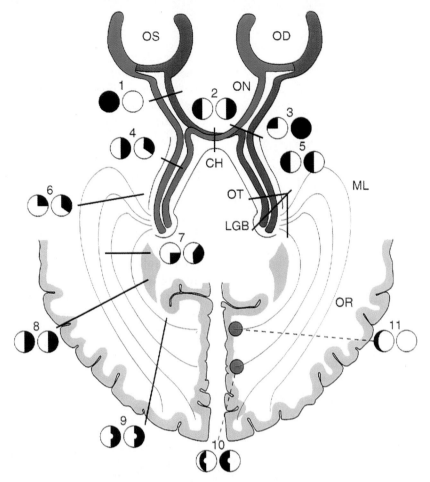

FIGURE 9.1. Schematic illustration of the visual pathway and visual field defects produced by lesions in various areas of the pathway. ON, optic nerve; CH, chiasm; OT, optic tract; LGB, lateral geniculate body; ML, Meyer's loop; OR, optic radiations.

1. Compromise of the left optic nerve results in a central scotoma in the left eye, with a normal right visual field.
2. A lesion of the optic chiasm may cause a bitemporal hemianopia.
3. A lesion at the junction of the right optic nerve and the chiasm results in a central scotoma in the right eye and a superior visual field defect that respects the vertical meridian in the left eye. This effect results from compromise of the inferior nasal crossing fibers from the left eye, which extend into the prechiasmal portion of the right optic nerve (i.e., Wilbrand's knee). The resulting visual field defect is known as a junctional scotoma, which is localized at the junction of the optic nerve and chiasm.
4. Complete interruption of the optic tract produces a homonymous hemianopic field defect. Subtotal lesions produce highly incongruous homonymous hemianopias.
5. Complete interruption of the optic tract, lateral geniculate body, and optic radiations results in a total contralateral homonymous hemianopia.
6. Fibers originating in the ipsilateral inferior temporal retina and the contralateral inferior nasal retina sweep anteriorly and laterally around the temporal horn (i.e., Meyer's loop) before transversing posteriorly. As a result, lesions of the temporal lobe characteristically produce superior, often incongruous homonymous quadrantanopias.
7. Parietal lobe lesions may interrupt visual pathway fibers from the superior retinas pursuing a more direct posterior course. This results in an inferior homonymous quadrantanopia.
8. Complete interruption of the optic radiations results in contralateral total homonymous hemianopia.
9. Posterior occipital lobe lesions result in homonymous hemianopic defects, which may spare the macula. Subtotal occipital lesions produce exquisitely congruous visual field defects because the fibers are more highly segregated in the occipital area.
10. Lesions affecting the posterior portion of the occipital lobe may spare the more anteriorly placed unpaired crossing peripheral nasal retinal fibers, resulting in a preserved temporal crescent in an otherwise congruous homonymous hemianopia.
11. Focal lesions involving the anterior-most portion of the occipital lobe may affect the receptive area for the unpaired crossing fibers from the contralateral nasal retina, resulting in a unilateral peripheral temporal visual field defect.

(Modified from Harrington DO, Drake MV. The visual fields: Text and atlas of clinical perimetry. 6th ed. St. Louis: CV Mosby; 1990, with permission.)

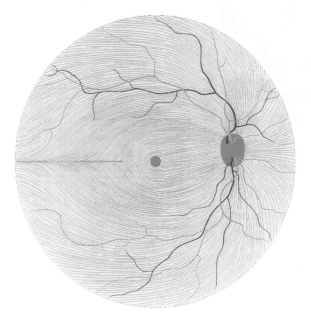

FIGURE 9.2. Schematic representation of the course of ganglion cell axons in the retina. The retinotopic origin of these nerve fibers is respected throughout the visual pathway. (Modified from Harrington DO, Drake MV. The visual fields. 6th ed. St. Louis: CV Mosby; 1990, with permission.)

scotoma is an area of decreased vision in the seeing field. A visual field defect may be relative or absolute. A *relative defect* varies in size or density according to the size, color, and intensity of the test stimulus, and an *absolute defect* is the same for all test targets. The term *homonymous* means the same side of the visual field is affected in each eye, and *hemi-*

anopia refers to one half of the field in which the defect obeys the vertical meridian. If the defect involves one fourth of the field and obeys the vertical meridian, the term *quadrantanopia* is used. A *homonymous* defect may be *congruous* (i.e., the same in each eye) or *incongruous* (i.e., shaped differently between the two eyes).

Prechiasmal Visual Field Defects

Axons of ganglion cells inferior to the horizontal raphe project into the inferior portion of the optic disc (Fig. 9.2). Those originating nasal to the fovea cross in the chiasm, and those from the temporal retina remain ipsilateral. Axons from ganglion cells superior to the horizontal course superiorly through the retina and tend to remain superior throughout the visual pathway. Axons in the papulomacular bundle pursue a more direct course into the temporal aspect of the disc but respect their retinotopic vertical and horizontal origin in the visual pathway.

A lesion of the retina or optic nerve can produce four types of monocular visual field loss: central or centrocecal scotoma; arcuate or altitudinal scotoma; nasal radial scotoma; and generalized depressions.

Central and Centrocecal Scotomas

A process that affects the macula or optic nerve may result in a *central scotoma* (Fig. 9.3). This scotoma may cross the vertical and horizontal midlines but does not extend to the blind spot.

A more extensive lesion of the papulomacular bundle or optic nerve produces a scotoma involving fixation and the

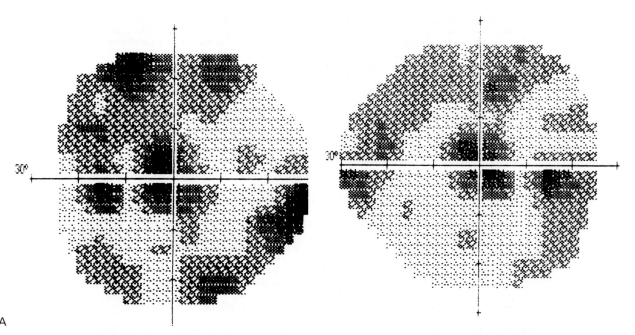

A

B

FIGURE 9.3. Bilateral central scotomas in a patient with nutritional optic neuropathy and with considerable depression throughout the tested field.

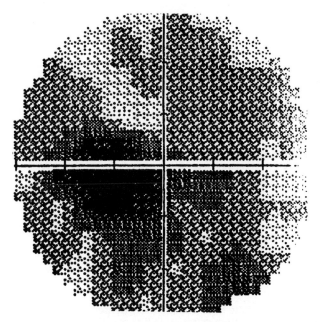

FIGURE 9.4. Centrocecal scotoma in the left eye of a 28-year-old woman with a sudden decrease in vision.

physiologic blind spot and is designated a *centrocecal scotoma* (Fig. 9.4).

Arcuate or Altitudinal Scotomas

Involvement of nerve fiber bundles produces an *arcuate scotoma* that extends from the blind spot to the horizontal

meridian, which is the perimetric representation of the horizontal raphe (Fig. 9.5A). An *altitudinal* defect may involve the superior or inferior portion of the visual field (Fig. 9.5B).

Temporal Wedge Scotoma

Because the nasal retinal nerve fibers reach the optic disc directly, any lesion involving these fibers produces a *wedge scotoma*.

Generalized Depression

Generalized depression is a nonlocalizing defect that may be produced by a variety of causes, including cataract, diffuse retinal disease, and optic nerve compression (Fig. 9.6).

Optic Chiasm Defects

The Optic Chiasm

The optic chiasm is a structure created by the joining of the optic nerves. The nerve fiber arrangement of the optic disc is essentially that of the retina, but as the fibers travel toward the optic chiasm, they rotate within the optic nerve and eventually line up along the vertical meridian. Because the optic nerve is essentially a cone projection system with most of the fibers subserving the papulomacular bundle, any lesion anterior to the chiasm that involves the optic nerve is likely to produce a central scotoma, although arcuate or altitudinal defects do occur.

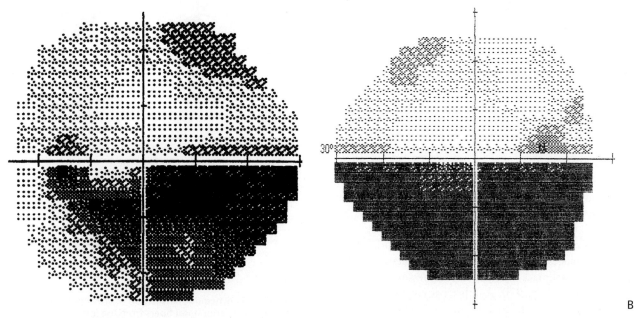

A   B

FIGURE 9.5. A: An inferior arcuate scotoma in the visual field of the left eye extends from the blind spot to the horizontal midline nasally. Glaucoma is the most common cause of arcuate scotomas, although any lesion of the optic nerve or retina can produce similar visual field defects. **B:** Inferior attitudinal scotoma in the right eye of a patient with nonarteritic anterior ischemic optic neuropathy.

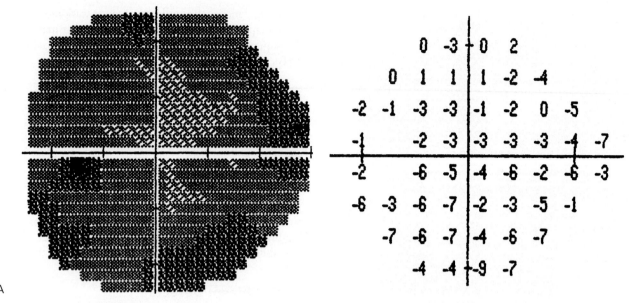

A

B

FIGURE 9.6. Generalized depression of the left visual field results from a moderately dense cataract and no other obvious ocular pathology. **A:** Gray scale. **B:** Pattern deviation fails to reveal any recognizable pattern of field loss.

As the optic nerves converge to form the optic chiasm, two important events occur: the fibers rotate to respect the vertical perimetric meridian, and the nasal retinal fibers of each eye cross to the opposite side. The fibers from the inferior nasal retina cross in the inferior portion of the optic chiasm, and those from the superior nasal retina remain superiorly. The inferior nasal fibers also extend forward into the contralateral optic nerve after crossing in the optic chiasm (i.e., Wilbrand's knee; Fig. 9.7). However, recently it has been suggested that Wilbrand's knee is an artifact of monocular enucleation as it has not been identified in the normal primate monkey, but shown to form gradually over a period of years following monocular enucleation.

The optic chiasm sits above the sella turcica, which houses the pituitary; the optic chiasm rests 10 mm above this gland. The result of this anatomic configuration is that only very large pituitary tumors are able to produce visual loss. Microadenomas do not cause chiasmal visual field abnormalities.

Clinical Features. More than 90% of chiasmal syndromes are produced by mass lesions, most commonly pituitary tumors, craniopharyngiomas, meningiomas, and gliomas. These tumors also may produce a variety of endocrine abnormalities. Involvement of the optic chiasm usually produces visual acuity loss and bilateral visual field defects. The hallmark of chiasmal compression is bitemporal hemianopia (Fig. 9.8). Another pattern, the junctional scotoma, is the most frequently encountered form of chiasmal visual field loss. A junctional scotoma occurs when a mass lesion may involve the optic chiasm and one of the optic nerves. This pattern of involvement produces a central scotoma in one eye with decreased central acuity and a su-

perior temporal depression that respects the vertical midline in the other eye. Traditionally this was said to be because of involvement of Wilbrand's knee (Figs. 9.1, 9.7). An alternative explanation is that it occurs because of combined compression of the optic chiasm and one (or both) optic nerves.

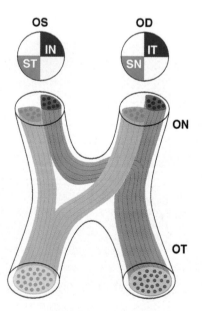

FIGURE 9.7. Schematic illustration of crossing fibers in the optic chiasm. The inferior nasal fibers from the left eye extend into the prechiasmal right optic nerve, forming Wilbrand's knee. ON, optic nerve; OT, optic tract; IN, inferior nasal; ST, superior temporal; IT, inferior temporal; SN, superior nasal. (Modified from Glaser JS. Anatomy of the visual sensory system. In: Tasman W, Jaeger EA, eds. Clinical ophthalmology, vol 2. 1994:4.)

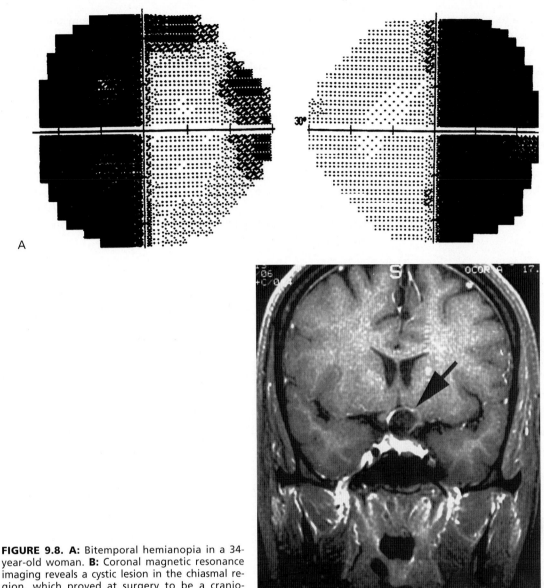

FIGURE 9.8. A: Bitemporal hemianopia in a 34-year-old woman. **B:** Coronal magnetic resonance imaging reveals a cystic lesion in the chiasmal region, which proved at surgery to be a craniopharyngioma.

These two defects—the bitemporal hemianopia and the junctional scotoma—exquisitely localize the lesion to the perichiasmal area.

Rarer types of scotomas may be encountered with chiasmal compression, depending on the anatomic variability of the chiasm in relation to the sella turcica. If the chiasm is postfixed, the intracranial optic nerves are longer, and upward expansion of a pituitary tumor impinges mainly on the perichiasmal optic nerves, producing bilateral central scotomas instead of a hemianopic defect. If the chiasm is prefixed, the posterior portion of the chiasm and a portion of the optic tracts rest over the sella turcica, and compression produces an incongruous homonymous hemianopia (i.e., optic tract syndrome).

Double vision may also be a sign of perichiasmal mass lesions. A type of double vision peculiar to chiasmal compression is the *hemifield slide phenomenon*. Affected patients complain of vertical displacement of columns of figures or lines on a printed page, because the bitemporal hemianopia destroys the interlocking mechanism for reading. Double vision may be produced by ocular misalignment, because pituitary tumors and other large perichiasmal mass lesions may also compromise the third, fourth, or sixth nerves in either cavernous sinus.

Management. Any patient presenting with a possible perichiasmal lesion must have a gadolinium-enhanced MRI scan. This is the best imaging technique for this area, and because 90% of chiasmal syndromes are produced by mass lesions, it is the first test to be ordered. Lesions other than tumors may produce chiasmal syndromes. If no mass is found, investigation for other causes, such as demyelinating disease, sarcoidosis, or trauma, should be undertaken.

Postchiasmal Visual Field Defects

The components of the postchiasmal visual pathway are the *optic tract, lateral geniculate body,* and the *optic radiations* (Fig. 9.1). The fibers originating in the ipsilateral temporal retina are joined by fibers from the contralateral nasal retina to form the postchiasmal pathway. Therefore, lesions of this portion of the visual pathway produce hemianopias in the visual fields of both eyes that are homonymous.

Complete interruption of the postchiasmal visual pathways at any point from the optic tract to the occipital lobe re-sults in a complete contralateral homonymous hemianopia. Complete hemianopias cannot be localized to a specific part of the visual pathway on the basis of the visual field alone. A visual field defect must be less than complete in order to be localizing to a specific area of the postchiasmal pathway.

Optic Tract

The optic tract is the continuation of the visual fibers be-tween the optic chiasm and the temporal lobe. An optic tract lesion is uncommon. Its characteristics depend on the cause. Two types of optic tract syndromes have been described.

Compressive optic tract syndrome most frequently is caused by a craniopharyngioma but may also result from pituitary tu-

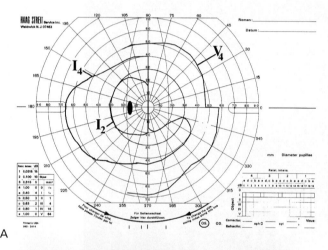

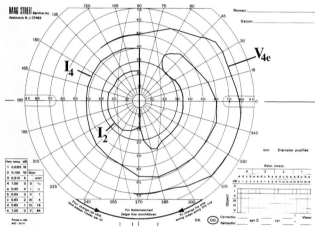

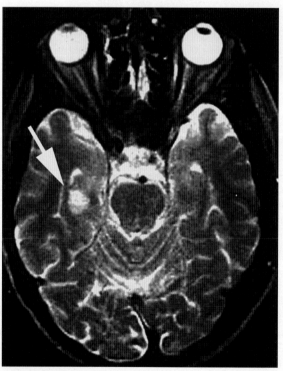

FIGURE 9.9. Highly incongruous right homonymous hemianopia re-sulting from a nonmass lesion at the junction of the chiasm and left op-tic tract. **A:** Left eye. **B:** Right eye. **C:** Contrast-enhanced axial magnetic resonance scan, showing an infarct in the area of the left optic tract *(ar-row).*

mors. The syndrome consists of a highly incongruous homonymous hemianopia contralateral to the side of the lesion, decreased acuity, and a relative afferent pupillary defect (RAPD) both ipsilateral to the side of the lesion and produced by compression of the optic chiasm and occasionally of the optic nerve.

An optic tract lesion produced by a demyelinating plaque, vascular occlusive phenomenon, or other *nonmass lesion* produces an incongruous homonymous hemianopia without decreased central acuity (Fig. 9.9). Patients do have an RAPD ipsilateral to the homonymous hemianopia (i.e., contralateral to the lesion), because the RAPD is on the side of the temporal visual field loss, which is greater than the nasal visual field loss in the contralateral eye.

Management. Any patient with a homonymous hemianopia requires MRI with gadolinium.

Optic Radiations

The optic radiation portion of the visual pathway extends from the lateral geniculate body to the occipital lobe. As the fibers leave the lateral geniculate body, they course anteriorly around the temporal horn to form *Meyer's loop* (Fig. 9.1). Involvement of this area produces a superior homonymous quadrantanopia (Fig. 9.1). Other nonocular signs of *temporal lobe dysfunction* include temporal lobe epilepsy and formed visual hallucinations.

As the visual fibers course toward the occipital lobe, they become more segregated, and the more posterior the lesion, the more congruous is the homonymous hemianopia. *Parietal lobe lesions* routinely produce inferior quadrantic visual field loss, which tends to be more congruous than that produced by temporal lobe lesions (Figs. 9.1, 9.10).

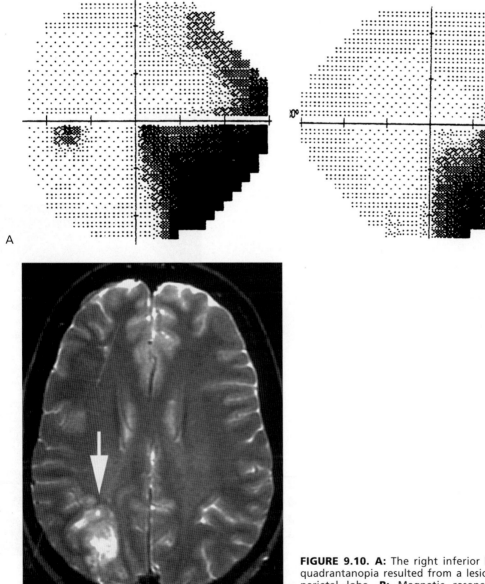

A

B

FIGURE 9.10. A: The right inferior homonymous quadrantanopia resulted from a lesion of the left parietal lobe. **B:** Magnetic resonance imaging demonstrates enhancement of an infarcted area in the left parietal lobe.

Occipital lobe lesions are often seen first by ophthalmologists, because patients may present only with visual problems and no other neurologic signs or symptoms. The hallmark of occipital lobe disease is the exquisitely congruous homonymous hemianopia (Fig 9.11). Two perimetric peculiarities are observed in some occipital lobe lesions. The first feature is preservation of the temporal crescent. An area in the anterior interhemispheric fissure contains an unpaired projection from the nasal retina. Lesions of the occipital lobe may spare this area, and the patient presents with an otherwise congruous hemianopia, but the crescent around the temporal portion of the visual field remains intact (Fig. 9.12). The temporal crescent is in the extreme temporal visual field. It is widest in the horizontal meridian where it extends from 60 degrees to approximately 90 degrees. Therefore, it cannot be identified on the 24-2 and 30-2 visual field tests. The second feature is macular sparing. Some homonymous hemianopias of occipital lobe origin appear not to involve a small area around fixation in the hemianopic field (Fig. 9.1). Although the exact mechanism for this finding is still controversial, it is not an artifact. It can be exquisitely localized to the occipital lobe.

Management. The most frequent occipital lobe lesion is ischemia, particularly in older patients. However, MRI with gadolinium is indicated for all patients with any newly discovered homonymous hemianopias.

OPTIC NERVE ABNORMALITIES

Optic Neuritis

The term optic neuritis signifies inflammation or demyelination of the optic nerves. It is a clinical syndrome that strictly may be applied to any inflammation (e.g., sarcoidosis, Lyme disease), but convention usually implies demyelination.

Clinical Features. Patients affected are almost invariably younger than 45 years of age. The visual changes are characterized by a sudden decrease in visual acuity, usually in one eye, preceded or accompanied by pain on movement of the eye. Pain on movement of the eye is an extremely important sign that occurs in more than 90% of patients with optic neuritis.

The visual acuity may be normal in optic neuritis, or it may be decreased to the level of no light perception. Visual field abnormalities in the form of a centrocecal scotoma or an altitudinal defect are common, as are acquired dyschromatopsia and an RAPD. The optic disc may be normal in the *retrobulbar* variety of optic neuritis or may be swollen with a few cells overlying the swollen disc in cases of *papillitis* (Fig. 9.13). Long-term disc appearance may be normal or may show optic nerve atrophy (Fig. 9.14).

Management. The Optic Neuritis Treatment Trial (ONTT) divided patients with acute optic neuritis into

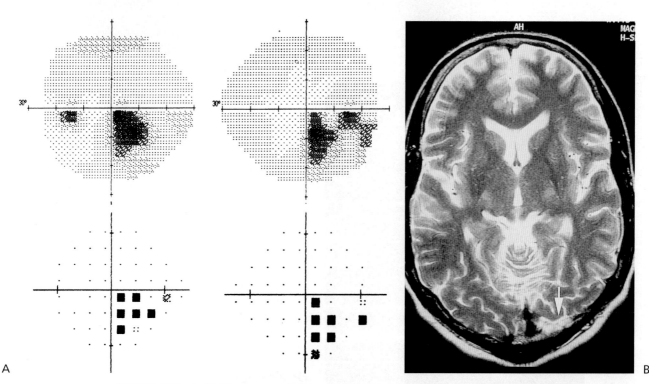

FIGURE 9.11. A: Right congruous inferior homonymous quadrantanopia. **B:** Magnetic resonance imaging demonstrates enhancement of an infarcted area of the left occipital lobe *(arrow)*.

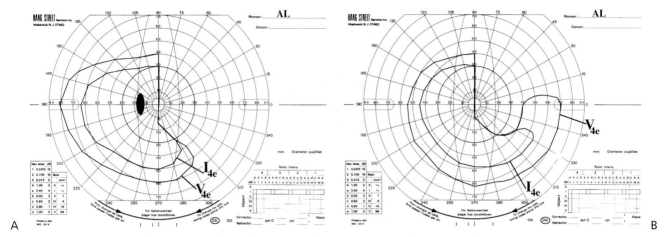

FIGURE 9.12. Temporal crescent. The patient has an incomplete right homonymous hemianopia, which appears incongruous but is very congruous except for a preserved temporal crescent to the I-4-E and V-4-E isopter in the right eye (i.e., Goldmann perimeter).

three treatment groups: intravenous methylprednisolone followed by oral taper; placebo; and oral prednisone alone. Isolated optic neuritis in its typical form requires no laboratory investigations. Cerebrospinal fluid (CSF) examination is also not mandatory in typical cases of optic neuritis.

Because of the high association of subsequent development of multiple sclerosis (MS) in patients with isolated optic neuritis who have abnormal MRI scans, an MRI scan may be done at the onset of the visual disturbance (Fig. 9.15). The 5-year follow-up results of the ONTT showed that the cumulative probability of developing clinically definite MS was 30% and did not differ by treatment group. However, the number of lesions on the brain MRI at study entry was a stronger predictor for the development of MS. If there were no MRI lesions, the 5-year risk of MS was 16%, but increased to 51% when three or more MRI lesions were present. Patients with no pain during the presentation of optic neuritis, mild visual acuity loss or optic disc swelling were identified as having a particularly low risk for the development of MS.

The ONTT has indicated that the ultimate recovery of vision is not affected by intravenous corticosteroid treatment. But treatment does hasten visual recovery. The only potential visual benefit would be in a one-eyed patient or a patient who desires rapid improvement in visual function. Oral corticosteroids alone should not be used because their use results in increased recurrences of optic neuritis in the same and fellow eye.

The Longitudinal Optic Nerve Study has shown that patients treated for acute optic neuritis with intravenous corticosteroids and who do have abnormal MRI scans have a much reduced risk of developing the signs and symptoms of MS over the 2 years following treatment. After this 2-year period, their risk approaches those of untreated patients (Table 9.1). It has been recommended that patients with

acute optic neuritis should be treated with high does of intravenous corticosteroids, although not for visual reasons but to provide short-term protection against the development of MS.

Anterior Ischemic Optic Neuropathy

Anterior ischemic optic neuropathy (AION) is the result of an infarction of the optic nerve head caused by compromise of the posterior ciliary artery circulation. Two general varieties of AION are recognized: a nonarteritic or idiopathic form and an arteritic form, secondary to giant cell arteritis.

Clinical Features. AION occurs in the vasculopathic age group and may result in decreased acuity, visual field defects, and a swollen, variably pale optic disc (Fig. 9.16).

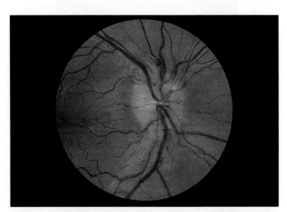

FIGURE 9.13. Papillitis. A 22-year-old woman noticed a sudden decrease in vision in her right eye and pain on eye movement. The disc is elevated and the margins blurred, with opacification of the nerve fiber layer inferiorly. The contralateral disc is normal.

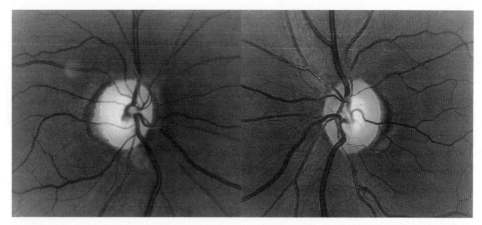

FIGURE 9.14. Optic nerve atrophy. A 30-year-old man developed retrobulbar neuritis in the right eye. His initial vision was 20/200. Four months later, temporal pallor of the right disc was seen *(left)*, but vision had improved to 20/25. The left disc was normal.

Nonarteritic AION occurs typically in patients older than 45 years of age, is sudden in onset, and is painless. The visual decrement can be mild to severe. Usually, the superior or inferior portion of the nerve is edematous and pale, and classically, there is a resultant altitudinal visual field defect (Fig. 9.17). Visual acuity is usually better preserved than in the arteritic variety, and the visual field defects tend to be stable. The fellow eye usually shows an optic disc with no cup, suggesting crowding of the retinal nerve fiber layer, which may contribute to the infarction process. The incidence of subsequent infarction in the second eye ranges from 14% to 35%. The risk of recurrent event to the same eye is 4%.

Arteritic AION results from giant cell (temporal) arteritis. The optic disc is usually paler than in the nonarteritic variety, and some areas of retinal ischemia may be seen (Fig. 9.18). The visual acuity is usually worse than in the nonarteritic variety, and the patients usually are older than 65 years of age. The symptoms associated with giant cell arteritis include those of polymyalgia rheumatica (e.g., stiffness and pain of the neck and shoulder muscles, weight loss, fever). Other common symptoms include pain in the jaw muscles on chewing, chronic headache, and tenderness in the forehead and temporal scalp areas. Sometimes an enlarged, nonpulsating temporal artery is palpable. A Westergren erythrocyte sedimentation rate (ESR) is usually elevated. Cupping of the optic disc is the most common end-stage disc appearance of arteritic AION, but occurs infrequently in nonarteritic AION (Fig 9.19).

Management. A Westergren ESR should be drawn immediately, and temporal artery biopsy should be performed if giant cell arteritis is suspected. The temporal artery does

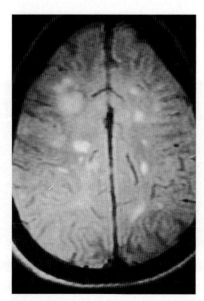

FIGURE 9.15. Magnetic resonance imaging shows typical white matter lesions that are indistinguishable from those seen in multiple sclerosis.

TABLE 9.1. CUMULATIVE PERCENTAGE OF PATIENTS WITH CLINICALLY DEFINITE MULTIPLE SCLEROSIS BY TREATMENT GROUP

Time Period (from enrollment)	Treatment Group (%)		
	Intravenous (n = 134)	Placebo (n = 134)	Oral Prednisone (n = 129)
6 mo	3.1	7.4	7.2
1 y	6.4	13.4	10.5
2 y	8.1	17.7	15.6
3 y	17.3	21.3	24.7
4 y*	24.7	26.9	29.8

*Four-year follow-up is not yet complete for all patients. From Beck RW, for the Optic Neuritis Study Group. The Optic Neuritis Treatment Trial: three-year follow-up results. *Arch Ophthalmol* 1995;113:136, with permission.

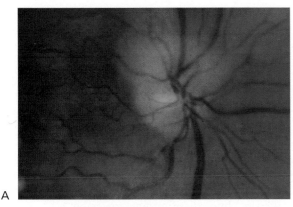
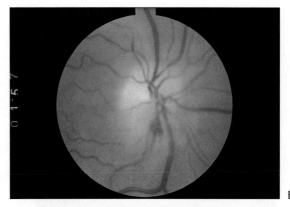

FIGURE 9.16. Nonarteritic anterior ischemic optic neuropathy. **A:** Acute onset of superior segmental swelling of the right optic disc, with 20/20 vision. **B:** Two weeks later, vision diminished to hand movements, the inferior disc was swollen, and the superior portion was becoming pale and atrophic. This type of second infarction in the same eye is rare, occurring in 4% of patients.

not need to show giant cells to establish the diagnosis, but it must show signs of inflammation (Fig. 9.20).

Systemic corticosteroids should be administered immediately in the arteritic form to prevent further visual loss, especially in the other eye. At least 80 to 100 mg of prednisone is required daily, and some physicians recommend high-dose intravenous steroids initially. The presence of AION and an elevated ESR are sufficient to institute steroid treatment. A temporal artery biopsy should be done as soon as possible, but treatment should not be delayed pending biopsy results, because the other eye is at risk. Steroid treatment must continue for months.

No treatment is useful for acute nonarteritic AION. A minority of patients may show progression of AION, with further loss of visual acuity or visual field.

Papilledema

Papilledema is bilateral optic disc elevation due to increased intracranial pressure. There is little or no true edema, because the disc elevation is caused by damming of the axoplasmic flow at the lamina cribrosa in response to increased perineural pressure. The exact mechanism by which increased intracranial pressure results in papilledema is unknown.

Clinical Features. Papilledema is divided into sequential stages. *Early or incipient papilledema* is characterized by minimal disc hyperemia, early nerve fiber layer opacification, and a loss of spontaneous venous pulsations (Fig. 9.21).

FIGURE 9.17. Inferior attitudinal defect in the right eye of the patient in Figure 9.16, as seen at initial presentation.

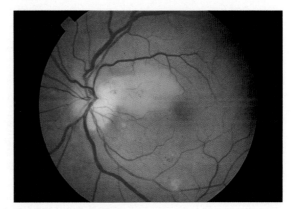

FIGURE 9.18. Arteritic anterior ischemic optic neuropathy. The optic disc is extremely pale, a sign of giant cell arteritis, and an adjacent area of the retina is infarcted.

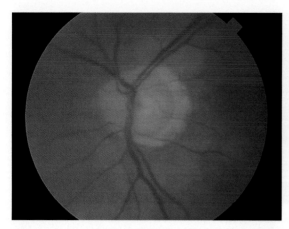

FIGURE 9.19. Cupping of the optic nerve in end-stage arteritic anterior ischemic optic neuropathy secondary to giant cell arteritis.

Acute or developed papilledema is expressed as peripapillary nerve fiber layer hemorrhages and, sometimes, as exudates (Figs. 9.22, 9.23). Disc elevation is more prominent than in the early form. In *chronic papilledema,* the hemorrhages and exudates disappear, and the disc develops a yellowish appearance (Fig. 9.24). Crystalline deposits that resemble disc drusen but are accumulations of axoplasmic debris may be present. Collateral circulatory channels in the form of optochoroidal shunt vessels may be seen. In *atrophic papilledema,* the optic disc is pale and flatter than in other stages. The nerve fiber layer is thinned, and concentric peripapillary pigment alterations indicate the boundaries of the previous disc edema (Fig. 9.25).

Patients with papilledema from any cause may experience several symptoms. *Transient visual loss* lasts for seconds in one or both eyes and frequently occurs when going from a supine to standing position. *Diplopia* related to a unilateral or bilateral cranial nerve VI palsy is a nonlocalizing sign of increased intracranial pressure. *Visual field defects* begin as enlarged blind spots, but with attrition of the nerve fiber layer arcuate defects similar to the progression of field loss in glaucoma may develop. A marked loss of peripheral vision is a late finding. *Visual acuity loss* occurs only late in the course of papilledema, after severe visual field loss has occurred. However, vision may decrease earlier if the patient has macular exudates, edema, or other retinal surface changes.

Management. Bilateral optic disc elevation, especially in the absence of signs of optic nerve dysfunction, must raise the possibility of papilledema due to increased intracranial pressure. Immediate imaging, preferably MRI, is performed to detect an intracranial mass lesion or hydrocephalus. If the result is normal, a lumbar puncture (LP) is performed to establish the diagnosis of increased intracranial pressure and to analyze the contents of the spinal fluid. Causes of papilledema other than intracranial mass lesions include pseudotumor cerebri and inflammatory, infectious, and malignant meningitis.

Idiopathic Intracranial Hypertension

Idiopathic intracranial hypertension (IIH) is a disorder with a strict group of clinical signs. Papilledema is usually present, but rarely the discs may appear normal. Neurologic imaging does not reveal a mass lesion or hydrocephalus. The CSF composition is normal, but opening pressure is increased. Other neurologic signs are absent, except for sixth nerve palsy. No underlying cause is found in IIH. When an underlying cause is identified, the disorder is called "pseudotumor cerebri due to . . ." (whatever the cause may be).

Clinical Features. Patients who have this condition may suffer from headaches, transient visual obscuration in one or

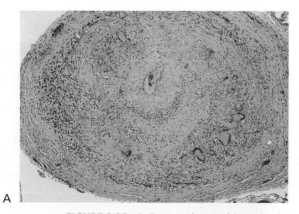

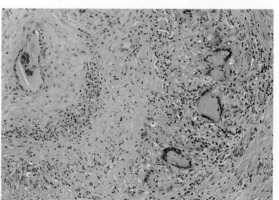

FIGURE 9.20. A: Temporal artery biopsy in giant cell arteritis reveals a chronically inflamed artery with marked narrowing of the lumen. (Hematoxylin and eosin stain; original magnification ×10). **B:** Higher magnification shows chronic inflammatory cells, including lymphocytes, epithelioid histiocytes, and giant cells in the wall of the thickened vessel. Segmental destruction of the muscularis and internal elastic lamina has occurred. The lumen is narrowed, and subintimal fibrosis is present (hematoxylin and eosin stain; original magnification ×25; photograph courtesy of Ralph C. Eagle Jr, M.D., Philadelphia, PA.)

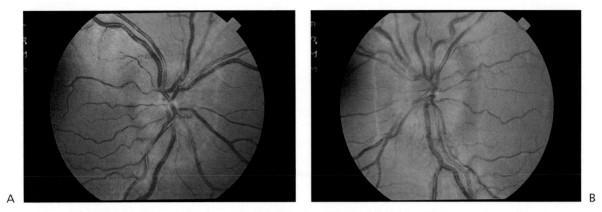

FIGURE 9.21. Early papilledema with disc elevation, blurring of the margins, hyperemia, and venous engorgement in the **(A)** right eye and **(B)** left eye.

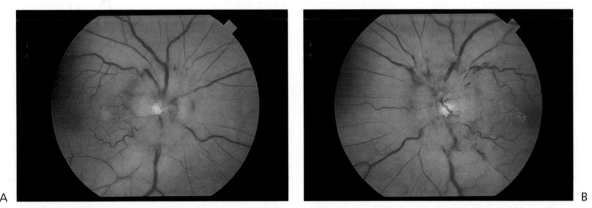

FIGURE 9.22. Acute papilledema with increased elevation and hemorrhages on the disc surface in the **(A)** right eye and **(B)** left eye.

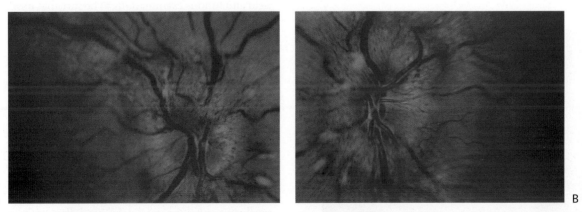

FIGURE 9.23. Acute papilledema with more extensive disc elevation and cotton-wool infarcts in the **(A)** right eye and **(B)** left eye. The left eye also has retinal folds developing between the disc and macula.

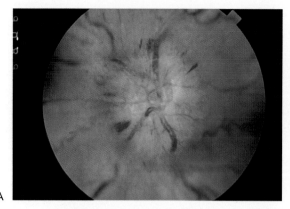
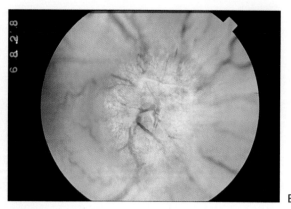

FIGURE 9.24. Chronic papilledema. **A:** Right eye, showing elevation and residual hemorrhages. **B:** The left disc is yellowish, and the hemorrhages have disappeared. Small shunt channels are developing on each disc.

both eyes that lasts for seconds, or double vision attributable to unilateral or bilateral sixth nerve palsies (Fig. 9.26).

IIH is found mostly in young obese women, although it may occur in children and in men. Pseudotumor cerebri can be produced by the administration or withdrawal of corticosteroids, excessive doses of vitamin A, tetracycline (including the semisynthetic varieties), NegGram, Cytoxan, and dural sinus thrombosis. In the absence of one of these or other causes, when the strict criteria for pseudotumor cerebri have been fulfilled, the disorder is said to be idiopathic.

The major permanent deficit these patients can suffer is visual loss. This occurs because of chronic papilledema, and the progression of the visual field loss is identical to that of glaucoma, commencing with only an enlarged blind spot and then progressing to arcuate defects, peripheral constriction of the field, and finally, marked constriction, leaving only a small central tunnel of vision. Acuity is lost late in the evolution of the chronic papilledema. In any patient with papilledema, even a morbidly obese young woman, imaging and LP are required to establish the diagnosis of IIH or pseudotumor cerebri.

Management. All patients suspected of having IIH need to have neuroimaging that excludes the presence of other intracranial pathology and an LP that should reveal normal CSF composition with an elevated opening pressure. If the CSF pressure is normal, but the clinical picture is suggestive of IIH, a repeat LP should be performed. A CT venogram or MRI venogram should be done to exclude dural sinus thrombosis.

Not all patients who have pseudotumor cerebri require treatment. If the patient is asymptomatic, the papilledema is relatively acute, but the patient has no visual field deficit, observation is permissible.

If weight loss does not result in resolution of the syndrome, progressive visual field loss occurs, or the optic discs are tending toward chronic papilledema, treatment with acetazolamide may be instituted. Acetazolamide, however, should be used in dosages of 2 to 5 g daily, depending on the patient's weight. If this medication does not relieve the syndrome, an operative procedure is indicated. Optic nerve sheath decompression is an excellent operation if the visual symptoms are paramount. Lumboperitoneal shunting may be more useful if headache is incapacitating.

The ophthalmologist's duty when following a patient with pseudotumor cerebri is to perform sequential visual field and fundus examinations to be sure that progressive visual field deterioration is not evolving.

Diabetic Papillopathy

Optic disc edema occurs in patients with type I or II diabetes mellitus.

Clinical Features. This is considered to be an atypical form of nonarteritic AION. Visual symptoms are usually minimal and resolve within several weeks, but may be severe and permanent. Although initially described in young insulin-dependent diabetics, it has been documented to occur as frequently in adult-onset diabetes mellitus. The disc swelling may be unilateral or bilateral. Eyes with diabetic papillopathy show a swollen, hyperemic disc with prominent, dilated, telangiectatic vessels over the disc that may mimic optic disc neovascularization (Fig. 9.27). Disc edema re-

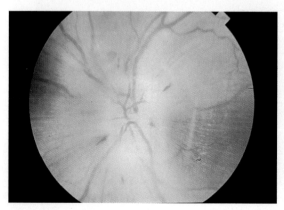

FIGURE 9.25. Atrophic papilledema. The optic disc is pale and flat. Concentric pigment alterations indicate the extent of the peripapillary edema.

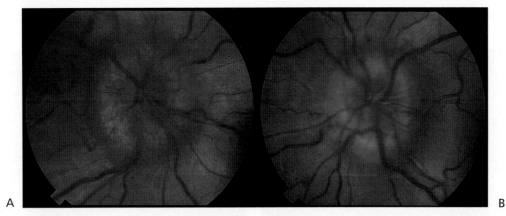

FIGURE 9.26. Pseudotumor cerebri. Papilledema in a 24-year-old, obese woman with severe headaches and obscuration of vision. The opening spinal fluid pressure was 600 mm H_2O. **A:** Right eye. **B:** Left eye.

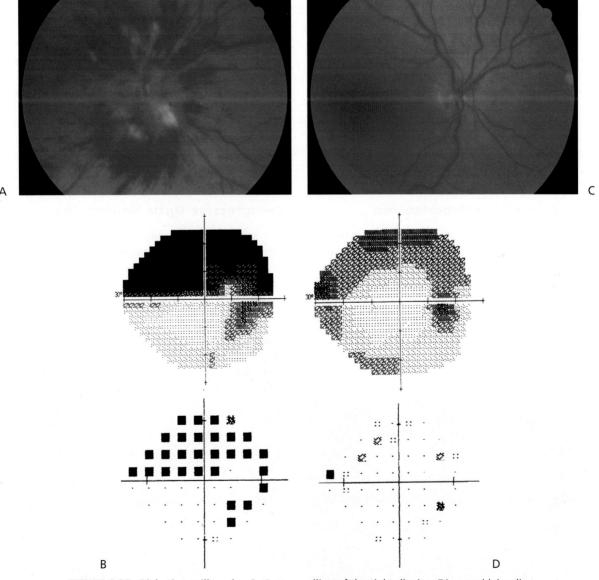

FIGURE 9.27. Diabetic papillopathy. **A:** Acute swelling of the right disc in a 74-year old, insulin-dependent diabetic of 25 years' duration. Hemorrhages, blurred disc margins, and optic disc edema are evident with **(B)** corresponding superior nerve fiber layer visual field defect seen on automated Humphrey perimetry. **C:** Same optic disc 3 months later shows significant resolution of the optic disc swelling with **(D)** improvement of the visual field.

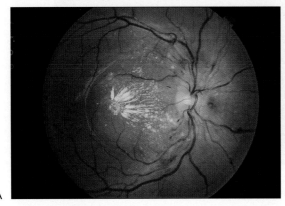
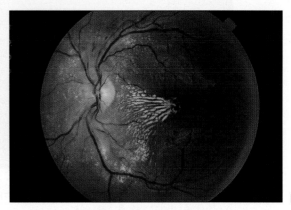

FIGURE 9.28. Hypertensive retinopathy in a 56-year-old woman with advanced renal disease and a blood pressure of 225/160 mm Hg. **A:** Right eye with edema of the disc, striated hemorrhages, edema residues in the form of a macular star, and vision limited to hand movements at 6 feet. **B:** The left eye has a macular star but minimal edema of the disc. Vision was 20/25. One year later, vision in the right eye improved to 20/40.

solves within 3 to 4 months, often without optic atrophy. The visual loss is mild and usually improves. Macular edema and background diabetic retinopathy frequently are present. Like patients with typical nonarteritic AION, patients with diabetic papillopathy seem to have a higher prevalence of "disc at risk" or small cup-to-disc ratios (<0.1).

Management. No specific treatment of the papillopathy is indicated.

Optic Neuropathy in Hypertension

Edema of the optic disc may be seen in patients with uncontrolled hypertension. Decreased visual acuity and visual field changes vary. The condition may be unilateral or bilateral. Cotton-wool spots, hard exudates, hemorrhage, and capillary drop-out may be associated with the disc swelling.

Other signs of hypertensive retinopathy are often present (Fig. 9.28).

Originally, edema of the optic discs in cases of severe hypertension was thought to be a sign of increased intracranial pressure. It is now considered to be a form of AION. Other theories postulated include a breakdown of the blood-retinal barrier and ischemia of the optic nerve head with resultant axoplasmic stasis.

Compressive Optic Neuropathy

The hallmark of any compressive optic neuropathy is a slowly progressive evolution of the signs of optic nerve disease, which include decreased acuity, dyschromatopsia, RAPD, and an optic nerve type of visual field defect. Ophthalmoscopically, the optic disc may appear swollen, normal, or atrophic.

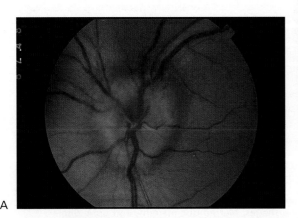
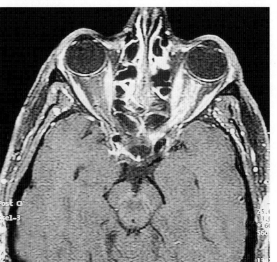

FIGURE 9.29. A: Unilateral disc edema in a 56-year-old woman with a meningioma involving the left optic nerve sheath. **B:** T1-weighted magnetic resonance imaging of orbit and brain demonstrating enhancement of the left optic nerve by an optic nerve meningioma.

Optic Nerve Tumors

Clinical Features. Optic nerve tumors may result in a swollen disc initially but optic nerve pallor eventually develops (Fig. 9.29). Optochoroidal shunt vessels may develop on the disc surface (Fig. 9.30). These vessels represent an alternative pathway for blood to egress the eye when the normal venous return is impaired.

The syndrome of optic atrophy and optochoroidal shunt vessels is usually caused by a *perioptic meningioma* in adults (usually middle-aged women) and a *glioma* in children. Proptosis and resistance to retropulsion of the globe may be evident with either tumor.

Management. Management is controversial for optic nerve meningiomas and gliomas. No treatment is indicated if the lesion is localized to one optic nerve and does not appear to be extending intracranially and if visual acuity is preserved. Any surgery on the optic nerve produces immediate loss of vision.

A few authors still advocate orbital exenteration for meningiomas in children and surgical extirpation of gliomas. Radiation therapy has been advocated to retard the growth of both tumors.

Orbital Optic Nerve Compression

Many orbital processes may produce a compressive optic neuropathy.

Clinical Features. The more common orbital conditions resulting in optic nerve compression include orbital inflammatory disease (e.g., pseudotumor), Graves' disease, and infections. Proptosis is a common feature. When ocular motility disturbances accompany decreased vision and proptosis, the term *orbital apex syndrome* is appropriate. The appearance of the optic nerve and visual field defects varies. If the process interferes with venous return, the optic nerve may be swollen. If the compression is slow to develop, as can occur with a tumor, optic atrophy may be seen.

The *optic neuropathy associated with Graves' disease* is the result of compression of the optic nerve at the orbital apex by markedly enlarged extraocular muscles (Fig. 9.31). Patients who develop this syndrome usually do not have marked proptosis but instead have dramatically increased resistance to retropulsion of the eyes.

Management. Imaging of the optic nerve is indicated when intraorbital optic nerve compression is suspected in Graves' disease. The management options for compressive optic neuropathy associated with Graves' disease with progressively decreasing visual function include low-dose orbital irradiation, systemic corticosteroids, and orbital decompression.

Intermittent Compression

Clinical Features. This unusual syndrome is produced when an orbital mass lesion causes optic nerve compression and decreased ocular blood flow in certain directions of gaze (Fig. 9.32). Directional gaze-induced amaurosis fugax is a sign of intraorbital optic nerve compression.

Management. Orbital imaging is indicated, and therapy usually consists of surgical removal of the mass.

Intracranial Compression

Clinical Features. This optic neuropathy is usually caused by perichiasmal mass lesions such as pituitary tumors, craniopharyngiomas, meningiomas, or aneurysms. Signs or symptoms of compression of other surrounding structures also may be present, such as chiasmal junctional syndrome or ocular misalignment due to cavernous sinus involvement. With intracranial compression, the optic disc usually is normal but becomes progressively swollen or atrophic. The sudden appearance of a chiasmal syndrome caused by rapid expansion of a pituitary tumor because of hemorrhage into or swelling of the tumor is called *pituitary apoplexy* (Fig. 9.33).

Management. MRI is superior to CT in diagnosing most

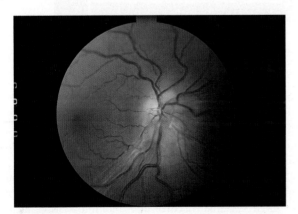

FIGURE 9.30. In a 12-year-old girl with an optic nerve glioma, the disc is becoming pale superiorly, with marked nerve fiber loss. An early shunt vessel is forming at 9 o'clock, off the central retinal vein.

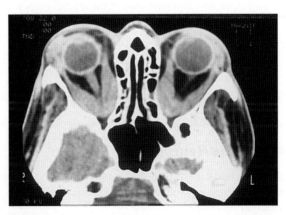

FIGURE 9.31. Graves' optic neuropathy. Axial computed tomography shows marked enlargement of the ocular muscles at the orbital apex. The medial walls of the orbit are bowed inward by the enlarged medial recti.

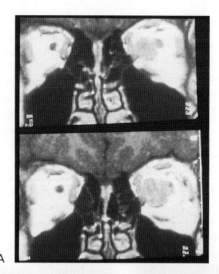

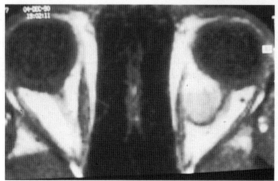

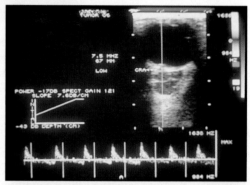

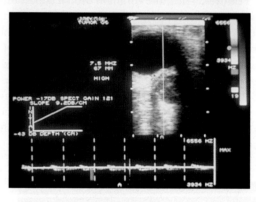

FIGURE 9.32. **A:** An orbital vascular mass lesion nasal to the right optic nerve is delineated by coronal magnetic resonance imaging. **B:** A mass lesion is visible in the medial portion of the right orbit. The left orbit is normal. On lateral gaze, the mass compressed the optic nerve, and vision fell to the level of no light perception, with an amaurotic pupil. **C:** Color Doppler orbital imaging shows a normal arterial flow and pulse wave in the central retinal artery in the primary position but **(D)** a complete lack of flow and flattening of the arterial pulse wave on lateral gaze.

instances of intracranial optic nerve or chiasmal compression.

Toxic Optic Neuropathy

The optic nerve may be adversely affected by toxic substances, including specific medications prescribed for nonocular conditions.

Clinical Features. Decreased acuity, dyschromatopsia, and bilateral central or centrocecal visual field defects are the hallmarks of toxic optic neuropathy. Bilaterality and relative symmetric involvement are the rules. The visual loss may be mild to severe and may be sudden in onset or slowly progressive. The fundus examination is usually normal, although disc edema may be observed. Optic atrophy subsequently develops in most cases.

Methanol (i.e., wood alcohol) is a commonly available substance with significant ocular neurotoxic effects (Fig. 9.34). The severe systemic effects of methanol intoxication, including acidosis and cerebral dysfunction, usually accompany the visual loss. Disc edema may be present. Toluene, used by glue sniffers, is another substance that is toxic to the optic nerve.

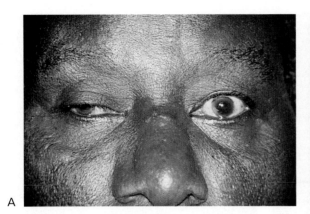

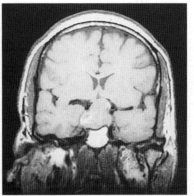

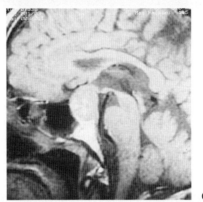

FIGURE 9.33. Pituitary apoplexy. **A:** Patient with a right cranial nerve III palsy. **B:** The coronal magnetic resonance scan shows a large pituitary tumor compressing the optic chiasm that caps the lesion. The tumor extends into the right cavernous sinus, causing the oculomotor problem. **C:** In this sagittal view [as well in coronal view **(B)**], blood appears as white areas in the tumor, indicating an acute hemorrhage.

Drugs with reported optic nerve toxicity include chloramphenicol, the halogenated hydroxyquinoline, and the antituberculosis agents isoniazid and ethambutol. The clinician should maintain a high degree of suspicion for a toxic optic neuropathy when a patient presents with bilateral centrocecal scotomas and no other obvious cause.

Management. The offending agent should be discontinued. There is no specific treatment for the optic neuropathy. Visual recovery is variable, but improvement occurs in many cases, with the exception of those associated with methanol ingestion. In methanol intoxication, reestablishment of the proper electrolyte balance and supportive measures are imperative.

Amiodarone Optic Neuropathy

Amiodarone has been documented to produce disc edema in a small percentage of patients. It has been documented to occur with treatment from 1 to 72 months, and the dosage varied from 200 to 1200 mg/day. Patients present with insidious unilateral or bilateral decreased vision that may gradually progress and is associated with optic nerve edema. The visual acuity and field loss tend to stabilize or improve following discontinuation of the medication. The major differences between nonarteritic AION and amiodarone optic neuropathy are that the visual loss is bilateral and insidious, and the optic disc swelling persists longer with amiodarone toxicity, tending to take months rather than weeks to resolve. The mechanism of amiodarone optic neuropathy is unknown, but histology has shown primary lipidosis of the optic nerve (Fig.9. 35).

FIGURE 9.34. The right fundus of a commercial sailor who had been at sea for 3 weeks and drank methanol from the ship's compass. He was comatose and had dilated pupils. Examination 2 days after ingestion showed the discs to be swollen and pale. Retinal edema was also present. The patient died 2 days later.

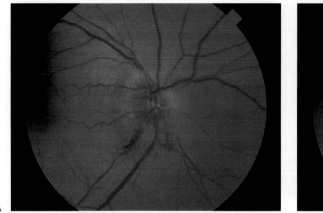
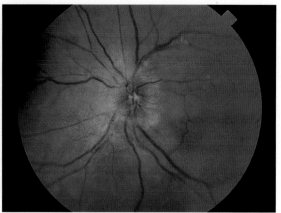

FIGURE 9.35. Amiodarone optic neuropathy. Bilateral disc edema with nerve fiber layer hemorrhages more prominent on the right disc.

Optic Neuropathy Associated With Nutritional Deficiency

Optic neuropathy has been associated with a deficiency of B-complex vitamins, particularly thiamine. Originally, this type of neuropathy was thought to be associated with chronic tobacco or alcohol abuse. However, most authorities now think that the nutritional deficiency is the underlying cause.

Clinical Features. The findings are those of a toxic optic neuropathy, with decreased acuity, dyschromatopsia, and bilateral centrocecal scotomas (Fig. 9.36). Initially, the fundus is normal, although instances of mild disc edema and hemorrhages have been reported. An affected patient with a longstanding nutritional deficiency has optic disc pallor.

Management. A return to a well-balanced diet with vitamin B complex supplements results in visual improvement

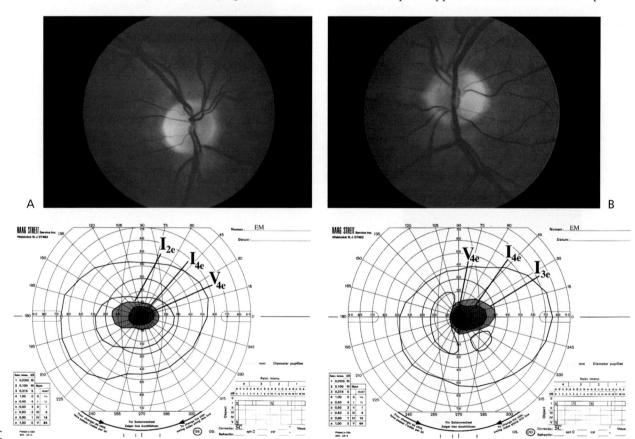

FIGURE 9.36. Nutritional-toxic optic neuropathy. A 36-year-old man noticed a gradual decrease in his vision over a 12-month period. He gave a history of serious alcohol abuse and poor dietary intake. Vision was 20/400 for the right eye and 20/200 for the left eye. Temporal pallor was seen in the **(A)** right disc and **(B)** left disc. **C:** Bilateral centrocecal scotomas were found on Goldmann visual field examination.

in some patients early in the course of the optic neuropathy. However, patients in whom optic disc pallor has developed rarely improve.

Traumatic Optic Neuropathy

The optic nerve may be injured by direct or indirect trauma to its intraocular, orbital, canalicular, or intracranial segment. Traumatic optic neuropathy is a true ocular emergency, and early recognition is crucial to effective management.

The optic nerve is anchored at the globe and chiasm and is tethered by the annulus of Zinn at the orbital apex and within the optic canal. However, within the orbit, the nerve assumes a sinusoidal pathway that is 7 mm longer than the globe to optic canal distance. This allows the globe to move freely and provides protection for the nerve, allowing it to be pushed aside by penetrating objects and permitting some degree of globe displacement without avulsing the nerve during blunt trauma.

Clinical Features. The presenting signs and symptoms of traumatic optic neuropathy depend on the circumstances of the injury. Typically, visual acuity is depressed to a level of 20/400 or less. Many patients are found to have light perception only or no light perception and an associated RAPD. The decrease in vision occurs with the injury in most cases, although a delayed worsening has been reported in fewer than 10% of cases.

Traumatic optic neuropathy may result from direct injury to the nerve within the orbit or indirectly from trauma to the face, globe, or head. *Direct trauma* to the optic nerve within the orbit can occur as the result of a missile or penetrating stab injury that may partially or completely transect the nerve. Intraorbital hemorrhage or hemorrhage within the optic nerve sheaths may produce a compressive type of optic neuropathy (Fig. 9.37). *Indirect injury* to the ocular portion of the nerve typically occurs as the result of a sudden rotation or anterior displacement of the globe, as can occur with a finger poke. Partial or complete avulsion of the nerve head may occur, resulting in the ophthalmoscopic appearance of a pit at the site of the papilla, surrounded by a ring of hemorrhage (Fig. 9.38). Central retinal artery or vein occlusion also may be seen ophthalmoscopically.

The most common form of traumatic optic neuropathy is the result of an indirect injury that affects the intracanalicular portion of the nerve. In a frontal head injury, the force is transmitted posteriorly through the orbital walls to the sphenoid bone and optic canal. Automobile, bicycle, and motorcycle accidents, along with falls and assaults, are the most common sources of trauma. Injury to the nerve may occur in several ways. In a frontal head impact with sudden deceleration, the orbital contents continue to move forward. The dura within the optic canal is anchored to the periosteum of the surrounding bone superiorly. The nerve is less firmly attached to its sheaths, creating a shearing motion that may damage the small pial vessels vital to the nutrient

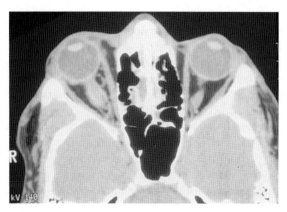

FIGURE 9.37. This patient poked himself in the right eye with a car antenna. Ptosis and rapidly progressive visual loss were experienced, and an entrance wound was found in the right upper lid. Axial computed tomography showed an enlarged optic nerve sheath consistent with optic nerve sheath hematoma. This was confirmed on surgical exploration. (Courtesy of John W. Shore, M.D., Boston, MA, and Jurij Bilyk, M.D., Philadelphia, PA.)

supply of the nerve in this area. Hemorrhage and edema within the optic canal may also compress the nerve, and fractures around the optic canal may result in bony fragments that may press on the nerve.

In cases of indirect trauma to the intracanalicular portion of the nerve, the ophthalmoscopic examination is normal. Injury to the intracranial portion of the optic nerve is rare but has been associated with closed head trauma.

Management. Traumatic optic neuropathy is primarily a clinical diagnosis. However, CT imaging is extremely helpful in evaluating the status of the orbit, the optic nerve, and the integrity of the surrounding bony structure. MRI may add information after it has been determined that no metallic foreign body is present.

There is no specific treatment for direct injury to the optic nerve. Compression on the nerve by intraorbital hemorrhage is treated by orbital decompression, and hemorrhage within the nerve sheath may be helped by an optic nerve sheath fenestration procedure. Generally, intraorbital for-

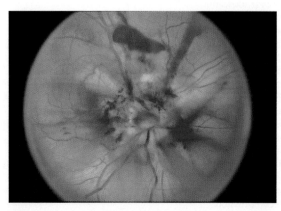

FIGURE 9.38. Avulsion of the optic nerve head, showing pit at the site of the papilla surrounded by a ring of hemorrhage. (Courtesy of William C. Benson, M.D., Philadelphia, PA.)

eign bodies should be removed, although some may be observed, depending on their composition and position in the orbit.

Treatment of posterior indirect traumatic optic neuropathy involving the intracanalicular portion of the nerve remains controversial (Table 9.2). Some clinicians recommend high doses of intravenous corticosteroids within the first 24 hours of injury, continuing for 2 to 3 days. Although there is some evidence that corticosteroids are helpful in spinal cord injuries, the efficacy of this treatment in traumatic optic neuropathy remains unproven, and the complications associated with corticosteroid therapy must be kept

in mind. Surgical depression of the optic canal is a treatment option in some cases but also remains controversial. The Traumatic Optic Neuropathy Treatment Trial is evaluating these treatment options.

Leber's Stellate Neuroretinitis

Leber's stellate neuroretinitis is the constellation of optic disc edema and a macular star due to any presumed or known inflammatory or infectious optic neuropathy. Cat-scratch disease caused by *Rochalimaea (Bartonella) henselae*, a gram-negative bacillus, is the most common infectious cause. Systemic symptoms are mild when present, but 50% of patients have a history of an antecedent viral infection. Ocular manifestations include Parinaud's oculoglandular syndrome, a unilateral granulomatous conjunctivitis with ipsilateral preauricular or submandibular lymphadenitis, uveitis, and retinal vasculitis. Diagnosis is facilitated by a history of a cat scratch combined with a high antibody (immunoglobulin G) titer to *R. henselae* in sera. The condition responds to several different antibiotics, including erythromycin, doxycycline, and ciprofloxacin (Fig 9.39). Other causes of neuroretinitis are idiopathic, viral (e.g., chickenpox, mumps, measles), spirochetal infections (secondary or tertiary syphilis), and Lyme disease (stage III).

Congenital Disc Anomalies

Pseudopapilledema

In patients with pseudopapilledema, the discs appear slightly elevated and the margins indistinct but without other signs of increased intracranial pressure.

Clinical Features. Normally optic discs are contiguous with the plane of the retina and possess a discernible optic cup. In some cases, discs may be elevated to simulate papilledema (Fig. 9.40). These discs do not have visible physiologic cups, and the large vessels appear to originate from the center of the discs. There are no dilated capillaries on the

TABLE 9.2. TREATMENT RECOMMENDATIONS FOR THE TWO MOST FREQUENT FORMS OF TRAUMATIC OPTIC NEUROPATHY

Optic Neuropathy Secondary to Orbital Hemorrhage (Orbital Compartment Syndrome)

Immediate lateral canthotomy and inferior cantholysis. Rule out any evidence of intraocular injury.

Methylprednisolone 250 mg IV q 6 hrs for 12–24 hrs, followed by rapid oral corticosteroid taper.

Frequent ice compresses (20 min on/20 min off for 6 hrs).

Topical therapy for markedly increased intraocular pressure (>45 mm Hg).

Consider IV mannitol.

Optic Neuropathy Secondary to Posterior Indirect Injury (Deceleration Injury)

Rule out any evidence of intraocular injury.

If no systemic contraindications are present:

Offer patient megadose IV corticosteroids (methylprednisolone load of 30 mg/kg, followed by 5.4 mg/hr continuous infusion for 48–72 hrs).

Counsel patient regarding the potential risks and side effects of systemic corticosteroid therapy.

Institute appropriate gastroesophageal protection (ranitidine, etc.).

If systemic contraindications are present (diabetes, immunosuppression, infection):

Obtain immediate medical consultation and proceed with corticosteroids, if allowed.

Obtain immediate CT imaging (NOT MRI!), with 1–1.5 mm axial and coronal sections of orbital apex, optic canal, and cavernous sinus.

If evidence of optic canal impingement by bony fragments is present, offer patient optic canal decompression. If optic canal appears normal or is fractured without impingement, continue with corticosteroids as above.

If optic nerve function deteriorates while on megadose corticosteroids, offer the patient optic canal decompression. If vision remains stable or improves, continue corticosteroids without surgical intervention.

After 48–72 hrs of megadose corticosteroids, discharge patient on oral taper of corticosteroid over 5–7 days, with close outpatient follow-up.

If vision deteriorates while on oral dose, reinstitute IV therapy with slower taper.

If optic neuropathy continues to progress, consider optic canal decompression.

CT, computerized tomography; IV, intravenous.

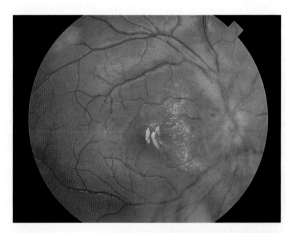

FIGURE 9.39. Neuroretinitis secondary to cat-scratch disease. The right optic disc is hyperemic and there is a macular star.

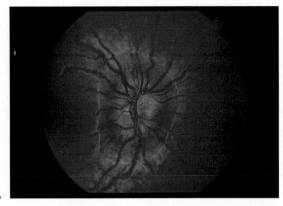
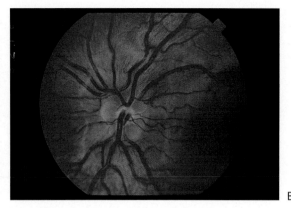

FIGURE 9.40. Pseudopapilledema. There is no cup in either nerve head, and the vessels egress from the center of the disc. There are no hemorrhages or exudates, and the nerve fiber layer is not opacified. The right disc **(A)** appears more elevated than the left **(B)**.

disc surface, and the nerve fiber layer is clear, without the opacification typical of papilledema. Hemorrhages and exudates are rarely present. In a significant percentage of these discs, the fullness is the result of visible or "buried" drusen.

Management. Pseudopapilledema usually is diagnosed during a routine eye examination or may be noticed on fundus examination as part of a workup for other medical problems. Follow-up to document the relative static appearance of the discs is helpful.

Drusen of the Optic Disc

Small, yellow-white formations in the optic nerve head anterior to the lamina cribrosa are known as hyaline bodies or, more commonly, *drusen.*

Clinical Features. The disc may appear elevated, with blurred margins and lacks a physiologic cup. The drusen are yellowish white and vary in size (Fig. 9.41). Sometimes, they are seen best in reflected light by directing the ophthalmoscopic beam at the disc margin. Drusen are presumed to be an accumulation of axoplasmic debris. They are invisible (i.e., buried) in early childhood but become more promi-

nent with age. They are bilateral in 66% of patients. Occasionally, optic nerve drusen may be associated with hemorrhages on the surface of the disc or in the peripapillary retinal or subretinal area (Fig. 9.42).

The visual field defects are highly variable but usually affect the nerve fiber bundle and may be progressive. There is no known method of halting or preventing progressive visual field loss. Visual acuity is rarely decreased. There is no unequivocal association with any systemic or ocular disease.

Pits of the Optic Nerve

Optic pits are congenital defects most frequently located temporally and inferiorly at the disc margin.

Clinical Features. Pits are sharply outlined and a deeper gray color compared with the remainder of the disc surface. The amount of excavation and the size are variable. A small, cilioretinal artery sometimes can be seen exiting at the pit margin. There may be adjacent chorioretinal atrophy. Visual acuity is usually good, but visual field changes in the form of nerve fiber bundle or altitudinal defects may be found. Evidence of serous retinal detachment in the macu-

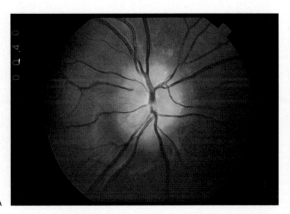
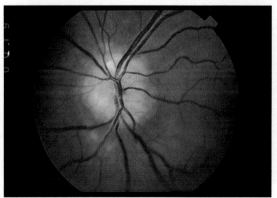

FIGURE 9.41. Drusen are visible as round, crystalline formations. The discs have a typical yellowish hue, and there are no cups. **A:** Right eye. **B:** Left eye.

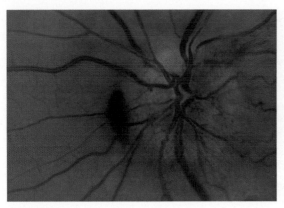

FIGURE 9.42. Right disc with visible drusen at the 11:30 position. Hemorrhages are seen on the disc surface and beneath the retinal pigment epithelium concentric to the disc.

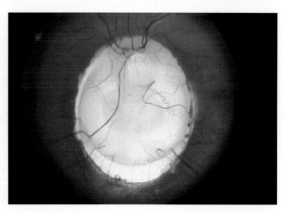

FIGURE 9.44. Large coloboma of the disc. This patient had a basal encephalocele due to a midline defect at the base of the skull.

lar area has been reported in 40% of eyes with congenital pits (Fig. 9.43). Chronic serous retinopathy may result in decreased vision. Fluorescein angiography is indicated if central serous retinopathy is suspected and cannot be confirmed by ophthalmoscopy alone.

Coloboma of the Optic Nerve

A larger congenital excavation of the optic nerve head is known as a coloboma and is related to a faulty closure of the fetal fissure.

Clinical Features. The disc is enlarged and appears white and excavated, typically in the inferior portion. The size of the coloboma varies, sometimes occupying most of the disc (Fig. 9.44). The vessels are located near the disc margin. Contiguous chorioretinal coloboma and peripapillary chorioretinal atrophy are common features. Visual acuity is often reduced from 20/100 to hand motions. As with pits, serous retinal detachments develop in a high percentage of eyes with disc colobomas. Disc malformations may be associated with other facial and skull defects, including basal encephaloceles.

Morning Glory Disc

Morning glory disc is a congenital disc anomaly characterized by an enlarged, funnel-shaped disc with a central core of white tissue surrounded by chorioretinal pigmentary changes, resulting in the ophthalmoscopic resemblance to the flower (Fig. 9.45).

Clinical Features. The disc is pale and enlarged to the extent that the reflex within the papillary space may be mistaken for a leukokoria. This disc is excavated, and the vessels are located at the periphery. The condition is unilateral. Vision is considerably reduced to the extent that an RAPD may be found. The cause remains controversial.

Oblique Insertion of the Optic Nerve

Optic discs that obliquely insert into the eye appear tilted on ophthalmoscopy (Fig. 9.46). The tilt may occur in any direction and is usually associated with a crescent adjacent to the disc. The association of congenitally tilted optic disc with an inferonasal scleral crescent is known as the *tilted disc syndrome.* Ectasia of the nasal and inferior fundus is seen in a high percentage of these patients and may produce a tem-

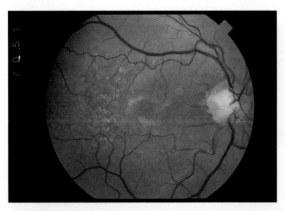

FIGURE 9.43. Typical edema residues in the macula of a patient with central serous chorioretinopathy associated with a pit of the right optic disc.

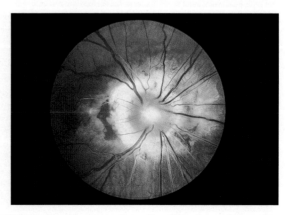

FIGURE 9.45. Morning glory disc. (Courtesy of Gary Brown, M.D., Philadelphia, PA.)

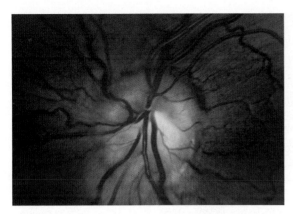

FIGURE 9.46. Tilted disc syndrome. The optic nerve appears to be tilted superiorly.

poral visual field defect. However, some of the field defects in tilted disc syndrome are "refractive scotomas," resulting from exaggerated astigmatism at an oblique axis, and they disappear with full lens correction.

Hypoplasia of the Optic Disc

A smaller than normal optic disc may be associated with delayed or incomplete physical growth, neuroendocrine disturbances, and central nervous system abnormalities.

Clinical Features. The disc is small, often pale, and may be surrounded by a yellow-white ring with variable pigmentation (Fig. 9.47). This appearance has been referred to as the *double ring sign*, with the peripheral margin of the encircling ring corresponding to the border of a normal-sized optic disc. The inner ring corresponds to the termination of the retina and retinal pigment epithelium. Vision may range from normal to the level of no light perception. Visual field defects are common but are not characteristic.

Hypoplasia of the optic disc has been associated with young maternal age, drug use during pregnancy, and maternal diabetes. Hypoplasia of the optic nerve may be associated with numerous and varied systemic developmental ab-

normalities. The association of an absence of the septum pellucidum, optic nerve hypoplasia, and pituitary dwarfism is known as septooptic dysplasia (*de Morsier's syndrome*).

Management. Children found to have decreased vision associated with hypoplasia of the optic nerve should have a trial of standard amblyopia therapy to determine if vision can be improved. Consultation with a pediatric endocrinologist is indicated to evaluate for growth and endocrine abnormalities.

Topless Optic Disc Syndrome

Topless optic disc syndrome or superior segmental optic hypoplasia is a congenital anomaly of the superior part of the disc. Patients usually have good visual acuity with an inferior altitudinal field defect. The disc appearance is characterized by pallor of the superior disc, a relative superior entrance of the central retinal artery, thinning of the superior peripapillary nerve fiber layer, and superior peripapillary scleral halo. It is most commonly seen in patients whose mothers had insulin-dependent diabetes (Fig 9.48).

Congenital Disc Sheathing

During embryonic development, glial cells surround the intravitreous hyaloid artery. This periarterial sheathing is known as *Bergmeister's papilla*. Late in fetal development, this papilla atrophies, and the degree to which it regresses determines in part the amount of physiologic cupping. However, if the regression is incomplete, residual amounts of glial tissue representing the former Bergmeister's papilla can be seen on the disc surface (Fig. 9.49). These formations also have been called prepapillary or congenital veils.

Patients with incomplete resolution of Bergmeister's papilla may present with a variety of other congenital optic disc abnormalities, including vascular loops, persistent hyperplastic primary vitreous, and morning glory disc anomaly.

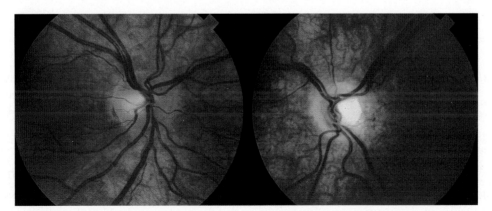

FIGURE 9.47. Hypoplasia of the optic nerve. The right optic disc is normal. A small nubbin of tissue is located nasally in the left disc. The rest of the disc is "empty," and a typical double ring sign is seen, particularly nasally. The nerve fiber layer is practically nonexistent.

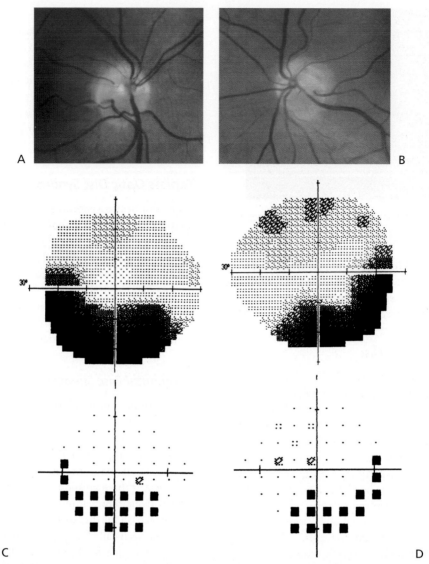

FIGURE 9.48. Topless disc syndrome (superior segmental optic disc hypoplasia). The optic disc is pale superiorly with a relative superior entrance of the central retinal artery, and superior peripapillary scleral halos. **A:** Right eye. **B:** Left eye. Humphrey automated perimetry shows bilateral inferior nerve fiber layer defects, worse in the left eye **(C)** than the right eye **(D)**, corresponding to the optic nerve appearance.

Persistent Hyaloid Artery

Occasionally, remnants of the primitive hyaloid artery are seen on the disc surface. The hyaloid artery enters the embryonic tissue at the 5-mm stage of development and reaches the posterior surface of the lens as part of the tunica vasculosa lentis. Regression of the hyaloid artery begins in the third month of gestation. Atrophy usually is complete by the eighth month, but portions of the artery may persist as atrophic, thread-like attachments or may be filled with blood (Fig. 9.50). The anterior attachment of the hyaloid artery to the posterior surface of the lens is known as a *Mittendorf's dot*, which persists as a small circular opacity in the inferior nasal aspect of the posterior lens capsule. Failure of the vascular system of the primary vitreous to regress leads to *persistent hyperplastic primary vitreous*.

Hereditary Optic Neuropathy

Leber's Hereditary Optic Neuropathy

Leber's hereditary optic neuropathy (LHON) is a hereditary syndrome characterized by bilateral visual loss, beginning in the second and third decades of life, and primarily affecting men.

Clinical Features. In the acute phase of the disease, there

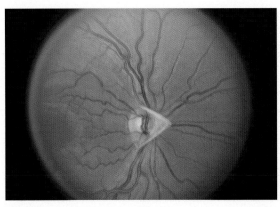

FIGURE 9.49. Bergmeister's papilla (i.e., congenital veil) is found typically on the nasal aspect of the disc.

is bilateral disc hyperemia and a characteristic peripapillary microangiopathy that may be present before visual symptoms are evident (Fig. 9.51). In the acute stage, the nerve fiber layer is opacified. As the acute phase recedes, the disc develops a pale, flat appearance. Vision is reduced to the range of 20/200 to finger counting.

Most of those affected are men. LHON is transmitted through the female line, although only 14% of affected individuals are women. An unaffected carrier mother transmits the disease to 50% of her sons. It has been advanced that all daughters of carrier mothers become carriers themselves. Men cannot transmit the disease to their progeny. The disease may be associated with pathogenic mutations of mitochondrial DNA at various nucleotide positions. These mitochondrial defects affect other systems, including skeletal and cardiac muscle. Cardiac conduction defects may be encountered.

LHON may be mistaken for optic neuritis because of the age of onset and the signs of an acute unilateral optic neuropathy, including a swollen optic disc. However, rapid involvement of the fellow eye, the peripapillary telangiectasia, the family history, and the lack of recovery in most cases should strongly suggest LHON. Other forms of inherited optic atrophy may produce decreased vision and pale discs in the young, and these forms may be dominant or recessive.

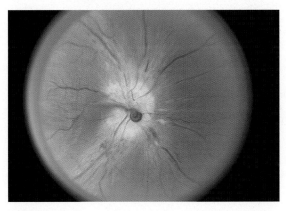

FIGURE 9.50. Blood-filled remnant of the hyaloid artery.

However, the hereditary optic atrophies are slowly progressive, without an acute phase.

Management. There is no treatment, although cases of spontaneous recovery to reasonable vision, even many years later, have been reported.

Dominant Optic Atrophy

Another optic nerve atrophy distinguishable from LHON is dominant optic atrophy. Visual acuity depression is mild in dominant optic atrophy.

Clinical Features. The onset of visual loss is insidious and occurs between 4 and 8 years of age. Vision is mildly to moderately depressed, usually in the range of 20/30 to 20/70. The condition is bilateral but may be asymmetric. Temporal pallor of the optic discs occurs (Fig. 9.52), dyschromatopsia may be present, and nystagmus has been reported in some pedigrees. Central scotomas are found on visual field examination. Vision remains stable in many cases, but a gradual decrease has been observed in others. Most patients do retain reasonably good visual function.

THE PUPIL

Innervation to the pupils is through the parasympathetic system, which produces pupillary constriction, and the sympathetic system, which produces pupillary dilation. A decrease in parasympathetic input produces pupillary mydriasis, and sympathetic lesions produce pupillary miosis. Because these abnormalities are usually unilateral, the presenting sign is anisocoria.

Anisocoria, a difference in size between the two pupils, is not necessarily a pathologic condition. It is estimated that approximately 20% of the normal population manifests clinically observable anisocoria (i.e., physiologic or simple anisocoria). The relative difference between pupillary size remains constant in dim and bright illumination in physiologic anisocoria. The degree of anisocoria due to sympathetic paresis is greater in dim illumination, and parasympathetic lesions produce anisocoria that is greater in bright light. Examination of the patient with anisocoria in different illumination levels is the first step in determining the cause of the pupillary disparity. Some pupillary abnormalities do not result in anisocoria but produce alterations in pupillary reactivity, shape, or position.

Pupillary reaction to light is decreased when a significant number of afferent visual fibers are not functioning, which may result from a disease process in the retina, optic nerve, optic chiasm, or optic tract. Lesions that destroy retinal function or involve the optic disc usually are visible with the ophthalmoscope, but for lesions of the retrobulbar optic nerve, the fundus examination initially may be normal. An abnormal pupil reaction to the swinging flashlight test is a *relative afferent pupillary defect* (Fig. 9.53). It provides objective evidence of anterior visual pathway dysfunction.

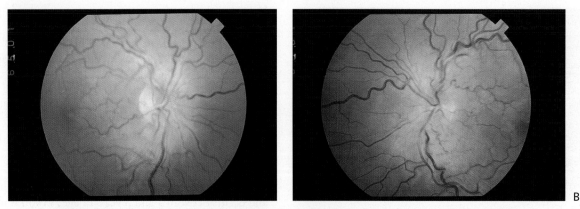

A

B

FIGURE 9.51. Acute Leber's hereditary optic neuropathy (LHON) in a 20-year-old man who tested positive for the 11778 mutation. **A:** The right eye was involved first. The nasal portion of the disc shows nerve fiber layer opacification, and pallor is developing in the papillomacular area of the optic nerve head. **B:** Later, the left eye became involved, with opacification of nerve fiber layer. Retinal peripapillary telangiectasis, a typical finding in LHON, is evident.

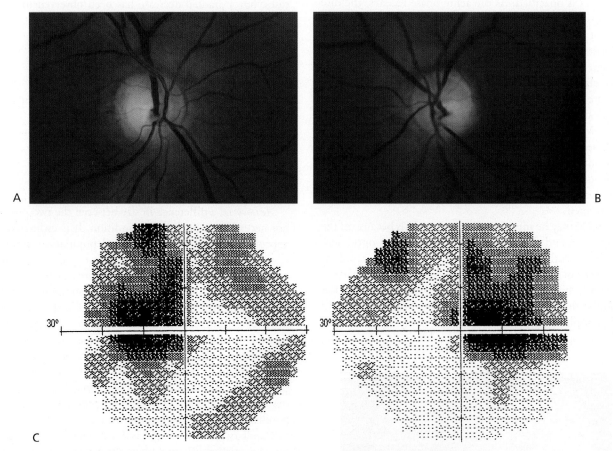

A

B

C

FIGURE 9.52. Dominant optic atrophy. Temporal pallor has occurred in the optic discs but has remained unchanged over 20 years of observation. **A:** Right eye. **B:** Left eye. **C:** Humphrey perimetry revealed typical pseudobitemporal hemianopia due to bilateral centrocecal scotomas.

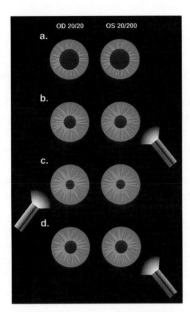

FIGURE 9.53. Relative afferent pupillary defect (RAPD). Vision in the right eye is 20/20, but vision in the left eye is 20/200 because of optic neuropathy. **A:** The pupils in dim light are equal. **B:** Light directed into the left eye results in a partial and sluggish contraction in each eye. **C:** Light directed into the right eye results in a brisk and normal reaction in each eye. **D:** The light quickly redirected into the left eye results in a dilatation of both pupils. It is possible to detect RAPD even in the presence of a dilated, dysfunctional pupil, as in a traumatic mydriasis or cranial nerve III palsy, by observing the other pupil.

Dilated Abnormal Pupil

When the larger pupil is the abnormal one, the anisocoria is more prominent in bright light, because the pupil cannot constrict normally. This condition may have neurologic or nonneurologic causes.

Pharmacologic Blockade

The unilateral instillation of a pupil-dilating medication produces anisocoria. This may occur inadvertently or may be purposely done for some secondary gain. A frequent accidental dilation of the pupil is produced by scopolamine-impregnated patches that are placed behind the ear to prevent motion sickness. Direct instillation of scopolamine to the eye surface by the patient's contaminated finger causes the pupillary dilation (Fig. 9.54).

To detect pharmacologic blockade as the cause of pupillary dilation, 1% pilocarpine is instilled in both eyes. The pupil constricts unless it is pharmacologically dilated or there is structural iris damage, which is visible on biomicroscopy.

Trauma

Traumatic mydriasis may be seen with or without iris sphincter ruptures. A history of trauma usually is elicited, or sphincter abnormalities are detected on slit lamp examination (Fig. 9.55). Pupillary excursions may be diminished. With time, the pupillary dilatation may lessen.

Tonic or Adie's Pupil

The patient is usually asymptomatic or has vague complaints of blurred reading vision. The pupil is dilated, constricts minimally or not at all in response to direct light, but does constrict slowly to sustained near effort (Fig. 9.56). The redilation phase is equally slow and tonic. Biomicroscopy of the iris sphincter shows areas of sector paresis that result in a characteristic slow, vermiform constriction of the pupil in response to bright light.

This condition may be isolated to the pupil or may be associated with decreased deep tendon reflexes in the lower extremities (i.e., Adie's syndrome). Adie's pupil is thought to result from a lesion in the ciliary ganglion, where the accommodative fibers far outnumber the fibers for the pupillary light reflex. Regeneration restores some accommodative pupillary movement but little light reaction.

Denervation hypersensitivity is demonstrated by pupillary constriction to weak (0.1%) pilocarpine solution. The exact

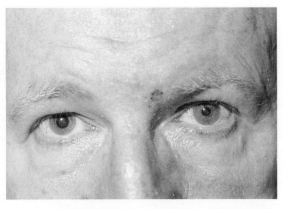
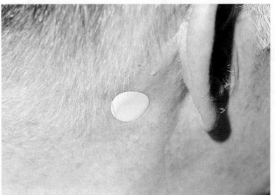

A   B

FIGURE 9.54. Pharmacologic mydriasis. **A:** The right pupil is dilated and does not constrict in response to 1% pilocarpine. **B:** The patient placed a scopalamine-impregnated patch for motion sickness behind the right ear and subsequently rubbed his right eye.

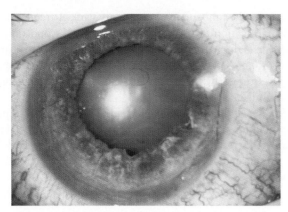

FIGURE 9.55. The right eye demonstrates iris sphincter tears from trauma induced by a bungee cord. (Photograph courtesy of John B. Jeffers, M.D., Philadelphia, PA.)

cause of or time for development of this denervation hypersensitivity is unknown. Before denervation hypersensitivity occurs, the pupil may not constrict even in response to 1% pilocarpine, causing confusion with pharmacologic blockade.

Over time, the Adie's pupil tends to become bilateral, and affected pupils become more miotic.

Parasympathetic Paresis

Pupillary dilation due to a parasympathetic lesion usually does not occur without other signs of cranial nerve III involvement, such as associated ocular muscle paresis and ptosis.

A cranial nerve III palsy with pupillary dilation is a medical emergency. The patient must be investigated for a compressive lesion, especially a posterior communicating artery aneurysm. Other compressive lesions, such as pituitary tumors, may produce this syndrome. An MRI scan is required, and if no mass is detected, immediate arteriography is necessary to rule out a posterior communicating artery aneurysm. Although the resolution of MRI or CT angiogra-

phy has improved, it has not eliminated the need for catheter angiography if MRI or CT is negative.

Dorsal Midbrain or Parinaud's Syndrome

Bilateral pupillary dilation with decreased reactivity to light but intact constriction to near effort (i.e., light near dissociation) is a hallmark of the dorsal midbrain syndrome. The pupils may also be eccentrically displaced, a condition called corectopia.

These patients are unable to look up voluntarily, and such an effort produces convergence retraction nystagmus (Fig. 9.57). Because this is a supranuclear disorder of upgaze, passive ductions (e.g., doll's head maneuver) produce more complete upgaze. Mass lesions in the pineal region are the most frequent cause of this syndrome, although nonmass lesions such as demyelinating disease and stroke can produce the dorsal midbrain syndrome.

Constricted Abnormal Pupils

Sympathetic Paresis or Horner's Syndrome

Sympathetic paresis of the eye produces *ptosis* because of decreased innervation of Müller's muscle and pupillary *miosis* (Fig. 9.58). Because the lower eyelid has an equivalent to

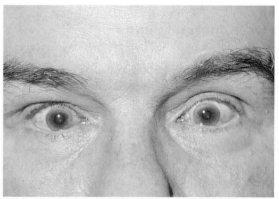

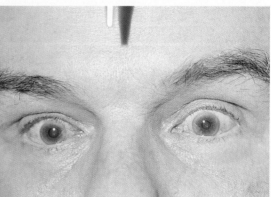

FIGURE 9.57. Dorsal midbrain syndrome (Parinaud's syndrome). The patient has **(A)** bilateral lid retraction, pupillary dilatation, and **(B)** the inability to look upward. The pupils do not react to light but do constrict to near effort.

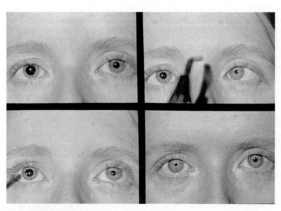

FIGURE 9.56. Adie's pupil. The right pupil *(upper left)* is dilated in standard light conditions, and it does not react to direct light *(lower left)* but does constrict slowly and tonically to near stimulus *(upper right)*. Marked miosis develops after instillation of 0.1% pilocarpine *(lower right)*.

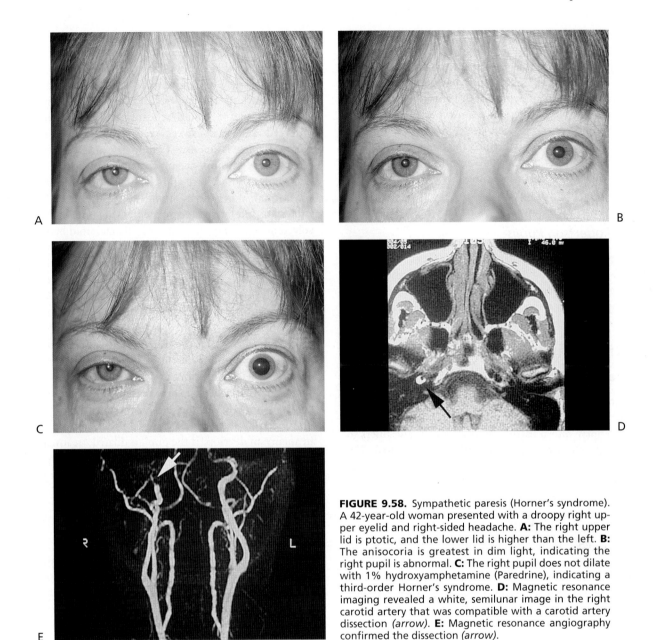

FIGURE 9.58. Sympathetic paresis (Horner's syndrome). A 42-year-old woman presented with a droopy right upper eyelid and right-sided headache. **A:** The right upper lid is ptotic, and the lower lid is higher than the left. **B:** The anisocoria is greatest in dim light, indicating the right pupil is abnormal. **C:** The right pupil does not dilate with 1% hydroxyamphetamine (Paredrine), indicating a third-order Horner's syndrome. **D:** Magnetic resonance imaging revealed a white, semilunar image in the right carotid artery that was compatible with a carotid artery dissection *(arrow)*. **E:** Magnetic resonance angiography confirmed the dissection *(arrow)*.

Müller's muscle (i.e., retractors of lower lid), the lower eyelid is higher on the side of the sympathetic paresis. Several inconsistent or transitory findings include decreased ipsilateral facial sweating, increased accommodation, and ocular hypotony. Iris heterochromia usually signifies congenital Horner's syndrome.

Horner's syndrome may occur with a lesion at any point along the three-neuron sympathetic chain. An isolated third-order Horner's syndrome is most likely to be caused by a benign condition and may be followed without investigation. Lesions of the first neuron usually produce other neurologic signs or symptoms, and second-order Horner's syndrome caused by superior pulmonary sulcus malignancies (i.e., Pancoast's syndrome) are accompanied by arm or scapular region pain.

The distinction between a preganglionic (i.e., first- and second-order Horner's syndrome) and a postganglionic (i.e., third-order Horner's syndrome) lesion can be made pharmacologically. Cocaine drops dilate normal pupils but not pupils with sympathetic paresis independent of the level of the lesion. Hydroxyamphetamine does not dilate the miotic pupil in Horner's disease if it results from a third-order neuron lesion but does dilate normal and first- and second-order Horner's pupils.

Management. The standard approach to investigating a patient with Horner's syndrome involves first pharmacologically confirming the diagnosis with topical cocaine (5% or 10%) and then localizing the lesion to the level of the neuron involved with hydroxyamphetamine 1%. An isolated postganglionic Horner's may be observed without investigation. If carotid dissection is suspected, an arteriogram is performed. Preganglionic Horner's is investigated with imaging along the course of the sympathetic chain. Another approach is to not rely on the pharmacologic testing as hydroxyamphetamine is neither 100% sensitive nor specific and postganglionic Horner's is not always benign. In this approach, all Horner's patients undergo MRI of the head and chest and magnetic resonance angiography (MRA) of the neck. For Horner's with heterochromia, if there is no evidence of birth trauma, imaging should be done to exclude cervical or mediastinal tumors.

Argyll-Robertson Pupils

The Argyll-Robertson pupillary abnormality usually is due to syphilis. Patients have bilateral pupillary miosis and a poor light reaction, despite possessing normal vision, but they have a normal near response (i.e., light near dissociation).

CRANIAL NERVE PALSIES

Cranial Nerve III Palsy

The third cranial nerve innervates the medial, inferior, and superior recti; the inferior oblique muscle, the levator palpebrae superioris, and it carries the parasympathetic fibers to the pupil. Signs of a cranial nerve III lesion are ptosis, decreased ocular elevation, depression and adduction, and occasionally, pupillary mydriasis.

Involvement of the third cranial nerve may represent a life-threatening situation. This condition, along with papilledema, is a true medical emergency.

Cranial nerve III arises in the midbrain from various subnuclear groupings. The lid and pupillary subnuclei are single-cell masses, and the subnuclei to the individual muscles innervated by cranial nerve III are paired. Another anatomic peculiarity of cranial nerve III is that the superior rectus fibers cross, with the right subnucleus giving rise to fibers innervating the left superior rectus and vice versa.

In the anterior cavernous sinus, cranial nerve III divides into a *superior division,* comprising lid and superior rectus fibers, and an *inferior division,* comprising medial and inferior rectus, inferior oblique muscles, and the parasympathetic pupillary fibers. However, partial, even divisional, involvement of cranial nerve III may occur at any point along its course.

Clinical Features. Cranial nerve III palsy produces ptosis and an inability to elevate, depress, or adduct the eye (Fig. 9.59). The pupil may be normal or dilated. Classically, isolated involvement of all portions of cranial nerve III without pupillary dilation is considered to be caused by infarction of cranial nerve III (i.e., vasculopathic mononeuropathy). Pupillary dilation, however, signifies a compressive lesion, and a posterior communicating artery aneurysm must be considered.

Management. Management of isolated cranial nerve III palsy in adults depends on whether the condition is total or partial and whether the pupil is normal or dilated.

For total palsy with a normal pupil, risk factors such as diabetes mellitus and hypertension in the appropriate age group (>45 years) should be identified. The patient can be observed and can expect recovery within 3 months. Neuroimaging is needed if the palsy progresses or other signs and symptoms occur. Patients between 10 and 40 years of age should have an MRI of the brain. If the results are normal, the patient should have a thorough medical evaluation and be observed closely. If the pupil becomes involved or signs and symptoms of subarachnoid hemorrhage develop, immediate arteriography is required.

For total palsy with a dilated pupil, the patient is admitted emergently. MRI is used to look for a compressive lesion, such as a pituitary tumor. If MRI is negative, arteriography is performed to search for a posterior communicating artery aneurysm.

For partial cranial nerve III paresis, the patient can be followed closely without treatment if the pupil is normal and the patient has risk factors that suggest a vasculopathic etiology. Alternatively, it is also reasonable to perform MRI followed by MRA if the MRI does not disclose a mass. Arteriography should be performed if symptoms or signs of an aneurysm develop. If the pupil is dilated, treatment is the same as for a patient with a total palsy and dilated pupil.

An isolated third cranial nerve palsy in younger patients may not be attributable to a vasculopathic process.

The suggested management of nontraumatic isolated cranial nerve III palsies in children follows:

Suspect ophthalmoplegic migraine in children.

Perform MRI for all children younger than 10 years of age, regardless of the state of the pupil. If the MR scan is negative, arteriography is not necessary because of the low likelihood of aneurysm.

Aberrant Regeneration

A peculiar ocular movement disorder may follow some cranial nerve III palsies (Fig. 9.60). This pattern is characterized by minimal or no ptosis in the primary position, eyelid elevation in attempted downgaze and adduction, restriction of vertical eye movements, and no pupillary constriction to light reflex but constriction on adduction. This pattern is seen most often after compressive III palsies, especially from posterior communicating artery aneurysms. It does not occur after vasculopathic III palsies.

The syndrome may be seen without a preceding apoplectic cranial nerve III palsy; this condition is called primary aberrant regeneration. This is an indication of a slowly growing mass lesion (e.g., meningioma, aneurysm) within the cavernous sinus.

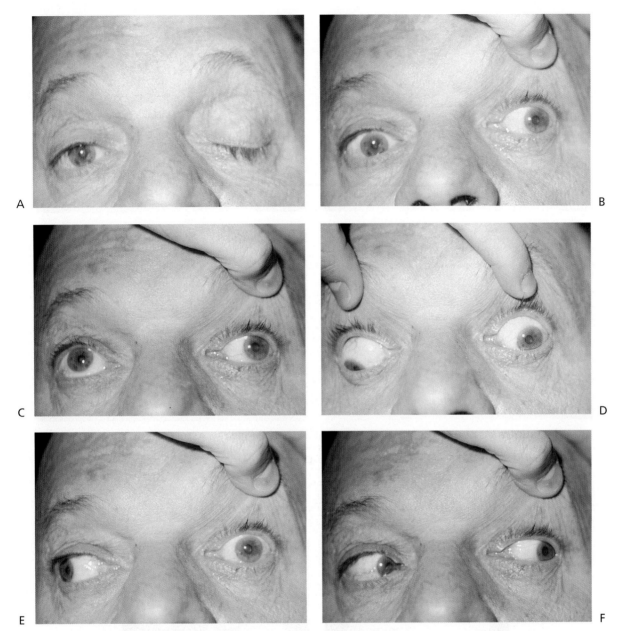

FIGURE 9.59. Third nerve palsy with relative pupil sparing. **A:** The patient has complete ptosis. **B:** In primary gaze, the affected left eye is deviated outwardly. The left pupil is only slightly larger than the right. The patient is unable to **(C)** elevate, **(D)** depress, or **(E)** adduct the eye. **F:** Abduction remains normal.

Cranial Nerve IV Palsy

The trochlear cranial nerve is the only cranial nerve to cross to the opposite side (i.e., the right nucleus becomes the left nerve) and to exit the brainstem dorsally. Because of its long intracranial course and its anatomic relation to the anterior medullary velum and the tip of the temporal lobe, it is vulnerable to a variety of insults, especially trauma.

Clinical Features. Paresis or paralysis of the trochlear nerve produces a hypertropia that is worse on gaze to the opposite side and on head tilt to the same side (Fig. 9.61).

Trauma is the most frequent cause of cranial nerve IV paresis. A blow to the top of the head can produce bilateral fourth nerve palsies characterized by alternating hypertropias on right and left gaze and by ocular torsion that may be as large as 15 degrees to 20 degrees. Unilateral cranial nerve IV paresis has a torsional component, but it is usually less than 5 degrees of excyclotorsion.

Patients may have cranial nerve IV weakness resulting from a congenital or longstanding insult. These patients usually have intermittent diplopia, because they have developed the ability to fuse abnormally large amounts of vertical

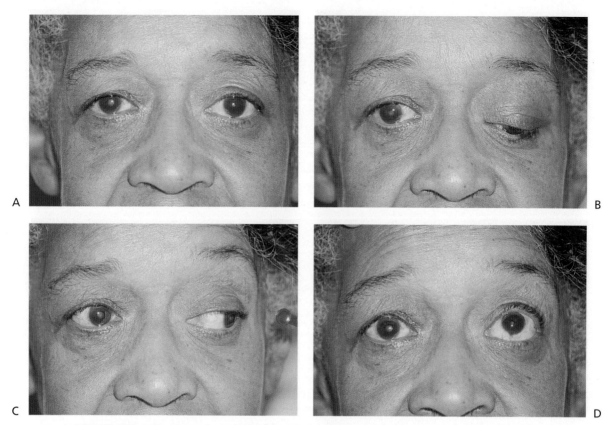

FIGURE 9.60. Aberrant regeneration after right cranial nerve III palsy. **A:** Four months after successful aneurysm surgery, there is minimal ptosis in primary gaze but retraction of the right upper lid develops on **(B)** downward and **(C)** left gaze. **D:** Superior gaze was also restricted.

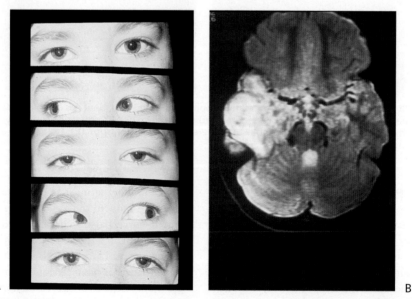

FIGURE 9.61. The patient is an 11-year-old boy with right cranial nerve IV palsy who has a right hypertropia, which is worse on left gaze. He has no history of trauma. **A:** On right head tilt *(top)*, the right eye elevates and the sclera below the inferior limbus is visible. On left head tilt *(bottom)*, the patient is orthotopic. He has normal vertical fusional amplitudes. **B:** Magnetic resonance scan of the same patient shows a large lesion of the right temporal lobe, which was a malignant glioma.

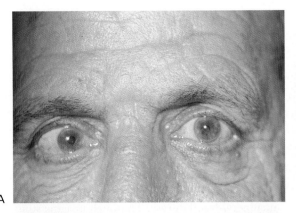
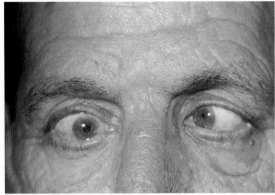

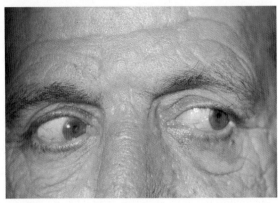

FIGURE 9.62. Right cranial nerve VI palsy. **A:** A right esotropia is demonstrated in the primary position. **B:** Right gaze reveals a complete abduction deficit. **C:** The patient was orthotopic on left gaze.

ocular misalignment. The finding of a *vertical fusional amplitude* greater than 5 prism diopters usually indicates a congenital cranial nerve IV paresis.

Management. Patients of all ages with large vertical fusional amplitudes need no further evaluation. They have decompensating congenital fourth nerve palsies.

In the absence of trauma, cranial nerve IV palsies that are isolated usually are vasculopathic in origin in patients older than 45 years of age. Under these circumstances, imaging may be deferred as long as the typical clinical course of a vasculopathic mononeuropathy is obeyed: no other structures involved, no progression after 1 week, and resolution usually within 3 months. Imaging is performed when deviation from this course occurs.

For patients who are in the nonvasculopathic age group without large vertical fusional amplitudes and for any patient with a motility disorder that is not quite classic or who demonstrates extraocular muscle fatigue, myasthenia gravis should be excluded. If the results are normal, MRI can rule out a posterior fossa tumor.

Cranial Nerve VI Palsy

The abducens nerve is often involved by intracranial processes because of its long course.

Clinical Features. Diplopia is the presenting symptom. There is decreased abduction of the involved eye, resulting in horizontal diplopia that is greatest on gaze to the affected side (Fig. 9.62). Cranial nerve VI palsy in an older adult is usu-

ally of vasculopathic origin if the palsy is isolated. If other signs or symptoms are present, further investigation (usually imaging) is directed at finding an intracranial lesion.

Unilateral or bilateral palsies may be a nonlocalizing sign of increased intracranial pressure from any cause. Any patient with sixth nerve palsies must have a fundus examination to rule out the presence of papilledema.

Other causes of abduction defects include spasm of the near reflex (Fig. 9.63); orbital muscle inflammation, such as

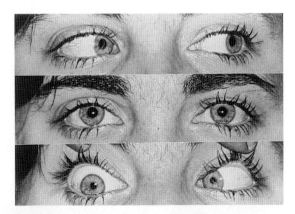

FIGURE 9.63. Spasm of the near reflex. The patient has a right abduction defect, but on right gaze *(lower photo)* the pupils are miotic compared with primary and left gazes. This indicates the patient is converging on "attempted" right gaze to simulate a right abduction defect. Pupillary miosis, which is part of the near triad along with convergence and accommodation, establishes the diagnosis. This complaint is usually nonphysiologic.

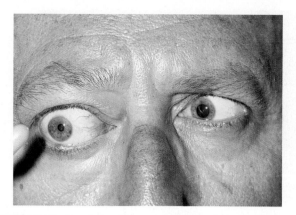

FIGURE 9.64. Restrictive myopathy. A right abduction defect is associated with right proptosis and lid retraction, unmistakable signs of thyroid-associated eye disease.

Graves' ophthalmopathy (Fig. 9.64); Duane's retraction syndrome (Fig. 9.65); medial rectus entrapment in the medial orbital wall following trauma, orbital, or sinus surgery (Fig. 9.66); and myasthenia gravis.

Management. A patient with an isolated unilateral nontraumatic sixth cranial nerve palsy who is younger than 14 years of age does not require imaging, because the condition is probably benign, unless the patient develops additional signs or symptoms of neurologic disease or has no history of a recent flu-like episode or vaccination. The physician should discuss with the parents the possibility of a compres-

sive lesion. If the parents are uncomfortable with not explicitly excluding the presence of a mass lesion, an MRI should be obtained.

Patients between 15 and 40 years of age represent a controversial management problem. Although in many of these patients the problem is benign, MRI is indicated. If the scan is negative, a thorough medical and neurologic examination and other laboratory studies are indicated to exclude entities such as hypertension, collagen vascular disease, MS, Lyme disease, and syphilis.

Children with bilateral sixth nerve palsies and no history of head trauma may have raised intracranial pressure or meningeal-based disease. Thorough imaging studies constitute the first step in the investigation.

For any infant or child with an ocular motor paresis, the diagnosis of battered child syndrome must be considered. The physician should seek other signs of maltreatment, such as bruises, a basilar skull fracture, long bone fractures, and retinal hemorrhages.

Multiple Cranial Nerve Palsies

Patients with more than one cranial nerve involved simultaneously or with other signs or symptoms require a different approach. The most frequent clinical syndromes are those of the cavernous sinus, superior orbital fissure, and orbital apex (Fig. 9.67). The anterior border of the cavernous sinus is the superior orbital fissure. Immediately anterior to the superior

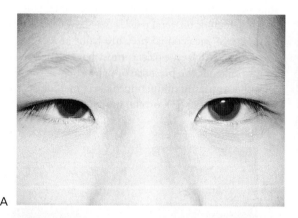

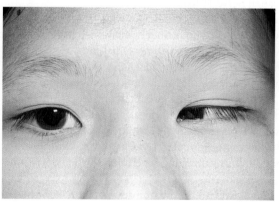

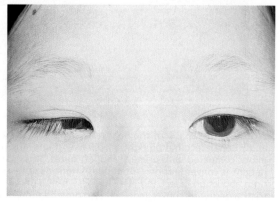

FIGURE 9.65. Duane's retraction syndrome. This child has bilateral abduction defects. **A:** A slight right esotropia is present in primary gaze. **B:** Right gaze shows a right abduction defect and narrowing of the left palpebral fissure. **C:** Left gaze shows similar defects.

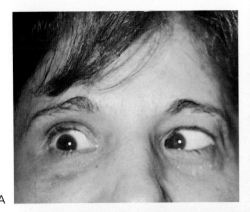
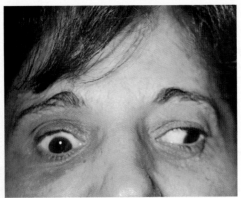

A

B

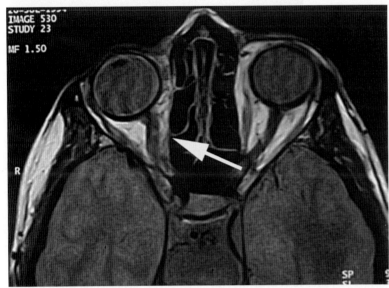

C

FIGURE 9.66. Medial rectus entrapment. This patient developed an abduction defect of the right eye after endoscopic sinus surgery. **A:** Right gaze shows a right abduction defect, and **(B)** left gaze demonstrates a restriction of the right medial rectus. **C:** Magnetic resonance reveals absence of the midportion of the right medial rectus muscle, with entrapment of the muscle stump and other tissue in the medial wall defect *(arrow)*. A forced duction test was markedly positive laterally.

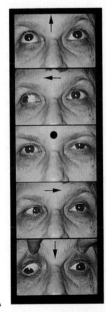

A

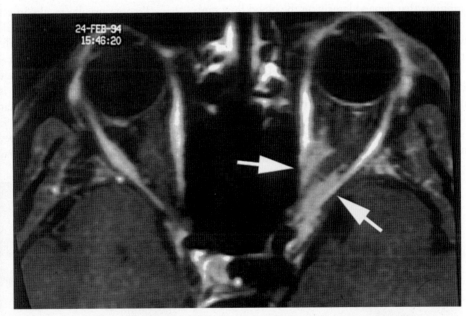

B

FIGURE 9.67. A 60-year-old woman with an inability to move the left eye and a swollen optic disc also had signs of an optic neuropathy. **A:** The eyes are orthotopic in primary gaze, although a left ptosis is evident. Right gaze reveals an adduction deficit in the left eye. In left gaze, the left eye cannot abduct, indicating multiple cranial nerve involvement. There is an inability to elevate and depress the left eye. **B:** Focused imaging revealed an enhancement at the orbital apex *(arrows)* that was later found to be lymphoma.

TABLE 9.3. LOCATION OF NERVES INVOLVED IN MULTIPLE CRANIAL NERVE PALSIES

Area of Nerve Lesions	Involved Cranial Nerves
Orbital apex	II, III, IV, VI
Superior orbital fissure	III, IV, V_1, VI
Cavernous sinus	III, IV, V_1, V_2, VI

orbital fissure is the orbital apex. The cranial nerves in each area are listed in Table 9.3.

Clinical Features. Any combination of deficits of the nerves contained in the cavernous sinus or superior orbital fissure may be produced by a variety of lesions. Mass lesions such as pituitary tumors, cavernous sinus meningiomas, or aneurysms; inflammatory process such as Tolosa-Hunt syndrome; or infiltrative lesions such as lymphoma can look the same clinically. Differentiation requires imaging and a variety of other investigations.

Management. The first study to be performed in the diagnosis of any patient with an orbital apex, superior orbital fissure, or cavernous sinus syndrome is MRI with gadolinium enhancement. Treatment depends on the nature of the lesion found.

CAVERNOUS SINUS ARTERIOVENOUS FISTULA

An abnormal communication between the arterial and venous circulation in the region of the cavernous sinus produces symptoms that depend largely on the blood flow rate within the fistula.

Clinical Features. Chemosis and dilated (arterialized) conjunctival blood vessels are the hallmark of this disorder. Double vision is produced by cranial nerve III, IV, or VI palsies. Proptosis is prominent with high-flow fistulas. The intraocular pressure may be elevated because of increased episcleral venous pressure. An orbital bruit may be heard and the vision decreased from the effects of macular edema or ischemia.

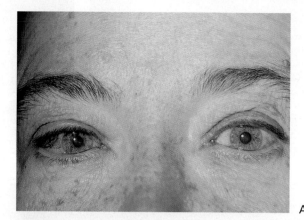
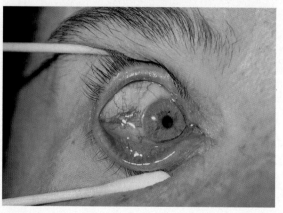

FIGURE 9.69. Low-flow fistula. **A:** The patient has right cranial nerve VI palsy with **(B)** "arterialized" conjunctival blood vessels.

Trauma usually results in a high-flow fistula because of tears in the intracavernous portion of the carotid artery (Fig. 9.68). Low-flow fistulas, with appreciably muted symptoms, occur as a result of dural arteriovenous malformations (Fig. 9.69). Because fistulas are treatable with interventional neuroradiologic techniques, it is important to classify them according to their specific anatomy, as has been done by Barrow and colleagues (Table 9.4).

Detection of a fistula can be made by imaging the superior ophthalmic vein with ultrasound. Documentation of a

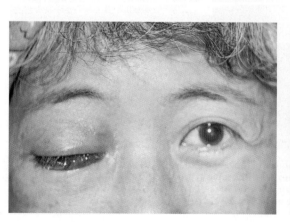
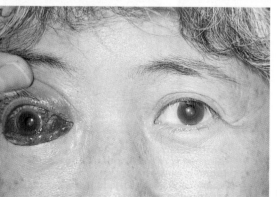

FIGURE 9.68. High-flow fistula. **A:** Ptosis and proptosis occurred in a 24-year-old woman after a car accident. **B:** Conjunctival chemosis, injection, and limitation of ocular movement are dramatic.

TABLE 9.4. CLASSIFICATION OF FISTULAS

Type	Description
Type A	Direct tears High flow Communication between ICA and CS
Type B	Dural AVM Slow flow Communication between meningeal branches of ICA and CS
Type C	Dural AVM Slow flow Communication between meningeal branches of ECA and CS
Type D	Dural AVM Slow flow Communication between meningeal branches of ICA, ECA, and CS

AVM, arteriovenous malformation; CS, cavernous sinus; ECA, external carotid artery; ICA, internal carotid artery.
From Barrow DL, Spector RH, Brown IF, et al. Classification and treatment of spontaneous carotid-cavernous sinus fistulas. *J Neurosurg* 1985;62:248, with permission.

reversal of blood flow in the superior ophthalmic vein establishes the presence of a fistula (Fig. 9.70). Arteriography is required to determine the precise communications if closure of the fistula is to be attempted.

Management. For high-flow fistulas, arteriography is employed to determine the area of communication. Treatment is achieved with interventional neuroradiologic occlusion of the communication.

For low-flow fistulas, treatment is less urgent and may be delayed. Intermittent carotid massage may cause spontaneous closure of the fistula, with resolution of the signs and symptoms. Arteriography is required if interventional closure of the fistula is to be performed.

A patient's orbital signs may become worse, seemingly indicating increased flow within the fistula. However, spontaneous closure of fistulas may produce a paradoxical worsening of signs and symptoms. This can be demonstrated by

color Doppler imaging, which shows decreased or no flow in the superior ophthalmic vein and not the increased flow expected. In this situation, observation of the patient is appropriate, anticipating eventual resolution of the orbital signs.

CHRONIC PROGRESSIVE EXTERNAL OPHTHALMOPLEGIA

Chronic progressive external ophthalmoplegia (CPEO) is a form of mitochondrial myopathy. It may be associated with multisystem dysfunction.

Clinical Features. Isolated CPEO is characterized by slowly progressive bilateral ptosis and decreased excursions (i.e., loss of saccades) of the eye in all directions (Fig. 9.71). Patients do not complain of diplopia, because ocular involvement is symmetric. The major limitation in these patients is caused by ptosis and not by the ophthalmoplegia. Lid elevation surgery should be undertaken cautiously because patients have no vertical eye movement (including Bell's phenomenon) and may suffer corneal exposure and decompensation after surgery.

Kearns-Sayre syndrome is a particular form of CPEO that occurs in children and is associated with peripheral *retinal pigment alternation* (Fig. 9.72) and *heart block*. The latter

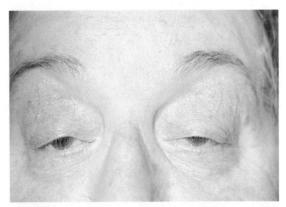
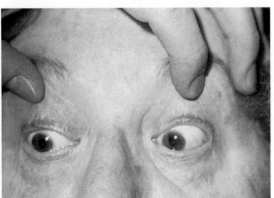

FIGURE 9.71. Chronic progressive external ophthalmoplegia. A 68-year-old woman had marked bilateral ptosis and limited excursions of eye movements in all directions: **(A)** straight forward gaze, **(B)** right gaze, *(continued)*

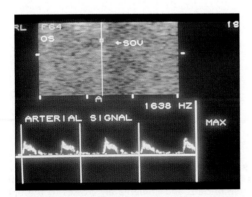

FIGURE 9.70. The color Doppler image reveals arterialized flow (red color) in the superior ophthalmic vein (SOV). Red color in the SOV indicates blood flow reversal from venous to arterial directions. Venous wave form *(bottom)* now has arterial spike characteristics.

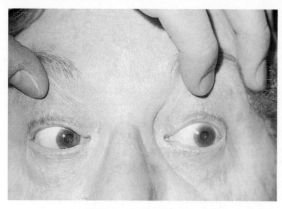
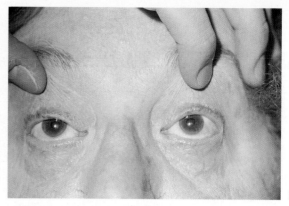

C

D

FIGURE 9.71. *Continued.* **(C)** left gaze, and **(D)** upgaze. Saccades were markedly slowed.

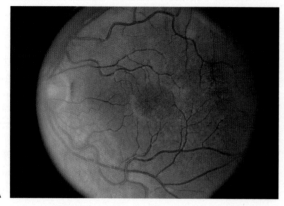
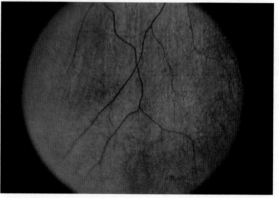

A

B

FIGURE 9.72. In the fundus of a 13-year-old girl with Kearns-Sayre syndrome, the typical pigmentary disturbances involve the **(A)** macula and **(B)** retinal periphery.

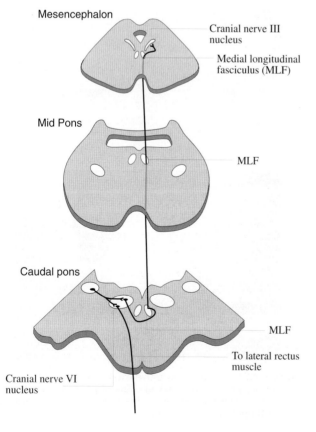

Mesencephalon

Cranial nerve III
nucleus

Medial longitudinal
fasciculus (MLF)

Mid Pons

MLF

Caudal pons

MLF

To lateral rectus
muscle

Cranial nerve VI
nucleus

FIGURE 9.73. Schematic diagram of the median longitudinal fasciculus (MLF) nerve fiber tract. The MLF begins in the left sixth cranial nerve nucleus and immediately crosses to the opposite side of the brainstem to ascend to the third nerve nucleus contralateral to the sixth nerve nucleus of origin. (Illustration courtesy of Neal H. Atebara, M.D.; adapted from Burde RM, Savino PJ, Trobe JD. Clinical decision in neuro-ophthalmology. 2nd ed. St. Louis: Mosby–Year Book; 1992:202, with permission.)

condition may be fatal unless the syndrome is recognized and a cardiac pacemaker inserted.

These patients may also have a variety of other problems, such as short stature that causes them to appear much younger than their age, increased CSF protein levels, cerebellar abnormalities, and electrolyte imbalances. These patients usually die in the second or third decade of life. There is no treatment.

PROGRESSIVE SUPRANUCLEAR PALSY

This disorder of ocular motility may resemble CPEO. However, progressive supranuclear palsy affects downgaze first, is associated with neck and truncal rigidity, and shows increased eye movement with a doll's head maneuver or caloric stimulation, indicating the supranuclear nature of the syndrome. The palsy is seen in patients in their sixth or seventh decade. These patients develop dementia and usually die of intercurrent pulmonary events. There is no effective treatment.

INTERNUCLEAR OPHTHALMOPLEGIA

The medial longitudinal fasciculus (MLF) is a nerve fiber tract in the brainstem that connects the sixth nerve nucleus with the contralateral third nerve nucleus, allowing conjugate eye movements to the right and left to be performed. The MLF arises in the sixth nerve nucleus, and the fibers almost immediately cross to the opposite side of the brainstem. They ascend from the pons to the midbrain, where they join the medial rectus subnuclei of the contralateral third nerve nucleus (Fig. 9.73). A lesion in the MLF produces a characteristic eye movement disorder called an internuclear ophthalmoplegia (INO).

Clinical Features. In its total form, the eye movement disorder is characterized by what appears to be an isolated medial rectus weakness ipsilateral to the side of the MLF lesion (e.g., a right adduction deficit is a right MLF lesion and a right INO). There is often an abducting nystagmus of the contralateral eye on gaze away from the affected side of the brainstem.

Patients often do not complain of double vision but complain of a strange visual phenomenon or of something being "wrong" with their vision.

In the case of complete INO, the adduction deficit is total, with the eye not moving inward past the midline. If the INO is incomplete (i.e., an ophthalmoparesis and not an ophthalmoplegia), the only abnormality may be a partial adduction deficit or no adduction deficit but a lag in the speed of the adducting saccade. This can be brought out in all forms of INO by having the patient look from extreme abduction quickly to the midline and documenting a saccadic "float" in the affected eye.

Any lesion involving the MLF may produce an INO. The most frequent causes of this disorder are MS and brainstem stroke. MS occurs mostly in young people, and the INO tends to be bilateral (Fig. 9.74). The INO from stroke usually occurs in older people and tends to be unilateral.

Management. Any patient who presents with an INO

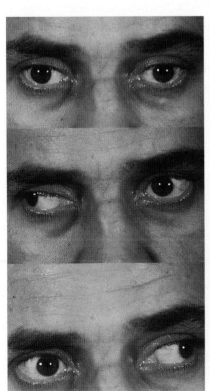
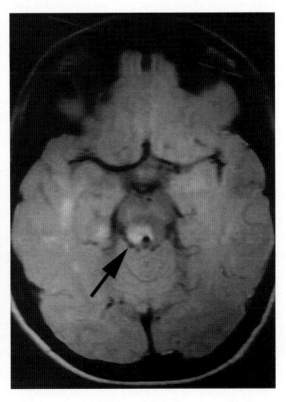

A,B

FIGURE 9.74. A: The patient has bilateral adduction deficits, but the eyes are straight in primary position *(top)*. **B:** The magnetic resonance scan shows a demyelinating plaque that crosses the midline at the brainstem, accounting for bilateral median longitudinal fasciculus lesions.

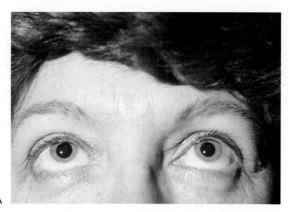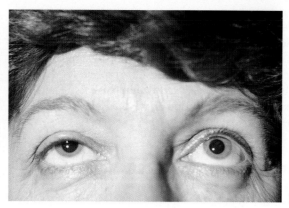

FIGURE 9.75. Myasthenia gravis. Slight right ptosis on initial upward gaze **(A)**, which increases after 1 minute **(B)**.

should have MRI of the brainstem performed. An INO represents intrinsic brainstem disease. The failure to image a lesion in the brainstem should not dissuade the examiner from making the diagnosis, because lesions in this area often are not seen, particularly if the imaging is less than ideal.

MYASTHENIA GRAVIS

Myasthenia gravis is an autoimmune disorder resulting in a decreased number of acetylcholine receptors at neuromuscular junctions.

Clinical Features. A drooping eyelid or double vision may be the initial ocular symptom of myasthenia gravis. Unilateral or bilateral ptosis, with or without other ocular signs, occurs as the initial manifestation of myasthenia in as many as 75% of patients. Myasthenic ptosis is absent or minimal on awakening but becomes more pronounced during waking hours. This fatigability may be demonstrated by having the patient look upward and waiting for increased ptosis to be exhibited (Fig. 9.75).

The hallmarks of myasthenic ptosis are variability, fatigability, and periods of exacerbation and remission. Ocular motility disorders may accompany the lid signs of myasthenia. Myasthenic ocular misalignment may simulate any pattern of neuro-ophthalmic strabismus.

Myasthenia gravis can be diagnosed by a variety of tests. The demonstration of elevated acetylcholine receptor antibodies establishes the diagnosis of myasthenia. Unfortunately, this test is positive for only 50% of patients with ocular myasthenia.

The Tensilon test consists of injecting up to 10 mg edrophonium chloride intravenously in divided doses and detecting improvement of ptosis. An unequivocal resolution of the ptosis is compelling evidence for myasthenia, although false-negative results occur (Fig. 9.76). False-positive test results are encountered more rarely. The ice test involves placing ice on a ptotic lid for 2 minutes. A 2-mm or greater improvement in ptosis has a 90% sensitivity and a 100% specificity for myasthenia gravis. Single fiber electromyography is positive in 88% to 92% of patients with ocular myasthenia (Fig 9.77).

Management. All newly diagnosed myasthenics must have chest imaging to search for thymic hyperplasia or thymoma and have thyroid function studies. The management of the disease is best left to neurologists or neuro-ophthalmologists.

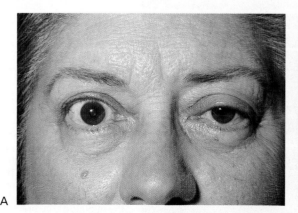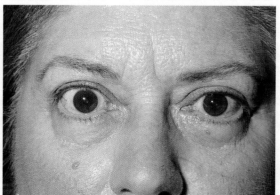

FIGURE 9.76. Patient with left ptosis **(A)**, which resolves on injection of intravenous edrophonium chloride (Tensilon) **(B)**.

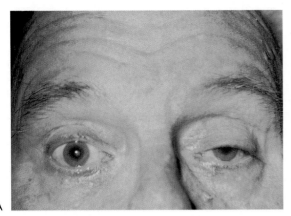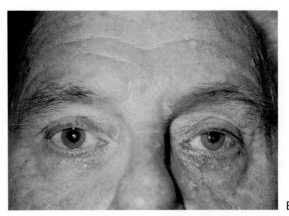

FIGURE 9.77. Patient with left ptosis **(A)**, which resolves after application of ice for 2 minutes **(B)**.

EYELID ABNORMALITIES

Lid Retraction

Lid retraction is present if the sclera is visible between the superior limbus and the upper lid. The most common cause of lid retraction is Graves' orbitopathy (Fig 9.78). Other causes of lid retraction include scarring following inflammation, dorsal midbrain syndrome, sympathetic irritation (Claude Bernard syndrome), metabolic disorders (e.g., cirrhosis), and volitional lid retraction.

Ptosis

A drooping eyelid may have neurogenic, muscular, or congenital causes and may be associated with several syndromes.

Clinical Features. All drooping of the upper eyelid is not true ptosis. Other causes include blepharospasm, apraxia of lid opening, and pseudoptosis from ocular misalignment. Other conditions involving the eyelid, such as chalazia, tumors, and preseptal cellulitis, may cause a ptotic lid.

Evaluation of the patient with ptosis should first determine if the condition is *congenital* or *acquired*. Old photographs are helpful in this regard. If acquired, a neuro-

ophthalmologic problem must be sought before the diagnosis of levator dehiscence is made. The most important neuro-ophthalmic entities are Horner's syndrome, cranial nerve III palsy, and myasthenia gravis.

Less frequently encountered causes of ptosis are Fisher's variant of the Guillain-Barré syndrome, botulism, and CPEO.

Essential Blepharospasm

Essential blepharospasm consists of bilateral, intermittent, uncontrollable spasm of the eyelids. The cause of essential blepharospasm is unknown.

Clinical Features. The clinical picture usually begins with frequent blinking but can progress until the patient must manually elevate one lid to see. This disorder is classified among the dystonias. It may be isolated, but if accompanied by other oral or facial movements, it is called *Meige's syndrome*.

Management. Medical treatment has been notoriously unsuccessful in treating blepharospasm. The first-line treatment consists of injection of botulinum toxin into the spastic orbicularis muscles. If the injections fail to relieve the symptoms, a variety of surgical options are available.

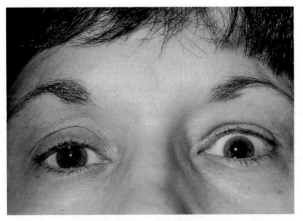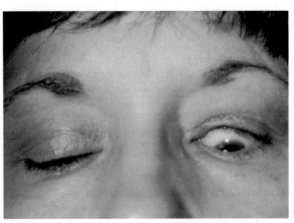

FIGURE 9.78. Lid retraction of the left eye in a 50-year-old woman with Graves' orbitopathy. **A:** Primary position. **B:** Lid retraction is still present in downgaze.

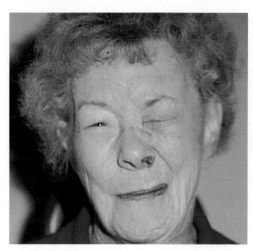

FIGURE 9.79. Hemifacial spasm in a 68-year-old woman. The condition is relieved for a period of months by botulinum injection.

Hemifacial Spasm

In this condition, sporadic, uncontrolled spasms occur on one side of the face.

Clinical Features. Hemifacial spasm presents initially as myokymic movements of the lower eyelid. When the disorder is fully developed, patients manifest unilateral spasm of one side of the face (Fig. 9.79). The spasm occurs unexpectedly, without an apparent precipitating cause. It lasts for seconds and then disappears. In the quiet phase, patients frequently show subtle signs of ipsilateral cranial nerve VII nerve weakness.

The likely causes are *idiopathic* or secondary to compression of cranial nerve VII by an aberrant loop of artery. Less frequent causes are MS and cerebellopontine angle tumors.

Management. The preferred treatment for hemifacial spasm is local injection of botulinum toxin.

BIBLIOGRAPHY

Adler CH, Zimmerman RA, Savino PJ, et al. Hemifacial spasm: evaluation by magnetic resonance imaging and magnetic resonance tomographic angiography. *Ann Neurol* 1992;32:502.

Anderson RL, Patrinely JR. Surgical management of blepharospasm. *Adv Neurol* 1988;49:501.

Barrow DL, Spector RH, Brown IF, et al. Classification and treatment of spontaneous carotid-cavernous sinus fistulas. *J Neurosurg* 1985;62:248.

Beck RW, Cleary PA, Anderson MM, et al. A randomized, controlled trial of corticosteroids in the treatment of acute optic neuritis. *N Engl J Med* 1992;326:581.

Beck RW, Cleary PA, Trobe JD, et al. The effect of corticosteroids for acute optic neuritis on the subsequent development of multiple sclerosis. *N Engl J Med* 1993;329:1764.

Beck RW, Cleary PA, and the Optic Neuritis Study Group. Optic Neuritis Treatment Trial: one-year follow-up results. *Arch Ophthalmol* 1993;111:773.

Beck RW, Savino PJ, Repka MX, et al. Optic disc structure in anterior ischemic optic neuropathy. *Ophthalmology* 1984;91:1334.

Beck RW, Savino PJ, Schatz NJ, et al. Anterior ischemic optic neuropathy: recurrent episodes in the same eye. *Br J Ophthalmol* 1983;67:705.

Beck RW, the Optic Neuritis Study Group. The Optic Neuritis Treatment Trial: three-year follow-up results. *Arch Ophthalmol* 1995;113:137.

Bilyk JR, Joseph MP. Traumatic optic neuropathy. *Semin Ophthalmol* 1994;9:200.

Boghen DR, Glaser JS. Ischaemic optic neuropathy. The clinical profile and history. *Brain* 1975;98:689.

Brown GB, Tasman W. Congenital anomalies of the optic disc. New York: Grune & Stratton; 1983:157.

Burde RM, Savino PJ, Trobe JD. Clinical decisions in neuro-ophthalmology. 2nd ed. St. Louis: CV Mosby; 1992:200.

Drachman DB. Myasthenia gravis. *N Engl J Med* 1994;330:1797.

Francis DA, Compston DA, Batchelor JR, et al. A reassessment of the risk of multiple sclerosis developing in patients with optic neuritis after extended follow up. *J Neurol Neurosurg Psychiatry* 1987;50:758.

Glaser JS. Topical diagnosis: prechiasmal visual pathways. In: Tasman W, Jaeger EA. Duane's clinical ophthalmology, vol 2. Philadelphia: JB Lippincott; 1994:7.

Hashimoto M, Ohtsuka K, Nakagawa T. Topless optic disk syndrome without maternal diabetes mellitus. *Am J Ophthalmol* 1999;128:111.

Horton JC. Wilbrand's knee of the primate optic chiasm is an artefact of monocular enucleation. *Trans Am Ophthalmol Soc* 1997;95:580.

Hoyt WF, Luis O. The primate chiasm. *Arch Ophthalmol* 1963;70:69.

Jacobson DM, Trobe JD. The emerging role of magnetic resonance angiography in the management of patients with third cranial nerve palsy. *Am J Ophthalmol* 1999;128:94.

Johns DR, Smith KH, Savino PJ, et al. Leber's hereditary optic neuropathy: clinical manifestations of the 15257 mutation. *Ophthalmology* 1993;100:981.

Kearns TP, Sayre GP. Retinitis pigmentosa, external ophthalmoplegia, and complete heart block; unusual syndrome with histologic study in one of two cases. *Arch Ophthalmol* 1958;60:280.

Keltner JL, Johnson CA, Spurr JO, et al. Visual field profile of optic neuritis: one year follow-up in the Optic Neuritis Treatment Trial. *Arch Ophthalmol* 1994;112:946.

Kissel JT, Burde RM, Klingele TG, et al. Pupil-sparing oculomotor palsies with internal carotid–posterior communicating artery aneurysm. *Ann Neurol* 1983;13:149.

Ksiazek SM, Repka MX, Maguire A, et al. Divisional oculomotor nerve paresis caused by intrinsic brain stem disease. *Ann Neurol* 1989;26:714.

Lam BL, Thompson HS, Corbett JJ. The prevalence of simple anisocoria. *Am J Ophthalmol* 1987;104:69.

Macaluso DC, Shultz WT, Fraunfelder FT. Features of amiodarone-induced optic neuropathy. *Am J Ophthalmol* 1999;127:610.

Moraes CT, DiMauro S, Zeviani M, et al. Mitochondrial DNA deletions in progressive external ophthalmoplegia and Kearns-Sayre syndrome. *N Engl J Med* 1989;320:1293.

Morrissey SP, Miller DH, Kendall BE, et al. The significance of brain magnetic resonance imaging abnormalities at presentation with clinically isolated syndromes suggestive of multiple sclerosis: a 5-year follow-up study. *Brain* 1993;116:135.

Optic Neuritis Study Group. The 5-year risk of MS after optic neuritis: experience of the Optic Neuritis Treatment Trial. *Neurology* 1997;49:1404.

Rivero A, Crovetto L, Lopez L, et al. Single fiber electromyography of extraocular muscles: a sensitive method for the diagnosis of ocular myasthenia gravis. *Muscle Nerve* 1995;18:943.

Regillo CD, Brown GC, Savino PJ, et al. Diabetic papillopathy: patient characteristics and fundus findings. *Arch Ophthalmol* 1995;113:889.

Rosenberg MA, Savino PJ, Glaser JS. A clinical analysis of pseudopapilledema. I. Population, laterality, acuity, refractive error, ophthalmoscopic characteristics, and coincident disease. *Arch Ophthalmol* 1979;97:65.

Savino PJ, Maus M. Botulinum toxin therapy. In: Breen LA. Neurologic clinics. Philadelphia: WB Saunders; 1991:205.

Savino PJ, Paris M, Schatz NJ, et al. Optic tract syndrome: a review of 21 patients. *Arch Ophthalmol* 1978;96:656.

Savino PJ, Sergott RC, Bosley TM, Schatz NJ. Hemifacial spasm treated with botulinum A toxin injection. *Arch Ophthalmol* 1985;103:1305.

Schatz NJ, Savino PJ, Corbett JJ. Primary aberrant oculomotor regeneration. A sign of intracavernous meningioma. *Arch Neurol* 1977;34:29.

Sergott RC, Cohen MS, Bosley TM, et al. Optic nerve decompression may improve the progressive form of non-arteritic ischemic optic neuropathy. *Arch Ophthalmol* 1989;107:1743.

Sergott RC, Grossman RI, Savino PJ, et al. The syndrome of para-

doxical worsening of dural cavernous sinus arteriovenous malformations. *Ophthalmology* 1986;94:205.

Steinsapir KD, Goldberg RA. Traumatic optic neuropathy. *Surv Ophthalmol* 1994;38:487.

Thompson HS. A classification of "tonic pupils." In: Thompson HS, Daroff R, Frisen L, et al. Topics in neuro-ophthalmology. Baltimore: Williams & Wilkins; 1979:95.

Van der Weil HL, Van Gijn J. Localization of Horner's syndrome: use and limitations of the hydroxyamphetamine test. *J Neurol Sci* 1983;59:229.

Vincent A, Newsom-Davis J. Acetylcholine receptor antibody as a diagnostic test for myasthenia gravis: results in 153 validated cases and 2067 diagnostic assays. *J Neurol Neurosurg Psychiatry* 1985;48:1246.

Wallace DC, Singh G, Lott MR, et al. Mitochondrial DNA mutation associated with Leber's hereditary optic neuropathy. *Science* 1988;242:1427.

CHAPTER 10

Oculoplastics

Joseph C. Flanagan
Robert A. Mazzoli
Edward H. Bedrossian, Jr.
Robert B. Penne
Mary A. Stefanyszyn

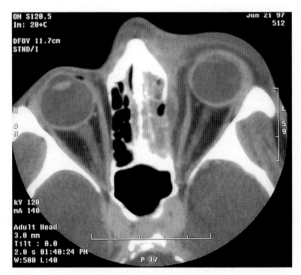 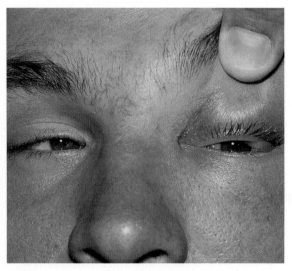

Orbital cellulitis in a 23-year-old male. Findings include left-sided proptosis, chemosis, orbital congestion, decreased ocular motility, and superficial inflammation. Computed tomography demonstrates ethmoid sinus opacification, with a medial subperiosteal abscess. Sinoorbital drainage is required.

ANATOMIC CONSIDERATIONS

CONGENITAL LID ABNORMALITIES

Ankyloblepharon and Cryptophthalmos
Blepharophimosis
Epicanthus, Telecanthus, and Teleorbitism
Euryblepharon, Congenital Ectropion, and Lid Coloboma
Epiblepharon, Distichiasis, and Congenital Entropion

ACQUIRED LID MALPOSITIONS

Entropion
Involutional Ectropion
Paralytic and Mechanical Ectropion

PTOSIS

Congenital and Acquired Ptosis
Dermatochalasis, Steatoblepharon and Blepharochalasis
Pseudoptosis
Neurogenic and Myogenic Ptosis and Myasthenia Gravis
Marcus-Gunn Jaw-Winking
Blepharospasm, Hemifacial Spasm, Myokymia, and Aberrant Regeneration

TUMORS

Xanthelasma, Histiocytoses, and Juvenile Xanthogranuloma
Hidrocystoma and Syringoma
Papilloma, Keratoacanthoma, Inverted Follicular Keratosis, and Seborrheic Keratosis
Capillary Hemangioma
Nevus Flammeus
Neurofibromatosis
Epidermal Inclusion Cysts and Milia
Hair Follicle Tumors
Nevocellular Nevi

Basal Cell Carcinoma
Squamous Cell Carcinoma
Sebaceous Cell Carcinoma
Malignant Melanoma, Eccrine Sweat Gland Carcinoma, and Merkel Cell Carcinoma
Other Malignant Tumors of the Skin

INFLAMMATIONS

Blepharitis, Chalazion, Hordeolum, and Molluscum Contagiosum
Vitiligo, Poliosis, Madarosis, and Trichotillomania
Sarcoidosis
Allergic and Atopic Dermatitis

LACRIMAL DRAINAGE DYSFUNCTION

Congenital Dacryostenosis, Dacryocystocele, and Dacryocystitis
Supernumerary Puncta, Lacrimal System Atresia, and Lacrimal Fistula
Acquired Dacryostenosis
Dacryocystitis
Lacrimal Sac Tumors

OCULOPLASTIC TRAUMA

Eyelid Trauma
Lacrimal System Trauma
Orbital Trauma

PROPTOSIS

Orbital Cellulitis
Fungal Infections
Orbital Inflammation
Histiocytosis X
Orbital Tumors
Secondary Tumors

ANATOMIC CONSIDERATIONS

The orbicularis oculi muscle is responsible for eyelid closure. This circular muscle is innervated by the seventh cranial nerve. The muscle is divided into three portions (Fig. 10.1A). The orbital portion is the thickest and is responsible for forcible lid closure. It inserts on the medial canthal tendon. The preseptal portion—as its name implies—overlies the orbital septum. It is important in eyelid closure, involuntary blinking, and the function of the lacrimal pump, aided by multiple insertions medially into the medial canthal tendon and around the lacrimal sac. These insertions contribute to the complicated lacrimal pump mechanism. Laterally, the muscle inserts into the lateral canthal tendon. The pretarsal orbicularis is the smallest portion and acts mainly in involuntary blinking and the lacrimal pump mechanism. Lateral and medial insertions are similar to those of the preseptal muscles.

The *frontalis muscle* supports the eyebrow and—along with the procerus and glabellar muscles—is responsible for its animation (Fig. 10.1B). It is also innervated by the seventh cranial nerve. The *orbital septum* originates from the orbital rim by a fibrous band called the *arcus marginalis*. Superiorly, the septum fuses with the *levator aponeurosis* variably above the superior tarsal border. This syncytial structure defines the entrance to the orbit proper. Anterior to the septum lies the preseptal orbicularis. Immediately posterior is the preaponeurotic fat, an important surgical landmark. It is convenient to consider this fat to be contained in two fat pockets superiorly, the nasal and central pads, while in the lower lid the fat is typically divided into three pockets: the nasal, central and lateral pockets. The inferior oblique muscle separates the nasal and central fat compartments in the lower lid, a critical anatomic relationship in lower lid and orbital surgery. The lacrimal gland occupies the lateral pocket in the upper lid, another key anatomic consideration. The levator complex lies immediately beneath the aponeurotic fat. The levator muscle originates posteriorly from the periorbita above the annulus of Zinn and extends anteriorly along the orbital roof, traveling above the superior rectus muscle. At the level of the equator of the globe, the muscle changes to aponeurosis and extends inferiorly over Whitnall's ligament to insert along the tarsus and medial and lateral rims (the levator horns). Attachments along the tarsus are complex. The main attachment is to the inferior two thirds of the anterior border of the tarsus, which effects opening the eyelid. In occidental lids, lesser attachments are made superficially through the *orbicularis muscle* to the skin near the superior border of the tarsus to form the upper eyelid crease. These attachments are significantly

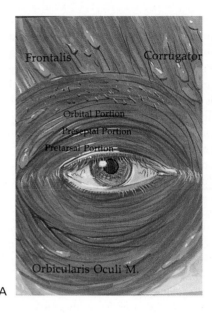

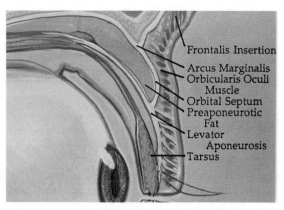

FIGURE 10.1. The musculature of the eyelid. **A:** The orbicularis oculi. **B:** The eyelid in cross section. (From Bosniak SL. Cosmetic blepharoplasty. New York: Raven Press; 1991:40, with permission.)

more diverse in Asian and oriental lids. The aponeurotic complex is innervated by the third cranial nerve. Not labeled in Figure 10.1 is *Müller's muscle,* which lies posterior to the levator aponeurosis. This is a sympathetically innervated muscle that attaches to the superior aspect of the tarsal plate and acts to elevate the lid. The *tarsal plate* is made of dense fibrous tissue and forms the structural framework of the eyelids. The upper tarsal plate is 25 mm long and 10 mm wide. The tarsal plates are attached to the lateral and medial orbital rims by the lateral and medial canthal tendons. The lid margin is rather flat anatomically, making critical landmarks relatively easily recognizable. Anteriorly, the *lashes* number approximately 100 in the upper lid and 50 in the lower. Posteriorly, 20 to 25 *meibomian glands* mark the area where the margin blends into the palpebral conjunctiva at the *mucocutaneous border.* Between the two sits the *gray line,* a superficial reflection of the muscle of Riolan (a small portion of the pretarsal orbicularis) visible in most patients.

CONGENITAL LID ABNORMALITIES

Ankyloblepharon and Cryptophthalmos

Embryologically, the eyelids develop from extensions of the frontonasal and maxillary processes, growing vertically over the developing globe during approximately the seventh week of gestation. The folds fuse along their horizontal margins and remain fused while the lid structures develop, until the fifth to seventh month, when the developed lids gradually separate. *Ankyloblepharon* (i.e., ankyloblepharon filiforme adnatum) describes a partial failure of the fused lids to separate, while the more severe condition *cryptophthalmos* is a complete failure of the lids to develop or separate (Fig. 10.2). The latter condition is almost uniformly associated with severe malformations of the globe, orbit, and adnexa, but ankyloblepharon may be an isolated condition. If the fusion is sufficiently extensive, amblyopia may develop, and medial fusion may obstruct the punctum.

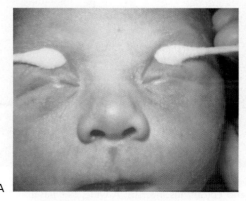

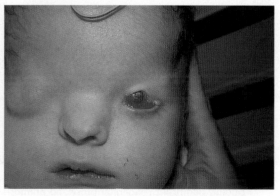

FIGURE 10.2. A: Ankyloblepharon. (Courtesy of Joseph Calhoun, M.D., Philadelphia, PA.) **B:** Cryptophthalmos. Patient with multiple developmental anomalies. The right eye demonstrates cryptophthalmos, and the left eye shows a large central lid coloboma.

Management. Ankyloblepharon is treated with simple lysis of the adhesive bands and reconstruction (e.g., punctoplasty), as needed. The adhesions do not generally recur. Treatment of cryptophthalmos can require extensive multidisciplinary reconstructive efforts.

Blepharophimosis

Blepharophimosis refers to an abnormally small palpebral fissure that is shortened both vertically and horizontally, but in which the lids themselves are normally developed (Fig. 10.3). Although it can be an associated finding in a variety of syndromes, as an isolated entity the condition is rare, transmitted as an autosomal-dominant trait. Characteristic features include severe congenital ptosis with poor levator function, epicanthus inversus, telecanthus, and an absolute shortage of skin in all four lids. Lateral ectropion, strabismus, motility disturbances, and nystagmus can also be associated features, as can flattening of the nasal bridge, and hyperteleorbitism. Though various degrees of mental deficiency have been reported, mental capacity is generally unaffected. Menstrual irregularities and infertility have also been reported in female patients. Differentiation from simple epicanthus, bilateral congenital ptosis, medial ankyloblepharon, and telecanthus requires close examination. The manifestations can vary from mild to severe.

Management. Patients should undergo a complete family history and physical examination to look for associated developmental anomalies. Radiographic images are obtained before surgical correction to rule out teleorbitism. Surgery is staged, beginning at 3 to 5 years of age, unless the ptosis is severe enough to warrant earlier intervention.

Epicanthus, Telecanthus, and Teleorbitism

Epicanthus (i.e., epicanthal folds) refers to prominent folds of skin in the inner canthus and is most prominent along the upper lid. Although it is a normal finding in those of Asian ancestry, it is abnormal in non-Asians (Fig. 10.4A). *Epicanthus inversus* exists if the fold extends predominantly from the lower lid to the upper lid; it is almost always an abnormal finding in all races and is associated with significant ptosis and poor levator function (Fig. 10.4B). If the fold is equally divided between the two lids, the condition is called *epicanthus palpebralis* (Fig. 10.4C). Although epicanthus commonly exists as an isolated finding, it can also be a component of several congenital conditions, such as blepharophimosis and Down's syndrome. The condition presents no particular ocular hazard. However, it often causes parental concern because of the appearance of or, more commonly, the semblance of *pseudoesotropia*. In the latter case, cover and cross-cover testing reveals orthophoria, and gentle distraction of the soft tissues of the nasal bridge reduces the webbed appearance of the medial canthi to reveal normal ocular alignment.

Telecanthus is a soft tissue abnormality defined as an abnormally widened separation of the medial canthi. As an isolated condition the interpupillary distance remains normal (Fig. 10.5). It is most often seen as a result of severe nasoorbital-ethmoid trauma in adults, but can occur congenitally, generally in conjunction with other ocular and facial anomalies. *Teleorbitism* (*hypertelorism,* or *hyperteleorbitism*) is a bony abnormality of the orbit wherein the medial walls are too widely separated (Fig. 10.6). In this condition, the interpupillary distance is abnormally widened. Soft tissue telecanthus is a secondary finding. The condition is almost invariably associated with other maldevelopments and is most often encountered in craniofacial dysmorphisms. *Hypoteleorbitism* describes abnormally close orbital walls.

Management. Rarely is surgery recommended for simple epicanthus. However, a variety of sliding flap techniques have been described for correction when performed for reconstruction of other abnormalities (e.g., blepharophimosis). Simple epicanthus normally resolves spontaneously as

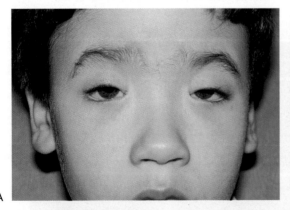
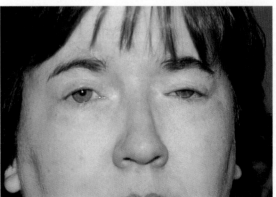

FIGURE 10.3. Blepharophimosis. **A:** Patient demonstrates typical findings of the condition, including significant congenital ptosis, lid phimosis, and epicanthus inversus. A wide, flat nasal bridge with telecanthus and pseudoesotropia are also present (Fig. 10.4B,C). The condition was inherited as a dominant trait. **B:** Mother of the patient in **(A)** after surgical correction as a child. Two of her brothers, her father, and maternal grandmother were also affected.

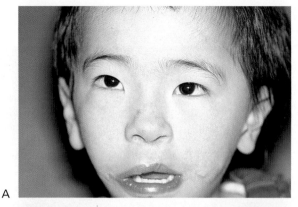

A

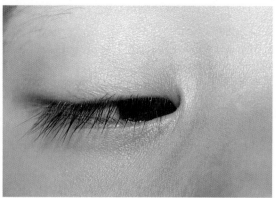

B

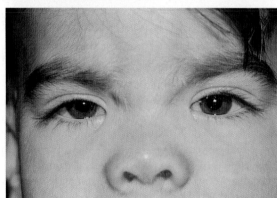

C

FIGURE 10.4. A: Epicanthus. Patient with Goldenhar's syndrome. The predominant fold extends from the upper lid. Telecanthus is also present (Fig. 10.5). **B:** Epicanthus inversus. The predominant fold is in the lower lid in this patient with blepharophimosis (Fig. 10.3A). **C:** Epicanthus palpebralis and pseudoesotropia. Patient with Cornelia de Lange syndrome. The lid fold is equally divided along the upper and lower lid. Pseudoesotropia is also apparent. However, the corneal light reflex demonstrates normal ocular alignment.

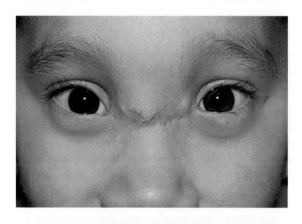

FIGURE 10.5. Telecanthus in a patient after surgical repair of frontal-nasal encephalocele. The lid malposition was congenital. The intercanthal distance is widened. However, the interpupillary distance is normal, indicating that the orbits themselves are not malpositioned.

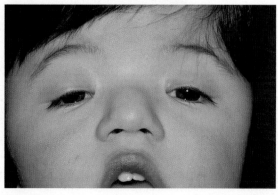

A

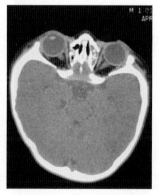

B

FIGURE 10.6. Teleorbitism. **A:** Patient with Crouzon's syndrome. The interpupillary distance is abnormally wide. **B:** Computed tomography demonstrates the widely separated medial walls and orbits.

the nasal bridge and midface develop. Pseudostrabismus resolves concomitantly.

Surgical correction of telecanthus necessitates resuspension of the medial canthal tendon, often requiring transnasal wiring. If teleorbitism coexists, as in the craniosynostoses, the bony medial walls must be narrowed as well. These procedures are best performed with the assistance of trained craniofacial surgeons.

Euryblepharon, Congenital Ectropion, and Lid Coloboma

Euryblepharon (i.e., megaloblepharon) is a rare congenital condition (Fig. 10.7). Contrasted to blepharophimosis—in which the lid apertures are too small (Fig. 10.3)—euryblepharon is characterized by palpebral fissures that are too wide. The eyelids are normally developed; however, the insertions of the canthal tendons appear to be too widely or anteriorly placed. This leads to poor apposition of the lid to the globe (lid stand-off) that is most marked laterally. *Congenital ectropion* may also occur. There may also be a downward dystopia of the canthus. The condition is most often isolated, but it may be inherited as an autosomal-dominant trait or may be associated with other congenital abnormalities. Microphthalmos or enophthalmos may give the appearance of euryblepharon but can be differentiated by a thorough examination.

Lid colobomas occur when the embryonic lids fail to fuse horizontally, producing a cleft in the lid margin (Fig. 10.8). Amniotic bands have been implicated, but colobomas are known to occur in conjunction with other anomalies of the head and face, particularly of the eyes. They occur commonly in the craniofacial clefting syndromes. Dermoids and dermolipomas are commonly found in proximity to the coloboma, most often at the apex. Large colobomas may af-

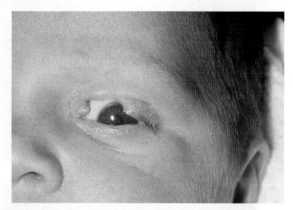

FIGURE 10.8. Upper lid coloboma was unassociated with other abnormalities. A dermoid is seen at the apex of the cleft.

fect the entire lid, simulating ablepharon. Lateral coloboma of the lower lid is a frequent finding in mandibulofacial dysostoses such as the Treacher Collins syndrome.

Management. If severe euryblepharon causes epiphora or exposure, resuspension of the lateral canthus using lateral tarsal strip may be contemplated. Small colobomas may be excised directly, with reconstruction of the affected lid through standard techniques. Larger colobomas require earlier intervention with more extensive reconstructive efforts to prevent corneal complications.

Epiblepharon, Distichiasis, and Congenital Entropion

True *congenital entropion* is a rare condition, occurring secondary to the absence, hypoplasia, or hypertrophy of the tarsal plate and pretarsal orbicularis (Fig. 10.9). In extreme cases, the tarsus may be bent permanently inward by amniotic bands, causing a "tarsal kink" that requires prompt surgical correction. More common, but still rare, are the con-

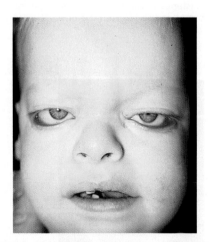

FIGURE 10.7. Euryblepharon with congenital ectropion. Notice the large lids, with downward and lateral dystopia of the lateral canthus, and poor globe apposition. There are other congenital anomalies.

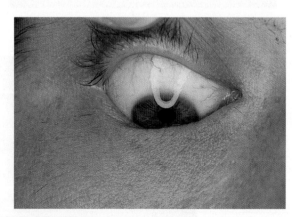

FIGURE 10.9. Congenital entropion. Adult patient with congenital, familial absence of lower lashes. Hypoplasia of the tarsal plate causes the lid margin to roll inward, especially during downgaze.

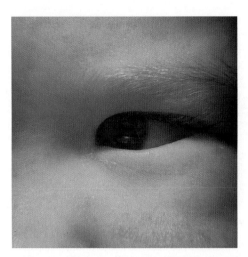

FIGURE 10.10. Epiblepharon. An extra roll of skin below the lashes can cause the lashes to roll inward, resulting in corneal irritation.

ditions of *epiblepharon* (Fig. 10.10), in which an extra fold of skin exists at the lid margin, occasionally causing a mechanical entropion, and *distichiasis* (Fig. 10.11), wherein an extra row of lashes grows toward the cornea from metaplastic meibomian gland orifices. This condition may be inherited, and often causes annoying corneal irritation, precipitating intervention.

Management. The conditions are generally isolated and well tolerated, but they may cause symptomatic corneal irritation. Treatment is supportive, with lubricants, unless keratitis exists, in which case surgery may be contemplated. Epiblepharon usually resolves with maturation and growth of the midface, although an elliptical skin and muscle excision is sometimes indicated to resolve the keratitis. Electrolysis or cryotherapy can be used to ablate distichiatic lashes. Rarely is a lid-splitting procedure required for this condition. True congenital entropion is treated by marginal rotation techniques.

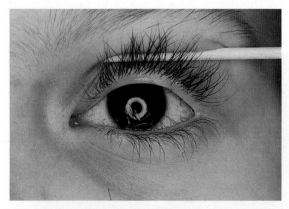

FIGURE 10.11. Distichiasis. A familial condition and congenital disorder in which extra lashes grow from the openings of metaplastic meibomian glands. The position of the lid margin is normal.

ACQUIRED LID MALPOSITIONS

Entropion

Involutional entropion is a common clinical finding. Laxity of the skin, orbicularis, and other supporting structures contribute to a lack of posterior lid support and tarsal stability, leading to inturning of the lid margin and lashes with resultant keratitis, conjunctivitis, and discomfort (Fig. 10.12A). The tissues can be lax at the lateral canthus, at the medial canthus, or in the horizontal length of the lid. Loss of the normal relation between the lower lid retractors and the tarsal base (i.e., lower lid retractor disinsertion) allows the preseptal orbicularis to override the lid margin, causing the lid to invert. Microvascular insufficiency may be a contributing factor. Involutional entropion is almost exclusively a phenomenon of the lower lid; upper lid entropion is more likely to be secondary to cicatricial changes. Although most cases are idiopathic, factors such as chronic irritation and eye rubbing (e.g., blepharitis, allergy), smoking, and familial tendencies toward skin laxity are undoubtedly contributing factors. The direction of the lashes at the lash border is usually anatomically normal, unlike the condition of *trichiasis*, in which the lid margin is typically stable but abnormal lashes are misdirected posteriorly (Fig. 10.12B). The two conditions may coexist.

Acute spastic entropion may result from various inflammations and irritations, or from trauma, such as cataract or lid surgery. *Cicatricial entropion* can occur as a result of surgery (e.g., tumor resection), reaction to medication, or chronic infectious or inflammatory diseases such as trachoma, pemphigoid, or Stevens-Johnson syndrome (Fig. 10.13). It may involve the upper or lower lids.

Management. Treatment is directed toward correcting the anatomic abnormality and removing inciting factors. Blepharoconjunctivitis is treated medically with warm compresses, antibiotic ointments, and lubricants. Canthal tendon laxity is corrected with plication procedures or resuspension (e.g., lateral tarsal strip). Horizontal laxity can be corrected with full-thickness wedge resection. Procedures to correct horizontally tight lids include excision of a base-down triangle from the posterior lamella, placement of fornix sutures (i.e., Quickert-Rathbun sutures), and suture plication of the orbital septum. Temporary measures for comfort may include taping the eyelid with lateral traction or placement of Quickert-Rathbun sutures at the bedside. Cicatricial changes of the posterior lamella often require grafting of spacer materials. Autogenous mucus membrane such as buccal mucosa or hard palate are excellent replacements. However, diseases such as Stevens-Johnson and pemphigoid, which affect the oral mucosa and the conjunctiva, may limit the feasibility of the mouth as a donor site. Other potential graft materials include fascia lata, processed human dermis, and banked sclera, although these materials may be especially irritating on the upper lid because of the

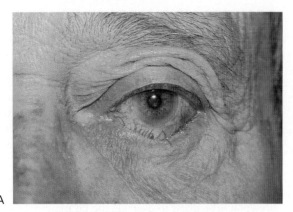 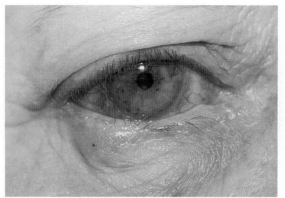

FIGURE 10.12. A: Involutional entropion. Significant lower lid laxity and detachment of the lower lid retractors allow the lid margin to rotate inward. Lashes can create chronic keratoconjunctivitis. When the lid margin is in a normal, everted position, the lash direction is anatomically normal. **B:** Trichiasis. Unlike entropion, the lid margin position is anatomically stable, but the lashes are misdirected. Corneal touch leads to chronic keratitis.

lack of mucosal surface. Marginal rotation and lash electrolysis may be required.

Involutional Ectropion

Involutional ectropion, like entropion, is common. It results from poor lid tone and horizontal laxity, allowing gravity and lid weight to pull the lower lid margin away from the globe (Fig. 10.14A). When the lid is pulled away from the globe, it fails to snap back into position as it does in younger patients. Symptoms include irritation and blepharoconjunctivitis. In severe cases, particularly if the lower lid retractors have become disinserted, frank tarsal eversion with severe keratinization of the conjunctiva can occur (Fig. 10.14B). Dysfunction of the lacrimal pump and punctal ectropion lead to symptomatic epiphora. Horizontal laxity is often exacerbated by excess skin and fat, called dermatochalasis. Occasionally, extreme dermatochalasis can produce "festoons" of the lower lid, also known as malar bags, secondary bags, and bags-on-bags.

Management. Treatment of involutional ectropion involves tightening of the lid sling (e.g., lateral tarsal strip,

wedge resection) and, if necessary, removal of redundant skin and fat with a modified Kuhnt-Szymanowski or lower lid blepharoplasty. Punctal eversion is corrected by a variety of punctoplasty techniques. Treatment of floppy eyelid syndrome requires lubrication and horizontal tightening of the upper and lower lids (Fig. 10.15). Aggravating conditions are treated concomitantly.

Paralytic and Mechanical Ectropion

Paralytic ectropion is a consequence of palsy or paralysis of the facial nerve (Fig. 10.16). Lid hypotonicity leads to marked ectropion, particularly in older adults, in whom involutional changes and laxity exacerbate the paralytic component. The palsy may be permanent or temporary, but it can lead to severe exposure keratopathy in either instance. Loss of normal lid position and function also leads to significant epiphora.

Mechanical ectropion can result from cicatricial changes of the anterior or middle lamella or tumor mass (Fig. 10.17). Any condition leading to scarring, including in-

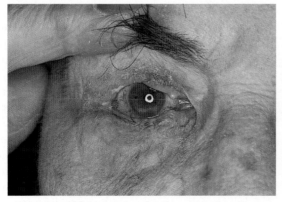 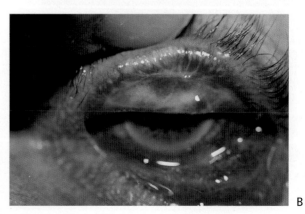

FIGURE 10.13. Cicatricial entropion. **A:** Multiple tumor resections of the upper lid resulted in cicatricial entropion and corneal irritation. **B:** Chronic glaucoma medication use led to cicatricial changes of the posterior lamella and entropion of both upper and lower lids.

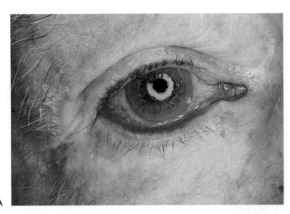
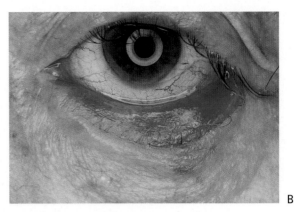

A

B

FIGURE 10.14. Involutional ectropion. **A:** Excess laxity and poor horizontal lid tone lead to sagging and eversion of the lid margin. Secondary mucus discharge and epiphora are not uncommon. **B:** In this severe case with retractor disinsertion and frank tarsal eversion, chronic exposure has led to secondary keratinization of the tarsal conjunctiva. Exposure changes usually resolve after correction of the ectropion.

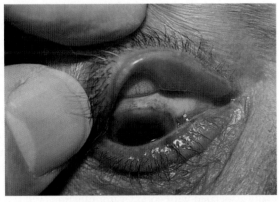
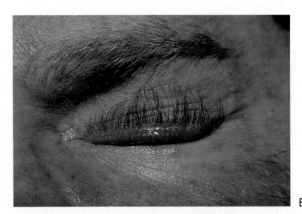

A

B

FIGURE 10.15. Floppy eyelid syndrome. **A:** The upper tarsus has begun to lose its natural rigidity and can be folded and everted easily. There is also significant laxity of the canthal ligaments. The velvety appearance of the conjunctiva is secondary to chronic papillary conjunctivitis. **B:** Aggravating conditions of floppy eyelid syndrome include overriding eyelids, which may contribute to chronic internal irritation. Associated physical conditions include obesity and obstructive sleep apnea.

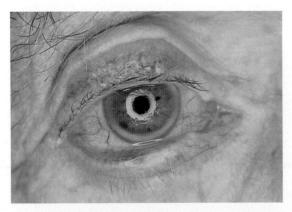
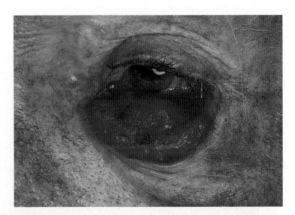

FIGURE 10.16. Paralytic ectropion. Patient after radical parotidectomy for mucoepidermoid carcinoma with subsequent facial palsy. Paralysis produces lagophthalmos and significant ectropion, with marked exposure keratopathy. Previous attempts at correction included implantation of auricular cartilage spacer in the lower lid and a gold weight in the upper lid, which is beginning to extrude at the inferonasal corner.

FIGURE 10.17. Mechanical ectropion: tumor. In a patient with metastatic prostate cancer, a mass of the lower lid physically pushes the lid margin away from globe.

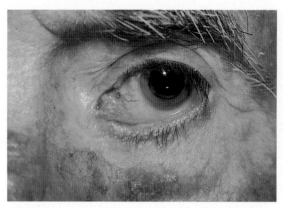

FIGURE 10.18. Mechanical ectropion: cicatrix. A patient with a cicatricial lower lid ectropion, most marked nasally, secondary to previous excision of skin cancer below the punctum.

flammation (e.g., atopic dermatitis), trauma (e.g., tumor resection, cosmetic surgery, laceration), and chemical or thermal burns, can cause abnormal foreshortening of the skin and muscle layer (Figs. 10.18, 10.19A). Contracture of the middle lamella and septum can result from orbital surgery (Fig. 10.19B). Large tumors of the lid and significant periocular edema can physically push the lid away from the globe.

Management. In the case of paralytic ectropion, the cause of the facial palsy must be investigated. Conditions such as herpes zoster infection (e.g., Ramsay Hunt syndrome), tumor (e.g., cranial nerve VII or VIII involvement), and trauma must be evaluated. Bell's palsy is an idiopathic palsy that resolves spontaneously and requires little more than supportive treatment. Other conditions, however, are best managed in conjunction with an otorhinolaryngologist. Ocular manifestations are treated with lower lid resuspension procedures such as the lateral tarsal strip operation. If exposure keratitis is severe, lateral or medial tarsorrhaphies may be needed, on either a temporary or permanent basis. Techniques for enhancing lid closure include insertion of a gold weight into the upper lid, wire springs and silicone slings, and nerve transplantation. The eye is kept well lubricated throughout the duration of the palsy.

If mechanical ectropion is caused by a lid mass, it is biopsied and managed as required. Cicatricial ectropion often requires lysis and revision of scar tissue, with placement of anterior lamellar skin grafts or middle lamellar spacer grafts as needed. Every attempt should be made to control inflammatory conditions such as dermatitis before any surgical intervention.

PTOSIS

Congenital and Acquired Ptosis

Congenital ptosis occurs most commonly as an isolated finding but also occurs in association with a myriad of other abnormalities and syndromes, such as blepharophimosis and Down's syndrome (Fig. 10.20). Strabismus may also be found. The ptosis is most often unilateral, but it may be bilateral in as many as 25% of cases. A familial inheritance pattern is not unusual. Unlike acquired ptosis, most cases of congenital ptosis are myogenic in origin and are often associated with poor levator and superior rectus muscle function (Fig. 10.21).

Pathologic studies have shown poor muscular development of the levator-superior rectus complex, with fibrous tissue replacing the normal musculature, and a paucity of muscle fibers. The degree of ptosis generally corresponds inversely to the degree of levator function; mild ptosis is generally associated with good levator function, and severe ptosis is indicative of poor levator function. An ill-defined or absent upper lid crease, downwardly directed lashes, and difficulty with lid eversion also imply poor levator development. The hallmark of congenital ptosis is lagophthalmos in downgaze, when the ptotic lid fails to fully follow the globe downward and assumes a higher position than the fellow lid (Fig. 10.22). Reduced ocular motility—especially in

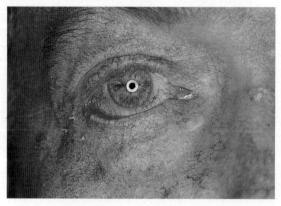

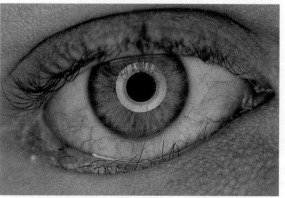

FIGURE 10.19. Mechanical ectropion: cicatrix. **A:** A patient with a cicatricial shortening of the anterior lamella secondary to chronic atopic dermatitis. **B:** An orbital trauma patient, status post orbital repair, with cicatricial contracture of the middle lamella and septum, leading to lower lid retraction. A previous unsuccessful attempt at correction included full-thickness wedge excision.

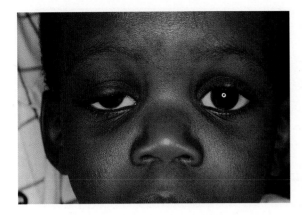

FIGURE 10.20. Significant congenital ptosis of the right upper lid encroaching into the visual axis. Such significant ptosis can lead to amblyopia, and should be repaired.

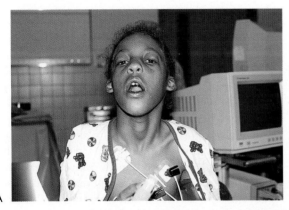

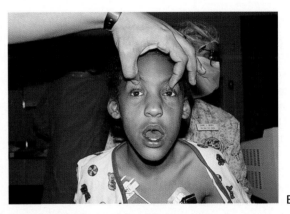

FIGURE 10.21. Congenital ptosis. **A:** Patient with incontinentia pigmenti. Ptosis is severe enough to cause her to assume a chin-up posture. This head position significantly compromises the inferior visual field, causing some patients to trip over objects on the floor. **B:** Elevating the lids manually shows good underlying ocular alignment.

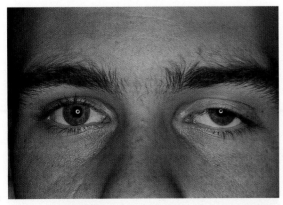

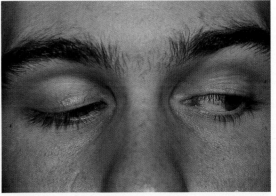

FIGURE 10.22. Congenital ptosis. **A:** Adult patient with mild left ptosis present since birth. **B:** Downgaze reveals characteristic lagophthalmos.

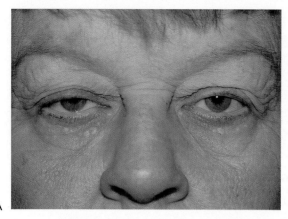
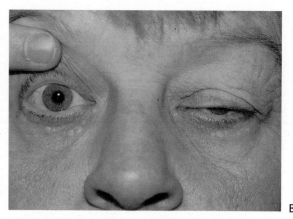

FIGURE 10.23. Acquired ptosis: aponeurotic. **A:** The patient shows several hallmarks of involutional ptosis, including moderate ptosis. The levator function was characteristically good. **B:** Manual elevation of one lid to an anatomically normal position causes the fellow eye to become more pronouncedly ptotic, a vivid demonstration of *Hering's law of equal innervation*. The same occurred when the left lid was manually lifted.

upgaze—and poor Bell's phenomenon can occur in 10% to 15% of patients, and 2% to 5% of patients may manifest the Marcus-Gunn jaw-winking phenomenon.

Acquired ptosis is most commonly secondary to pathology of the levator aponeurosis. *Aponeurotic ptosis* can occur with dehiscence, fatty degeneration, or frank disinsertion of the tissues (Fig. 10.23). Involutional atrophy is the most common underlying cause, although inflammation, repeated edema, and ocular surgery can also result in separation of the aponeurosis from its tarsal attachments. Chronic use of contact lenses and some topical medications have also been implicated. The hallmarks of aponeurotic pathology include mild-to-moderate ptosis with preservation of good levator function and upward migration of the normal lid crease (Fig. 10.24A). In contrast to the lagophthalmos in downgaze, which is characteristic of congenital ptosis, the lid with an aponeurotic defect often shows greater than normal depression on downgaze. The tissues are sometimes so attenuated that the underlying iris is almost visible through the thin lid skin (Fig. 10.24B). Most cases occur in older

adults, but the condition can occur in younger patients with underlying susceptibilities, such as atopy or fatty degeneration. Because the levator subnucleus is a single subnucleus of CN III, equal innervation is sent to both levators. Consequently, elevation of a ptotic lid may result in worsening—or unmasking—of ptosis in the fellow lid, a demonstration of Hering's law (Fig. 10.23).

Traumatic ptosis can occur with any damage to the levator or its aponeurosis (Fig. 10.25). Lid lacerations should be evaluated for levator involvement. Subperiosteal hematomas and blow-out fractures of the roof may induce transient or permanent ptosis. *Mechanical ptosis* (Fig. 10.26) can also result from trauma (e.g., lid edema, hematoma, emphysema, cicatrix), infection (e.g., preseptal or orbital cellulitis), tumor, and dermatochalasis.

Management. The evaluation of congenital or acquired ptosis is directed to identifying the cause. Neurologic and myogenic causes must be eliminated before surgical correction, and they may require referral to appropriate subspecialists. The height of the palpebral fissures and posi-

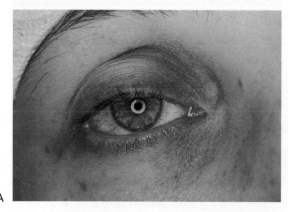
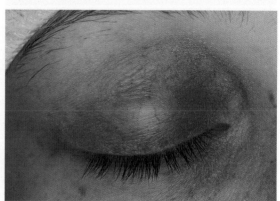

FIGURE 10.24. Acquired ptosis: aponeurotic. **A:** The patient has a high lid crease and moderate lid droop. **B:** The iris is visible through the thin lid skin above the tarsal base.

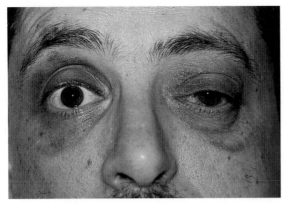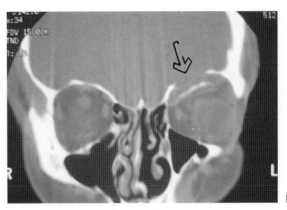

A   B

FIGURE 10.25. Acquired ptosis: traumatic. **A:** The patient suffered a left frontal skull fracture involving the orbital roof secondary to a motor vehicle accident. Other findings included numbness of the forehead (cranial nerve V₁), restriction of elevation, and pulsatile exophthalmos. **B:** Computed tomography shows a depressed roof fracture *(arrow)* and subperiosteal hematoma. Open reduction through a craniotomy resolved all findings.

tion of lid margins should be inspected to determine if a true ptosis exists instead of secondary ptosis or pseudoptosis. In cases of true ptosis, evaluation of levator function is critical in planning appropriate surgical correction. Minimal ptosis can be corrected by internal (e.g., conjunctival mullerectomy, tarsal-conjunctival mullerectomy) or external (e.g., external levator resection) approaches. Moderate ptosis often requires levator aponeurotic reconstruction, but severe ptosis usually demands frontalis fixation or ptosis crutches.

Dermatochalasis, Steatoblepharon, and Blepharochalasis

Dermatochalasis is a common aging change characterized by excess skin of the lids. The baggy eyelid skin may be sufficient to cause a *secondary* or *mechanical ptosis* of the upper lids or ectropion of the lower lids (Fig. 10.26). Herniating orbital fat (*steatoblepharon*) can magnify the problem. *Blepharochalasis* is characterized by recurrent bouts of bilateral angioneurotic edema, which secondarily distends the overlying skin tissues. The lid becomes thinned and takes on a crenulated or "cigarette-paper" texture. Women are affected more commonly than are men. The condition may last for several years, but it appears to be self-limited. The condition is benign, but the skin changes may remain (Fig. 10.27).

Management. The conditions are benign. If the excess skin is sufficient to create secondary ptosis of the upper lid and compromise visual function, or to create ectropion of the lower lid, blepharoplasty can be considered. A variety of techniques have been suggested to manage festoons, including extended blepharoplasty, orbicularis suspension, and direct excision.

Pseudoptosis

Pseudoptosis is the appearance of ptosis although true ptosis does not exist. It can be caused by enophthalmos of any cause including anophthalmos, socket contracture, traumatic orbital blow-out fracture, phthisis, and involutional

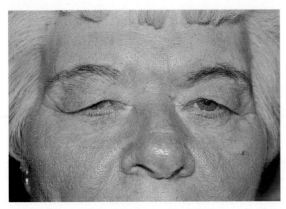

FIGURE 10.26. Dermatochalasis: secondary ptosis. The patient has excessive upper lid skin, creating a mechanical ptosis that interferes with the upper visual field (both eyes).

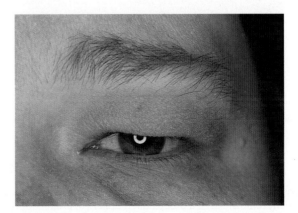

FIGURE 10.27. Blepharochalasis. The patient had recurrent bouts of upper lid swelling. Chronic changes of distended and thinned "cigarette-paper" skin remain.

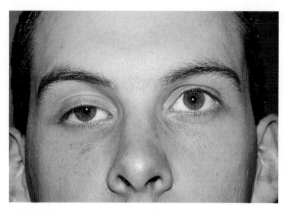

FIGURE 10.28. Pseudoptosis: enophthalmos secondary to an orbital blow-out fracture (right eye).

atrophy (Fig. 10.28). Contralateral lid retraction, overcorrection of contralateral ptosis, and contralateral proptosis can also create the appearance of lid droop (Fig. 10.29).

Management. Enophthalmos can occur after trauma, erosion of the orbit by tumors or chronic sinusitis, and atrophy of the orbital tissues because of trauma, involutional atrophy, nutritional deficits, or cachexia. Evaluation includes appropriate history taking, testing for infraorbital dysesthesia, and radiologic evaluation as required. Contralateral lid retraction (e.g., thyroid retraction) should always be looked for and appropriate laboratory tests ordered. Management is directed at correcting the identified defect. For example, enophthalmos secondary to recent orbital trauma is repaired by reduction of the orbital fracture. Thyroid eye disease is treated with topical lubricants, and surgical lowering of the retracted eyelids if needed. Cicatricial and mechanical retraction is treated by releasing the cicatricial bands and placement of spacer grafts to the skin or posterior lamella, as necessary.

Neurogenic and Myogenic Ptosis and Myasthenia Gravis

The neurogenic causes of ptosis include *oculomotor palsy* and *Horner's syndrome.*

Cranial nerve III palsy also affects ocular motility and may also affect the pupil (Fig. 10.30). The underlying causes include tumors, infection, inflammation, and vascular and metabolic disorders. This paralytic ptosis is generally severe, with little or no levator function. Aberrant regeneration may cause abnormal lid elevation with attempted ocular movements.

Horner's syndrome results from sympathetic denervation to the lid and orbit. Classic findings include mild ptosis with excellent levator function and miotic anisocoria, which is more apparent in darkness (Fig. 10.31). Lower lid elevation (i.e., reverse ptosis) is often present, resulting in narrowing of the palpebral fissure and apparent enophthalmos. Ipsilateral anhidrosis results from involvement of the sudomotor fibers. Heterochromia is a sign of congenital or infantile onset. The causes include trauma, vascular insult, tumors (particularly those of the pulmonary apex), and intracavernous lesions. The mild ptosis reverses with instillation of Neo-Synephrine.

Acquired myogenic ptosis results from several degenerative conditions affecting the levator and oculomotor muscles. *Chronic progressive external ophthalmoplegia* (CPEO) encompasses a spectrum of mitochondrially inherited muscular dystrophies that also affect ocular motility and levator function (Fig. 10.32). Patients slowly develop progressively severe ptosis with poor levator function, little or no ocular movement, and poor Bell's phenomenon. A characteristic exotropia is manifested in advanced stages, although patients seldom complain of diplopia. Larger and more distal structures away from the head and neck can be variably af-

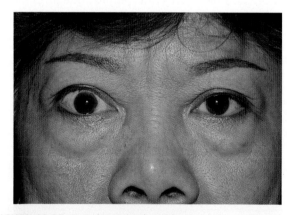

FIGURE 10.29. Pseudoptosis: thyroid eye disease. A 50-year-old patient complained of a drooping left upper lid. Examination revealed proptosis and lid retraction of the right eye. Laboratory studies revealed the presence of thyroid disease.

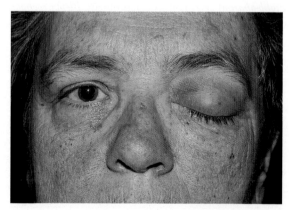

FIGURE 10.30. Neurogenic ptosis: oculomotor palsy. Metastatic paratracheal adenocarcinoma produced a complete orbital apex syndrome. Oculomotor palsy and ptosis were complete. Note the downwardly directed lashes and the loss of the natural lid crease. Other findings include proptosis and significant orbital congestion.

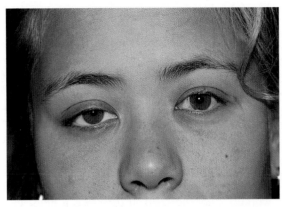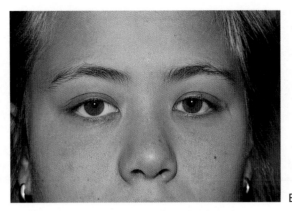

FIGURE 10.31. Horner's syndrome. **A:** Before Neo-Synephrine. A 17-year-old patient developed Horner's syndrome after resection of a lymphangioma from the right pulmonary apex. Findings include mild ptosis and miosis. **B:** Ptosis resolves after instillation of Neo-Synephrine.

fected, depending on the specific disorder. In oropharyngeal dystrophy, chewing and swallowing are affected, and in myotonic dystrophy, muscles and genitalia are involved. Ocular manifestations are protean, ranging from pigmentary retinopathy (e.g., Kearns-Sayre syndrome [KSS] or "CPEO plus"; Fig. 10.33), to polychromatophilic cataract (e.g., myotonic dystrophy). Cardiac conduction delays (KSS) and peripheral nerve disorders can also occur in mitochondrial encephalopathies. Biopsy of skeletal muscle often shows "ragged red fibers" that reflect an abnormal number of mitochondria. Although the pigmentary retinopathy of KSS is often referred to as "pseudo-retinitis pigmentosa," or "RP-like," the visual course and prognosis of the two conditions is not similar. These conditions are often diagnosed clinically, but may require extensive chromosomal and neurologic testing as well as muscle biopsy.

Myasthenia gravis is a disorder of adults affecting the neuromuscular endplate, altering the synaptic transmission of acetylcholine. Findings can be multiple, depending on the muscle complex affected, but ocular findings, including in-

termittent diplopia and ptosis, often arise primarily (Fig. 10.34). The ptosis characteristically varies through the day, depending on the fatigue of the levator. There is a well-recognized association with thyroid dysfunction and thymoma. The condition may be confirmed via edrophonium injection (Tensilon) and ice-pack tests, which can quickly and temporarily reverse ptosis, and by antibody testing. However, both false-positive and false-negative results are known to occur, making the diagnosis still a clinical one.

Management. Patients with new-onset ptosis thought to be of neurogenic or myogenic origin or with Horner's syndrome should undergo full evaluation, including laboratory analysis and radiologic and pharmacologic testing, to determine the cause. Patients suspected of having CPEO should undergo routine electrocardiogram testing. Referral to a neuroophthalmologist may be warranted. Treatment of any

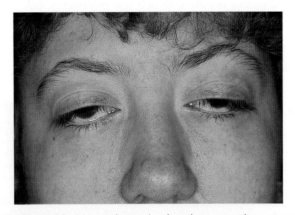

FIGURE 10.33. Myogenic ptosis: chronic progressive external ophthalmoplegia (Kearns-Sayre syndrome). The patient manifests severe ptosis with characteristic facies of longstanding external ophthalmoplegia. The ocular motility is severely limited, and levator function is extremely poor. The patient also has significant visual field defects secondary to pigmentary retinopathy but has not developed cardiac conduction delays. The patient complained of progressive ptosis that interfered with daily functions, requiring her to manually elevate her lids.

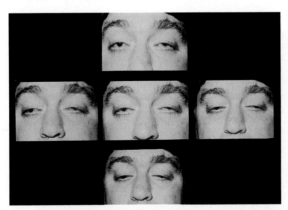

FIGURE 10.32. Myogenic ptosis: chronic progressive external ophthalmoplegia. The composite photograph shows the decrease in ocular motility characteristic of myopathic processes.

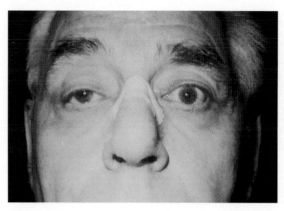

FIGURE 10.34. Myasthenia gravis. The patient noticed gradual worsening of moderate ptosis (right eye). He also complained particularly of having to use his forehead to lift his eyes. Questioning disclosed a history of intermittent diplopia.

associated ptosis should be approached with caution and depends on the severity of the condition, the degree of visual impairment, and the amount of levator function. Treatment options include conjunctival mullerectomy, levator resection, frontalis suspension, and ptosis crutches. These patients are at risk for postoperative exposure keratitis.

Marcus-Gunn Jaw-Winking

In 1833, Marcus-Gunn described a patient with unilateral congenital ptosis that elevated with jaw movements. The *Marcus-Gunn jaw-winking* phenomenon is thought to result from an abnormal synkinetic connection between cranial nerves V and III. Branches from the motor root of cranial nerve V destined for the ipsilateral lateral pterygoid muscle (or less commonly, the inner pterygoid) innervate the ipsilateral levator muscle such that jaw movements, especially those to the opposite side, cause elevation of the lid (Fig. 10.35). Jaw-winking may occur in 2% to 5% of patients with congenital ptosis. Familial patterns are not uncommon, and rare bilateral cases have been described. The sever-

ity of the disorder appears to lessen with time and age, but this may reflect adaptation to the condition and the ability to suppress the motions that trigger obvious lid retraction. The condition can be confused with *aberrant regeneration of cranial nerve VII* (i.e., winking jaw of Wartenberg; Fig. 10.36). In this latter, acquired condition, motor fibers originally innervating the orofacial musculature are redirected abnormally to the orbicularis fibers, causing synkinetic closure of the lid with ipsilateral facial movements. It is common after trauma to cranial nerve VII.

Management. The Marcus-Gunn jaw-winking phenomenon is an isolated neurologic finding, and further workup is not indicated. If the ptosis is mild, and the jaw-winking is of little cosmetic concern, the condition may be observed indefinitely. If surgery is contemplated, levator disinsertion with subsequent frontalis suspension is generally recommended. Some ophthalmologists recommend the procedure be done bilaterally to avoid postoperative asymmetry.

Blepharospasm, Hemifacial Spasm, Myokymia, and Aberrant Regeneration

Hyperkinetic dystonias of cranial nerve VII are characterized by involuntary contractures of the muscles subserved by the facial nerve. In *blepharospasm*, the spasms are bilateral and most often involve the eyelids and brows, but they sometimes extend to the lower face and neck (Fig. 10.37). The spasms can be severe enough to impair daily activities. The disorder begins between 40 and 60 years of age and affects women three times more often than men. Patients often learn "tricks" that defeat the spasms, such as yawning, whistling, or other facial movements. The spasms can be stress-related but are characteristically absent during sleep. *Essential blepharospasm* is generally idiopathic, but many factors may cause *reflex blepharospasm*.

Hemifacial spasm is often caused by compression and irritation of the facial nerve root by an intracranial tumor or

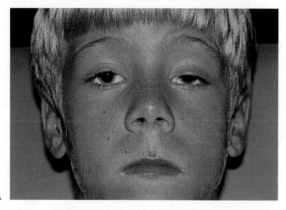
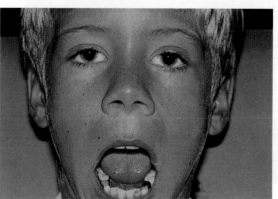

A   B

FIGURE 10.35. Marcus-Gunn jaw-winking. **A:** Significant ptosis of the left eye at rest. **B:** The lid elevates with jaw movement, reflecting the synkinesis between the pterygoid and levator muscles (cranial nerves V and III).

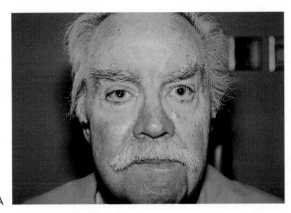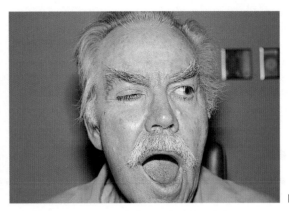

A   B

FIGURE 10.36. Aberrant regeneration of cranial nerve VII. **A:** Patient after extensive right parotidectomy for malignant oncocytic carcinoma with secondary right facial palsy. The lid is in a normal position while at rest. **B:** Aberrantly directed nerve fibers from the lower face now innervate the orbicularis and cause the lid to close with facial movement.

aberrant vessel, or after facial nerve palsy of any cause (Fig. 10.38). Most cases, however, are idiopathic. The spasms affect only one side of the face, are unaffected by tricks, and persist through sleep, often awakening those so afflicted. The age of onset is later than in blepharospasm.

Aberrant regeneration typically occurs after traumatic injury of the seventh nerve. Unlike blepharospasm and hemifacial spasm, these facial contractures are not involuntary spasms but are coincident with facial movements. Involuntary eyelid closure with smiling, chewing, or grinning results from misdirected nerve fibers originally destined for lower facial musculature regenerating into the orbicularis. Consequently, the eyelid spasms occur only with facial expression. Similarly, upper fibers initially innervating the eyelids can reinnervate the lower oral musculature, resulting in oral spasms on blinking. Salivary fibers may reinnervate the lacrimal gland, resulting in gustatory epiphora, or "crocodile tears."

Intermittent, rapid-frequency, fine-motor fasciculations are known as *myokymia*. The condition is benign, is more transitory than any of the other conditions, and is often related to stress.

Management. Patients with facial hyperkinesis should be thoroughly questioned for a history of facial nerve disorders, previous trauma, or palsy. Dizziness, vertigo, decreased hearing and tinnitus suggest eighth cranial nerve pathology, which may contiguously induce hemifacial spasm. An audible bruit may indicate vascular compression of the nerve root. All patients with hemifacial spasm should undergo radiologic imaging of the cerebellopontine angle to rule out intracranial pathology. Medical management of these disorders is generally ineffective. Anxiolytics, antidepressants, antiparkinsonians, and neuroleptics have all been tried without much success. Local chemodenervation with *Clostridium botulinum* toxin type A (BoTox) and other medications has proven to be successful in controlling the spasms, but the effects are temporary, and retreatment is often required. The length of effect is generally longer for

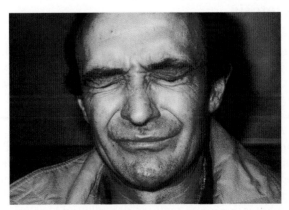

FIGURE 10.37. Essential blepharospasm. Severe involuntary spasms of the eyelids can significantly impede daily functions such as driving, essentially incapacitating the patient.

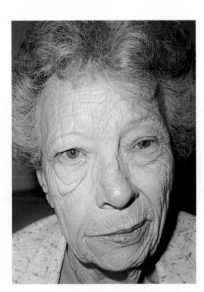

FIGURE 10.38. Patient with left hemifacial spasm. The spasms extend into the neck, as evidenced by the significant platysmal band. The neurologic evaluation was negative.

hemifacial spasm than for blepharospasm. Denervation is less widely used because of its poor record of success. Some patients may benefit from wide orbicularis myectomy, which requires meticulous extirpation of the involved muscles. Neurosurgical decompression of the facial canal with interposition of a sponge between the nerve root and an encroaching vessel can be successful in selected patients.

TUMORS

Xanthelasma, Histiocytoses, and Juvenile Xanthogranuloma

Xanthelasmas are the most common form of cutaneous xanthoma, typically arising in middle-aged and older women. They appear as flat, plaque-like, creamy yellow lesions and are the result of abnormal lipid deposition within the dermis (Fig. 10.39). The medial aspect of the lids is most commonly affected. Although there is no firm association with hyperlipidemia, they can occur in diabetes and in hyperlipidemic or hereditary conditions, particularly in younger patients. The lesion is benign, but it can be cosmetically disfiguring.

The common xanthelasma is not associated with the more uncommon conditions of *histiocytosis* (e.g., Hand-Schüller-Christian disease, Letterer-Siwe disease, or eosinophilic granuloma), in which the lesions usually occur in childhood, are more nodular, involve deeper structures, and produce lytic bony lesions. These latter conditions are often associated with significant multisystem disease and can be profoundly morbid or fatal.

Juvenile xanthogranuloma is a benign condition that arises in childhood. The typical lesion is a yellow-orange, solid nodule, but the mass can also take on a deeper color (Fig. 10.40). Although the lesion is typically located on the skin, it can occur intraocularly or, more uncommonly, in the orbit. Spontaneous hyphema has been reported from rupture of the vessels in iris lesions.

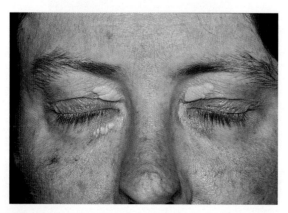

FIGURE 10.39. This otherwise healthy woman has creamy yellow plaques in the dermis of all four lids, which is typical of xanthelasma.

Management. Xanthelasmas are benign growths and are best managed conservatively. Although the association with hyperlipidemia is rare, if the lesion appears in a young patient, lipid evaluation is warranted. Otherwise, no workup is needed. If the lesion is significantly large or cosmetically disfiguring, simple excision is curative. However, the lesion may recur. Some lesions may be amenable to treatment with cutaneous laser.

Patients suffering from the histiocytoses should be referred for further evaluation and care. Eosinophilic granuloma can be excised locally or treated with irradiation. The lesion sometimes involutes spontaneously. Juvenile xanthogranuloma is a benign condition. Lesions typically resolve spontaneously. The eyes should be thoroughly examined to rule out intraocular involvement.

Hidrocystoma and Syringoma

Hidrocystomas (i.e., sudoriferous cysts, sweat gland cysts, eccrine hydrocystomas) are apocrine or eccrine in origin. They often arise on the lid margin as single or multiple translucent cystic nodules. On incision, a clear or milky fluid is expressed from a smooth-walled cavity (Fig. 10.41). Cystic basal cell carcinoma is often initially misdiagnosed as hidrocystoma.

Syringoma are solid nodules that resemble milia. They are more common in young female patients and typically arise on the lower lids as multiple, irregular nodules, although they may also arise on the cheeks and forehead (Fig. 10.42). The nodule may contain keratin. The masses are probably eccrine in origin.

Management. These lesions are benign and require no further workup. Simple excision of the mass, including the cyst wall, is generally curative. However, because rare malignant counterparts have been reported, large or recurrent lesions should be sent for biopsy.

Papilloma, Keratoacanthoma, Inverted Follicular Keratosis, and Seborrheic Keratosis

Several benign epithelial tumors of the lid are common. *Squamous papillomas* are by far the most common. They may be single or multiple and tend to involve the lid margin. They are typically sessile or pedunculated, with many finger-like projections containing fibrovascular cores (Fig. 10.43).

Keratoacanthoma is a rapidly growing, dome-shaped lesion with elevated, rolled edges and a central keratin-filled crater (Fig. 10.44). These lesions typically grow over a period of 2 months or less, are generally painless, and often regress spontaneously but may leave a scar. The lesion is benign but is sometimes confused clinically and histologically with squamous cell carcinoma.

Inverted follicular keratosis often presents as a cutaneous

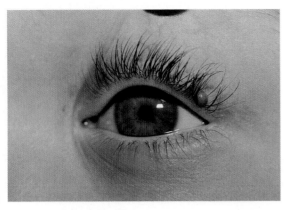
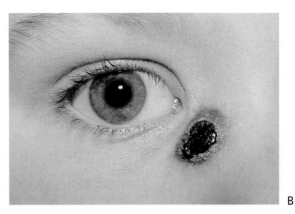

A

B

FIGURE 10.40. Juvenile xanthogranuloma (JXG). **A:** Characteristic yellow-orange, solid tissue nodule arose on the lid margin of this 2-year-old boy. This was the sole tumor found on the patient. The ocular examination was normal. **B:** Another patient with a JXG lesion on the side of the nose. Its color is somewhat darker than that of the tumor in **A**. Biopsy specimens of each patient showed characteristic Touton giant cells and foamy histiocytes.

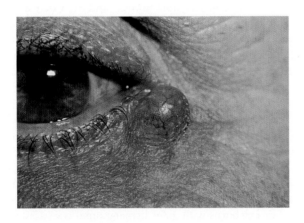

FIGURE 10.41. Hidrocystoma is a nontender cyst of the lid. The lesion is well circumscribed and translucent.

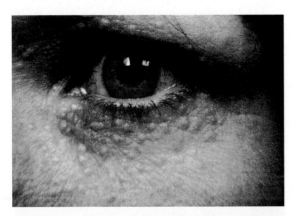

FIGURE 10.42. Syringoma. These are small solid nodules that resemble milia and are more common in young women.

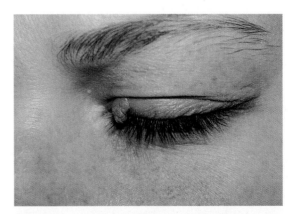

FIGURE 10.43. Squamous papilloma. A sessile, fleshy nodule with finger-like projections and fibrovascular cores.

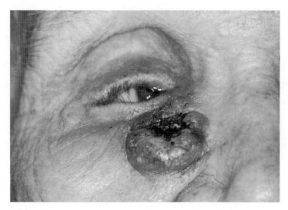

FIGURE 10.44. Keratoacanthoma. This dome-shaped lesion arose over a matter of months. A central, keratin-filled crater can be seen.

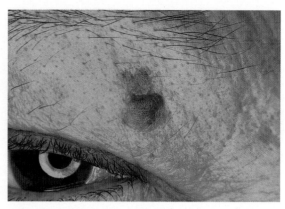

FIGURE 10.46. Seborrheic keratosis. Typical appearance of a flat, elevated plaque that appears "stuck on." The lesion does not have deep extensions through the skin.

horn at the lid margin (Fig. 10.45). It tends to grow rapidly, often in less than 3 months. Most physicians think the lesion represents an irritated seborrheic keratosis.

Seborrheic keratosis is common in older persons. It appears as a flatly elevated, verrucous growth of variable pigmentation. It is typically well demarcated, appears stuck on the skin, and may have a friable surface (Fig. 10.46).

Management. These benign skin lesions can be managed by single excision. Because of their similarity to cancerous lesions, submission for pathologic examination should be considered.

Capillary Hemangioma

Capillary hemangioma (i.e., strawberry nevus, benign hemangioendothelioma) is the most common primary orbital and cutaneous tumor of childhood. Only rarely is the lesion seen at birth; it usually arises shortly thereafter as a red, irregularly dimpled, raised lesion, called a *strawberry nevus* (Fig. 10.47). The lesion characteristically goes through a period of rapid growth over the first 6 to 12 months, with gradual spontaneous involution. Most regress by 3 years of age. Before involution, hemangiomas may be tender to

touch and may swell with crying (without significantly changing color), but with regression, the mass becomes less tender, much smaller, more fibrotic, and less vascular, making surgical excision less hemorrhagic and possibly less difficult. The overlying skin remains abnormal, with mild atrophic changes and pallor and developing a crepe paper texture. Unlike the port wine stain angioma of Sturge-Weber, capillary hemangiomas are raised and irregular, are redder than port wine nevi, and blanch with pressure. Feeder vessels can often be identified. If the tumor is primarily orbital or deeper in the dermis, the cutaneous appearance takes on a more bluish hue (Fig. 10.48).

The lesion is benign with no tendency for malignant transformation. However, a generalized bleeding disorder secondary to profound thrombocytopenia has been associated in newborns with giant hemangiomas (i.e., Kasabach-Merritt syndrome). If a periorbital mass is large enough, it may induce a mechanical ptosis or astigmatism, resulting in amblyopia. Most lesions are solitary, but as many as 20% of patients may have multiple foci. The head and neck region is most commonly affected, but visceral, central nervous sys-

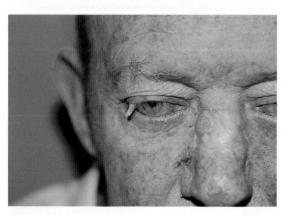

FIGURE 10.45. Inverted follicular keratosis. The lesion at the lid margin has a cutaneous horn.

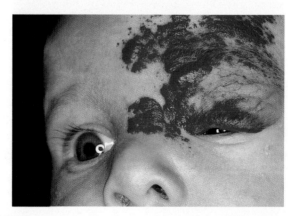

FIGURE 10.47. Capillary hemangioma. A large, diffuse lesion of the left face. The surface is raised and irregular, with a bright red color characteristic of superficial hemangiomas. Significant ptosis can produce occlusion amblyopia.

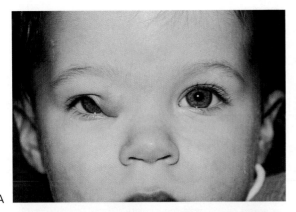

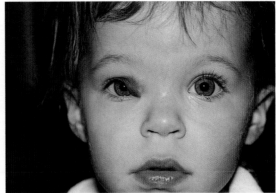

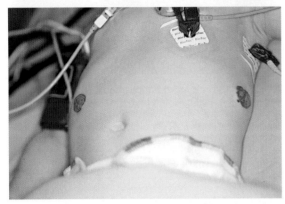

FIGURE 10.48. Capillary hemangioma. **A:** The lesion of the upper lid is large enough to partially occlude the visual axis and induced a significant astigmatic error and strong visual preference for the left eye, requiring occlusion therapy. Cycloplegic refraction: OD, +5.50 × 030 degrees; OS, +1.75 sph. Because it is located in the deeper tissue layers, this hemangioma appears more bluish than more superficially located lesions. **B:** Three days after intralesional steroid injection, the hemangioma has shrunk out of the visual axis. **C:** The patient also had more peripheral lesions on the trunk.

tem (CNS), and lymphatic hemangiomas have also been described (Fig. 10.48C). Emotional and cosmetic considerations are often the overwhelming parental concerns.

Management. The desire for intervention should be tempered with knowledge of the natural history of spontaneous involution. Patients must be closely followed for development of ptosis or amblyopia. If the lesion is small and inconsequential, observation is recommended. The parents should be queried about the presence of other lesions. Although the precise mechanism of action is not well understood, intralesional corticosteroid injection is the most common treatment. Complications have included systemic corticosteroid absorption, eyelid necrosis, and central retinal artery occlusion. The fundus should be examined immediately after injection. Systemic and topical steroids, irradiation, cryotherapy, and injectable sclerosing agents have also been used with variable success. However, each carries its own risks. If surgical excision is contemplated, it should be postponed until the lesion has involuted. Because of the vascularity of the tumor, laser scalpels may be useful.

Nevus Flammeus

Nevus flammeus (i.e., port wine stain, claret stain, Sturge-Weber syndrome, encephalotrigeminal syndrome) is a large, flat, violaceous, vascular malformation characterized by diffusely ectatic, cavernous vascular spaces and channels in the upper layers of the dermis. Unlike capillary hemangioma, which usually arises just after birth, nevus flammeus is well circumscribed and grows with the patient throughout life. The tumor typically follows the distribution along the branches of the trigeminal nerve (Fig. 10.49), but it commonly crosses the midline or is bilateral. It often occurs away from the head and neck region. Unlike capillary hemangioma, it neither regresses nor involutes with age, nor does it blanch with pressure. It is more violaceous (i.e., port wine) than strawberry red, which is perhaps a reflection of the blood moving slower through the tumor, and the color often deepens with crying or a Valsalva's maneuver. Feeder vessels are uncommon. If the tumor is nodular, it is softer and more compressible than a hemangioma, feeling somewhat spongier than the firmer counterpart. With time, the mass often becomes more nodular and fibrotic (Fig. 10.50).

The tumor may be associated with other vascular malformations, such as the Klippel-Trénaunay-Weber syndrome, in which venous and lymphatic malformations coexist on the trunk and extremities, and the Sturge-Weber syndrome. The latter condition, one of the phakomatoses, is the most well-known abnormality associated with facial nevus flammeus. Associated findings include diffuse choroidal hemangioma, retinal detachment, and glaucoma. Ocular involvement is more frequent if the malformation affects the upper trigeminal distributions (i.e., V1 and V2). Central anomalies include vascular malformations of the ipsilateral lep-

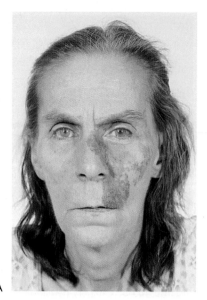 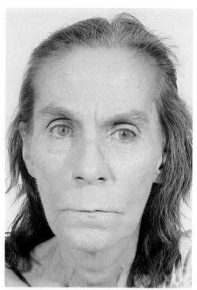

FIGURE 10.49. Nevus flammeus. **A:** Without makeup. The lesion is much darker than a capillary hemangioma. **B:** Many patients are able to disguise the lesion well by using heavy makeup.

tomeninges, with calcification of the underlying cortex and consequent risk of seizure disorders, and various degrees of mental retardation.

Management. Because of the risk of glaucoma and retinal detachment, patients require full examinations at routine intervals, especially if the lid, forehead, and globe are involved. Glaucoma may develop at any age and is difficult to treat. Patients with lesions of the head and neck should also be referred for neurologic evaluation and imaging, because seizures and mental retardation are not uncommon. Treatment of the lesion itself is often frustrating, because the overlying soft tissue and underlying skeleton are often malformed. Facial stains may be covered conservatively with heavy makeup. Although surgery may be considered for older patients whose lesions have become nodular, advances with dermatologic lasers have made photocoagulation a popular alternative in all ages.

Neurofibromatosis

Plexiform neurofibromas are a hallmark of *neurofibromatosis*, also called von Recklinghausen's syndrome. They occur along peripheral nerves of the lid and orbit but are infiltrative rather than isolated or encapsulated. Arising in the first decade, they present a typical appearance that diffusely involves all tissues of the lid and can extend into the orbit (Fig. 10.51). The normal architecture is distorted, often with the loss of most soft tissue landmarks. Diffuse soft tissue involvement typically creates a secondary ptosis, often worse laterally, which pro-

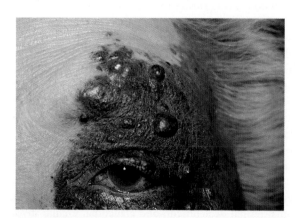

FIGURE 10.50. Chronic Sturge-Weber syndrome. The lesion shows the typical nodularity and pedunculation of chronicity. As suspected from the eyelid and conjunctival involvement, the patient also suffers from unilateral glaucoma.

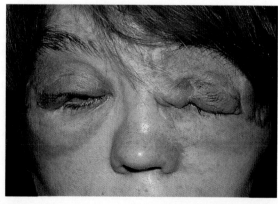

FIGURE 10.51. Neurofibromatosis. The upper lids are diffusely involved with plexiform neurofibromas. The patient is anophthalmic (left eye), having lost the eye to massive proptosis and exposure secondary to an optic nerve glioma. She has had multiple debulking procedures.

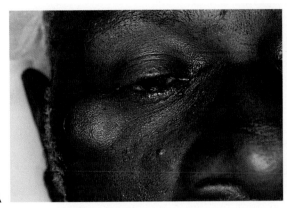
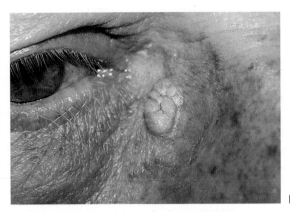

A   B

FIGURE 10.52. Epidermal inclusion cyst. **A:** A slowly growing mass over the right zygoma with normal overlying skin. The mass is nontender and is attached to the overlying skin but has no deep attachments. **B:** A more superficial lesion shows the typical characteristics of yellow color and telangiectasis, which can lead to an erroneous diagnosis of sebaceous cyst.

duces a "lazy S" configuration. The infiltrative nature of these benign tumors can massively enlarge the lid, giving a "bag of worms" sensation. The lid and lash margins are often abnormal, and ocular function can be compromised.

Patients with neurofibromatosis (especially Type II) are at increased risk of CNS tumors such as optic nerve glioma and acoustic neuroma, as well as congenital glaucoma.

Management. Because plexiform neurofibromas are pathognomonic for neurofibromatosis, the patient should undergo a thorough ocular and physical examination, including radiographs of the head. Large, unsightly lid masses may be debulked for cosmetic reasons, with reconstruction dictated by the extent of excision. Because of the infiltrative nature of the tumor, the lesions typically recur, necessitating multiple procedures.

Epidermal Inclusion Cysts and Milia

Inspissation of the hair follicle, with subcutaneous entrapment of keratin produces a freely movable dermal or subcutaneous nodule known as an *epidermal inclusion cyst* or a *sebaceous cyst* (Fig. 10.52A). The color of the mass depends on the location within the dermis. Deep lesions are covered by normal skin, and more superficial lesions may appear yellow or fatty, with overlying telangiectatic vessels, leading to the common misnomer of *sebaceous cyst* (Fig. 10.52B). The mass is often attached to the skin but is not anchored to deep structures. The cyst may rupture, leading to secondary inflammation and scarring. Epidermal inclusion cysts can occur anywhere on the body, including upper and lower lids and the brows. If allowed to enlarge, upper lid lesions can create a mechanical ptosis.

Milia are very small superficial keratin cysts, approximately 1 to 4 mm in diameter, that can arise in large numbers. Their creamy yellow or white color is characteristic of their location in the superficial dermis (Fig. 10.53). They can occur spontaneously or secondary to lid trauma and can

be thought of as miniature epidermal inclusion cysts. They are benign.

Management. Epidermal inclusion cysts can be effectively managed by excision of the mass and entire cyst wall. This can be done through a skin incision over the lesion, with subcutaneous dissection of the cyst, or by simple excision and closure of the entire mass.

Milia can be treated by decapitating the mass or incising the overlying skin with a hypodermic tip or razor blade scalpel. The keratin cyst is expressed with gentle pressure.

Hair Follicle Tumors

Hair follicle tumors, including trichoepithelioma, tricholemmoma, trichofolliculoma, and pilomatrixoma, are benign, with little malignant potential. Most occur as solitary masses or nodules that have a marked predilection for the face, head, and neck. Many simulate basal cell carcinoma, intradermal nevus, neurofibroma, and other adnexal tumors, and they may be difficult to differentiate clinically. Most arise in adulthood.

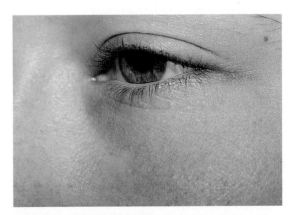

FIGURE 10.53. Milia are multiple, small, yellow lesions of the superficial skin. The patient had similar lesions on all eyelids.

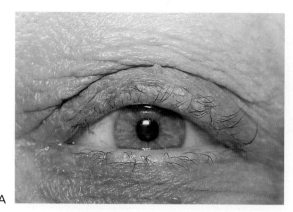
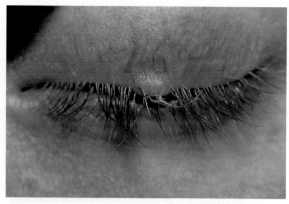

A   B

FIGURE 10.54. A: Trichoepithelioma. A 65-year-old woman was observed incidentally to have nodular growths on all eyelids. The lesions were painless and had been present for an unknown length of time. Biopsy specimens revealed them to be trichoepithelioma. **B:** Trichofolliculoma. Fine white hairs growing from a central pore typify trichofolliculoma. A painless mass was present for several months in this 25-year-old man.

Trichoepithelioma presents as a solitary, flesh-colored, dome-shaped papule (Fig. 10.54A). It may be particularly difficult to differentiate from basal cell carcinoma clinically and histologically. An autosomal-dominant form (i.e., Brooke's tumor) begins in adolescence with multiple tumors, associated with multiple cylindromas and syringomas. Tricholemmoma can also present as multiple lesions but most commonly appears as a solitary, flesh-colored growth in later adulthood. However, the lesion is sometimes pearl gray, leading to confusion with basal cell carcinoma. Multiple tricholemmomas of the face, head, and hands are associated with an increased risk of breast, thyroid, and gastrointestinal cancers and with other fibrous hamartomas (e.g., Cowden disease). *Trichofolliculoma* is the most highly differentiated hair follicle tumor. It is characterized by fine white hairs growing from a central pore in a flesh-colored papule. (Fig. 10.54B)

Unlike the previous entities, which typically arise in adulthood, *pilomatrixoma* (i.e., calcifying epithelioma of Malherbe) arises primarily in childhood and adolescence. The typical lesion is a solitary, firm, subcutaneous nodule, which is mobile under the skin. Telangiectatic vessels are common, as is a pink or violaceous color.

Management. The lesions are benign and have little malignant potential. However, they can be cosmetically disfiguring. Because of the similarity in appearance with other skin malignancies, biopsy should be considered to rule out more significant pathology. Treatment is by simple excision. Dermabrasion and laser vaporization may also be effective in treating lesions away from the eyes.

Nevocellular Nevi

The skin contains a large number of melanocytes, dendritic cells of neural crest origin that produce melanin. Nevus cells are thought to be a specialized form of melanocyte that possesses the ability to form nests and aggregations within the skin. Nevocellular or melanocytic nevi are categorized according to the histologic location of the cells within the dermis. *Junctional nevi* occur at the junction of the dermis and epidermis. They appear most commonly in childhood as round or ovoid, flat macules. Pigmentation varies from light to dark brown. They often enlarge and become darker during childhood and adolescence, becoming raised, pigmented nodules, called *compound nevi* (Fig. 10.55). Hair growth is common. These lesions have characteristics of junctional and intradermal nevi. Malignant transformation can occur with junctional and compound nevi. As the name suggests, *intradermal nevi* are primarily located purely within the dermis. They are raised nodules and may be minimally pigmented (Fig. 10.56). Malignant transformation is unusual.

Management. Nevi are benign but may be cosmetically unsightly. Excision is usually curative, although the lesion may recur if incompletely removed. Subsequent differentiation from melanoma may be difficult. Any excised pigmented lesion should be sent for pathologic examination.

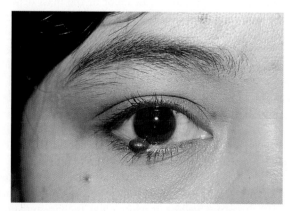

FIGURE 10.55. This compound nevus grew slowly over years from a previously flat "mole" that had been present since childhood.

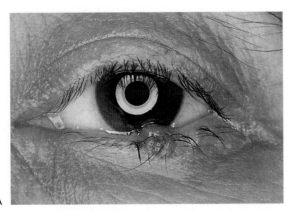 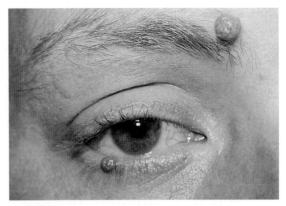

FIGURE 10.56. Intradermal nevus. **A:** Verrucous appearance of a flesh-colored, lightly pigmented, elevated mass that had been present for longer than 4 years. **B:** Multiple intradermal nevi.

Other methods of destruction, such as cryotherapy or electrodesiccation, should not be used.

Basal Cell Carcinoma

Basal cell carcinoma is the most common skin malignancy. It is more common in the lower lid than the upper, but it can occur anywhere on the ocular adnexal skin (Fig. 10.57). Although it has low metastatic potential and is generally well controlled by local excision, significant morbidity can occur through neglect, recurrence, or inadequate surgical treatment. Chronic sun exposure is known to be a risk factor, as are age and fair skin. Skin cancers of all types are uncommon in darkly pigmented populations.

The tumor starts in the epithelium but can extend into the deeper tissues to involve the orbit or lacrimal drainage system. Several clinical types are recognized, though the distinction is often made at the pathologist's microscope. Although the nodular and sclerosing types of tumor are generally well circumscribed, the morphea type may be poorly demarcated, with multilevel finger-like projections and extensions. Basal cell carcinoma may also take on a cystic or nevoid appearance, sometimes mimicking hidrocystoma or pigmented lesions such as melanoma. Basosquamous carcinoma may be more aggressive than the nodular type. Clinically, the lesions appear as firm masses on the epithelium with variable, deep extensions. The edges of the lesion are typically raised, with the rolled edges forming a central crater of pearl gray tissue (Fig. 10.58). Inherent vascularity and easy excoriation may cause chronic ulceration and bleeding. A lesion at the lid margin often causes lash loss. The most common lesion is found in older adults. However, multiple tumors can arise in the second decade as part of the *basal cell nevus syndrome*. In this autosomal-dominant condition, multiple basal cells of the skin arise from ordinary-looking nevi, predominantly on the face and eyelids. The lesions, especially those around the nose and eyes, behave more aggressively than most. Other associated systemic findings include prognathism with mandibular bone cysts,

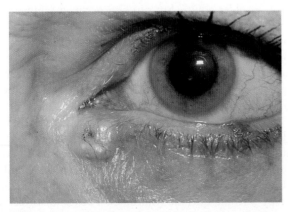 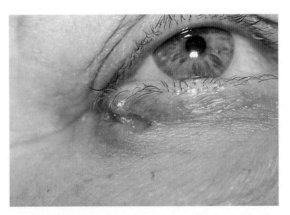

FIGURE 10.57. Basal cell carcinoma. Well-circumscribed, pearly gray tumor of the epithelium, with raised, rolled edges and central ulceration. An independent vascular pattern is also visible. Lesions of the medial canthal area can easily involve the lacrimal drainage system and orbit.

FIGURE 10.58. Basal cell carcinoma. A well-defined, firm mass of the lateral canthus with a deep central crater and markedly rolled edges, although the mass is not characteristically pearly gray. A biopsy confirmed basal cell carcinoma. Like lesions of the medial canthus, the tumors of the lateral canthal region can give rise to deep orbital extension.

skull and skeletal anomalies, teleorbitism, partial agenesis of the corpus callosum, and medulloblastoma.

Basal cell carcinoma must be differentiated from chronic chalazion, keratoacanthoma, dermal nevus, and other skin malignancies.

Management. Evaluation should include inspection and palpation of the deeper tissues and orbit. If basal cell carcinoma is suspected, an incisional biopsy in the office can provide the diagnosis. Particular attention should be paid to lesions of the medial and lateral canthi, as these sites offer easy entrance of tumor cells into the deep orbit. After the diagnosis is established, complete excision by Mohs' micrographic technique or frozen-section control and reconstruction is curative, because the lesion has little metastatic potential. However, the patient must be continually monitored for recurrences and the development of new tumors. Although cryotherapy is often used on other cutaneous sites, it should not routinely be a primary treatment for tumors of the lid and adnexa because of the inability to guarantee complete excision. Lesions of the medial and lateral canthal regions require careful attention because of the proximity of the lacrimal drainage system, the increased tendency to deep orbital extension, and the difficulty in reconstruction of these areas. Patients should be advised of the need for sun protection.

Squamous Cell Carcinoma

Squamous cell carcinoma occurs much more commonly on the conjunctiva, cornea, and mucus membranes than on the lid. Like squamous cell carcinoma elsewhere, lid lesions are much more aggressive than the more common basal cell carcinoma. They have a much greater potential for local extension and regional and widespread metastasis, although the overall incidence of metastasis is still low and the risk of death rare. Primary lesions of the lid are less likely to metastasize than those that arise in other locations. The tumor occurs most commonly in older patients. However, patients with underlying skin diseases such as xeroderma pigmentosum, discoid lupus, and lupus vulgaris are commonly affected at an earlier age. Actinic keratosis is the most common precursor lesion. However, the tumor may arise in other areas of chronic irritation and trauma, such as ulcers, scars, burns, previous irradiation sites, and keloids. While a lesion of the upper lid is more likely to be a squamous cell carcinoma than a basal cell carcinoma, the lower lid is still more commonly involved than the upper. But both cancers can occur anywhere along the adnexa. The squamous cell lesion tends to be more infiltrative and less nodular than basal cell carcinoma, with more keratinization and less distinct margins (Fig. 10.59). Lash loss is common if the lid margin is involved. The lesion grows less rapidly than keratoacanthoma—with which it shares some pathologic features—but it grows more rapidly than basal cell carcinoma. The potential for deep invasion, orbital extension, and metastasis is

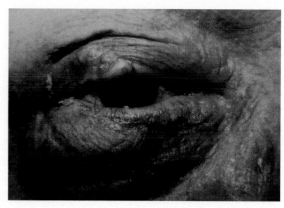

FIGURE 10.59. Squamous cell carcinoma. A firm mass of the upper lid with marked lash loss and destruction of the normal lid margin. Incisional biopsy showed squamous cell carcinoma, which was subsequently excised with clear frozen-section margins.

higher than for basal cell carcinoma. Squamous cell carcinoma must be included in the differential diagnosis of any form of nontender lid lesion.

Management. Incisional biopsy of any suspicious or recurrent lesion is diagnostic. After the diagnosis is made, wide, full-thickness excision with surgical margin control is recommended. Close follow-up is mandatory because of the risk for deep or orbital invasion and metastasis. Orbital exenteration may be required if orbital extension or deep perineural involvement is confirmed.

Sebaceous Cell Carcinoma

This highly malignant tumor may arise from any of the sebaceous components of the lid, including the meibomian glands and the glands of Zeis of the lashes, brow, and caruncle. Although it is an uncommon tumor, it is certainly not rare, accounting for more than 3% of eyelid malignancies. Some reports show it to be the second most common skin cancer of the lid. Like most epithelial tumors, it occurs primarily in older adults, but can also occur in younger patients, especially those who have received prior orbital radiotherapy. *Sebaceous carcinomas* of the ocular adnexa are more common and more aggressive than those arising elsewhere on the body. The mass may be subcutaneous and therefore be confused with chalazion, although sebaceous cell carcinoma tends to be firmer, yellow, and involves the lid margin more frequently than the tarsal surface, leading to lash loss (Fig. 10.60). The tumor often spreads superficially along the epithelium (i.e., pagetoid spread), with crusting, ulceration, and the appearance of chronic, unilateral blepharoconjunctivitis that is unresponsive to medical therapy (i.e., masquerade syndrome). The tumor is very often multicentric, with skip areas that may involve other areas of the lid, the conjunctiva, or the cornea before the tumor becomes clinically evident. These characteristics often lead to unfortunate delays in diagnosis and treatment.

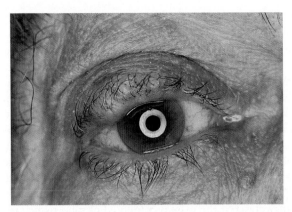

FIGURE 10.60. Sebaceous cell carcinoma. A large, firm, painless mass of the right upper lid. Although this lesion does not show the loss of lashes associated with carcinoma, the mass is still suspected of being malignant. As an irregular mass of the lid border with suggestions of a firm, nodular mass or as a diffusely indurated and thickened lid, the tumor typically grows slowly, with a minimal amount of epithelial involvement, but it may invade deep tissues and orbital structures early, requiring aggressive surgical excision.

Although the long-term survival rate has dramatically increased, the overall mortality rate of the disease still approaches 20%, with local recurrences common and lymphatic metastasis occurring in roughly 25% of patients. The lung and liver are often involved.

Management. The effective treatment of sebaceous cell carcinoma rests with early detection and wide excision, coupled with close follow-up for local, regional, and distant metastasis. A high index of suspicion is needed when evaluating a solid mass in the elderly, because a delay of even 6 months may prove fatal. Chalazia that recur after excision, any solid tissue tumor, or a mass that is in any way atypical, particularly if associated with lash loss, should be biopsied for examination. Wide excision with frozen-section control is required for the primary lesion. However, because of multicentric growth, negative frozen section margins are not definitive. Consequently, map biopsies should also be submitted from other areas of the lids, conjunctiva, and possibly the globe. Orbital exenteration may be required in cases of orbital or diffuse eyelid involvement. Regional lymph nodes should be palpated before surgery, and if enlarged, should be biopsied as well. The role of sentinel lymph node dissection in this tumor is not yet clear. Patients must be followed closely for the development of lymphatic metastases. Adjunctive radiotherapy may be of some benefit for diffuse disease.

Malignant Melanoma, Eccrine Sweat Gland Carcinoma, and Merkel Cell Carcinoma

Like *malignant melanoma* elsewhere, lesions arising on the lids are rare but potentially lethal, with a great tendency for widespread hematogenous and lymphatic spread. Although

the tumor accounts for less than 1% of all skin tumors, it is responsible for more than 60% of all skin cancer deaths. The incidence of melanoma has increased dramatically over the last 2 decades. There may be a hereditary component. The tumor tends to arise in older individuals, is more common in the fair-skinned and less common in the darker-pigmented population, and may arise from preexisting nevi that have undergone malignant change. Although solar exposure is thought to increase the risk of melanoma, absence of actinic history is not protective against the tumor, particularly the superficial, spreading variety. Most melanomas appear as flat pigmented lesions of various colors, but they may be nodular and melanotic (Fig. 10.61). Prognosis is correlated to depth of invasion. Because of the thin skin of the lids, conventional staging schemes such as the Clark and Breslow systems are not accurate predictors of prognosis. Patients having one lesion are at risk of developing other lesions and require lifetime follow-up.

Several malignant tumors arise in the deeper subcutaneous tissues of the lid, without the epithelial surface changes that are characteristic of the more common skin cancers. Typical of these tumors, the uncommon incidence is inversely related to their ease of diagnosis and malignant potential. Benign tumors of eccrine sweat glands of the lids are rather common, including syringoma, hidrocystoma, spiradenoma, acrospiroma, and chondroid syringoma. *Eccrine sweat gland carcinoma* is unusual but often very highly malignant, with a potential for local recurrence, deep invasion, and regional or distant lymphatic and visceral metastasis. The tumor typically arises predominantly in middle-aged to elderly men as a discrete, firm, nodular mass or as a diffusely indurated and thickened lid (Fig. 10.62). The tumor typically grows slowly, with a minimal amount of epithelial involvement, but it may invade deep tissues and

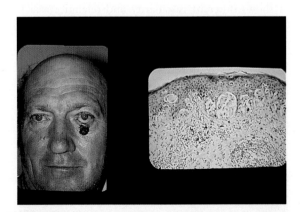

FIGURE 10.61. Malignant melanoma. This darkly pigmented lobular lesion with irregular borders was diagnosed on biopsy to be a malignant melanoma. Two thirds of the lower lid was resected and reconstruction was accomplished with a two-stage Hughes procedure including a full-thickness skin graft. Low magnification photomicrograph *(right)* showing junctional nests of tumor cells with extension into the dermis (hematoxylin and eosin ×10).

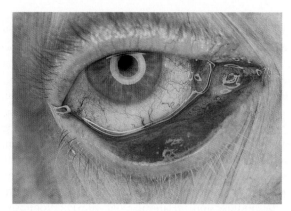

FIGURE 10.62. Eccrine sweat gland carcinoma. The patient was referred for evaluation of mechanical ectropion secondary to possible basal cell carcinoma. Inspection revealed the epithelium to be normal. However, a large, firm mass was palpable subcutaneously. It did not respect the tarsus and had deep extensions medially in the area of the medial canthus. Biopsy revealed sweat gland carcinoma, requiring eventual orbital exenteration.

orbital structures early, requiring aggressive surgical excision.

Merkel cells are neuroepithelial cells in the deep dermis that contribute to sensation. Their potential for malignant transformation is low, but when malignancy occurs, the tumor is exceptionally aggressive, with a capacity for lymphatic spread to regional and distant sites, particularly the liver and spleen. The tumor is potentially highly lethal, just as malignant melanoma. It is most common in older adults, and although an actinic history may be found, it is not a well established risk factor. Because of the rarity of the tumor, delay in diagnosis is common. As a rapidly growing, violaceous, painless mass, it is most commonly mistaken for chalazion. Unlike many other skin malignancies, alopecia is not a common finding. The mass is firm but not nontender and often shows inherent vascularity and telangiectasia (Fig. 10.63). Without a biopsy, the diagnosis is invariably missed,

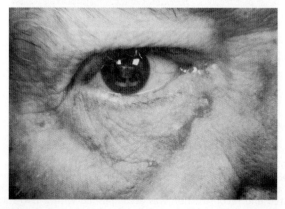

FIGURE 10.63. Merkel cell carcinoma. The lesion was initially treated as a chalazion. Subsequently, biopsy disclosed a Merkel cell carcinoma. This is an aggressive tumor with a high rate of metastasis.

but even histologic analysis presents difficulty, because it is commonly confused with other small cell tumors such as lymphoma and metastatic oat cell lung cancer. Special neuroendocrine stains are needed for accurate diagnosis.

Management. Because of the very highly malignant and lethal potential, a high index of suspicion is necessary when evaluating pigmented or subcutaneous tumors. Pigmented tumors arising from longstanding skin lesions, particularly those demonstrating any change in color, size, or shape, should be considered for biopsy. Any subcutaneous mass, whether typical for chalazion or not, should also be regarded suspiciously, particularly if the lid shows any evidence of telangiectasia, if the mass is composed of solid tissue rather than typical lipogranulomatous material on biopsy, or if the mass recurs after initial excision. Aggressive, early treatment by wide resection is recommended. Unfortunately, because of the aggressive nature of these tumors, frozen section control is not definitive, though it is still recommended. The role of sentinel node dissection and biopsy in these tumors is being investigated, and may play a part in advancing survival. Adjunctive radiotherapy may be of benefit, and lifetime follow-up is required. The prognosis is guarded, both for the eye and for life.

Other Malignant Tumors of the Skin

Several malignancies are commonly found in the lid. These tumors tend to affect the deeper tissues of the lids rather than the epithelium and clinically appear as subcutaneous or deep nodules with variable mobility. Most masses are well circumscribed and painless, and they arise over the course of weeks to months, with gradual enlargement. They are often misdiagnosed as chalazion or epidermal inclusion cysts before biopsy.

Although *metastases* are more common to the orbit than the lid, the adnexal tissues can also be affected. The most common primary sites are breast, lung, colon, and prostate, although many other primary tumors have been known to metastasize. Although most patients have a known history of primary cancer, a lid mass may be the presenting symptom.

Hemangiopericytoma is a potentially malignant tumor that more commonly affects the orbit than the lid. It arises primarily in adults in the fourth and fifth decades, but it has been known to occur in younger and older patients. The tumor is most often benign, but it has a well-known potential for local recurrence, malignant transformation, widespread metastasis, and death.

Fibrous histiocytoma can arise anywhere on the body. In the ocular adnexa, it is most commonly found in the orbit, but it may arise within the lid tissues as well. The tumor's behavior in either site is similar; it varies from frankly benign, to locally aggressive, to frankly malignant. The tumor arises as a well-circumscribed, painless mass and may be confused with several neural tumors, including heman-

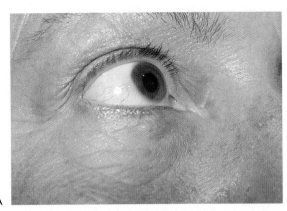
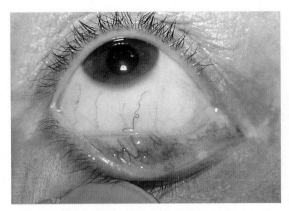

FIGURE 10.64. Chalazion. **A:** Painless mass of the tarsus, unresponsive to warm compresses. **B:** A conjunctival component is visible on lid eversion.

giopericytoma, neurilemmoma, and fibrosarcoma. The tumor may recur locally, usually as a result of incomplete excision, but it can metastasize with lethal results. Local extension of aggressive tumors is common.

Management. Because of the potential for oversight and misdiagnosis, any discrete lid mass unresponsive to conventional, conservative measures should be considered for excisional biopsy. Simple incision and curettage should be used cautiously, opting instead for pathologic examination of any suspicious lesion. Before excisional biopsy, a photograph or drawing of the lesion should be made to facilitate relocation of the mass if further excision is required. Masses should be excised completely, with adequate surrounding tissue removed to ensure clear margins.

INFLAMMATIONS

Blepharitis, Chalazion, Hordeolum, and Molluscum Contagiosum

Blepharitis is a nonspecific inflammation of the eyelids, generally involving the lid margin and typically arising sec-

ondary to staphylococcal colonization. Seborrhea, acne rosacea, and *Demodex folliculorum* infection are additional etiologic agents. The classic findings include redness of the lid margin, collarette formation, scurf accumulation, irregularity of the lid margin, and inspissation of the meibomian gland orifices. *Chalazion* occurs if the meibomian gland duct is obstructed, with subsequent extrusion of the lipid into the adjacent soft tissues, stimulating lipogranulomatous inflammation and fibrosis (Fig. 10.64A). The lesion is localized to the tarsus and often is tender initially but resolves to become nontender. A conjunctival component is typically evident on lid eversion (Fig. 10.64B). Incision and drainage of the lesion produces a characteristic yellow gelatinous material (lipogranuloma) surrounded by dense fibrous tissue (Fig. 10.65). *Hordeolum* is an acute infection of any gland of the lid, e.g., meibomian, Zeis, or Moll (Fig. 10.66). "Styes" are painful, tender masses that arise abruptly and that may incite a surrounding cellulitis. Incision and drainage produces a purulent discharge. *Molluscum contagiosum* characteristically produces painless, pearly nodules with central umbilications (Fig. 10.67). An accompanying follicular conjunctivitis attests to the viral etiology.

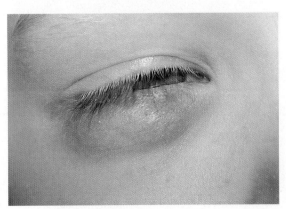
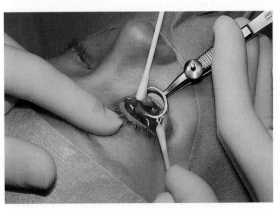

FIGURE 10.65. Chalazion. **A:** Large, painless mass that grew slowly over 4 months affected the entire lower lid of this 7-year-old boy. **B:** Incision and drainage revealed a lipogranulomatous material characteristic of chalazion.

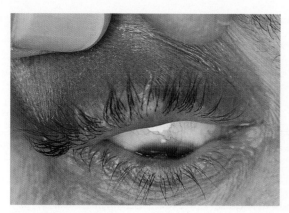

FIGURE 10.66. Hordeolum. A tender mass of the right upper lid is seen with surrounding cellulitis. A chalazion of the central lower lid is also present.

Management. Because of the ubiquity of staphylococcal lid disease and the commonplace nature of blepharitis, typical chalazion and hordeolum pose little diagnostic or therapeutic challenge. However, clinicians should be suspicious of atypical characteristics that would warrant further evaluation. Asymmetry of blepharitis involvement or unilateral "conjunctivitis"—especially if unresponsive to routine therapeutic measures—should call to mind alternative diagnoses such as a masquerading condition like sebaceous cell or Merkel cell tumor, particularly if there is lid thickening, induration, and lash loss. Atypical locations of chalazia and hordeola, such as the base of the tarsus or exclusively at the lash margin—especially if there is no identifiable internal component—may prompt the clinician to send any incision and drainage specimens for biopsy, particularly if the chalazion has recurred after prior excision or if the characteristic lipogranulomatous debris is not expressed. Rare tumors with grave prognoses, such as sebaceous cell and Merkel cell carcinomas, are often initially misdiagnosed as chalazion.

Vitiligo, Poliosis, Madarosis, and Trichotillomania

Vitiligo is characterized by progressive, patchy loss of skin pigmentation. It is uncommon but can be associated with other autoimmune disorders, such as alopecia areata, thyroid dysfunction, Vogt-Koyanagi-Harada syndrome, and sympathetic ophthalmia. It has also occurred secondary to the use of topical medications, steroid injections, and as postinflammatory or posttraumatic sequela. *Poliosis* (progressive whitening of the lashes) and *madarosis* (loss of lashes) occur with regularity in patients with alopecia areata and dysthyroidism (Fig. 10.68A,B). Madarosis in the face of a lid mass should provoke a search for malignancy, such as squamous cell, sebaceous cell, or Merkel cell carcinoma. However, not all malignancies will cause lash loss.

Trichotillomania is the act of intentionally pulling out one's lashes. It may be the result of nervous tic, habit, or excess anxiety (Fig. 10.68C). When asked, most patients will admit to voluntarily pulling their lashes.

Management. Because of the strong association with other autoimmune disorders, patients with poliosis, madarosis, or vitiligo should undergo thorough ocular and medical evaluation, including thyroid function testing. Referral to specialists in retina-vitreous-uveitis, rheumatology, and dermatology may be appropriate. Alopecia areata is often treated with intralesional corticosteroid. However, involvement of the brows and eyelashes portend poor long-term prognosis for hair regrowth. Systemic steroids are rarely used.

Sarcoidosis

Sarcoidosis is a multisystem granulomatous disorder predominantly affecting young adults. Ocular involvement can be found in as many as 40% of persons of African descent and 20% of Caucasians with the condition. The most common

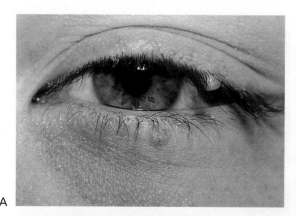
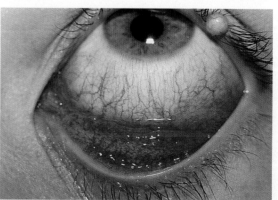

FIGURE 10.67. Molluscum contagiosum. **A:** A 13-year-old boy was referred for evaluation of lid masses of the left eye. Central umbilication of these pearly nodules is characteristic of molluscum contagiosum. **B:** Examination also revealed unilateral follicular conjunctivitis.

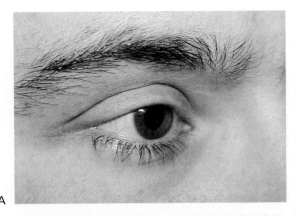

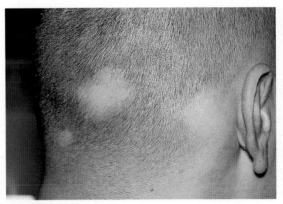

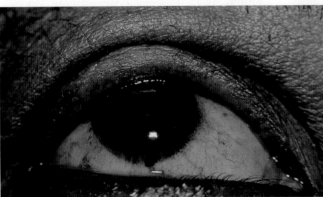

FIGURE 10.68. Madarosis, poliosis, alopecia areata, and trichotillomania. **A:** The patient complained of a loss of lashes from the right upper lid over 2 years. There was no history of intraocular inflammation. There was a loss of approximately 50% of lashes from the lid, with poliosis of the remaining lashes. **B:** The patient's scalp shows areas of patchy alopecia and whitening of the remaining hair. The patient had previously undergone treatments for alopecia areata with intralesional corticosteroid injections without success. Metabolic evaluation revealed undiagnosed primary hypothyroidism. **C:** This patient was asymptomatic, and admitted to intentionally plucking her eyelashes.

ocular finding is granulomatous anterior uveitis. Various skin and lid lesions can be found in approximately 30% of patients with chronic disease. Erythema nodosum, "millet seed" subcutaneous nodules, and confluent violaceous nodules of the midface (lupus pernio) are all seen. The most common skin findings are slightly raised, granulomatous plaques and nodules that are brown to yellow (Fig. 10.69).

Most patients with sarcoidosis present with intraocular

or other orbital findings, such as a lacrimal gland mass. Occasionally, superficial manifestations may be the presenting problem. Ocular evaluation should include examination of the lids, lacrimal glands, and salivary glands. If the diagnosis has not been confirmed, biopsy of a superficial lesion can be performed quickly. Patients with known histories of sarcoidosis should be biopsied to rule out other processes and malignancies.

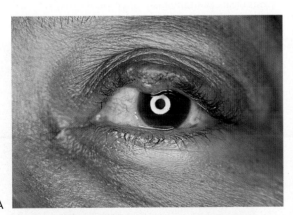

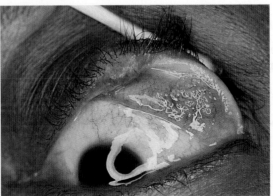

FIGURE 10.69. Sarcoid granuloma. **A:** A patient with known pulmonary sarcoid noticed irregular lid masses of both eyes that enlarged over 2 years. **B:** Eversion shows large, yellow granulomas of the tarsal conjunctiva. There were similar lesions on the right eye. The patient had no other ocular or orbital findings, except dry eyes.

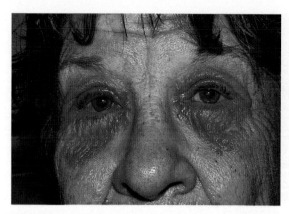

FIGURE 10.70. Allergic dermatitis. The patient had acute onset of redness, swelling, and itching of all lids. The patient had been using neomycin ophthalmic ointment. After discontinuing the ointment, she was treated with cool compresses and a mild topical steroid ointment, producing prompt resolution of her symptoms.

Allergic and Atopic Dermatitis

A variety of agents can incite *allergic dermatitis* of the eyelids. Seasonal allergens and pollens, fumes, cosmetics, and medications can trigger allergic and toxic reactions. The condition is characterized by marked edema, erythema, intense itching, and excoriation of the lids (Fig. 10.70). The remainder of the skin, face, and hands may be unaffected. *Atopic dermatitis* also manifests with pruritus, swelling, and erythema, but the onset is earlier in childhood, and there is generally a family history of other atopic conditions such as hay fever, asthma, or atopic dermatitis. With repeated insults and chronic inflammation, the skin becomes thickened and excoriated, causing induration of all layers of the skin. Cicatricial changes can lead to lid retraction and ectropion.

Management. Avoidance and discontinuation of known aggravating factors is key in the management of both conditions. Antihistamines may help seasonal factors. Topical steroids may help control the inflammatory component. Surgery may be needed if cicatricial changes occur.

LACRIMAL DRAINAGE DYSFUNCTION

Congenital Dacryostenosis, Dacryocystocele, and Dacryocystitis

Although as many as 73% of term stillborn fetuses have been shown to have lacrimal obstruction, only 6% of children have symptomatic *congenital dacryostenosis*. The obstruction most commonly occurs at the distal end of the tear duct, in the area of the valve of Hasner, but can occur anywhere along the lacrimal drainage system. Symptoms include epiphora and chronic crusting and mattering of the eyelids (Fig. 10.71). Pressure over the nasolacrimal sac may produce reflux of mucopurulent matter. The incidence of dacryostenosis is significantly higher in the presence of craniofacial abnormalities such as cleft lip and palate, and the

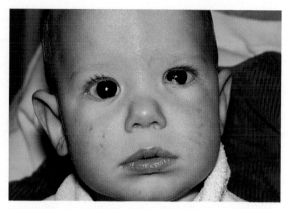

FIGURE 10.71. Congenital dacryostenosis. The child's parents complained of epiphora of both eyes since the child's birth. The right eye cleared spontaneously, but the left eye continued to tear, with morning crusting and heavy mattering.

clefting and synostotic syndromes. *Congenital dacryocystocele* presents at birth or shortly thereafter as a nontender, soft, bluish mass below the medial canthal tendon (Fig. 10.72). In addition to distal obstruction, proximal obstruction in the area of the common internal punctum prevents outward reflux and decompression, and pressure over the sac is therefore nonproductive. When aspirated or expressed, the contents are generally thick and mucoid, but they may be xanthochromic and viscous. The contents are most often sterile, but if bacteria are sequestered, the condition can develop into frank dacryocystitis. *Infantile dacryocystitis* is uncommon, but signs and symptoms are similar to those in adults, with painful, tender swelling of the inferior medial canthal area and surrounding cellulitis (Fig. 10.73).

Management. Because epiphora and photophobia are often presenting symptoms of congenital glaucoma, patients should be completely examined to rule out this grave entity. After eliminating the possibility of glaucoma, the treatment of dacryostenosis includes warm compresses and antibiotic drops and ointments. Gentle downward massage over the nasolacrimal sac may be added. Most symptomatic obstructions clear spontaneously. If epiphora persists until the child

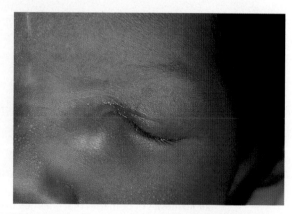

FIGURE 10.72. Congenital dacryocystocele. The painless, uninflamed bluish mass is located below the medial canthal tendon.

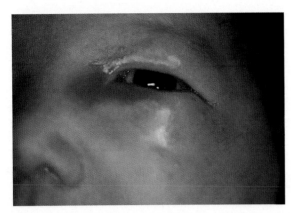

FIGURE 10.73. Infantile dacryocystitis is a painful, tender swelling of the inferior medial canthal area, with surrounding cellulitis. At birth, the child's parents had noticed a nontender, bluish mass in this area, which probably represents an underlying dacryocystocele that had become infected.

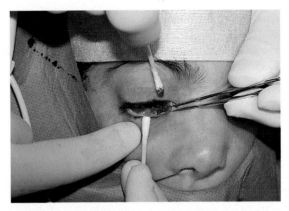

FIGURE 10.74. Punctal and canalicular atresia. A 3-year-old child with Nager's syndrome, a variation of Treacher Collins syndrome, presented with tearing of the right eye since birth. Examination with the patient under anesthesia revealed an absence of upper and lower puncta in the right eye. Cut-down of the lower lid revealed complete absence of the canaliculus. The nasolacrimal sac and duct were also found to be poorly developed.

is 9 to 12 months of age, probing and irrigation are recommended. Some clinicians advocate early probing in the office, using light sedation. Additional measures include medialization of the inferior nasal turbinate, balloon catheter dilation of the duct, and silicone intubation under general anesthesia.

Spontaneous resolution of dacryocystocele is uncommon. Early treatment with probing, irrigation, and decompression is recommended. Percutaneous aspiration provides temporary relief but does nothing to correct the causal obstructions. Dacryocystitis should be treated aggressively with topical and systemic antibiotics, with particular attention given to adequate coverage of *Haemophilus influenzae*. Hospitalization is usually required. Incision and drainage are sometimes necessary. After the infection is controlled, probing and irrigation should be performed promptly. Occasionally, dacryocystorhinostomy may be required for recurrent or anomalous cases.

Supernumerary Puncta, Lacrimal System Atresia, and Lacrimal Fistula

Congenital anomalies of the lacrimal system are uncommon. *Supernumerary puncta* are multiple openings into a single canaliculus. However, not all puncta are always patent. The punctal promontory may be poorly developed or atretic or may be occluded by imperforate membranes. Although imperforate puncta generally overlie otherwise intact drainage systems, severe *punctal atresia* often indicates significant underlying pathology, such as *canalicular atresia* (Fig. 10.74). This represents a complete failure of the canalicular system to develop and may be associated with other significant lacrimal drainage anomalies. Complete atresia of the lacrimal sac and duct is rare and represents agenesis or malformation of the distal aspect of the lacrimal anlage. This condition can be an associated finding in malformations of the midface. *Congenital fistulae of the lacrimal*

sac are epithelial tracts that extend from the sac to the skin surface (Fig. 10.75). They may be unilateral or bilateral and may be completely patent or end as a blind sac. If the fistula is patent, tears or mucopurulent drainage can be found at the skin ostium, usually located just inferior and lateral to the inferior punctum.

Management. As with congenital dacryostenosis, epiphora is the most common presenting complaint. If a fistula is present, parents may complain of tears or discharge on the skin or along the nose. The lacrimal drainage system should be inspected thoroughly in the office to identify atretic or imperforate structures. Atretic or imperforate puncta can be opened easily with a simple incision, after which the canaliculus is probed and irrigated to ensure distal patency. Atretic canaliculi require canalicular reconstruc-

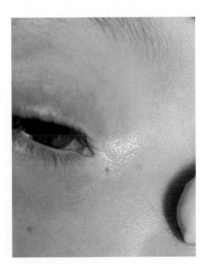

FIGURE 10.75. Congenital lacrimal fistula inferior to the medial canthus. There was a positive paternal family history of similar fistulas. The fistula did not connect to the sac and was excised completely.

tion or conjunctivodacryocystorhinostomy. Unlike acquired lacrimal fistulae, which heal spontaneously, congenital lacrimal fistulae must be excised and closed surgically.

Acquired Dacryostenosis

Obstruction of the tear drainage system can occur at any age. *Punctal* and *canalicular stenosis* can develop secondary to chronic irritation and inflammation, autoimmune disorders such as Stevens-Johnson syndrome or pemphigoid, viral infections, or trauma, and as a sequela of topical and systemic medications such as antivirals and antineoplastics (Fig. 10.76). *Canaliculitis,* an acute infection of the canaliculi, can be caused by a host of organisms, but *Actinomyces israelii* is the most common pathogen (Fig. 10.77). Canalicular stones and abscesses can form, requiring incision and curettage removal. *Acquired dacryostenosis* (i.e., obstruction of the lacrimal sac and nasolacrimal duct) occurs most commonly as an idiopathic entity, although biopsy specimens may show chronic inflammatory changes consistent with chronic, indolent, or subacute dacryocystitis. Fungal hyphae may also form dacryoliths, stones, and casts of the sac. Midfacial trauma and prior sinus surgery can cause secondary compression and scarring of the duct. Occult tumors of the sac or sinuses are rare but must always be considered. Patients with dacryostenosis complain of epiphora, often of sufficient magnitude to require keeping a tissue (Fig. 10.78). Chronic mattering, morning crusting, and mucopurulent discharge with chronic blepharoconjunctivitis can also occur. Evaluation may require diagnostic imaging.

Patients complaining of epiphora should be evaluated for reflex hypersecretion (e.g., keratitis sicca) and underlying lid position abnormalities (e.g., entropion, ectropion). Particular attention should be given to the medial canthal drainage structures. Punctal stenosis may be treated with one- or two-snip punctoplasty. If associated with canalicu-

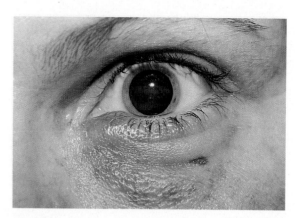

FIGURE 10.77. Canaliculitis. A 32-year-old woman had an acute onset of painful swelling of the inner canthal region. Inspection revealed painful induration and erythema of the punctum and canaliculus.

lar stenosis secondary to chronic inflammation or medications, canalicular reconstruction may be necessary, including management with warm compresses and topical antibiotics. Occasionally, canaliculotomy must be performed to remove stones or drain abscesses. Dacryostenosis is most commonly diagnosed by office probing and irrigation (Fig. 10.79A). The cannula should not be advanced beyond the lacrimal sac, because this area is difficult to anesthetize adequately. The area of the lacrimal sac should be palpated for masses. Imaging may be useful in cases of trauma or if underlying stones or tumors are suspected (Fig. 10.79B,C). Dacryocystorhinostomy can successfully treat acquired dacryostenosis.

Dacryocystitis

Acute dacryocystitis can occur at any age. However, it is more common as an acquired condition among middle-aged or older adults. A variety of conditions can lead to dacryostenosis, which predisposes to stagnation of tears and bacterial overgrowth, which can then fulminate into an acute infection. Midfacial trauma, sinus surgery, oral-maxillofacial surgery, dacryoliths, tumors, and chronic indolent dacryocystitis have been associated with acute dacryocystitis. Often, no underlying condition is identified. The patients typically have a history of epiphora or chronic blepharoconjunctivitis, with mucopurulent discharge and crusting (Fig. 10.80). A history of bloody tears or a mass above the medial canthus should heighten suspicion of a lacrimal sac tumor. Patients present with acute onset of a painful mass in the medial canthal area, which is swollen, tender, erythematous, and warm to the touch, with a surrounding cellulitis. Often, an abscess is located medially below the medial canthal tendon. With spontaneous drainage, a fistula may form to the sac (Fig. 10.81).

Management. Acute dacryocystitis requires aggressive treatment with intravenous and oral antibiotics. Abscesses, if not draining spontaneously, must be incised and drained.

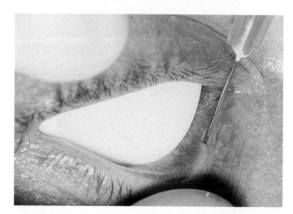

FIGURE 10.76. Punctal stenosis. An adult patient previously treated with 5-fluorouracil developed epiphora secondary to punctal and canalicular stenosis. The punctum had completely closed and was reopened with an incision.

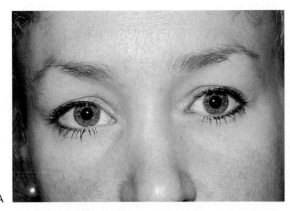
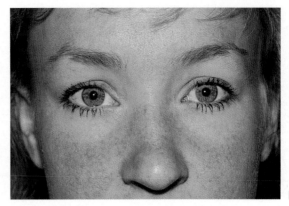

FIGURE 10.78. Acquired dacryostenosis. **A:** A 24-year-old patient presented with constant epiphora of the left eye which caused her to keep tissues on hand. The fluorescein dye disappearance test is markedly delayed. Irrigation revealed 100% obstruction of the nasolacrimal duct. **B:** Six months after dacryocystorhinostomy with silicone intubation, the patient is asymptomatic and has a normal result with the dye disappearance test.

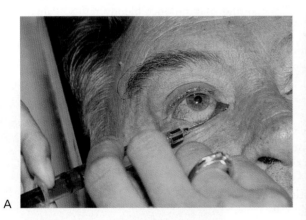

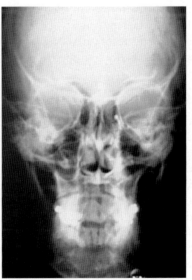

FIGURE 10.79. Diagnosis of dacryostenosis. **A:** Reflux on irrigation of the lacrimal system can indicate significant obstruction. Bloody reflux is highly suggestive of tumor. Palpation of the nasolacrimal sac can disclose tumor masses. **B:** Irrigation with contrast dye can disclose physical obstructions and irregularities of the lumen. In this plain film dacryocystography (DCG), a dacryolith is visible as an irregular outline in the left nasolacrimal system. DCG can also be performed with a computed tomography scan. **C:** With dacryoscintigraphy, the instillation of a radioisotope (technetium 99) can be useful in evaluating tear flow physiology and demonstrating occlusions. This scan reveals distal obstruction of the right duct.

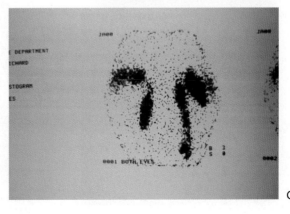

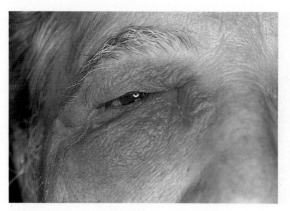

FIGURE 10.80. Acute dacryocystitis is evidenced by a large, tender, swollen, fluctuant erythematous mass arising in the medial canthal area.

Although most clinically significant dacryostenosis can be diagnosed on the basis of clinical history and simple irrigation, a computed tomography (CT) scan is often performed to identify tumors, bony erosion and landmarks, or stones. Irrigation should not be performed in the setting of acute dacryocystitis. Definitive therapy consists of dacryocystorhinostomy. Submission of tissue for pathologic examination is highly recommended to look for unsuspected pathology.

Lacrimal Sac Tumors

Tumors of the lacrimal sac are rare. Approximately 25% are inflammatory lesions, including granulomatous disease. The remainder are true neoplasms, most of which are malignancies of epithelial origin (e.g., squamous cell). Nonepithelial tumors (e.g., lymphoma, fibrous histiocytoma) have been described as well (Fig. 10.82). The clinical presentation varies, but the presence of bloody tears or a painless, noncompressible mass above the medial canthus is highly suspicious for tumor. Although benign lesions may have slower growth, with longer symptoms of epiphora or

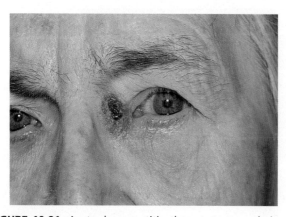

FIGURE 10.81. Acute dacryocystitis, the spontaneous drainage of a sac abscess, may lead to fistula formation. Unlike congenital fistulas of the sac, acquired fistulas generally close spontaneously.

recurrent dacryocystitis than malignancies, such histories do not rule out malignancies. A history of pain, rapid growth, and bloody discharge suggests a tumor. A history of chronic sinusitis, sinus surgery, or midfacial trauma may indicate mucocele formation.

Palpation generally reveals a firm, irreducible mass in the area of the medial canthus. Irrigation may not be obstructed (Fig. 10.83). The CT scan may show a mass in the area of the lacrimal sac, bony erosion, local extension into the orbit, or diffuse infiltration, depending on the nature of the tumor. Many epithelial tumors (e.g., squamous, inverted squamous, transitional papillomas) may arise primarily or concurrently in the sinuses. Such tumors may be prone to recurrence. Tumors may extend into and protrude through the canaliculi (Fig. 10.84).

Management. Patients complaining of epiphora should be questioned closely about a history of bloody tears and prior sinus surgery or disease, as well as of systemic diseases such as Wegener's granulomatosis, sarcoid, and lymphoma. Office irrigation may reveal partial or complete obstruction and may produce bloody reflux. Palpation of the medial canthus may disclose a firm, irreducible mass. Inspection and palpation of regional lymph nodes are recommended. If

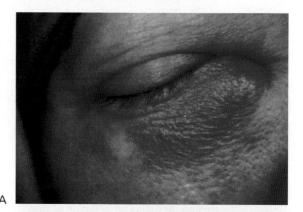

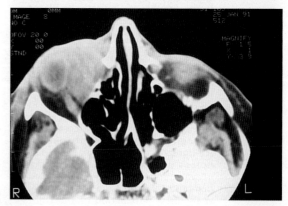

FIGURE 10.82. Lymphoma. **A:** The patient presented with acute dacryocystitis and a 4-month history of tearing. **B:** Computed tomography shows a diffuse, infiltrative mass conforming to the orbital walls without bony erosion. The globe is markedly indented. The area of the sac is also infiltrated. Biopsy confirmed the clinical suspicion of orbital lymphoma.

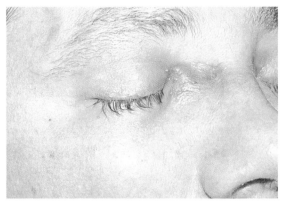

FIGURE 10.83. A firm mass above the medial canthus was of recent onset. Computed tomography showed underlying bony erosion and a mass in the area. Biopsy revealed squamous cell carcinoma.

there is a strong suspicion of tumor or stone, radiologic imaging is recommended. CT is preferred to evaluate bony integrity. Dacryocystography can be performed concurrently. Surgical management depends on the history and CT findings and can include incisional biopsy, excisional biopsy, dacryocystectomy, or wide excision. Extensive

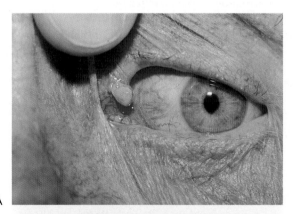

A

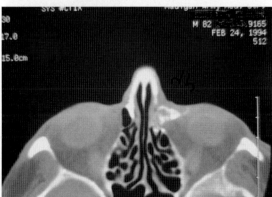

B

FIGURE 10.84. Squamous papilloma. **A:** The patient presented with epiphora of a 5-year duration and a papillomatous growth from the upper canaliculus. Biopsy revealed squamous papilloma. **B:** Computed tomography dacryocystogram shows involvement in the sac *(arrow)*.

surgery should be based on pathology. Combined procedures with an ear, nose, and throat surgeon may be necessary. Because of the small possibility of occult tumors of the sac, some surgeons routinely send biopsy specimens from routine dacryocystorhinostomies for histologic evaluation.

OCULOPLASTIC TRAUMA

Eyelid Trauma

Blunt Trauma

Blunt trauma or contusion to the eyelids is a nonpenetrating injury by an external force that does not break or lacerate the epidermis or dermis (Fig. 10.85).

Management. Patients deserve careful history taking and an examination, including slit lamp and dilated ophthalmoscopy, to rule out associated intraocular involvement. Care should be taken to ensure that the globe has not been ruptured. Plain radiographs and CT scans are often necessary to rule out orbital fractures. Ten-minute ice compresses every 2 hours can reduce posttraumatic edema if applied within the first 2 days of injury.

Penetrating Trauma

Lacerations Not Involving the Lid Margin
These lacerations penetrate the skin and deeper structures but do not involve the eyelid margin (Fig 10.86). They can be caused by blunt or sharp objects, including human fingernails or animal paws.

Management. A complete history and physical examination should be performed to rule out intraocular involvement. Surgical repair is performed, using an anatomic ap-

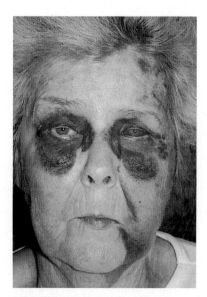

FIGURE 10.85. Ecchymosis and edema are the most common presenting signs of blunt trauma.

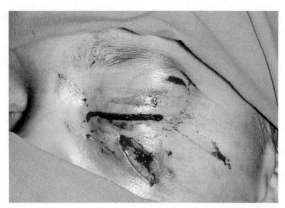

FIGURE 10.86. This 3-year-old boy was hit on the left side of his face by a dog's paw. The superficial lacerations were debrided, irrigated, and examined for foreign bodies. They were then closed in an anatomic fashion using 6-0 plain gut sutures.

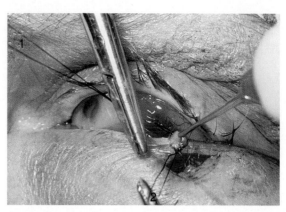

FIGURE 10.88. The tarsal suture *(suture no. 1)* and lash line *(suture no. 2)* have been placed. *Suture no. 3* is being placed through the gray line. These three sutures together were then incorporated in the superior-most skin suture to prevent corneal irritation.

proach to correct any associated levator muscle involvement. Imbedded foreign bodies should be removed, and necrotic tissue should be debrided. The use of 6-0 absorbable or nonabsorbable sutures, eversion of the wound edges, and early suture removal can reduce posttraumatic scarring.

Lacerations Involving the Lid Margin
Full-thickness lacerations extend through the eyelid margin and may be regular or irregular (Fig. 10.87).

Management. The eyelid margin is closed using a three-suture technique. Suture no. 1 is placed through the tarsus of one wound edge and then through the tarsus of the other wound edge, avoiding the palpebral conjunctiva. The suture is secured and cut long. Suture no. 2 is passed in the eyelash line through both wound edges. It is secured and left long. With the eyelid held on stretch by pulling on the first two sutures, suture no. 3 (Fig. 10.88) is then passed through the gray line of one wound edge and then through the gray line of the other wound edge. This suture is then secured and cut

long. Associated lacerations of the eyelid are then closed in a layered fashion. The tarsus is closed with 5-0 chromic or Vicryl sutures without passing through the conjunctiva. The skin and orbicularis are then closed with a 6-0 silk or nylon suture. The long ends of the three eyelid margin sutures are incorporated in the superior-most skin suture to prevent corneal irritation by the margin sutures.

Lacerations Involving the Medial Canthal Tendon
The superficial heads of the pretarsal orbicularis oculi muscle unite to form the medial canthal tendon. Often, transmarginal lacerations that involve the canaliculus also sever the superficial head of the medial canthal tendon.

Management. Lacerations in the medial canthal angle (Fig. 10.89) demand evaluation of the upper and lower

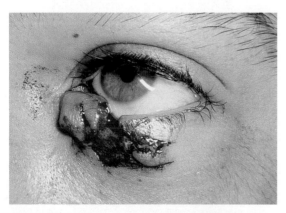

FIGURE 10.87. This 11-year-old boy fell on a shelf bracket, suffering an irregular, full-thickness lid laceration. The eye was not involved.

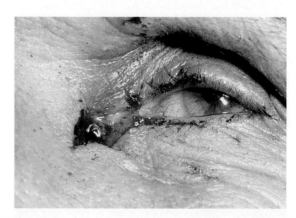

FIGURE 10.89. This 59-year-old man was hit in the left medial canthus with a meat hook. The skin, orbicularis oculi muscle, and anterior head of the inferior horn of the medial canthal tendon were severed. The canalicular system was intact. The inferior horn of the medial canthal tendon was reattached to its stump at the periosteum using 5-0 chromic sutures. The overlying orbicularis oculi muscle was closed with 5-0 chromic sutures. The skin was closed with 6-0 silk sutures.

canaliculus, the nasolacrimal sac and duct, and the medial canthal tendon. Involvement is usually confirmed by inspection. The integrity of the inferior and superior limbs of the medial canthal tendon can be assessed by grasping each lid with forceps or fingers and tugging the lid laterally. Disinsertion can be palpated with the finger from the other hand or can be visualized by temporal displacement of the punctum beyond the nasal limbus.

Treatment of medial canthal tendon evulsion depends on the nature of the evulsion. If the upper and lower anterior limbs are evulsed but the posterior attachment of the tendon is intact, the evulsed limbs may be sutured to its stump or to the periosteum overlying the anterior lacrimal crest with 5-0 chromic cat gut. The overlying skin is closed with interrupted 6-0 silk or nylon sutures. If the posterior limb of the medial canthal tendon is evulsed, then transnasal wiring may be necessary.

Lacerations of the Lateral Canthal Tendon

Isolated lacerations of the lateral canthal tendon are relatively rare and less complicated than those involving the medial canthal tendon. Although the medial canthal angle is slightly rounded, the lateral canthal angle is sharp. Recognizing this difference helps to achieve good postoperative cosmetic and functional results.

Management. The integrity of the inferior and superior limbs of the lateral canthal tendon can be assessed by grasping each lid and pulling it medially (Fig. 10.90). Disinsertion of the tendon can be seen by an almond-shaped deformity or "rounding" of the lateral canthal angle. The cut end of the lateral canthal tendon should be reattached to the lateral canthal tendon stump in the area of the lateral orbital tubercle. This is performed with 5-0 double-arm absorbable or nonabsorbable sutures. The lid margin is then closed using the three-suture technique previously described.

Burns

Patients who sustain burns of the eyelid are often critically ill or injured. Injury may be in the form of thermal (Fig. 10.91), chemical, or radiation burns. Protection of the eyeball to avoid corneal exposure, ulceration, and infection must be of primary consideration. Burns are caused by the application of heat to the body through direct contact or indirectly by radiant heat. The resultant burns vary only in degree, depending on the intensity and duration of application. Burns are classified as first, second, and third degree.

First-degree burns are characterized by erythema of the skin and only microscopic destruction of superficial layers of the epidermis. This is typical of a mild sunburn or when the head of a match strikes the eyelid skin.

Second-degree burns demonstrate greater tissue destruction in the epidermis and superficial layers of the adjacent dermis. Because regeneration occurs from remaining epithelial elements, second-degree burns are described as partial-thickness burns. These burns can be caused by boiling water or direct contact with a hot piece of metal or flame. This results in an erythematous, weeping, painful lesion associated with blisters and bullae. Superficial layers of the skin can be readily wiped away. The remaining skin appears waxy, white, and dry.

Third-degree burns are characterized by total, irreversible destruction of the epidermis and dermis. Because spontaneous regeneration of the epithelium is not possible, third-degree burns are known as full-thickness burns. Clinically, the skin appears dry, hard, and inelastic. These burns are caused by direct flame contact, by immersion in scalding water, or by direct chemical or electrical contact.

Thermal Burns

A common mild thermal burn is caused by the head of a match or cigarette ashes that strike the skin of the eyelids.

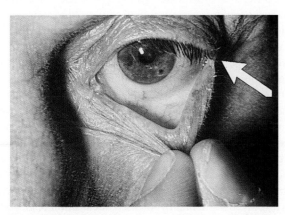

FIGURE 10.90. Disinsertion of the lateral canthal tendon is demonstrated by "rounding" of the lateral canthal angle as the lid is pulled medially. Medial canthal tendon laxity is also demonstrated by lateral displacement of the punctum tangent to the medial limbus.

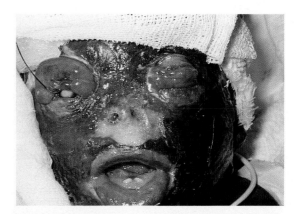

FIGURE 10.91. An 8-month-old boy, who was a victim of a domestic fire, received third-degree burns to his entire face, resulting in complete ectropion of both upper lids. Conservative treatment with moist chambers and lubrication was initiated while he was being stabilized medically. The patient died before definitive surgical repair could be initiated.

Although it is quickly cooled, it results in local destruction and coagulation of proteins, usually in the epidermis. The local pink or white discoloration usually resolves as the epidermis regenerates.

More severe thermal burns (Fig. 10.91) are caused by prolonged contact with a high temperature heat source or fire. In some situations, total destruction is the final result. However, some portion of the eye or eyelids is usually salvaged.

Management. Severe burns of the eyelid are treated conservatively by keeping the exposed area free from contamination. If destruction of the tissues is so extensive that the cornea is exposed, immediate steps are taken to protect the eye. These include lubricating drops, antibiotic drops and ointments, moist chambers, and temporary tarsorrhaphies. After cicatricial changes occur in the eyelids, there is often a rapid deterioration of the patient's ocular status. With the progression of cicatrization, more aggressive treatment may be necessary. Permanent tarsorrhaphies should be more extensive than seem necessary. In the past, skin grafting was usually delayed until cicatricial changes stabilized. However, the use of full-thickness skin grafts from the opposite eyelid or split-thickness skin grafts from a hairless portion of the extremities may be necessary early in the course to reduce ocular morbidity.

Late treatment of thermal burns involves excision of the cicatrix with the use of split- or full-thickness skin grafts. The recipient lid should be placed on stretch to increase the area to be grafted. The use of tissue expanders may also be helpful.

Chemical Burns

The severity of chemical burns of the eyelids is determined by the substance, its concentration, and the duration of contact. Acid burns (Fig. 10.92) are usually self-limited and not as destructive as alkali burns (Fig. 10.93). Clinical signs of

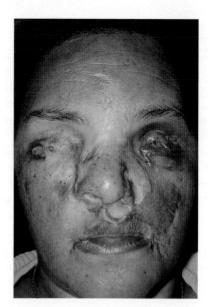

FIGURE 10.93. A 50-year-old woman had received lye burns to her face at 3 years of age. She lost function of both her eyes. Notice the residual ectropion of her left lower lid despite numerous skin grafts.

mild-to-moderate chemical burns include mild eyelid edema and hyperemia of the periocular skin. Ocular signs include corneal epithelial defects, focal areas of conjunctival chemosis, hyperemia, and a mild anterior chamber reaction. Evidence of more severe chemical burns includes pronounced chemosis, perilimbal blanching, corneal edema, moderate-to-severe anterior chamber reaction, increased intraocular pressure, and local necrotic retinopathy.

Management. An accurate history is necessary to determine the time of injury, the nature of the chemical, and the duration of exposure before irrigation. Emergent treatment includes copious irrigation of the eyelids, preferably with saline or Ringer's lactated solution for at least 30 minutes. If neither of these is available, nonsterile water should be used. The lower and upper fornices should be irrigated if possible. Manual use of intravenous tubing connected to an irrigation solution facilitates the irrigation process. Five minutes after ceasing irrigation, litmus paper should be touched to the inferior fornix. If the pH is not neutral (pH = 7), irrigation should be continued. After irrigation, the fornices should be further examined, and any sequestered particles of caustic material and necrotic conjunctiva should be removed. Similarly, the periocular skin should be cleaned. Sequestered particles should be removed and necrotic skin debrided. Silvadene cream or similar antibiotics can be applied to the skin. Therapy for uveitis (e.g., 0.25% scopolamine), along with mild topical antibiotic ointments (e.g., erythromycin) and oral hypotensive medication (e.g., acetazolamide) and oral pain medication are used as needed. Management of more severe ocular burns may require hospitalization for close monitoring of intraocular pressure and corneal healing. Lysis of early conjunctival adhesions using

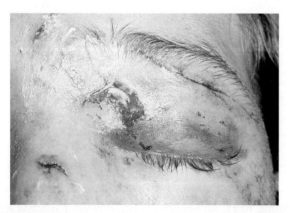

FIGURE 10.92. A 19-year-old car mechanic had a battery explode in his face. Mild hyperemia and edema of the eyelids are associated with areas of necrotic skin. Fortunately, the eye was not involved. The lids were irrigated, and necrotic tissue was debrided. He healed with minimal local scar formation.

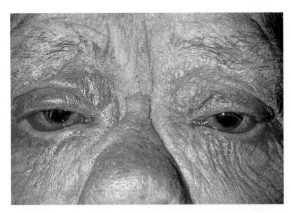

FIGURE 10.94. A 70-year-old man underwent 4 weeks of radiotherapy for a malignant ethmoid tumor. The point source of radiation was located over the bridge of his nose. Notice the local erythema, dry scaly skin, and bilateral lower lid ectropion.

a glass rod may be necessary. If symblepharon forms despite attempted lysis, the use of a scleral shell, therapeutic contact lens, or ring conformer may be necessary.

Late surgical treatment of chemical burns involves various procedures. A mucous membrane graft or conjunctival graft may be necessary to reconstruct the fornices and repair symblepharon. Full-thickness or split-thickness skin grafting may be necessary to correct eyelid ectropion resulting from loss of the anterior lamella of the eyelids.

Radiation Burns

Unlike thermal burns, the burns from an ionizing radiation source (Fig. 10.94) do not initially appear to be severe. If the lids are exposed to high does of radiation, erythema is the only early sign. Later, the skin may atrophy or undergo chronic ulceration. Massive doses cause areas of necrosis. Fortunately, the tarsus is resistant to this type of damage, but it may become distorted by superficial cicatrization. Corneal compromise or cataracts may develop months or years after irradiation. Basal cell carcinoma or squamous cell carcinoma may develop in areas of intense irradiation. This

presents an unfavorable situation for surgical revision and repair.

Management. Early management is similar to that of thermal burns with respect to protection of the eye. Mild radiation burns of the skin can be treated conservatively with mild antibiotic ointments, digital massage, and topical antibiotic ointments, if necessary. Delayed surgical treatment for ectropion and cicatrization follow the same principles of lid reconstruction discussed for thermal burns.

Lacrimal System Trauma

Canalicular trauma can be in the form of burns, toxic medication, autoimmune disease, infections, or mechanical injury. Chemical, thermal, or radiation burns can damage the lacrimal system. Toxic medications, including antiviral agents (e.g., adenine arabinoside), antineoplastic agents (5-fluorouracil), cholinergic drugs (e.g., pilocarpine), anticholinergic drugs (e.g., eserine, phospholine iodide), and adrenergic drugs (e.g., epinephrine), can cause punctal or canalicular stenosis. Autoimmune diseases, including ocular pemphigoid and Stevens-Johnson syndrome, can cause punctal occlusion. Fungal, viral, bacterial, and chlamydial infections can cause canaliculitis. Mechanical injury includes repeat canalicular and nasolacrimal probings, ocular or adnexal surgery involving the canaliculus, and canalicular lacerations.

Canaliculitis

The patient with canaliculitis presents with epiphora and localized pain over the canaliculus. There is an associated "fish mouth" or dilated punctum (Fig. 10.95A). The most common cause of canaliculitis is *A. israelii* (*Streptothrix*). This bacterium is a filamentous, gram-positive rod (Fig. 10.95B).

Management. Medical treatment consists of warm compresses; expression of concretions, which may have a "cottage cheese" texture; and topical antibiotics such as peni-

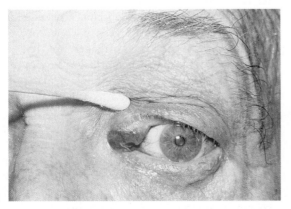

A

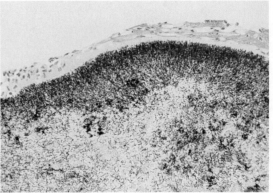

B

FIGURE 10.95. A: Canaliculitis with local edema and erythema of the left upper canaliculus. **B:** High-power, hematoxylin-and-eosin preparation of a canalicular stone shows filamentous, gram-positive rods.

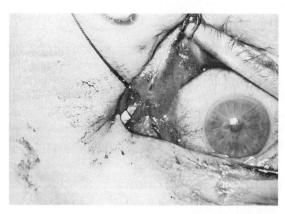

FIGURE 10.96. Canaliculotomy with canalicular stones.

cillin (100,000 U/mL, one drop qid for 2 weeks). Sulfonamides or erythromycin are acceptable alternatives. Chronic canaliculitis requires curettage alone or in combination with canaliculotomy (Fig. 10.96) to remove canaliculoliths. Dacryocystorhinostomy may be required.

Canalicular Lacerations

Periocular trauma may involve one canaliculus (i.e., single canalicular laceration) or the upper and the lower canaliculi (i.e., bicanalicular lacerations). The diagnosis is made by careful inspection, with diagnostic probing and irrigation when necessary. Primary repair is desired within 24 to 48 hours of injury.

Management. The choice of general or local anesthesia depends on the age of the patient, associated ocular trauma, lid lacerations, medial canthal tendon avulsions, and nasolacrimal fractures (Fig. 10.97). General anesthesia is preferred for children, for anxious adults, and for placement of a bicanalicular stent. Identification of the severed ends of the canaliculi is facilitated by using the operating microscope.

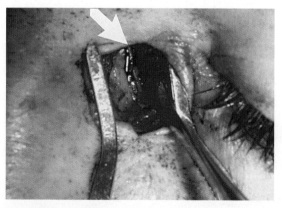

FIGURE 10.97. An 18-year-old boy had persistent epiphora 3 months after the repair of a canalicular laceration. Lacrimal irrigation confirmed a nasolacrimal duct obstruction. A fracture of the nasolacrimal bone was confirmed by a computed tomography scan. A fracture is seen through the left nasolacrimal bone during the dacryocystorhinostomy.

Anastomosis of the cut ends of the canaliculi, with two or three preplaced 9-0 nylon sutures and two or three preplaced 5-0 chromic paracanalicular sutures, is performed over a stent (Fig. 10.98A). The chromic sutures are secured before the nylon sutures to reduce tension on the wound. Numerous stent materials exist, including Veirs rods, Johnson rods, or silicone tubing. Silicone is preferred because it is soft, flexible, and comfortable. It is less likely to cause corneal irritation and may be left in place for 6 months or longer, if necessary.

Monocanalicular stents are preferred for monocanalicular lacerations, avoiding damage to the normal canaliculus. One end of the silicone tube is allowed to coil in the nasolacrimal sac while the other end is passed through the punctum and secured to the eyelid (Fig. 10.98B). Newer monocanalicular tubes have attached punctal plugs to allow stabilization of the tube in the punctum (Figs. 10.98C,D).

Bicanalicular intubation is necessary for repair of bicanalicular lacerations. The loose ends can be tied under the inferior turbinate in the nose. Alternatively, a Beyer pigtail probe can be used cautiously to pass the loose ends of the silicone tubing into the palpebral fissures; the ends are then tied near the caruncle. Associated medial canthal tendon lacerations, skin lacerations, or lid margin lacerations are then closed appropriately.

Orbital Trauma

Retrobulbar Hemorrhage

A retrobulbar hemorrhage (Fig. 10.99) is a hemorrhage into the orbital cavity, anteriorly bound by the orbital septum and canthal tendons. Limited increases in orbital volume result in anterior displacement of the septum and the globe. A retrobulbar hemorrhage also can result in increased intraorbital and intraocular pressure. The most common causes of retrobulbar hemorrhage are blunt trauma and penetrating injury by the entry of foreign bodies. Retrobulbar hemorrhage from surgery of the eyelids and orbit has occurred after retrobulbar injection, blepharoplasty, dacryocystorhinostomy, palpebral dacryoadenectomy, repair of orbital and facial fractures, and sinus surgery.

Idiopathic orbital hemorrhages are less common. Spontaneous retrobulbar hemorrhages have occurred with orbital lymphangiomas, cavernous hemangiomas, and aneurysms of the ophthalmic artery. Blood disorders associated with spontaneous orbital hemorrhage include hemophilia, leukemia, vitamin K deficiency, anemia, hypertension, scurvy, and von Willebrand's disease.

Clinical Features. Sudden orbital and ocular pain and decreased vision associated with a recent history of trauma to the eye or orbit are frequent complaints. Lid ecchymosis, chemosis, proptosis with resistance to retropulsion, diffuse subconjunctival hemorrhage with nonvisible sclera posterior to the subconjunctival hemorrhage, limited motility in any or all fields of gaze, and elevated intraocular pressure are

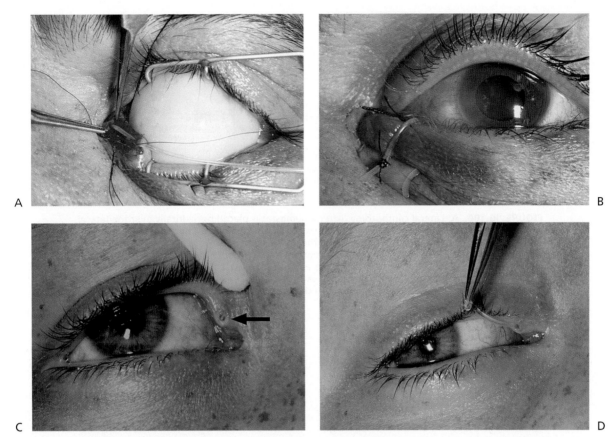

FIGURE 10.98. A: Preplaced 9-0 nylon canalicular sutures and preplaced 5-0 chromic paracanalicular sutures are shown. The Silastic intubation tube is coiled in the nasolacrimal sac. **B:** The completed monocanalicular repair. The Silastic tube exiting from the punctum is secured to the eyelid with a full-thickness lid suture on a bolster. **C:** Monocanalicular intubation tube with attached punctal plug (mini-minoka tube) is seen in right upper punctum of this 11-year-old boy who is 6 months status post repair of canalicular laceration. **D:** The mini-minoka tube is easily removed from the patient in Figure 10.98C with jeweler's forceps.

clinical signs. Progressive deterioration of vision and the visual fields, dyschromatopsia, and an afferent pupillary defect signify optic nerve dysfunction. Disc edema and choroidal folds may be seen.

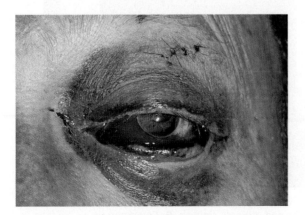

FIGURE 10.99. A 59-year-old man was hit in the left eye with a wrench and suffered a retrobulbar hemorrhage. His decreased vision, increased intraocular pressure, lid edema, ecchymosis, proptosis, and a subconjunctival hemorrhage improved with conservative treatment.

The differential diagnosis includes orbital cellulitis; orbital fractures; ruptured globe; subperiosteal hemorrhage; and optic nerve sheath hemorrhage.

Management. A complete ophthalmic examination should check for signs of threatened vision, such as decreased visual acuity, an afferent pupillary defect, loss of color vision, elevated or decreased intraocular pressure, central artery pulsations, and choroidal folds.

Treatment of retrobulbar hemorrhages is reserved for patients with visual loss or marked increases in intraocular pressure. If vision is threatened, CT scans of the orbit, including axial and coronal views, should be delayed until initial treatment has been instituted. Initial measures for the treatment of increased intraocular pressure associated with threatened vision include carbonic anhydrase inhibitors (500 mg of acetazolamide, taken orally), topical β-blockers (0.5% timolol, every 30 minutes for 2 doses), hyperosmotic agents (20% mannitol, 1 to 2 g/kg, administered intravenously for 45 minutes), and a lateral canthotomy with superior and inferior cantholysis (Fig. 10.100). Patients with mildly elevated intraocular pressure or mild proptosis who do not have visual deficits may be observed, because hemor-

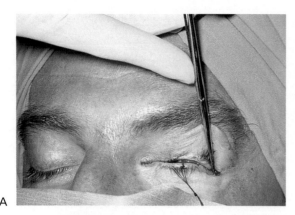
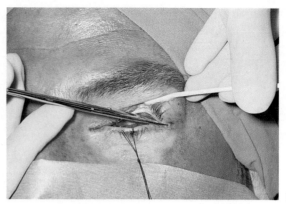

A   B

FIGURE 10.100. A: Lateral canthotomy. After a hemostat is placed horizontally over the lateral canthus for 1 minute, it is released, and sterile scissors are used to make a horizontal incision 1 cm toward the lateral orbital rim. **B:** Cantholysis of the inferior arm of the lateral canthal tendon. The scissors are redirected from 45 degrees to 90 degrees, and the skin and conjunctiva of the initial incision are separated so the scissors can be placed with the posterior blade anterior to the conjunctiva and the anterior blade posterior to the skin, engaging only the inferior arm of the lateral canthal tendon. Release of tension is felt when the inferior arm of the lateral canthal tendon is cut.

rhages usually resolve in several weeks. If vision remains threatened after the treatment, emergent orbital decompression may be required if the optic nerve becomes compromised. The retrobulbar hemorrhage may be drained directly through a lateral or medial orbitotomy, depending on the location of the hemorrhage. A subperiosteal hemorrhage (Fig. 10.101) is drained after the periosteum is elevated with a Freer elevator and the clot evacuated. Bone removal in either situation is usually unnecessary.

Patients who fail to respond to these measures may require a two-wall orbital decompression to remove the orbital floor and medial wall. Visual loss secondary to hemorrhage within the intraorbital portion of the optic nerve sheath should be treated with optic nerve sheath decompression.

Pulse therapy with corticosteroid therapy is often used concomitantly. A regimen of 250 mg of methylpred-

nisolone, administered intravenously every 6 hours for 12 doses, is followed by 80 mg taken orally daily for 1 week.

Intraorbital Foreign Bodies

Intraorbital foreign bodies are composed of inorganic, organic, or mixed materials. Inorganic foreign bodies include stone, plastic, glass, iron, lead, steel, aluminum, and most other metals (Fig. 10.102). These are usually well tolerated in the absence of infection. Pure copper foreign bodies may create a noninfectious, suppurative response requiring removal. Copper alloys with less than 85% copper (i.e., brass, bronze) are fairly well tolerated and usually do not generate such a response. Organic material such as wood and vegetable matter typically produce an acute suppurative infection, subacute infection, or a delayed granulomatous reac-

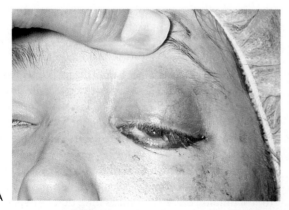
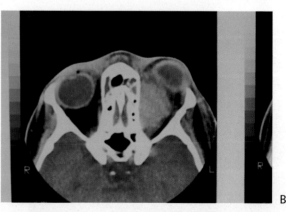

A   B

FIGURE 10.101. A: This 19-year-old woman suddenly developed proptosis and no light perception in her left eye after 2 weeks of preseptal cellulitis and ethmoid sinusitis. **B:** Computed tomography demonstrates a large subperiosteal hemorrhage along the medial orbital wall, compressing the optic nerve and distorting the globe. Blood was surgically drained through a supranasal orbitotomy. Six weeks after surgery, her vision returned to 20/25.

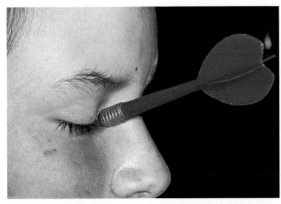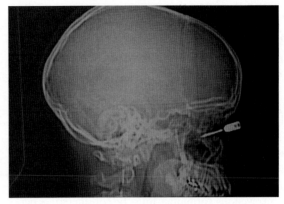

FIGURE 10.102. A: This 12-year-old boy was struck in the right orbit with a dart. The entry site on the right lower lid was inferior to the canaliculus. The results of his eye examination were normal. **B:** Sagittal computed tomography scan of the patient.

tion, mimicking an expanding orbital mass. Intraorbital foreign bodies should be removed if they are composed of vegetable matter, if they are anterior in the orbit, or if they have sharp edges. Intraorbital foreign bodies may be safely observed without surgery if they are inert, have smooth edges, and are located in the posterior orbit and not compromising the optic nerve.

Clinical Features. Symptoms vary from none to decreased vision, pain, lid edema, and diplopia. There may be no signs of an inert orbital foreign body, or there may be a palpable orbital mass, limitation of ocular motility, propto-

sis, edema, ecchymosis of the eyelids or conjunctiva, and the presence of an entry site (Fig. 10.103A). An afferent pupillary defect may be present in the case of traumatic optic neuropathy.

Management. A detailed history should determine the composition of the foreign body, the circumstances of the injury, the period since the original injury, and the degree of symptoms. Ocular injury, optic nerve injury, and CNS involvement must be ruled out.

CT scanning is the most useful modality for imaging metallic intraorbital foreign bodies. Magnetic resonance

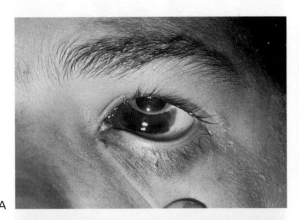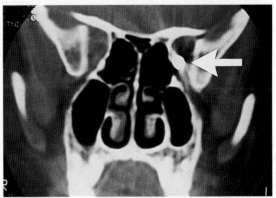

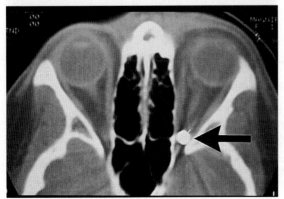

FIGURE 10.103. A: This 10-year-old boy suffered a BB injury to the left eye and orbit. The entry site is below the inferior canaliculus and extends through the caruncle. **B:** A coronal computed tomography (CT) scan shows the BB in the left orbital apex, inferomedial to the optic nerve. **C:** An axial CT scan shows the intraorbital BB at the orbital apex, inferior to the optic nerve. This patient was managed conservatively. His visual acuity, optic nerve, color vision, and pupillary reflexes have remained stable 4 years after the trauma.

imaging (MRI) is useful for imaging inorganic foreign bodies and glass without lead. Axial and coronal views (Fig. 10.103B,C) should be ordered for foreign body localization and to rule out a ruptured globe, optic nerve, CNS involvement, or associated sinus involvement. MRI is contraindicated if a metallic foreign body is suspected. A-scan ultrasonography is helpful for localizing intraocular foreign bodies, but it is less helpful in detecting or localizing small intraorbital foreign bodies.

Treatment of intraorbital foreign bodies involves culturing the wound or object from which the foreign body arose and tetanus prophylaxis. If the patient is febrile, hospitalization and intravenous antibiotics must be considered. A perforation or a ruptured globe should be repaired. Secondary enucleation is indicated if there is no useful vision or a risk of sympathetic ophthalmia exists. Organic foreign bodies (Fig. 10.104A,B) should be removed in toto. The risk of residual wood foreign bodies exists, and additional surgery may be required (Fig. 10.104C,D). Surgical removal along the entry tract is most desirable. The use of a small-diameter endoscope may improve visualization. A close working relationship with an otolaryngologist, neurosurgeon, and neuroradiologist is necessary when adjacent structures are involved.

Fractures

Orbital Floor Fractures

Orbital floor fractures are classified as direct fractures or indirect fractures. Direct fractures (Fig. 10.105) are posterior extensions of inferior orbital rim fractures. Direct fractures are caused by a compressive force at the inferior rim that leads to buckling of the orbital floor. Indirect fractures (Fig. 10.106) of the orbital floor are not associated with an inferior orbital rim fracture, and are commonly known as blow-out fractures. The term *blow-out fracture* was developed in 1957 by Smith and Regan when they proposed that indirect fractures resulted from a sudden increase in intraorbital

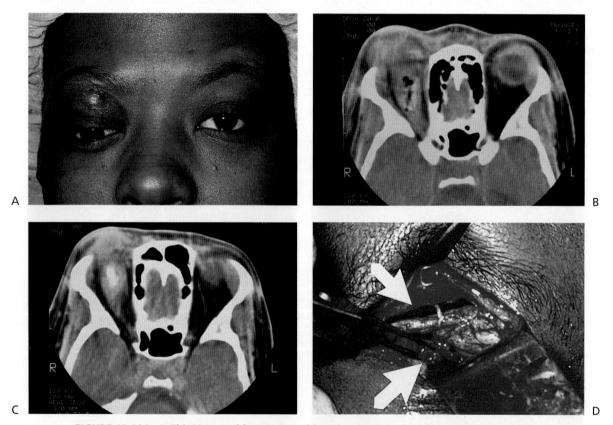

FIGURE 10.104. A: This 29-year-old woman was hit with a tree branch in the right orbit 8 months before this photograph. At that time, her right orbit was explored, and a small wooden foreign body was removed. She was lost to follow-up but returned 8 months later with an inferiorly displaced right globe, proptosis, and a tense right upper lid, as seen here. **B:** Computed tomography (CT) at the time of initial injury shows a soft tissue density and air in the superior aspect of the right orbit. No obvious foreign body is seen. **C:** The repeat CT scan of the patient 8 months later shows fibrous encapsulation of a residual piece of wood in the superior aspect of the right orbit. **D:** A superior orbitotomy was performed. The wooden foreign body was retrieved from the peripheral surgical space *(bottom arrow)*. The subperiosteal space was void of any foreign body *(top arrow)*.

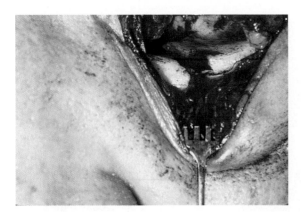

FIGURE 10.105. A direct fracture of the orbital floor extends from the infraorbital rim.

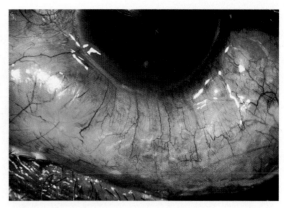

FIGURE 10.107. Subconjunctival emphysema in a patient with a medial orbital wall fracture who blew his nose.

pressure caused by the force created by an object that was greater than the diameter of the orbital entrance. The orbital contents are compressed, and the intraorbital bones break at their weakest points, the medial wall (0.25 mm thick) and the posterior medial aspect of the orbital floor (0.50 mm thick). The degree of increased intraorbital pressure determines whether or not orbital tissue herniates through these fractures to become entrapped. Most isolated medial wall fractures are asymptomatic unless the patient has orbital or eyelid emphysema.

Clinical Features. Patients with a recent history of orbital trauma, commonly with objects larger than the orbital entrance such as a fist, a soft ball, or a dash board injury, may complain of pain on attempted vertical eye movements, local point tenderness at the infraorbital rim, binocular diplopia, or lid swelling, particularly after nose blowing. Signs include ecchymosis and edema of the eyelids, limited vertical movement of the globe, orbital emphysema, subcutaneous emphysema, or subconjunctival emphysema (Fig. 10.107), hypesthesia in the distribution of the ipsilateral infraorbital nerve, enophthalmos, and globe ptosis.

Management. A thorough ophthalmologic examination should include visual acuity, pupillary reactions, adnexal

evaluation, orbital palpation, extraocular motility (Fig. 10.108A), slit lamp examination, ophthalmoscopy, and a traction or forced duction test. A neurologic evaluation is indicated if there is a history of loss of consciousness. Severe intraocular damage, such as a ruptured globe, is rarely associated with blow-out fractures. Traumatic iritis, hyphema, and retinal edema are more common associated findings. Loss of vision may result from an associated injury to the optic nerve.

Orbital floor fractures are radiographically well demonstrated by CT scans of the orbit with coronal (Fig. 10.108B) and sagittal views. They detail the extent of the fracture and associated prolapse of orbital contents. Although plain films of the orbit, specifically a Waters' view, are useful as a screening test, CT scans more accurately demonstrate the fracture size and involvement of the extraocular muscles, which help the surgeon with management decisions.

Small floor fractures with no significant entrapment of orbital tissues may be managed conservatively. This includes nasal decongestants (e.g., Afrin nasal spray, twice daily) for 10 to 14 days, broad-spectrum oral antibiotics (e.g., 250 to 500 mg of cephalexin, taken orally four times daily or 250 to 500 mg of erythromycin, taken orally four times daily) for 10 to 14 days, avoidance of nose blowing, and application of ice compresses to the orbit every 2 hours for the first 48 hours. Some surgeons use prednisone (60 to 80 mg, taken daily for 5 days), beginning during the first 48 hours after injury. Diplopia caused by edema of the muscles resolves more quickly with steroids, but diplopia associated with muscle entrapment does not improve. The use of steroids may allow the surgeon to make an earlier decision concerning the need for surgery. Enophthalmos that was not evident initially may become more apparent as orbital edema subsides.

Surgical indications are controversial but include entrapment of the orbital contents, causing diplopia within 30 degrees of the primary position, confirmed by a positive forced duction test and radiologic evidence of entrapment; cosmetically unacceptable enophthalmos; and fractures involving

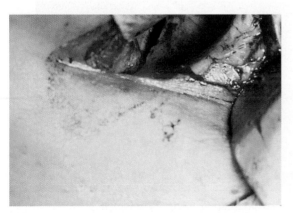

FIGURE 10.106. Indirect or blow-out fracture of the orbital floor. The entrapped orbital contents have been released.

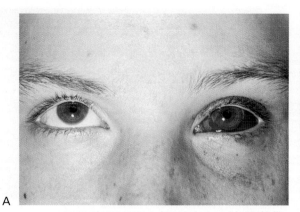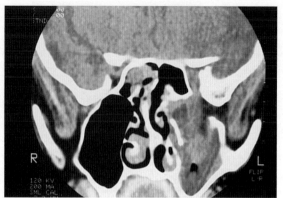

FIGURE 10.108. A: A 17-year-old boy with limited upgaze of the left eye 10 days after being hit with a lacrosse stick. **B:** The computed tomography scan shows a large orbital floor fracture with a free-floating bone fragment in the maxillary sinus.

one half of the orbital floor particularly when associated with large medial wall fractures (Fig. 10.109), which may lead to subsequent fibrosis and contracture of the prolapsed tissue.

Surgical repair of blow-out fractures is usually delayed 10 to 14 days, a period that permits subsidence of orbital edema and reevaluation of the clinical findings. Commonly, a transconjunctival (i.e., inferior fornix) incision is combined with a lateral cantholysis, or an infraciliary incision is combined with a skin-muscle flap to expose the infraorbital rim. After prolapsed soft tissue is released from the fracture site, a synthetic or homoplastic orbital floor implant is usually placed.

Potential complications of fracture surgery include persistent diplopia, infraorbital nerve dysfunction, enophthalmos, exophthalmos, eyelid malposition, infection, implant extrusion (Fig. 10.110), and, rarely, visual loss.

Tripod Fractures

A tripod fracture is a fracture involving the zygomatic bone. As the name implies, it classically involves fractures at three

sites: the zygomaticofrontal suture, the zygomaticomaxillary suture, and the zygomatic arch. With displaced zygomatic fractures, there is usually a fourth or fifth fracture site: the orbital floor or the anterior wall of the maxillary sinus. The name *tripod* may be a misnomer. The zygomatic bone is responsible for the prominence of the cheek and is an important feature in the facial skeleton. It helps to protect orbital contents from traumatic forces. The lateral canthal tendon and Lockwood's ligament are attached to the zygomatic bone at the lateral orbital tubercle. Patients with fractures and displacement of the zygomatic bone may present with cosmetic deformities involving malar flattening, inferior displacement of the lateral canthal angle, and globe ptosis. The anatomic relations of the zygomatic bone (Fig. 10.111), the zygomatic arch, the mandible, and the temporalis and masseter muscles govern normal movement of the mandible. Tripod fractures can disturb these structural associations and interfere with normal mastication.

Tripod fractures are classified according to the type of displacement of the zygomatic bone. The direction of displacement depends on the direction of the traumatic forces.

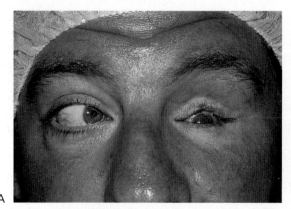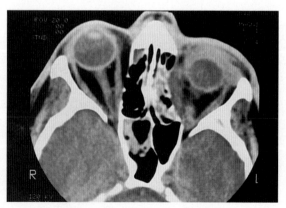

FIGURE 10.109. A: This 35-year-old man was kicked in the left orbit. He has ptosis of his left upper eyelid, 4 mm of left globe ptosis, and limited abduction of the left eye. **B:** The computed tomography scan shows a large medial wall fracture that has entrapped the medial rectus muscle.

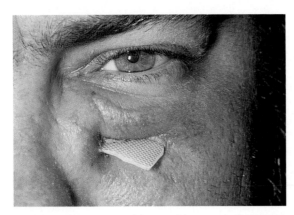

FIGURE 10.110. A 37-year-old man with an extruding alloplastic orbital floor implant.

Forces from above can cause downward displacement of the zygoma, creating a gap deformity at the lateral orbital rim, inferior displacement of the lateral canthal angle (Fig. 10.112), retraction of the lower lid, and a step deformity of the inferior orbital rim. Forces from below can cause superior displacement and "telescoping" of bone fragments of the lateral orbital rim. An inwardly displaced fracture of the zygomatic arch may impinge on the coronoid process, limiting movement of the mandible to cause pain or jaw movement.

Clinical Features. Patients frequently complain of numbness of the cheek, nasolabial fold, upper lip, and gingiva around the upper teeth on the injured side. The hypesthesia results from trauma to the infraorbital and alveolar nerves. They may also have pain on movement of the jaw. In addition to the signs seen with orbital floor fractures, patients with tripod fractures may also demonstrate malar flattening, inferior displacement of the lateral canthal angle and telescoping, or gap deformities at the lateral orbital rim.

Management. Life-threatening injuries may be associated with facial trauma. Systemic and neurologic evaluation takes precedence over ophthalmologic assessment. Because the zygomatic bone absorbs the impact of trauma and protects the globe, the frequency and severity of ophthalmic injuries are somewhat less in tripod fractures than with orbital floor fractures. Nevertheless, ocular injury is associated with facial trauma in 11% to 40% of cases. A complete ophthalmologic evaluation is necessary and should include assessment of visual acuity, pupillary reaction, extraocular motility, sensory nerves, and dentition with orbital palpation, slit lamp examination, ophthalmoscopy, forced duction testing, exophthalmometry, and tonometry. Visual loss may be associated with a contusion or transection of the optic nerve.

Tripod features are radiographically well demonstrated on a Waters' view radiograph. The zygomatic arch can be evaluated with the submental-vertex view. CT scans of the orbit with coronal (Fig. 10.113) and axial views provide the most detail of the zygomatic bone and other orbital fractures.

Nondisplaced tripod fractures with no significant entrapment of orbital contents, malar flattening, or impingement of the coronoid process of the mandible can be managed conservatively. This includes the use of nasal decongestants, broad-spectrum oral antibiotics, avoidance of nose blowing, application of ice compresses, and the use of systemic prednisone. Surgical indications include persistent pain on mastication, inferior displacement of the lateral canthal tendon and Lockwood's ligament, persistent diplopia with muscle entrapment, and cosmetically unacceptable malar flattening.

Surgical repair can be done within 24 to 48 hours if the deformities are pronounced. In less dramatic cases, surgical repair of tripod fractures can be delayed 7 to 10 days to allow orbital edema to decrease. The transconjunctival approach combined with a lateral cantholysis allows good exposure of the zygomatic bone, the orbital rim, and the orbital floor. Optimal results are obtained with open reduction and internal fixation of bone fragments using interosseous wires or microplates (Fig. 10.114). If necessary,

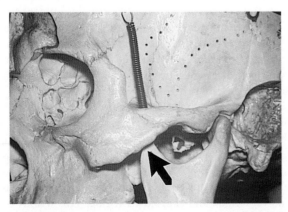

FIGURE 10.111. This skull demonstrates the close relation of the coronoid process *(arrow)* of the mandible with the zygomatic arch. Inward displacement of the zygomatic arch impinges on the coronoid process of the mandible, resulting in pain on movement of the jaw.

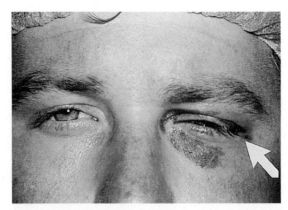

FIGURE 10.112. Inferior displacement of the left lateral canthal angle is seen in this 37-year-old man with a left lateral wall fracture and inferior displacement of the zygomatic bone.

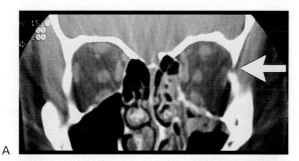

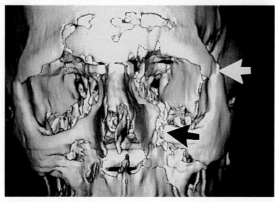

FIGURE 10.113. A: The coronal computed tomography (CT) scan shows a nondisplaced floor fracture and disarticulation of the zygomaticofrontal suture *(arrow)*. **B:** This three-dimensional CT scan of a tripod fracture from another patient demonstrates disarticulation of the zygomaticofrontal suture *(white arrow)* and the zygomaticomaxillary suture *(black arrow)*, with inferior displacement of the zygomatic bone.

an orbital floor implant is placed to prevent recurrent prolapse of the orbital contents.

PROPTOSIS

Orbital Cellulitis

Orbital cellulitis is a bacterial infection of the orbit most often associated with sinus disease. Patients present with a 1-

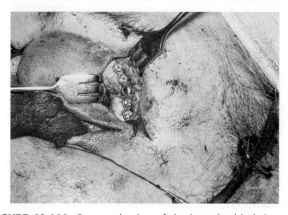

FIGURE 10.114. Open reduction of the lateral orbital rim and internal fixation with microplates and screws.

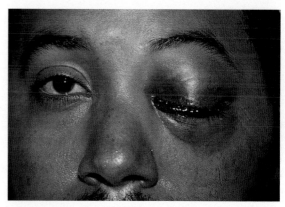

FIGURE 10.115. Orbital cellulitis presenting with massive swelling, chemosis, erythema, and poor ocular motility.

to 2-day history of progressive redness and swelling of the periorbital areas.

Clinical Features. Preseptal and orbital cellulitis present with swollen, red, and warm lids, possibly with a fever and an elevated leukocyte count. Orbital cellulitis is differentiated from preseptal cellulitis by orbital signs that may include chemosis, limited motility, proptosis, orbital resistance to retropulsion, an afferent pupillary defect, and decreased vision (Fig. 10.115). The onset of infection may have been preceded by an upper respiratory infection, especially in children. Fever and leukocytosis are more common in children but not always present. Associated sinus disease is thought to cause 85% of cases. Other causes include external wounds or bites, recent dental work, and dacryocystitis. A CT scan is required for patients with orbital cellulitis to rule out an orbital abscess or mass and to assess the paranasal sinuses (Fig. 10.116).

Gram-positive organisms are the most common cause of infection, with *Staphylococcus aureus* and *Streptococcus* species often identified as the offending organism. In children younger than 5 years of age, *H. influenzae* must be considered. Blood cultures are often negative, especially in adults, and the exact organism often remains unidentified.

If a patient is not responding to appropriate antibiotic coverage, an orbital abscess must be suspected. This can be identified with repeat CT scans and is most commonly seen as a subperiosteal collection (Fig. 10.117). The identified abscess requires immediate surgical drainage.

Cavernous sinus thrombosis is the feared complication of orbital cellulitis. The infection travels either by extension or through venous drainage into the cavernous sinus, setting up a potentially fatal intracranial infection. Clinically, this is seen by the sudden onset of bilateral chemosis, pain, proptosis, lid injection, fever, malaise, severe headache, and optic nerve, retinal, and choroidal swelling. This serious condition carries a significant risk of death.

Orbital pseudotumor is a condition that may be difficult to differentiate from orbital cellulitis. Orbital pseudotumor is more commonly associated with pain or pain with eye

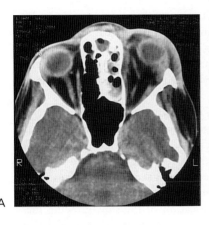
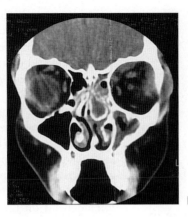

A   B

FIGURE 10.116. Axial **(A)** and coronal **(B)** computed tomography scans show pansinusitis and diffuse orbital swelling of left side consistent with orbital cellulitis.

movement. Pseudotumors can have an acute presentation, but they commonly occur subacutely, becoming more noticeable over several days. A fever or leukocytosis points toward orbital cellulitis but, especially in children, can be associated with orbital pseudotumor.

Management. Differentiation between preseptal cellulitis and orbital cellulitis is key in the management of this condition. Preseptal cellulitis in adults can be treated with a broad-spectrum oral antibiotic, with follow-up examination the next day. If the condition continues to worsen over 48 hours or develops signs of orbital cellulitis, admission to the hospital for intravenous antibiotics and a CT scan is required. Management of children with preseptal cellulitis is somewhat controversial. Some institutions admit all children with preseptal cellulitis for intravenous antibiotics. Children who can adequately be examined and have no evidence of orbital involvement or signs of systemic toxicity can be placed on broad-spectrum oral antibiotics and be seen the next day.

Children and adults with orbital cellulitis need immediate broad-spectrum intravenous antibiotics, an orbital CT scan, and a complete blood count and differential.

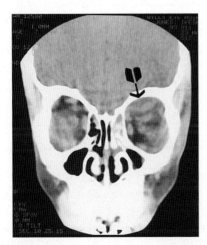

FIGURE 10.117. Coronal computed tomography scan showing subperiosteal abscess formation *(arrow)* in the left superior nasal orbit.

Antibiotics should be instituted quickly and not delayed while the patient is admitted and tested. Once on intravenous antibiotics, there should be some noticeable improvement within 48 hours. Any significant associated sinus disease needs to be evaluated, with possible drainage if the patient is not improving. If no improvement is seen, an orbital abscess should be suspected, and a repeat CT scan may be required.

Orbital cellulitis generally requires 5 to 7 days of intravenous antibiotics, depending on the clinical response. This is usually followed by 10 to 14 days of oral treatment.

Fungal Infections

Mucormycosis

This aggressive, opportunistic fungal infection is generally an infection of uncontrolled diabetics or immunocompromised patients. Patients present soon after the onset of deep, boring pain, which is followed by progressive proptosis, sudden visual loss, and orbital apex syndrome. Successful treatment depends on early recognition of mucormycosis and an aggressive medical and surgical approach.

Clinical Features. The fungal pathogen, *Phycomycetes mucorlais,* occurs naturally in soil, air, skin, and food. The organism gains entrance through the nasopharynx or sinuses and, in a person with normal cellular defenses, the organism is controlled by the cellular immune system. In an immunocompromised patient, the organism proliferates in the sinus or nasopharynx. The orbit is invaded secondarily, with the organism causing vascular necrosis and infarction as it progressively invades blood vessels. Early signs are deep, boring pain and sinusitis. *Mucormycosis* is often initially treated as a bacterial sinusitis, but it must be suspected in any immunocompromised patient with sinusitis and orbital disease. Later in the progression, cellulitis, proptosis, apical neuropathies, and intracranial spread develops. The classic black scar usually develops late in the disease. Without prompt recognition and treatment, the disease is often fatal.

The CT scan usually shows sinus disease with or without bony destruction and adjacent orbital involvement. The CT

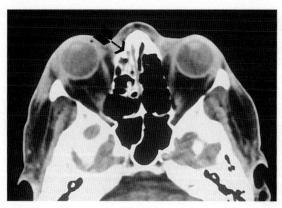

FIGURE 10.118. The axial computed tomography scan of patient with mucormycosis shows clouding and mucosal thickening in the left ethmoid sinus *(arrow)*.

findings can be subtle in early disease and can cause a delay in diagnosis (Fig. 10.118).

Management. The key to treatment is early recognition. There is significant potential for a fatal outcome with this disease in these often very sick patients. Once suspected and confirmed with a tissue diagnosis, treatment must be aggressively aimed at controlling the systemic disease, using systemic amphotericin B and surgical excision of involved tissues. This must be done in a hospital with a well-coordinated team effort. The role of hyperbaric oxygen in this disease continues to be debated.

Aspergillosis

Aspergillus is ubiquitous and occurs as an opportunistic infection. The orbital disease occurs in two forms. One form occurs in debilitated patients, and the second occurs in healthy persons who often have a history of sinus disease, polyps, or living in hot, humid areas.

Clinical Features. The diffuse form is often seen in patients with some immune compromise. A history of chronic sinus disease is common. *Aspergillus* organisms invade the orbital vessels, causing arteritis, thrombosis, and occlusion of the vessels. This leads to a progressive destruction of the

orbital bones and infiltration of the optic nerve and orbital contents. This condition usually presents as slowly progressive, unilateral proptosis, ocular pain, and visual loss. Late signs include lid edema, chemosis, fever, and leukocytosis. This infection may even lead to an endophthalmitis and death.

The localized form develops as a slow-growing sclerotic mass that generally begins in the sinuses and extends secondarily into the orbit (Fig. 10.119). There may be an associated allergic component with an IgE-mediated antibody-antigen reaction to specific fungal antigens. This is seen in healthy people who live in hot, humid climates. The symptoms depend on the location of the slow-growing mass. More interior masses present as proptosis and globe displacement, while posterior masses present with visual loss and dysmotility.

Management. Once suspected and confirmed with orbital imaging, the diagnosis must be made pathologically. The primary treatment is then complete drainage and debridement of all areas involved, if possible. The diffuse form is more often fatal but if drained early, the localized form often does well. Amphotericin B and other antifungal agents may be helpful in treating the diffuse form.

Orbital Inflammation

Orbital Pseudotumor

Orbital pseudotumor comprises a wide spectrum of inflammatory syndromes. These vary in their location in the orbit and in onset. They all present with various degrees of pain, proptosis, swelling, and injection of the orbit or globe. Once diagnosed, they respond to corticosteroid treatment.

Clinical Features. This group of disorders is marked by the acute or subacute onset of orbital inflammatory disease. Histologically, these include infiltration by a polymorphous group of inflammatory cells, including neutrophils, lymphocytes, plasma cells, macrophages, and fibrocytes. Clinically, the onset is associated with pain, swelling, erythema, and orbital dysfunction (Fig. 10.120). The exact symptoms depend on the location of the process. The in-

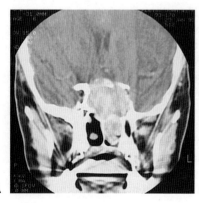
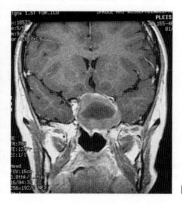

A   B

FIGURE 10.119. Allergic noninvasive form of aspergillosis shown by **(A)** computed tomography and **(B)** magnetic resonance imaging (MRI). MRI demonstrates the central hypodense fungal ball surrounded by mucin.

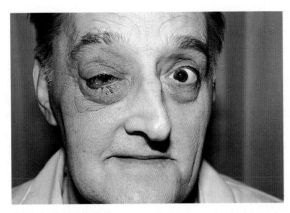

FIGURE 10.120. A patient with orbital pseudotumor presented with swelling, redness, pain, and limited motility.

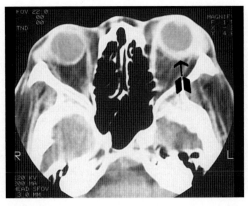

FIGURE 10.122. An axial computed tomography scan shows diffuse scleral thickening *(arrow)* and anterior orbital inflammation that are consistent with orbital scleritis.

flammation may be anterior, diffusely involving the orbit, apical, lacrimal, a myositis, or any combination. Anterior processes present with pain, redness, and swelling of the lids and anterior orbit. If the process is apical, there may be few external signs but intense pain with loss of vision and motility. Myositis includes pain, proptosis, swelling, and loss of function of the affected muscle. Lacrimal gland involvement presents as swelling and pain of the lacrimal gland and upper lid. This can sometimes be subacute or even chronic, with less pain and a mass effect.

Possible ocular findings include uveitis, scleritis, papillitis, and exudative retinal detachment. In children, the disease is more likely to be bilateral and have ocular involvement, and there may be an elevated sedimentation rate and CSF pleocytosis. Children may also have a fever associated with orbital pseudotumor.

CT scanning usually shows diffuse thickening of the involved structures without any bony changes (Figs. 10.121–10.123). The combination of acute onset of pain along with this CT picture usually make the diagnosis straightforward.

Management. The diagnosis is based on clinical examination and orbital imaging, and pseudotumor is treated with systemic steroids. Depending on the patient's medical condition, the usual adult dose is 60 to 80 mg of oral prednisone per day. Most patients have a noticeable reduction in pain and swelling in 24 to 48 hours. If the condition has been more chronic, it may take longer to notice a response. After the condition has improved, the steroids can be tapered over 4 to 5 weeks. If there is a poor response to prednisone or a flare condition on tapering the medication, the clinical diagnosis must be suspected. In these cases, an orbital biopsy is done to establish or confirm the diagnosis, because some tumors can mimic pseudotumor.

Inflammation primarily involving the lacrimal gland is more likely to be associated with other conditions such as viral or bacterial dacryoadenitis, sarcoidosis, lymphoid proliferation, and Sjögren's syndrome. Some clinicians suggest routine biopsy of any process primarily involving the lacrimal glands. Lacrimal gland processes must be biopsied if there is not a rapid response to steroids.

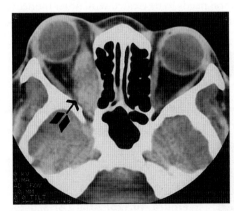

FIGURE 10.121. The axial computed tomography scan of orbital myositis demonstrates an enlarged right medial rectus muscle *(arrow)*.

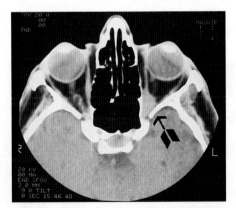

FIGURE 10.123. An axial computed tomography scan shows localized orbital inflammation at the left globe orbital apex, which resulted in decreased vision and dysmotility, with minimal external signs of inflammation.

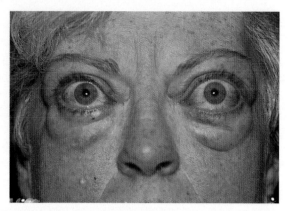

FIGURE 10.124. Thyroid-related ophthalmopathy with proptosis, lid retraction, and limited motility.

Thyroid-Related Ophthalmopathy

Thyroid-related ophthalmopathy is an immune-mediated process that results in orbital inflammation and scarring. It occurs four to five times more commonly in women than men and is most common in middle age. The results may be mild swelling of the orbit, or it can result in severe proptosis, lid retraction, corneal exposure, motility disturbances, or visual loss secondary to optic nerve compression. Ninety percent of patients have or have had a systemic thyroid abnormality.

Clinical Features. Thyroid-related ophthalmopathy is characterized by chronic orbital inflammation and scarring. Usually, this is a bilateral process, but it can be asymmetric. This autoimmune process results in infiltration of extraocular muscles and orbital fat by inflammatory cells in the short term and by mucopolysaccharide and collagen in the long term. The disease process is marked by early inflammation and long-term fibrosis and scarring.

Early manifestations of the disease can often be subtle, with nonspecific redness, irritation, chemosis, and eyelid swelling. The presence of a systemic thyroid imbalance is helpful in establishing the diagnosis but not necessary to make the diagnosis, because 10% of the patients are euthyroid. Early signs of lid retraction, lid lag, or evidence of any

systemic thyroid imbalance help confirm the diagnosis. As the disease process progresses, eyelid retraction and lid lag become more obvious, and corneal exposure must be watched for. Proptosis and restriction of motility are also later signs (Fig. 10.124). The inferior rectus muscle is the most commonly involved muscle, followed by the medial rectus, making restricted upgaze and lateral gaze the most common motility disturbances. The CT scan shows involvement of the muscle bellies and sparing of the tendons (Fig. 10.125). If extraocular muscle involvement progresses, the optic nerve may become compressed at the orbital apex by these swollen muscles. Visual acuity, color vision, visual fields, and presence of an afferent pupillary defect must all be monitored in these patients to rule out optic nerve compression.

A patient typically goes through a period of 6 to 24 months of active disease. During this period, there is active inflammation, and the ocular manifestations are changing. After this phase is completed, the eye typically remains stable, despite the residual scarring of the muscles and orbit.

Management. Management of thyroid-related ophthalmology is complicated by the wide variability of disease manifestations and by a lack of consensus about the best treatment. Initial assessment of the patient requires determination of disease activity, which is important in making decisions about management. All patients require an evaluation and monitoring of their thyroid status. Patients may be euthyroid on presentation, but their thyroid status must be followed over time. Careful evaluation for optic nerve compression or significant corneal exposure must be done. All patients will benefit from lubrication of the eyes. Good patient education about thyroid-related ophthalmopathy and what the patient can expect is invaluable.

Patients with active disease are candidates for orbital irradiation. Irradiation appears to stop progression of thyroid-related ophthalmopathy in a significant percentage of patients. Irradiation does not reverse the scarring already present from the disease. Irradiation takes up to 6 months to have full effect, so any acute problem such as optic nerve compression needs to be treated with other modalities, often in conjunction with irradiation. Patients with active disease

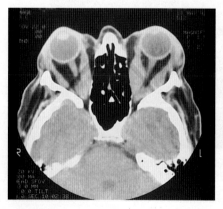

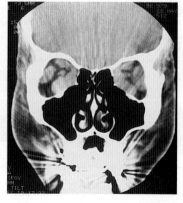

A   B

Figure 10.125. Axial **(A)** and coronal **(B)** computed tomography scans show enlargement of all extraocular muscles in a patient with thyroid-related ophthalmopathy.

will require an orbital CT scan. This helps assess muscle size, activity, and may later assess response.

Patients with inactive disease are without active inflammation and are unlikely to benefit from irradiation. Treatment includes observation, lubrication, and possible surgery to correct changes caused by thyroid-related ophthalmopathy. These patients do not require imaging unless the diagnosis is in question or decompressive surgery is being considered.

Systemic steroids are indicated for short-term management of the inflammation from thyroid-related ophthalmopathy. The exact mechanism of action is unclear but steroids are effective in decreasing inflammation. This is especially helpful in optic nerve compression or severe corneal exposure. Irradiation itself takes weeks to work, so the addition of steroids gives rapid, short-term treatment. Long-term use of steroids is limited by side effects.

Surgical management, which often involves multiple stages and treatments over months to years, may include orbital decompression, eye muscle surgery, and eyelid surgery. The need for acute surgical management of severe disease has decreased with the use of irradiation. There still are the rare patients who will require acute orbital decompression for optic nerve compression. More often, surgery is required to try and reverse the results of the chronic orbital scarring form thyroid-related ophthalmology.

Langerhans Cell Histiocytosis

Langerhans cell histiocytosis, formerly known as histiocytosis X, is a rare collection of disorders of the mononuclear phagocytic system. The former terms eosinophilic granuloma of the bone, Letterer-Siwe disease, and Hand-Schüller-Christian disease are being replaced by the terms unifocal and multifocal eosinophilic granuloma of bone, and diffuse soft-tissue histiocytosis.

Clinical Features. The nature of involvement and long-term prognosis of this disease appears to be related to the patient's age and the extent of disease. Children younger than 2 years of age have a mortality rate of 55% to 60%, compared with 15% for older children. The extent of the disease is usually apparent early in its course. The diffuse soft tissue disease tends to produce fulminant systemic involvement in very young children. The unifocal disease tends to be in older children and has the best prognosis.

Systemic involvement can vary greatly but may include fever, localized infections, skin lesions, hepatosplenomegaly, lymphadenopathy, and possibly bone marrow involvement.

Orbital disease characteristically involves the superotemporal area. Bony involvement can be quite limited or extensive. Soft tissue involvement alone is rare and is usually secondary to extension from the surrounding bone. This pattern of disease results in a mass effect on the globe or orbital structures. The bony lesions may be sclerotic or have a lytic appearance, with secondary expansion to surrounding

tissues seen on CT scans. This bony involvement can lead to the described triad of diabetes insipidus, exophthalmos, and bony lesions.

Management. Suspected isolated orbital lesions must be biopsied. If the biopsy confirms the diagnosis, local curettage is often curative. However, low-dose irradiation may be considered if growth continues. Evidence of multifocal bony involvement or systemic involvement should be looked for in these patients. Diffuse systemic involvement or multifocal involvement requires aggressive treatment by a pediatric oncologist. This may include irradiation, chemotherapeutic agents, and steroids.

Orbital Tumors

Lymphoid Tumors

Lymphoid tumors comprise a spectrum from benign to highly malignant lesions. The presentation of these lesions can vary greatly. They are the most common primary orbital malignancy in adulthood. Lymphoid orbital tumors respond very well to radiation therapy. A tumor in the orbit should alert the clinician to the possibility of lymphoma elsewhere in the body.

Clinical Features. Patients with lymphoproliferative disease of the orbit classically present with a painless mass and its secondary mass effect. Inflammatory signs are rarely present and the onset of lymphoid inflammation is insidious. Lymphoid lesions may present subconjunctivally (Fig. 10.126) with a visible, fleshy mass, in the orbit with globe displacement and dysfunction, or with an enlarged lacrimal gland. The anterior, subconjunctival lesions are more likely to be benign than the more posterior tumors. The orbital involvement is usually extraconal. Patients may have a history of lymphoid disease elsewhere in the body.

CT scans reveal a mass that usually molds around the globe, orbit, and orbital structures rather than causing direct displacement (Fig. 10.127). Bony involvement is rare, and as many as 25% of cases may have bilateral involvement of the orbits.

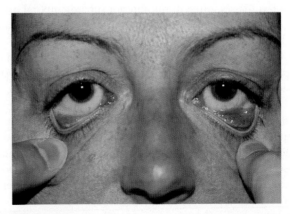

FIGURE 10.126. Bilateral lymphoid infiltrates of the inferior conjunctival fornix.

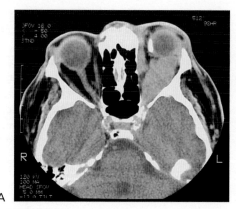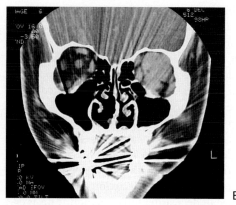

FIGURE 10.127. Diffuse infiltration by a lymphoma of the left orbit. Lymphoid tumors tend to mold around orbital structures rather than displacing them. **A:** Axial view. **B:** Coronal view.

Management. Management generally involves a team approach of pathology, oncology, and radiation oncology specialists along with the ophthalmologist. After an orbital mass is identified and lymphoma is suspected, tissue is needed to identify the lesion as lymphoid and stage its degree of malignancy. An aggressive systemic workup is also needed to look for any evidence of systemic lymphoid disease. The extent of systemic disease and the histopathologic diagnosis need to be taken into account when deciding upon treatment for each patient. Cases that are localized to the orbit are often treated with orbital irradiation, but systemic involvement by malignant lymphoma usually requires some form of chemotherapy. Even benign lymphoid hyperplasia localized to the orbit implies the patient is at risk of developing lymphoma elsewhere in the body in the future, and long-term follow-up is necessary.

Dermoid and Epidermoid Cysts

These benign cystic lesions comprise about 5% of orbital lesions. They are choristomas that probably arise from sequestration of epidermal tissue in deeper layers during embryonal development. The superficial lesions typically present in the first few years of life as firm, slow-growing, painless masses, often in the anterior superotemporal orbit. Deeper lesions are less common and typically present later in life.

Clinical Features. Dermoid and epidermoid cysts can be separated into superficial and deep lesions. Both are cystic lesions, but epidermoids are keratin-filled cysts lined by epidermis and without dermal appendages. These lesions are more common in the skin and less common in the orbit. A dermoid cyst contains dermal appendages in its wall and is filled with keratin, but it may also contain hairs. Dermoid cysts typically involve the orbit and are thought to arise from ectodermal tissue pinched off in a bony suture during embryonic development.

The superficial lesions are typically recognized early in childhood, often in the first year. They are classically located

in the superotemporal orbit, adjacent to the orbital rim (Fig. 10.128), but they can occur in other locations. They grow slowly, are painless, and may be attached to the orbital rim. CT scans reveal a well-defined mass with a lucent center. There may be some bony fossa formation but not true bony erosion.

Deep orbital lesions typically present later because of their deep location and very slow, painless growth. These lesions can arise from virtually any orbital suture and are typically discovered because of their secondary mass effect within the orbit (Fig. 10.129). These deeper dermoids must be differentiated from the superficial lesions, because the dermoid cyst is much more difficult to remove and can sometimes extend intracranially.

Rarely, if the cyst ruptures from trauma or spontaneously, significant orbital inflammation and scarring can result. An incompletely excised cyst can also result in chronic orbital inflammation and scarring from continued leakage of the cyst's contents.

Management. Treatment of these lesions involves excision. The only debate is when and, in the deep cases, how to approach removal. Superficial dermoids tend to grow slowly, and as the child becomes more active, the risk of rup-

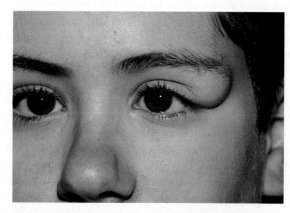

FIGURE 10.128. Superficial dermoid cyst with a classic superotemporal location.

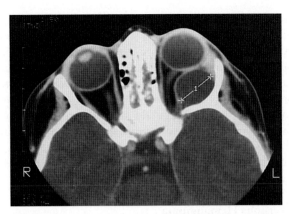

FIGURE 10.129. An axial computed tomography scan of a deep orbital dermoid demonstrates molding of the lateral orbital wall.

ture increases, making excision a consideration. These lesions should be completely excised sometime between the ages of 1 and 5 years. If there is any question during the preoperative examination that the lesion is more than superficial, a CT scan should be done to document the lesion's full extent. Superficial lesions can usually be excised through a lid crease approach. Complete excision of the entire cyst, with attempted destruction of any small tail that is attached to a bony suture, is important. Deeper lesions require more extensive surgery and, rarely, a combined neurosurgical procedure. The key is complete excision of the entire lesion, because any remnants left in the orbit can result in chronic orbital inflammation and scarring.

Vascular Tumors

Capillary Hemangioma

Capillary hemangiomas are abnormal proliferations of endothelial cells forming capillary-like vessels. These lesions typically present in the first few months of life. Rapid growth during the first few weeks is followed by spontaneous regression over months to years. Patients often have other hemangiomas elsewhere on their bodies. Amblyopia, because of astigmatism or occlusion and severe proptosis, may necessitate treatment.

Clinical Features. Capillary hemangiomas can be divided into the superficial form that involves skin or conjunctiva and the deep form that is located in the orbit. Patients can also present with a combined form.

Superficial lesions, called strawberry nevi, can be located anywhere on the body. These lesions are located in the dermis and rarely require treatment.

Deep orbital lesions typically present with a mass effect in the orbit, causing proptosis and globe displacement (Fig. 10.130). Orbital imaging shows a variable lesion from well circumscribed to infiltrating. MRI reveals characteristics of blood flow to and within the lesion. This information may be more helpful than CT in treating this lesion.

Combined lesions that are superficial and deep cause the most clinical problems. These lesions can grow and impinge on the visual axis, possibly causing amblyopia. They may press on the globe, causing astigmatic changes. Like the superficial lesions, these tend to grow during the first year of life and then regress with time.

Management. With time, these lesions regress on their own, and if possible, close observation is the therapy of choice. Treatment is required for lesions causing amblyopia or severe proptosis, although the best form of treatment is not clear. Intralesional corticosteroid deposition, systemic corticosteroid therapy, or surgical excision seem to be the most helpful modalities, combined with aggressive treatment of the amblyopia.

Lymphangioma

Lymphangiomas are vascular lesions containing endothelium-lined channels that are isolated from the vascular system of the surrounding structures. These lesions develop in childhood but are often not recognized until early adulthood.

Clinical Features. Lymphangiomas are composed of multiple serous-filled vascular channels, accumulations of lymphocytes, a collagen network, areas of smooth muscle, old hemorrhage, and dysplastic vessels. These lesions are sometimes confused with venous anomalies, but lymphangiomas are isolated from the vascular system.

Lymphangiomas can occur superficially, deep in the orbit, or in a combined form. The superficial lesions present in childhood as clear cystic structures with some blood-filled or partially blood-filled cysts (Fig. 10.131). Deeper lesions often present with a deep orbital hemorrhage and sudden onset of proptosis, pain, and possibly, decreased vision. If the orbital hemorrhage results in visual loss or corneal exposure, drainage of the blood-filled cyst, along with attempted excision of the vascular anomaly causing the bleeding, is required. The surrounding structures are often scarred, and complete excision is usually impossible.

Combined lesions are usually recognized in childhood because of their superficial components. These can be very

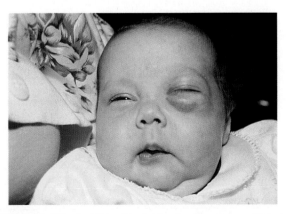

FIGURE 10.130. A child with right subcutaneous capillary hemangioma without the usual strawberry appearance.

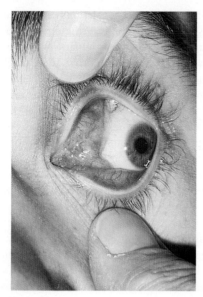

FIGURE 10.131. A patient with lymphangioma of the left orbit presented with a mass involving the medial upper eyelid. Notice the cystic spaces involving the conjunctiva.

large, cause significant cosmetic deformity, and threaten vision because of optic neuropathy or amblyopia. These lesions may require surgical management on an urgent basis because of a hemorrhage or elective surgery because of the progressive enlargement of the lesion. Because lymphangiomas have an infiltrative growth pattern, complete excision is almost impossible. They are often debulked but continue to grow. It has been suggested that the risk of subsequent hemorrhage is increased after the initial debulking surgery.

CT scans show a poorly defined, infiltrative lesion with various densities (Fig. 10.132). MRI is often better at identifying these lesions with their cystic areas of blood in patients of different ages.

Management. Management of lymphangiomas is difficult. The slowly progressive course and the infiltrative na-

ture of these lesions make most treatments less than satisfying. After the lesion is identified as a lymphangioma, observation should be the first choice. Some lesions subsequently come to attention because of a spontaneous orbital hemorrhage that may need to be drained if causing visual loss or corneal exposure. Other lesions may need to be debulked in time as they slowly enlarge and infiltrate the orbit. Because of the infiltrative nature of lymphangiomas, complete surgical excision is usually impossible without damaging vital structures. Ultimately, some patients are left with poorly functioning or blind eyes.

Cavernous Hemangioma

Cavernous hemangiomas are benign, well-circumscribed, intraconal lesions that typically present in adulthood with slowly progressive proptosis. These lesions are successfully treated by surgical excision.

Clinical Features. Cavernous hemangiomas typically present with slowly progressive proptosis that, once noticed, is often identified in old pictures from previous years. These patients present for diagnosis or treatment when they are 20 to 70 years of age. The presenting symptoms depend on the position of the lesion and the size. In addition to proptosis, the symptoms include orbital pain, diplopia, optic nerve compression, and distortion of the globe. The CT scan typically shows a well-circumscribed, intraconal mass that displaces orbital structures (Fig. 10.133). These lesions are low-flow vascular lesions with variable enhancement patterns seen on CT scans.

Management. Management involves surgical excision. Once isolated, these lesions are usually very easily separated from surrounding orbital structures and removed. Bleeding is usually not a problem, because cavernous hemangiomas are low-flow lesions. Cavernous hemangiomas enlarge with time, and once symptomatic should be excised. Asymptomatic lesions may be removed to rule out tumors with malignant potential such as hemangiopericytomas or fibrous histiocytomas.

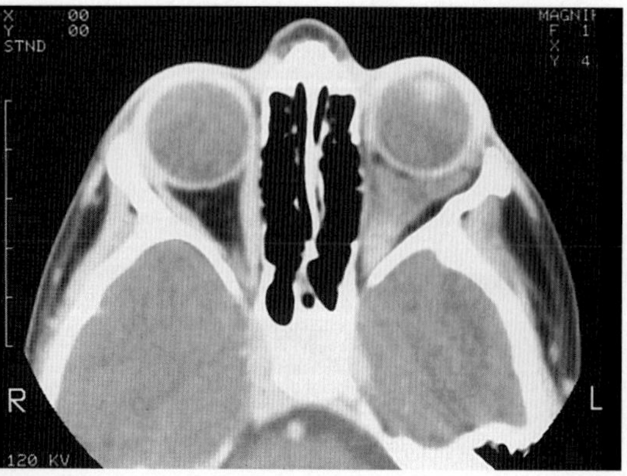

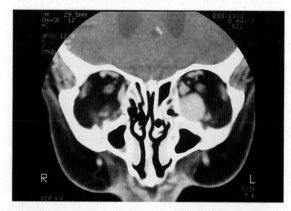

FIGURE 10.132. An axial computed tomography scan shows deep orbital infiltration by a lymphangioma.

FIGURE 10.133. Computed tomography scan of a cavernous hemangioma, demonstrating a well-encapsulated, contrast-enhanced tumor of the left orbit.

Hemangiopericytoma

Hemangiopericytomas are rare vascular orbital tumors that originate from pericytes. The lesion classically presents in the superior orbit as a growing, well-circumscribed mass.

Clinical Features. Hemangiopericytomas present similarly to cavernous hemangioma, with symptoms secondary to mass effect. Unlike cavernous hemangioma, these are more likely to grow in less than 1 year. A CT scan shows a well-circumscribed mass in the retrobulbar orbit. These lesions are often moderately vascular.

Management. Management is complete surgical excision. These lesions are usually well circumscribed, without infiltration, but they may have associated draining vessels. Pathologic evaluation of these lesions is important. The lesions are divided into benign, intermediate, and malignant tumors. The literature indicates that as many as 30% of these lesions recur, and 10% to 15% metastasize. Local recurrence is more common after incomplete or piecemeal excision and by malignant lesions. Metastasis is also more likely for malignant lesions but has been seen in benign tumors. Because local recurrence and metastasis can occur years later, these patients need to be followed on a long-term basis.

Vascular Abnormalities

Arteriovenous Malformation

An arteriovenous malformation is the result of an abnormal connection between an artery and the venous system draining the orbit. Symptoms vary with the amount of arterial flow from mild vascular engorgement to severe pulsatile proptosis, chemosis, and elevated intraocular pressure.

Clinical Features. Arteriovenous malformations are divided into high-flow and low-flow abnormalities. The malformation is an abnormal connection between an artery and venous system, typically the cavernous sinus. The size of the artery that arteriolizes the venous system determines the symptoms associated with this abnormality.

Low-flow malformations typically occur spontaneously and are thought to be related to venous thrombosis within the cavernous sinus. The theory is that, as the sinus recanalizes, small arteries in the wall of the cavernous sinus enlarge to form a shunt into the venous system. Symptoms typically consist of mild swelling of the orbit and engorgement of the veins. Symptoms may wax and wane, and as many as 40% of cases spontaneously resolve.

High-flow malformations are most often related to head trauma resulting in a tear in the cavernous sinus portion of the internal carotid artery. This sets up a high flow of blood into the cavernous sinus and arterialization of the orbital and ocular venous system. Patients often have an audible bruit, pulsatile exophthalmos, chemosis, orbital swelling, episcleral vascular engorgement, and increased intraocular pressure (Fig. 10.134). The CT scan shows diffuse engorgement of orbital structures, enlarged muscles, and an en-

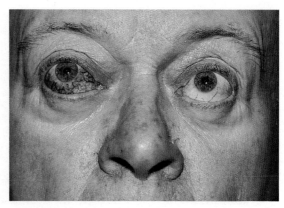

FIGURE 10.134. External photograph of a patient with an arteriovenous malformation with dilated, tortuous episcleral vessels of the right eye.

larged superior ophthalmic vein. Color Doppler ultrasonography of the orbit shows flow reversal in the venous system.

Management. Treatment involves intravascular embolization of the shunt. Almost all high-flow systems require embolization. Because there is a significant chance the low-flow systems will spontaneously thrombose, observation is indicated unless there is impending visual loss, uncontrollable intraocular pressure, severe pain, swelling, or corneal exposure.

Venous Anomalies

Venous anomalies are composed of segments of dilated venous system. Their manifestations depend on the degree of connection with a functional venous system. Superficially, they appear as distended venous areas; deep lesions can lead to spontaneous orbit hemorrhage.

Clinical Features. These lesions are more understandable if divided into a distensible form and a nondistensible form or varix. Nondistensible venous anomalies are typically isolated from the venous system. When located deep in the orbit, these present with a sudden onset of pain and proptosis associated with an acute hemorrhage. Superficial lesions present with swelling and distortion of the lids and anterior orbital structures that can be quite disfiguring (Fig. 10.135).

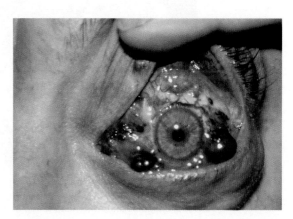

FIGURE 10.135. Extensive varices of the orbit and lids.

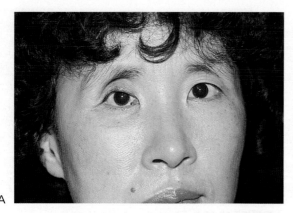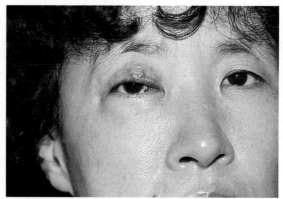

FIGURE 10.136. The patient is shown to have a deep orbital varix with an enophthalmic right eye **(A)** and proptosis after Valsalva's maneuver **(B)**.

The distensible form usually presents in the first decade of life. Typically, these lesions enlarge with increased jugular pressure, because they have a direct connection with the venous system. Patients with deep lesions typically present with enophthalmos secondary to an enlarged orbit and fat atrophy from the chronic, intermittent venous distension (Fig. 10.136). If the lesion is located anteriorly, venous engorgement occurs with increased venous pressure. Valsalva's maneuvers or placing the patient's head in a dependent position can demonstrate the venous engorgement. When comparing the axial and corolla views on CT scans, a significant difference in the lesion size is noticed because of the dependent position of the head during the coronal views (Fig. 10.137).

Management. Observation is generally the rule for these lesions. Severe orbital hemorrhage with severe pain or visual loss may require drainage of the blood. The venous anomaly is usually not able to be identified or removed. The anterior lesions causing extreme disfigurement can be treated with a YAG contact or CO_2 laser with some degree of success.

Neural Tumors

Optic Nerve Glioma

Clinical Features. Gliomas of the orbital portion of the optic nerve are diagnosed in preschool children with a loss of vision, proptosis, papilledema, optic atrophy, and strabismus. Visual loss is usually the first symptom, which is often picked up on routine screening. Proptosis can be minimal to massive, producing an axial and downward displacement of the globe (Fig. 10.138). Between 25% and 50% of children with optic nerve gliomas have neurofibromatosis. The CT scan demonstrates a fusiform enlargement of the optic nerve and, if the tumor extends intracranially, enlargement of the optic canal (Fig. 10.139). MRI is helpful in delineating the intracranial extent of the tumor. Gliomas are well-circumscribed astrocytic tumors derived from interstitial cells, astroglia, and oligodendroglia. The tumor can be primarily astrocytic with eosinophilic inclusions called Rosenthal fibers, or it can be myxomatous with cystic areas that can expand rapidly.

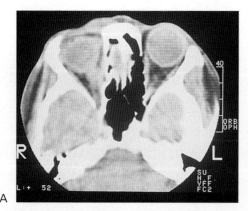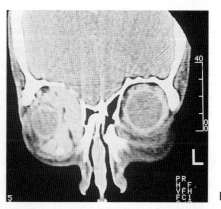

FIGURE 10.137. Axial **(A)** and coronal **(B)** computed tomography scans of the patient with an orbital varix (Fig. 10.136). There is a significant increase in the size of the varix when filming the coronal image because the head is in a dependent position.

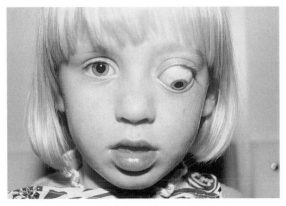

FIGURE 10.138. Child with massive proptosis and downward displacement of the left globe secondary to an optic nerve glioma.

Management. Treatment of orbital gliomas is controversial, ranging from observation to aggressive intracranial and orbital surgery. If the tumor is restricted to the orbit, vision is good, and proptosis is minimal, careful follow-up with repeated assessment of visual acuity, color vision, proptosis, visual fields, visual evoked response, and repeat CT or MRI scans is indicated. If vision is compromised, tumor growth

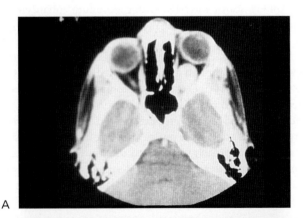

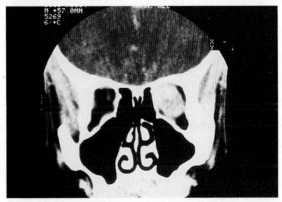

FIGURE 10.139. Axial **(A)** and coronal **(B)** computed tomography scans demonstrate fusiform enlargement of the optic nerve caused by a well-circumscribed optic nerve glioma.

documented, and the chiasm or other side are not involved, neurosurgical resection of the optic nerve from the chiasm to its insertion into the globe is the treatment of choice. In bilateral cases or those involving the chiasm, surgery is restricted to orbital resection for massively proptotic blind eyes or ventricular shunting to relieve hydrocephalus. The efficacy of irradiation or chemotherapy for this tumor is questionable.

Neurofibroma

Clinical Features. Neurofibromas can occur as solitary tumors or as manifestations of systemic neurofibromatosis. Pathologically, they are composed of intertwining bundles of Schwann cells within the nerve sheaths, endoneural fibroblasts, and axons. In contrast to the solitary neurofibromas that occur in the second decade, the diffuse and plexiform lesions present in the early years. Early plexiform neurofibromas present with ptosis and eyelid thickening; however, the globe itself, including sclera, iris, ciliary body, cornea, and choroid, may be infiltrated, resulting in glaucoma and buphthalmos (Fig. 10.140). Visual loss may occur as a result of occlusion amblyopia, orbital and ocular infiltration, or glaucoma. Neurofibromatosis is associated with café-au-lait spots, axillary freckling, fibroma molluscum, dysplasia of the orbital walls, congenital glaucoma, iris nodules, optic nerve gliomas, and perioptic meningiomas. Absence of portions of the sphenoid wing can cause pulsating exophthalmos (Fig. 10.141).

Neurofibromatosis is inherited as an autosomal-dominant gene with irregular penetrance. Two forms of the disease, central and peripheral, occur, and they rarely overlap. Peripheral neurofibromatosis is heralded by the development of café-au-lait spots, associated with visceral neurofibromas, pheochromocytomas, and neurilemomas, and various skeletal abnormalities, including absence of the sphenoid wing. Central neurofibromatosis is characterized by development of tumors in the CNS, including astrocytomas, meningiomas, schwannomas, and ependymomas.

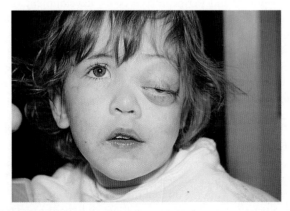

FIGURE 10.140. Neurofibroma of the left orbit results in proptosis, downward displacement of the globe, ptosis, and glaucoma secondary to ocular involvement.

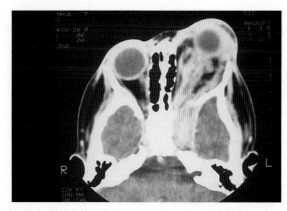

FIGURE 10.141. An axial computed tomography scan shows a diffuse neurofibroma of the left orbit and intracranial extension.

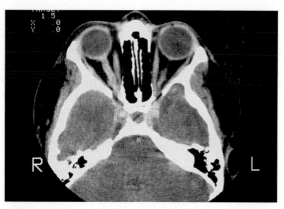

FIGURE 10.142. An axial scan of an optic nerve sheath meningioma of the right optic nerve. Notice the "railroad-track" sign of a central lucent optic nerve surrounded by tumor.

Management. Solitary neurofibromas are rare. However, they can be easily excised. Plexiform lesions are difficult to treat, because they infiltrate normal tissues and recurrent debulking procedures may not be cosmetically satisfactory. Some surgeons suggest that debulking procedures are unacceptable and that, in the cases of major orbital involvement, only exenteration can produce an effective result.

Meningiomas

Meningiomas arise from the meningothelial cap cells of the arachnoid villi. They most commonly occur in middle-aged women, and the symptoms depend on the lesion's location. In addition to meningiomas of the optic nerve, intracranial meningiomas can affect orbital and visual structures, especially suprasellar, sphenoid ridge, and olfactory groove tumors.

Clinical Features. *Optic nerve sheath meningiomas* initially cause visual disturbances that are usually associated with minimal proptosis. Color vision abnormalities and visual field changes such as enlargement of the blind spot or a contracted visual field precede the loss of visual acuity. The optic nerve undergoes progressive edema, with engorgement of papillary and peripapillary vessels, development of optociliary shunt vessels, and eventual optic atrophy. CT scans and MRI studies are helpful in the diagnosis and follow-up (Fig. 10.142). The intracranial extent of the tumor can be best visualized on gadolinium-enhanced MRI scans. The tumor can appear as a tubular, fusiform enlargement or as a globular thickening. *Psammomatous meningiomas* are calcified and can demonstrate by a "railroad track" sign on the CT scan, with a lucent optic nerve surrounded by high-density tumor.

The *sphenoid wing meningioma* is the most common intracranial meningioma to present with orbital findings. This tumor arises from the dura of the sphenoid bone, grows in a plaque pattern, is infiltrative, and causes hyperostosis, making total excision difficult and recurrence common. Vision is often not affected, and early findings can be subtle. Unilateral eyelid edema, temporal fullness, and proptosis

may be evident in the absence of cranial nerve palsies and visual deficits (Fig. 10.143). Vision is eventually threatened from optic nerve compression by the tumor or hyperostosis. Visual loss can slowly progress, and similar to the findings in optic nerve sheath tumors, color vision and field loss can precede changes in visual acuity. A combination of CT scans and MRI studies can delineate the extent of the tumor. Hyperostosis and psammomatous calcifications are easily seen on CT scans, and MRI with gadolinium enhancement better delineates the soft tissue extent of the tumor (Figs. 10.144, 10.145).

Management. Patients with good vision and slowly progressive lesional growth can be observed with repeated CT or MRI studies to document the progression of optic nerve sheath meningiomas. Aggressive tumors or those with intracranial spread require surgical excision. After the tumor is suspected of entering the optic canal, a combined neurosurgical orbital approach is indicated to ensure complete excision and prevent recurrence and spread to the chiasm. Radiotherapy is reserved for certain bilateral cases, and its efficacy is controversial. Chemotherapy is ineffective.

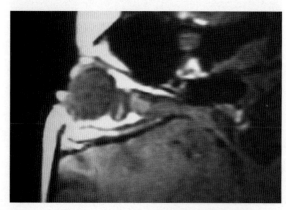

FIGURE 10.143. The T1-weighted magnetic resonance image demonstrates the intracranial extension of an optic nerve sheath meningioma.

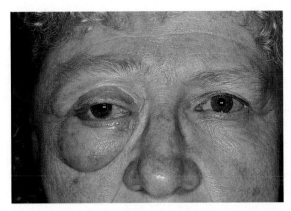

FIGURE 10.144. A patient with a sphenoid wing meningioma presented with massive proptosis, swelling of the eyelids, and fullness in the right temporalis fossa. Vision and globe motility were intact.

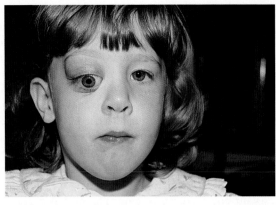

FIGURE 10.146. A child presented with rapidly evolving proptosis, downward displacement of the globe, and erythema of the eyelids.

Observation or surgical excision are the primary options in the treatment of sphenoid wing meningiomas. Slowly progressive lesions in older women can be observed for long periods, until cosmesis is unacceptable and vision is deteriorating. Bony invasion and involvement of vital structures may prevent complete excision; however, major debulking with removal of tumor and hyperostotic bone can decrease proptosis and decrease compressive symptoms, with some reversal of vision. Although radiotherapy is recommended after incomplete excision, its efficacy is questionable.

Mesenchymal Tumors

Rhabdomyosarcoma
Clinical Features. Rhabdomyosarcoma is the most common primary orbital malignancy of childhood. The tumor arises from the pluripotential mesenchyme that normally differentiates into striated muscle. The well-differentiated form is rare, with the embryonal and alveolar type being most common. Rhabdomyosarcoma presents with rapidly evolving exophthalmos associated with eyelid injection and

swelling (Fig. 10.146). The tumor is most commonly found in superior and retrobulbar locations, and it can erode through the orbital bones into the sinuses, causing nasal stuffiness or nosebleeds. On CT scans, the mass can be circumscribed or poorly defined and homogeneous in density; it can destroy bone (Fig. 10.147). The differential diagnosis includes neuroblastoma, chloroma (i.e., granulocytic sarcoma), pseudotumor, lymphangioma, and hemangioma.

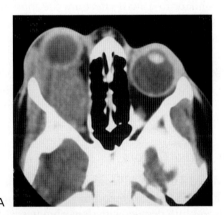

A

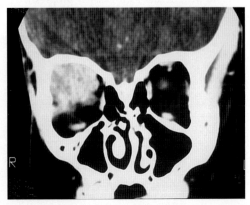

B

FIGURE 10.147. Axial **(A)** and coronal **(B)** computed tomography scans of a rhabdomyosarcoma reveal a large, homogenous mass in the superior aspect of the right orbit.

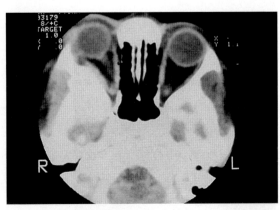

FIGURE 10.145. An axial computed tomography scan of a sphenoid wing meningioma demonstrates massive hyperostosis of the right sphenoid wing.

Management. Treatment consists of immediate biopsy and excision, followed by irradiation and chemotherapy. The radiation dose varies from 4000 to 6000 cGy units, depending on the amount of residual tumor and age of the child. After irradiation, visual loss secondary to corneal changes, cataracts, and retinal problems are very common. Enophthalmos, ptosis, lacrimal duct stenosis, facial asymmetry, and bone hypoplasia can also occur. Chemotherapy consists of vincristine, actinomycin, and cyclophosphamide. Some centers are now advocating excision followed by chemotherapy without irradiation, especially in younger children. Exenteration is reserved for the rare radioresistant and recurrent tumor. The overall 5-year survival rate is 95% for cases of orbital rhabdomyosarcoma, much better than for rhabdomyosarcomas elsewhere in the body. All children should be referred to a pediatric oncology center, where a complete workup for metastases and staging of the disease is done before commencing appropriate treatment.

Fibrous Histiocytoma
Clinical Features. The most common mesenchymal orbital tumor of adults is the fibrous histiocytoma. The tumor consists of fibrous-appearing histiocytic cells and usually presents in middle life, occurs equally in men and women, and has a variable growth pattern. Proptosis and visual disturbances secondary to a mass effect are the most common findings. On CT scans, the mass is usually well circumscribed and can resemble other tumors such as a cavernous hemangioma and hemangiopericytoma.

Management. Complete tumor excision is the treatment of choice. However, if the lesion is recurrent and aggressive, a limited exenteration may be necessary to eliminate the disease. Radiotherapy has not been effective.

Lacrimal Gland Tumors

Benign Mixed Tumor or Pleomorphic Adenoma
Clinical Features. The pleomorphic adenoma presents in the fourth and fifth decades with slowly progressive proptosis and displacement of the globe downward and medially. At the time of presentation, the symptoms have usually existed for a few or more months. The tumor is usually not painful unless it has undergone malignant change or corneal exposure has occurred. On CT scans, it appears as a globular, well-circumscribed mass, and pressure may have expanded the lacrimal fossa (Fig. 10.148).

Management. Complete excision without biopsy is the treatment of choice. If the tumor is not completely excised, it can recur and rarely undergoes malignant change. Similarly, longstanding pleomorphic adenomas that are not removed can undergo malignant change, heralded by increasing symptoms, especially pain.

Adenoid Cystic Carcinoma
Clinical Features. Adenoid cystic carcinoma is the most common epithelial malignancy of the lacrimal gland. Its incidence peaks in the fourth and second decades. Misdiagnosis is most common in the younger age group, because the tumor is not suspected. The tumor usually occurs as a rapidly developing mass in the lacrimal fossa. Because of its propensity for perineural spread, it can be associated with pain or paresthesia. On CT scans, the tumor can be well circumscribed. However, bony destruction, calcification, or extension toward the orbital apex are more often diagnostic (Fig. 10.149). The course of the disease can vary from rapid progression to a more indolent course, with long periods of remission followed by recurrent disease locally or metastasis to the lungs. The 5-year survival rate is approximately 50%, with a continuing decline to less than 20% in 15 years. The relentlessly fatal course despite long disease-free intervals necessitates aggressive long-term follow-up.

Management. Exenteration followed by radical radiotherapy was regarded as the treatment of choice for adenoid cystic carcinoma. Wide resection followed by radiotherapy does not seem to negatively alter the prognosis and is the current treatment of choice. The dismal prognosis may be related to the escape of the tumor past the surgical margins of resection by early perineural or bony spread before diagnosis.

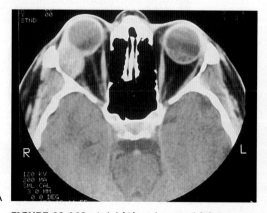 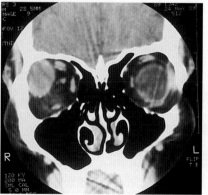

FIGURE 10.148. Axial **(A)** and coronal **(B)** computed tomography scans demonstrate a globular, well-circumscribed mass in the right lacrimal fossa, which is typical of a benign mixed tumor.

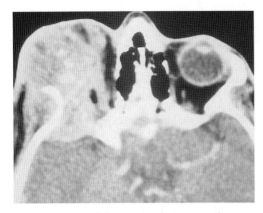

FIGURE 10.149. An axial computed tomography scan shows adenoid cystic carcinoma of the lacrimal gland with intracranial invasion. Notice the bone destruction and calcification.

Secondary Tumors

Metastatic Tumors

Metastases to the orbit can be categorized as those appearing in the pediatric or the adult group. In children, the most common metastases include neuroblastoma, leukemia, and Ewing's sarcoma. Breast, lung, genitourinary, gastrointestinal, prostate, thyroid, carcinoid, and renal metastases occur in the adult population. Adult metastatic disease can present with inflammatory findings, diplopia, and pain. The development of enophthalmos rather than proptosis secondary to tumor-induced cicatrization is most commonly seen in sclerosing breast carcinoma. However, it can occur in lung, prostate, and gastrointestinal carcinomas.

Neuroblastoma

Clinical Features. Neuroblastoma arises from the primitive neuroblasts of the sympathetic system, most commonly from the retroperitoneal abdominal region near the adrenal gland, followed by the thorax, cervix, and pelvis. Orbital involvement occurs late in the disease and presents with abrupt ecchymotic unilateral or bilateral proptosis, ptosis, and periorbital swelling. Other ocular manifestations include opsoclonus-myoclonus and Horner's syndrome secondary to mediastinal involvement. CT scans reveal involvement of the superolateral orbit and zygoma with areas of bony destruction and lucency secondary to necrosis.

Management. Treatment consists of aggressive chemotherapy with or without local irradiation. Disease-free survival after 2 years is less than 10%. Total-body irradiation followed by bone marrow rescue has had encouraging results.

Breast Carcinoma

Clinical Features. Breast carcinoma is the most common orbital metastasis in women. It usually occurs a few years after mastectomy, but it can be the presenting symptom or occur some 20 years later. The tumor causes a firm infiltration of the orbit and has a predilection for extraocular muscles, resulting in diplopia. The sclerosing cicatricial breast carci-

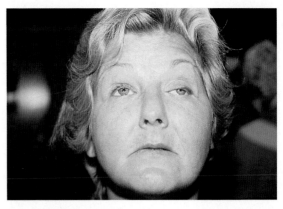

FIGURE 10.150. The patient has breast metastases to the left superior orbit, resulting in ptosis, decreased elevation of the left globe, and enophthalmos.

noma results in enophthalmos, ptosis, and restricted motility (Fig. 10.150). CT scans reveal a diffuse, infiltrative, reticulated pattern and involvement of the muscles. On MRI, the lesions often are hyperdense on the T2-weighted image (Fig. 10.151).

Management. The treatment of orbital breast carcinoma is primarily radiation therapy, with adjunctive hormonal manipulation if indicated. The indication for chemotherapy is a rapidly progressing systemic disease, especially in an estrogen receptor–negative tumor. The purpose of the treatment is palliative, because even the most aggressive treatment does not usually increase survival after the disease is metastatic.

Mucocele

Clinical Features. Mucoceles are cystic lesions arising most commonly from the frontal and ethmoidal sinuses. Obstruction of the normal sinus ostia results in entrapment of secretory epithelium, expansion of the sinus, thinning of the bony walls, and eventual erosion into the orbit. Patients with frontoethmoidal mucoceles present with a downward and lateral displacement of the globe. Maxillary mucoceles can cause an upward or downward displacement of the globe, depending on the destruction of the orbital floor and

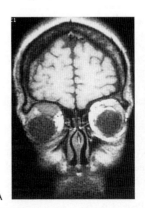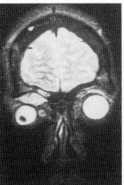

A   B

FIGURE 10.151. T1-weighted **(A)** and T2-weighted **(B)** magnetic resonance images of a breast carcinoma metastasis in the right superior orbit. Notice the hyperdense lesion on the T2-weighted scan.

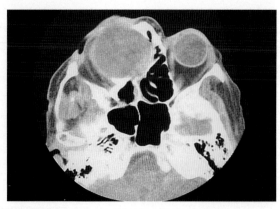

FIGURE 10.152. Computed tomography scan of a large, globular frontoethmoidal mucocele.

size of the cyst. Mucoceles of the sphenoid and posterior ethmoid sinus can cause functional visual problems such as a loss of vision and diplopia secondary to compression of the optic nerve, apical structures, and cavernous sinus. The diagnosis is easily made on CT scans, which demonstrate an expanded, opacified sinus filled with a soft tissue density mass with well-defined margins and with erosion and sclerosis of bone (Fig. 10.152).

Management. Treatment is complete removal of the mass and secretory epithelium with reestablishment of normal sinus drainage or obliteration of the sinus with a fat implant. External and endoscopic surgical approaches are used.

BIBLIOGRAPHY

Abramson DH, Ellsworth RM, Tretter P, et al. The treatment of orbital rhabdomyosarcoma with radiation and chemotherapy. *Ophthalmology* 1979;86:1330.

Abramson DH, Jereb B. Radiation treatment of malignant ophthalmic neoplasms. In: Smith BC. Ophthalmic plastic and reconstructive surgery, vol 2. St. Louis: CV Mosby; 1987:1165.

Alper MG. Management of primary optic nerve sheath meningiomas. Current status-therapy in controversy. *J Clin Neuroophthalmol* 1981;1:101.

Arndt KA. Manual of dermatologic therapeutics. Boston: Little Brown & Co; 1978.

Arthurs B, Silverstone P, Della Rocca RC. Medial wall fractures. In: Bosniak SL, Smith BC. Advances in ophthalmic plastic and reconstructive surgery, vol 6. New York: Pergamon Press; 1987:393.

Baghdassarian SA, Shammas HF. Eosinophilic granuloma of the orbit. *Ann Ophthalmol* 1977;9:1247.

Ballen PH. Thermal chemical and radiation burns. In: Steward WB. American Academy of Ophthalmology manual on ophthalmic plastic and reconstructive surgery. San Francisco: American Academy of Ophthalmology; 1984:280.

Beard C. Ptosis. 3rd ed. St. Louis: CV Mosby; 1981.

Bedrossian EH Jr. Eyelid trauma repair. In: Albert DM. Ophthalmic surgery: Principles and techniques. Blackwell Science; 1999:1155.

Bedrossian EH Jr. Evaluation of orbital injuries. In: Bosniak SL, Smith BC. Advances in ophthalmic plastic and reconstructive surgery. New York: Pergamon Press; 1987:37.

Bedrossian EH Jr. Banked fascia lata as an orbital floor implant. *Ophthal Plast Reconstr Surg* 1993;1:66.

Berlin AJ. Acute adnexal trauma. In: Stewart WB. Ophthalmic plastic

and reconstructive surgery. Academy manuals program. San Francisco: American Academy of Ophthalmology; 1984:273.

Bosniak SL. Ectropion. In: Smith BC. Ophthalmic plastic and reconstructive surgery. St. Louis: CV Mosby; 1987:562.

Boyd MJ, Collin O Jr. Capillary hemangiomas: an approach to their management. *Br J Ophthalmol* 1991;75:298.

Bullock JD, Warwar RE, Bartley GB, et al. Unusual orbital foreign bodies. *Ophthal Plast Reconstr Surg* 1999;15:44-51.

Bullock JD, Yanes B. Ophthalmic manifestations of metastatic breast cancer. *Ophthalmology* 1980;87:961.

Caronni EP. Craniofacial surgery. Boston: Little Brown & Co; 1985.

Cassady JV. Developmental anatomy of the nasolacrimal duct. *Arch Ophthalmol* 1952;47:141.

Castronuovo S, Prokhel GB. Orbital hemorrhage. In: Linberg JV. Oculoplastic and orbital emergencies. East Norwalk, CT: Appleton & Lange; 1990:145.

Char DH. Thyroid eye disease. 2nd ed. New York: Churchill-Livingstone; 1990.

Collin JR. Entropion and trichiasis. In: Stewart WB. Ophthalmic plastic and reconstructive surgery. San Francisco: American Academy of Ophthalmology; 1984:131.

Crawford JS, Pashby RC, Apt RK. Embryology and congenital anomalies. In: Stewart WB. Ophthalmic plastic and reconstructive surgery. San Francisco: American Academy of Ophthalmology; 1984:90.

Della Rocca RC, Bedrossian EH Jr. Orbital floor fractures. In: Clayman HM. Atlas of contemporary ophthalmic surgery. St. Louis: CV Mosby; 1980;899.

Della Rocca RC, Bedrossian EH Jr. Zygomaticomaxillary fractures. In: Clayman HM. Atlas of contemporary ophthalmic surgery. St. Louis: CV Mosby; 1980:909.

Demant E, Hurwitz JJ. Canaliculitis: review of twelve cases. *Can J Ophthalmol* 1980;15:73.

Dortzbach RK, Segrest DR. Orbital aspergillosis. *Ophthal Surg* 1983;14:240.

Duke-Elder S. Congenital anomalies of the ocular adnexa. In: Duke-Elder S. System of ophthalmology, vol 3. St. Louis: CV Mosby; 1963:827.

Ellis JH, Banks PM, Campbell J, et al. Lymphoid tumor of the ocular adnexa. *Ophthalmology* 1985;92:1311.

Engrav LH, Heimbach DM, Walkinshaw MD, et al. Excision of burns of the face. *Plast Reconstr Surg* 1986;77:744.

Ferry AP, Abedi S. Diagnosis and management of rhino-orbital-cerebral mucormycosis (phycomycosis): a report of 16 personally observed cases. *Ophthalmology* 1983;90:1096.

Flanagan JC, Mauriello JA. Management of lacrimal sac tumors. *Adv Ophthal Plast Reconstr Surg* 1984;3:399.

Flanagan JC, Stokes DP. Lacrimal sac tumors. *Ophthalmology* 1985;85:1282.

Font RF, Ferry AP. Carcinoma metastatic to the eye and orbit: III. A clinicopathologic study of 28 cases metastatic to the orbit. *Cancer* 1976;38:1326.

Font RL, Gamel JW. Adenoid cystic carcinoma of the lacrimal gland. A clinicopathologic study of 79 cases. In: Nicholson DH. Ocular pathology update. New York: Masson Publishing USA; 1980:277.

Font RL, Gamel JW. Epithelial tumors of the lacrimal gland: an analysis of 265 cases. In: Jakobiec FA. Ocular and adnexal tumors. Birmingham: Aesculapius; 1978:787.

Font RL, Hidayat AA. Fibrous histiocytoma of the orbit: a clinicopathologic study of 150 cases. *Hum Pathol* 1982;13:199.

Font RL. Eyelids and lacrimal drainage system. In: Spencer WH. Ophthalmic pathology. 3rd ed. Philadelphia: WB Saunders; 1986:2141.

Frank A, Wachtel T. The early treatment and reconstruction of eyelid burns. *J Trauma* 1983;23:874.

Friedberg MD, Rapuano CJ. Wills Eye Hospital office and emergency room diagnosis and treatment of eye disease. Philadelphia: JB Lippincott; 1990:17.

Garber PF, MacDonald D, Beyer-Machale CK. Management of trauma to the eyelids. In: Smith BC. Ophthalmic plastic and reconstructive surgery. St. Louis: CV Mosby; 1987:437.

Garber PF. Management of injuries to the lacrimal system. In: Bosniak SL, Smith BC. Advances in ophthalmic plastic and reconstructive surgery, vol 3. New York: Pergamon Press; 1984:1175.

Geeraetes WJ. Ocular syndromes. 3rd ed. Philadelphia: Lea & Febiger; 1976.

Glaser JS. Infranuclear disorders of eye movement. In: Tasman W, Jaeger EA. Duane's clinical ophthalmology, vol 2. Philadelphia: JB Lippincott; 1993.

Glassburn JR, Klionsky M, Brady LW. Radiation therapy for metastatic disease involving the orbit. *Am J Clin Oncol* 1984;7:145.

Griffith DG, Salasche SJ, Clemons DE. Cutaneous abnormalities of the eyelid and face. New York: McGraw-Hill; 1987.

Grove AS, McCord CD. Orbital disorders: diagnosis and management. In: McCord CD, Tannenbaum M. Oculoplastic surgery. New York: Raven Press; 1987.

Grove AS. Giant dermoid cysts of the orbit. *Ophthalmology* 1979;86:1513.

Haik BG, Carroll GS, Kilmer SL. Periocular hemangiomas. In: Mannis MJ, Macsai MS, Huntley AC. Eye and skin disease. Philadelphia: Lippincott-Raven; 1996.

Haik BG, Karcioglu ZA, Pechous BP. Capillary hemangioma (infantile periocular hemangioma). *Surv Ophthalmol* 1994;38:399.

Hanneken AM, Miller NR, et al. Treatment of carotid-cavernous sinus fistulas using a detachable balloon catheter through the superior ophthalmic vein. *Arch Ophthalmol* 1989;107:87.

Harris GJ, Sakol PJ, et al. An analysis of thirty cases of orbital lymphangioma: pathophysiologic considerations and management recommendations. *Ophthalmology* 1990;97:1583.

Harris GJ, Will BR. Orbital aspergillosis. *Ophthal Plast Reconstr Surg* 1989;5:207.

Harris GT, DiClementi D. Congenital dacryocystocele. *Arch Ophthalmol* 1982;100:1763.

Hawes MJ. Canalicular lacerations. In: Linberg JV. Oculoplastic and orbital emergencies. East Norwalk, CT: Appleton & Lange; 1990:15.

Houle TV, Ellis PP. Aspergillosis of the orbit with immunosuppressive therapy. *Surv Ophthalmol* 1975;20:35.

Hoyt C, Lambert S. Lids. In: Taylor D. Pediatric ophthalmology. Boston: Blackwell Scientific Publications; 1990:141.

Hoyt WF, Baghdassarian SA. Optic glioma of childhood. Natural history and rationale for conservative management. *Br J Ophthalmol* 1969;53:793.

Iliff CE. Mucoceles in the orbit. *Arch Ophthalmol* 1973;89:392.

Imes RK, Hoyt WF. Childhood chiasmal gliomas: update on the fate of patients in the 1969 San Francisco study. *Br J Ophthalmol* 1986;70:179.

Jackson IT, Laws ER, Martin RD. The surgical management of orbital neurofibromatosis. *Reconstr Surg* 1983;71:751.

Jakobiec FA, Depot MJ, Kennerdell JS, et al. Combined clinical and computed tomographic diagnosis of orbital glioma and meningioma. *Ophthalmology* 1984;91:137.

Jakobiec FA, Iwamoto T, Patell M, et al. Ocular adnexal monoclonal lymphoid tumors with a favorable prognosis. *Ophthalmology* 1986;93:1547.

Jakobiec FA, Jones IS. Neurogenic tumors. In: Duane's clinical ophthalmology, vol 2. Philadelphia: JB Lippincott; 1992.

Jakobiec FA, Jones IS. Vascular tumors, malformation, and degenerations. In: Tasman W, Jaeger EA. Duane's clinical ophthalmology, vol 2. Philadelphia: JB Lippincott; 1992:6.

Jakobiec FA, Rootman J, Jones IS. Secondary and metastatic tumors of the orbit. In: Tasman W, Jaeger EA. Duane's clinical ophthalmology, vol 2. Philadelphia: JB Lippincott; 1992.

Janetta PJ. Hemifacial spasm. In: Samili M, Janetta PJ. The cranial nerves. Berlin: Springer-Verlag; 1981:484.

Jones DB, Steinkuller PG. Microbial preseptal and orbital cellulitis. In: Duane TD. Clinical ophthalmology, vol 4. Philadelphia: JB Lippincott; 1989.

Jones HM. Some orbital complications of nose and throat conditions. *J R Med Soc* 1981;74:409.

Jones KL. Smith's recognizable patterns of human malformation. 5th ed. Philadelphia: WB Saunders; 1997.

Jordan DR, Patrinely JR, Anderson RL, et al. Essential blepharospasm and related dystonias. *Surv Ophthalmol* 1989;34:123.

Katowitz JA, Low JE. Lacrimal drainage surgery. In: Tasman W, Jaeger EA. Duane's clinical ophthalmology, vol 6. Philadelphia: JB Lippincott; 1993.

Kennerdell JS, Dresner SC. The nonspecific orbital inflammatory syndromes. *Surv Ophthalmol* 1981;29:93.

Kilmer SL. Adnexal tumors. In: Mannis MJ, Macsai MS, Huntley AC. Eye and skin disease. Philadelphia: Lippincott-Raven; 1996.

Kingston JE, McElwain TJ, Malpas JS. Childhood rhabdomyosarcoma: experience of the children's solid tumor group. *Br J Cancer* 1983;48:195.

Kivela T, Tarkkanen A. The merkel cell and associated neoplasms in the eyelids and periocular region. *Surv Ophthalmol* 1990;35:171.

Kobalter AS, Roth A. Benign epithelial neoplasms. In: Mannis MJ, Macsai MS, Huntley AC. Eye and skin disease. Philadelphia: Lippincott-Raven; 1996.

Kobryn JL, Blodi FC, Weingeist TA. Ocular and orbital manifestations of neurofibromatosis. *Surv Ophthalmol* 1979;24:45.

Kohn R. Hepler Management of limited rhino-orbital mucormycosis without exenteration. *Ophthalmology* 1985;92:1440.

Kulwin D. Acute eyelid and periocular burns. In: Linberg JV. Oculoplastic and orbital emergencies. East Norwalk, CT: Appleton & Lange; 1990:39.

Kulwin D. Modern management of ophthalmic burns. *Highlights Ophthalmol* 1990;30:1.

Kulwin D. Treatment of periorbital burns. In: Bosniak SL. Advances in ophthalmic plastic and reconstructive surgery, vol 7. New York: Pergamon Press; 1987:167.

Kuper Smith MJ, Berenstein A, et al. Management of nontraumatic vascular shunts involving the cavernous sinus. *Ophthalmology* 1988;95:121.

Kushner BJ. Congenital nasolacrimal system obstruction. *Arch Ophthalmol* 1982;100:597.

Kushner BJ. Intralesional corticosteroid injection for infantile adnexal hemangiomas. *Am J Ophthalmol* 1982;93:496.

Lee DA, Campbell JR, Waller RR, et al. A clinicopathologic study of primary adenoid cystic carcinoma of the lacrimal gland. *Ophthalmology* 1985;92:128.

Leone CR, Lloyd WC. Treatment protocol for orbital inflammatory disease. *Ophthalmology* 1985;92:1325.

Leone CR. The management of ophthalmic Graves' disease. *Ophthalmology* 1984;91:770.

Leone CR. The management of pediatric lacrimal problems. *Ophthal Plast Reconstr Surg* 1989;5:34.

Lewis RA, Gerson LP, Axelson KA, et al. Von Recklinghausen neurofibromatosis. II. Incidence of optic gliomata. *Ophthalmology* 1984;91:929.

Long JA. A method of monocanalicular silicone intubation. *Opthalmic Surg* 1988;3:204.

Lowry JC, Bartley GB. Complications of blepharoplasty. *Surv Ophthalmol* 1994;38:327.

Mansour AM, Cheng KP, et al. Congenital dacryocystocele; a collaborative review. *Ophthalmology* 1991;98:1744.

Maurer H, Foulkes M, Gehan E. Intergroup Rhabdomyosarcoma Study II, preliminary report. *Proc Am Soc Clin Oncol* 1983;2:70.

Mauriello JA, Flanagan JC. Management of orbital and ocular adnexal tumors and inflammations. New York: Field and Wood Medical Publishers; 1990:226.

McCord CD, Tanenbaum M, Dryden RM, et al. Eyelid malpositions. In: McCord CD, Tanenbaum M. Oculoplastic surgery. New York: Raven Press; 1987:279.

McCord CD, Tannenbaum M. Oculoplastic surgery. New York: Raven Press; 1987.

McNab AA, Colin D Jr. Eyelid and canthal lacerations. In: Linberg JV. Oculoplastic and orbital emergencies. East Norwalk, CT: Appleton & Lange; 1990:1.

Moster ML. CPEO, MERRF and MELAS. In: Abstracts from the North American Neuro-ophthalmology Society 18th Annual Meeting; 1992.

Mulliken JB, Young AE. Vascular birthmarks: hemangiomas and malformations. Philadelphia: WB Saunders; 1988.

Musarella MA, Chen HSL, DeBoer G, et al. Ocular involvement in neuroblastoma: prognostic implications. *Ophthalmology* 1984; 91:936.

Nelson CC, Oestriecher J. Eyelid trauma. In: Focal points. San Francisco: American Academy of Ophthalmology; 1991:10.

Nunery WR, Martin RT. Zygoma and complex facial fractures. In: Linberg JV. Oculoplastic and orbital emergencies. East Norwalk, CT: Appleton & Lange; 1990:1167.

Nunery WR, Wilson FM. Suppurative canaliculitis. In: Bosniak SL, Smith BC. Advances in ophthalmic plastic and reconstructive surgery, vol 3. New York: Pergamon Press; 1984:157.

Orcutt JC. Orbital foreign bodies. In: Linberg JV. Oculoplastic and orbital emergencies. East Norwalk, CT: Appleton & Lange; 1990:183.

Osher RH, Schatz NJ, Duane TD. Acquired orbital retraction syndrome. *Arch Ophthalmol* 1980;98:1798.

Paris GL, Bullock JD, Lauring L. Ectropion. In: Stewart WB. Ophthalmic plastic and reconstructive surgery. San Francisco: American Academy of Ophthalmology; 1984:143.

Peterson RA, Robb RM. The natural course of congenital obstruction of the nasolacrimal duct. *J Pediatr Ophthalmol Strabismus* 1978;15:246.

Petro J, Tooze FM, Bales CR, et al. Ocular injuries associated with periorbital fracture. *J Trauma* 1979;19:730.

Reifler DM. Orbital metastases with enophthalmos: a review of the literature. *Henry Ford Hosp Med J* 1985;33:171.

Rice CD, Kersten RC, Mrak RE. An orbital hemangiopericytoma recurrent after 30 years. *Arch Ophthalmol* 1989;107:552.

Rootman J, Hay E, Graeb D, Miller R. Orbital-adnexal lymphangiomas. A spectrum of hemodynamically isolated vascular hamartomas. *Ophthalmology* 1986;93:1558.

Rootman J, Nugent R. The classification and management of acute orbital pseudotumors. *Ophthalmology* 1982;89:1040.

Rootman J, Robertson WJ. Tumors. In: Rootman J. Diseases of the orbit. Philadelphia: JB Lippincott; 1988.

Rootman J. Diseases of the orbit. Philadelphia: JB Lippincott; 1988:231.

Roy FH. Ocular differential diagnosis. 3rd ed. Philadelphia: Lea & Febiger; 1984.

Ryan SJ, Font RC. Primary epithelial neoplasms of the lacrimal sac. *Am J Ophthalmol* 1973;76:73.

Sauer GC. Manual of skin diseases. 6th ed. Philadelphia: JB Lippincott; 1991.

Scott AB. Botulinum treatment for blepharospasm. In: Smith BC. Ophthalmic plastic and reconstructive surgery. St. Louis: CV Mosby; 1987:609.

Sergott RC, Grossman RI, Savino PJ, Bosley TM, Schatz NJ. The syndrome of worsening of dural cavernous sinus arteriovenous malformation. *Ophthalmology* 1987;94:205.

Setzkorn RK, Lee DJ, Iliff NT, Green WR. Hemangiopericytoma of the orbit treated with conservative surgery and radiotherapy. *Arch Ophthalmol* 1987;105:1103.

Sherman RP, Rootman J, Lapointe JS. Orbital dermoids: clinical presentation and management. *Br J Ophthalmol* 1984;68:642.

Shore JW, McCord CD, Popham JK. Surgery of the eyelids. In: Duane's clinical ophthalmology, vol 6. Philadelphia: JB Lippincott; 1992.

Silver, Bernard, et al. Ophthalmic plastic surgery: a manual prepared for the use of graduates in medicine. San Francisco: American Academy of Ophthalmology; 1977:242.

Slamovits TL, Glaser JS. The pupils and accommodation. In: Tasman W, Jaeger EA. Duane's clinical ophthalmology, vol 2. Philadelphia: JB Lippincott; 1993.

Slamovits TL. External disease and cornea. Basic clinical science course, sect 8. San Francisco: American Academy of Ophthalmology; 1993:87.

Slamovits TL. Neuro-ophthalmology. Basic clinical science course, sect 5. San Francisco: American Academy of Ophthalmology; 1993:119.

Slamovits TL. Orbit, eyelid and lacrimal system. Basic clinical science course, sect 7. San Francisco: American Academy of Ophthalmology; 1993:96.

Smit TJ, Mouritis MP. Monocanalicular lesions: to reconstruct or not. *Ophthalmology* 1999;106:1310.

Smith B, Regan WF Jr. Blowout fractures of the orbit: mechanism and correction of internal orbital fracture. *Am J Ophthalmol* 1957;44:733.

Smith BC. Ophthalmic plastic and reconstructive surgery. St. Louis: CV Mosby; 1987.

Smith BC, Nesi FA. Practical techniques in ophthalmic surgery. St. Louis: CV Mosby; 1981:50.

Sutula FC, Glover AT. Eyelid necrosis following intralesional corticosteroid injection for capillary hemangioma. *Ophthalmic Surg* 1987;24:103.

Tanenbaum M, McCord CD. The lacrimal drainage system. In: Tasman W, Jaeger EA. Duane's clinical ophthalmology, vol 4. Philadelphia: JB Lippincott; 1993.

Vinken PJ, Bruy GW. Handbook of clinical neurology, vol 42, part 1. Amsterdam: North Holland Publishing; 1981:319.

Vogintzks KV. Lymphoid tumors of the orbit and ocular adnexa: a long-term follow-up. *Ann Ophthalmol* 1984;16:1046.

Weinstein GS, Anderson RL. Diagnosis and treatment of blepharospasm. In: Smith BC. Ophthalmic plastic and reconstructive surgery. St. Louis: CV Mosby; 1987:600.

Weiss A, Friendly D, Eglin K, et al. Bacterial periorbital and orbital cellulitis in childhood. *Ophthalmology* 1983;90:195.

Wharam M, Beltangady M, Hays D, et al. Localized orbital rhabdomyosarcoma. An interim report of the Intergroup Rhabdomyosarcoma Study Committee. *Ophthalmology* 1987;94:251.

Wilson ME, Parker PL, Chavis RM. Conservative management of childhood orbital lymphangioma. *Ophthalmology* 1989;96:484.

Wilson WB, Gordon M, Lehman RAW. Meningiomas confined to the optic canal and foramina. *Surg Neurol* 1979;12:21.

Woog JJ, Albert DM, Solt LC, et al. Neurofibromatosis of the eyelid and orbit. *Int Ophthalmol Clin* 1982;22:157.

Wright JE. Orbital vascular anomalies. *Trans Am Acad Ophthalmol* 1974;78:OP606.

Wright JE, Call NB, Liaricos S. Primary optic nerve meningioma. *Br J Ophthalmol* 1980;64:553.

Wright JE, McDonald WI, Call NB. Management of optic nerve gliomas. *Br J Ophthalmol* 1980;64:545.

Wright JE. Factors affecting the survival of patients with lacrimal gland tumors. *Can J Ophthalmol* 1982;17:3.

Wright JE. Primary malignant neoplasms of the lacrimal gland. *Br J Ophthalmol* 1992;76:401.

Wright JE. Primary optic nerve meningiomas: clinical presentation and management. *Trans Am Acad Ophthalmol Otolaryngol* 1977;83:617.

Zimmerman RA, Bilaniuk LT, Metzger RA, et al. Computed tomography of orbital facial neurofibromatosis. *Radiology* 1983;146: 113.

Pediatric Ophthalmology

Bruce M. Schnall
Joseph H. Calhoun

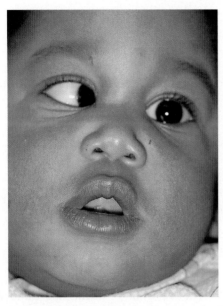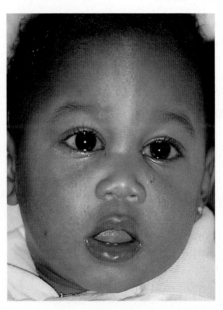

A: Eight-month-old with infantile esotropia. *B:* Two days status post recession of both medial recti 7.0 mm.

VISUAL DEVELOPMENT

Healthy infants are born with the potential, not the ability, to see clearly and normally if the proper conditions are met. The eyes must be anatomically normal. The media must be optically clear, without opacities of the cornea, lens, and vitreous. The infant must have visual input of some kind. The normal environment of the home is more than adequate to satisfy that requirement. The light or visual input coming from the environment must be at least moderately well focused on the retina for good vision to develop. If binocular function is to develop, the eyes must be aligned so that each eye receives similar images. If the eyes are not aligned but are otherwise normal, each eye learns to see independently of its mate.

At birth, the normal visual responses to the family or an examiner are rather meager, with the neonate perhaps responding just to light or bright objects. Within several weeks, a normal baby follows faces and, by several months, small objects, toys, and fingers if those objects are presented reasonably close to the infant (usually within several feet). A normal 6-month-old child is interested in the world within his reach or within several feet, and he is less interested or uninterested in objects 10 feet or more away. To judge how well such an infant sees, the examiner should test using small objects within the close range. The infant's world of visual interest gradually expands, and by 1 year of age, the normal child is attentive to interesting, new, moving, or noisy objects 10 to 20 feet away. By 2.5 years, some children recognize Allen pictures equivalent in size to 20/20 Snellen let-

ters. By 3 years of age, most children can recognize and respond to this size of target.

DIAGNOSTIC TESTS

The evaluation of infants and children is similar in many ways to the evaluation of adults. The retinoscope, ophthalmoscope, and slit lamp are used for all patients. However, there are some major differences in the information needed and the techniques required to get that information.

Evaluation of Vision

The evaluation of vision in normal children older than 3 years of age is similar to the assessment of vision in adults. A target is presented, and the patient is asked whether he or she sees it. For children 3 to 5 years of age, Allen pictures can be used. For children 4 to 6 years of age, the tumbling E is satisfactory. For many children older than 5 and for most older than 7 years of age, the alphabet can be used, as it is for adults.

For the preverbal child, usually younger than 3 years of age, the assessment of vision is somewhat more problematic. The assessment can be divided into three phases: history from the family, clinical visual testing, and ocular examination.

By asking the right questions of the family, useful information can be obtained about how the child sees at home with both eyes open. Less information can be obtained about how one eye sees relative to the other. A child several months of age should look at the mother when feeding, should follow the parent's face, and should smile when the parents approach. A child 6 to 12 months of age should easily pick up small objects, can pick up or reach for small finger foods, and can crawl or walk to find toys or other interesting objects across the room. By 12 months of age, most children can walk. They should be able to move around well in a strange environment, such as a different house or the yard. Sitting close to the television or holding things close is not, in isolation, a sign of poor vision.

The patient's *history* sometimes indicates that one eye sees better or worse than the other, but the degree of difference cannot be assessed. If one eye always turns in or out, that eye is the poorer seeing eye, but how much poorer requires further testing.

Clinical visual testing in the preverbal child requires first and foremost that the examiner get the child interested in something and then make it progressively more difficult for the child to see. For example, the examiner could use a lollipop or a toy to get the child's interest and then hide more and more of it behind the hand or move it farther away. Once the child is interested in an object, he or she should be equally interested if one eye is covered.

The *clinical examination* can detect a variety of abnormalities that can modify the assessment of the vision. From the combination of these three sources, a reasonably accurate judgment about the vision can be made. In some cases, it is a judgment of exclusion. If the eyes are normal, the vision is almost certainly normal. No child is too young to have an assessment of vision.

Evaluation of Strabismus

The diagnosis and quantification of strabismus is the other major area of the pediatric ophthalmologic examination.

The diagnosis of strabismus is made by inspection when the deviation is large and apparent by the cover test or its variations when the deviation is small.

The cover for the cover test can be the traditional black paddle or occluder, but often it is less frightening for infants if the examiner uses two fingers or a thumb (with the rest of the hand on the infant's forehead). If each eye is covered in turn, and the opposite eye does not move, the eyes are straight with both eyes open. If either moves, a tropia exists. If neither moves, indicating straight eyes with both open, but both move when alternately covering each eye, the patient has a phoria. The direction of movement determines whether the deviation is eso-, exo-, or hyper-.

Quantifying the angle or degree of strabismus is most conveniently performed with prisms of graded sizes in combination with alternately covering each eye; this is the prism alternate cover test. Alternately covering each eye, noting the movement of the eyes, and introducing prisms of known size until the movement is eliminated can measure the size of the angle of the strabismus, whether the deviation is a phoria or a tropia. The determination of whether the strabismus is a phoria or tropia has previously been made by the cover-uncover test. This test requires that the patient fix on a target for a sufficiently long time for the examiner to neutralize or eliminate the deviation with prisms.

In less cooperative patients, Krimsky's test can be used (Fig. 11.1). The patient fixes on a light while the examiner introduces prisms of sufficient size to center the corneal light reflex on the middle of each pupil. This method is less accurate than the prism alternate cover test and is useful only for a tropia, not a phoria.

Even less accurate is the Hirschberg light reflex test. It assumes that there is a deviation of 7 degrees for each 1 mm the corneal light reflex is displaced from the center of the pupil. By knowing that the normal cornea is about 11 mm in its horizontal diameter, the examiner can calculate the

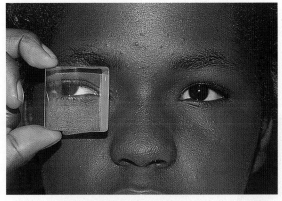
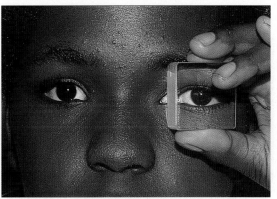

A   B

FIGURE 11.1. Krimsky's test. **A:** The patient looks at a point light source. A prism of sufficient strength is placed before the deviating eye until the corneal light reflexes are in the same location in front of each pupil. **B:** A variation of Krimsky's test is to place a prism of sufficient strength before the fixing eye until the deviating eye appears to be in the straight-ahead position. For this method to be accurate, the extraocular movements must be normal in each eye.

distance of the light reflex from the center of the pupil. This method gives the results in degrees, not prism diopters as in the previous two methods.

Any of these methods can be used to quantify the deviation at any fixation distance. Clinically, it is most useful to observe the deviation when the patient is fixing at a distance (≥4 m) or near (0.3 m). Any of these methods can be used in any position or direction of gaze, traditionally in the nine cardinal positions for clinically useful information.

TYPES OF STRABISMUS

Esotropia

Congenital Esotropia

Infants with congenital esotropia develop a large angle of esotropia at several months of age (Fig. 11.2). Because it is not present at birth, some ophthalmologists prefer to name this condition infantile esotropia. The cause is unknown. It occurs in otherwise normal infants, but it is more common in infants with developmental delay and in infants with hydrocephalus.

The angle of deviation is usually larger than 30 prism diopters and may be as large as 90 prism diopters. About half of these infants see equally well with each eye, and these infants alternately fix or look with either eye. In the infants with equal vision, fixation to either side is accomplished with the adducting eye, fixing across the nose (Fig. 11.3). This is called cross fixation. In this situation, because of the esotropia, the abducting eye does not reach the lateral canthus or may reach only the midline. This may simulate a bilateral lateral rectus or abducens palsy. However, bilateral abducens palsy does not occur in otherwise healthy infants. Normal abduction can be demonstrated, usually with marked gaze evoked or end point nystagmus, if the adducting eye can be covered and the infant can be induced to look laterally. The infant often looks at something straight ahead

with either eye in an adducted position, assuming a horizontal face or head turn toward the side of the fixing eye.

In about half of these infants, one eye sees better than the other. There is amblyopia in the nonpreferred eye. In these infants, the better eye is used for fixation in all gazes, and in gaze to the side of the better eye, that eye abducts fully. In gaze to the other side, the better eye fixes in adduction, and the poorer seeing eye does not abduct fully because of esotropia. This can look like a unilateral abducens palsy or a type 1 Duane's syndrome. If the examiner recognizes the difference in vision, confusion is unlikely. The amblyopia must be treated by patching until the vision is equal, as determined by the infant spontaneously fixing with either eye.

The refractive errors, as determined by cycloplegic refraction, in these infants are the normal refractive errors of this age. Most have low degrees of hyperopia, some have moderate degrees of hyperopia, and few are myopic.

The treatment for this condition is surgery. Most physicians recess each medial rectus muscle a graded amount, depending on the angle of deviation. Some also resect one or both lateral rectus muscles for large deviations. Most agree that surgery should be performed before 2 years of age to enhance the chance for the infant to gain some binocular function, and most perform surgery any time after the child is 6 months of age if the vision is equal, the child is healthy, and the proper facilities for safe anesthesia are available.

The success rate for surgery in the short term is quite high. Most of the infants have aligned eyes after surgery, but in months to several years, many of these children have a recurrence of the esotropia. Often, the recurrent esotropia is accommodative and can be treated with glasses for the hyperopia, determined with cycloplegic refraction. On average, the hyperopia is less than the average hyperopia in later-onset accommodative esotropia, but many children need additional surgery for recurrent esotropia. The second surgery is usually a resection of one or both lateral rectus muscles.

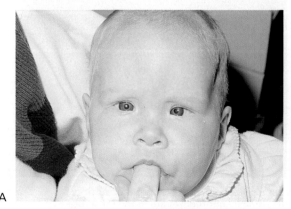
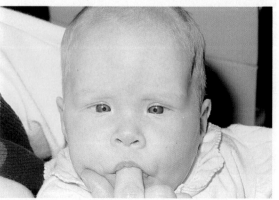

A   B

FIGURE 11.2. Congenital esotropia in a 3-month-old infant. **A:** The right eye is being used for fixation. **B:** The left eye is being used for fixation. The infant is spontaneously alternating fixation, indicating equal vision in each eye.

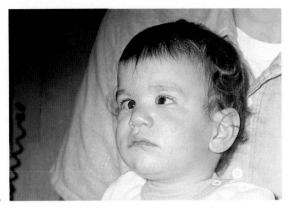
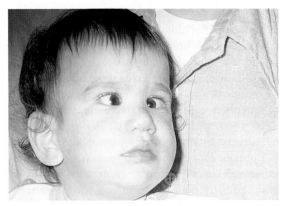

FIGURE 11.3. Congenital esotropia with a larger angle of deviation. **A:** The infant fixates with the right eye in adduction with his face turned to the right. **B:** The infant fixates with the left eye in adduction with his face turned to the left.

Many of these children develop overaction of the inferior oblique muscles or dissociated vertical deviations, which may warrant surgical correction. A few infants may have either of these conditions at the time the esotropia is diagnosed. Some of these children develop an abnormal head position: a face turn or a head tilt to either side. For most of these children, no cause can be found for the abnormal head position.

Latent nystagmus is commonly seen in children who have had congenital esotropia and who may or may not have had surgery for it. Manifest nystagmus is less commonly

seen. Both conditions may persist throughout life, although the amplitude of the nystagmus decreases with time.

A-Pattern Esotropia. One subtype of congenital esotropia is A-pattern congenital esotropia. It is much less common than the typical congenital esotropia described previously. In A-pattern esotropia, the eyes are straight in downgaze but develop progressively larger esotropia in primary or straight-ahead gaze and even more esotropia in upgaze (Fig. 11.4). As the infant acquires head control, it is apparent that he or she prefers a chin-up or head-back position to look at things, because it places the eyes in a position

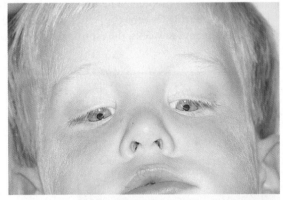
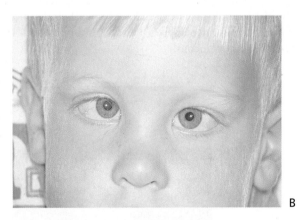
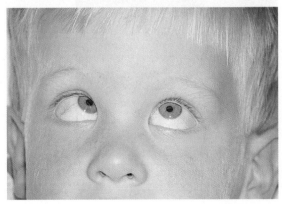

FIGURE 11.4. Congenital esotropia with A pattern. **A:** The preferred chin-up position in which the eyes are aligned. **B, C:** The esotropia becomes progressively larger as the gaze is elevated.

in which they are aligned. In most of these infants, there is overaction of the superior oblique muscles. This observation is often difficult to elicit because it requires that the infant look down and to the side. Sometimes, overaction of the superior oblique muscles can be observed if the infant is lying down in the arms of one of the parents. Another clue to overaction is to observe intorsion of the fundus with the indirect ophthalmoscope. If the divergence in downgaze, the A pattern, is secondary to the superior oblique overaction, the superior oblique function must be weakened surgically, along with recession of the medial rectus muscles for the esotropia in the primary position. In infants with A-pattern esotropia but without overaction of the superior oblique muscles, the accepted surgical treatment is to recess each medial rectus muscle and offset the muscle insertion up by as much as one-half tendon width.

Pseudoesotropia. Pseudoesotropia, the illusion of esotropia, is a common reason infants are referred to ophthalmologists. Normal infants have a flat nasal bridge that often causes the medial canthus to be displaced over the nasal conjunctiva (Fig. 11.5). As the infant looks straight ahead, less nasal conjunctiva is visible compared with the temporal conjunctiva, and it may appear to the observer, the parents, or the primary care physician that either or both eyes are turned inward. This illusion is aggravated in side gaze, in which the cornea of the adducting eye can be partially covered by the nasal bridge at the medial canthus. As the child grows, the distance between the eyes increases and the nasal bridge grows forward, effectively pulling each medial canthus toward the midline. The pseudoesotropia then disappears. This underlies the old wives' tale that esotropia in infancy goes away spontaneously.

Accommodative Esotropia

Accommodative esotropia is the most common type of esotropia. It is an esotropia that is produced by or caused by accommodation. Accommodation is always accompanied by convergence, called accommodative convergence. In the normal person, accommodation on a near target produces a convergence of both eyes such that the near target is seen clearly and singly. There is a normal relation between the accommodation on the near target and the accommodative convergence (i.e., normal AC/A ratio). When a normal person who is a little farsighted or hyperopic looks at a distant object, accommodation brings the image of the object of interest to a sharp focus on the retina.

There are two main types of accommodative esotropia, but there are combinations and variations of these two types. In the more common type, there is a normal AC/A ratio, but the accommodation needed is excessive because of abnormally large hyperopia. This is called the refractive type of accommodative esotropia (Fig. 11.6). In the less common type, the accommodation or hyperopia is normal, but the convergence response, the AC/A ratio, is abnormally high. This type may be called the nonrefractive, the high AC/A, or the convergence excess type.

The average age of onset for either type of accommodative esotropia is 2.5 years, with a range of 6 months to 6 years of age. When either type begins before 1 year of age, it may be confused with congenital esotropia.

In the refractive type, the degree of hyperopia, as determined by cycloplegic refraction, is abnormally high, on average about 4 to 5 diopters. The onset may be intermittent, initially occurring when the child is fatigued or ill. Typically, in days to weeks, the esotropia becomes constant.

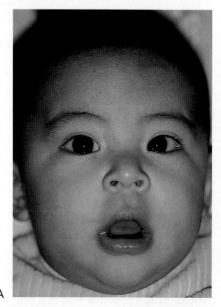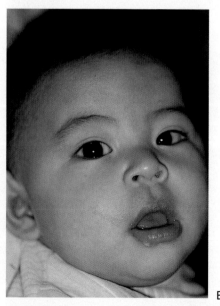

FIGURE 11.5. Pseudoesotropia. **A:** Much more conjunctiva is visible on the temporal side of the cornea in this normal infant. The light reflex is centered in both eyes. **B:** The illusion of pseudoesotropia is even greater in side gaze.

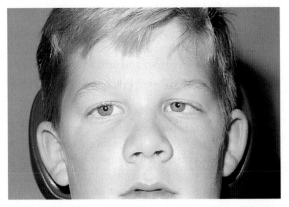
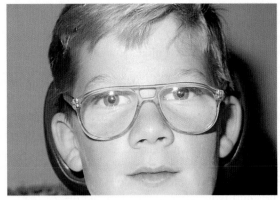

FIGURE 11.6. A: Refractive-type accommodative esotropia. **B:** A left esotropia is eliminated with the use of glasses.

Amblyopia is common in this type of esotropia. The child usually prefers to fix with the less hyperopic eye and turn in the more hyperopic eye. The child may experience diplopia in the first days to weeks after the onset and may close one eye to avoid the second image. After that, a suppression scotoma in the deviating eye eliminates the awareness of diplopia. In this type of esotropia, the angle of the deviation is the same at distant and near fixation. The size of the deviation can be 15 to 50 prism diopters.

For any new esotropia at any age, a lateral rectus muscle or abducens nerve palsy must be excluded. In accommodative esotropia, the angle of deviation is concomitant; the deviation is the same in primary, left, and right gaze at any given fixation distance. In a patient with a lateral rectus weakness, the angle of the deviation increases in gaze to the side of the weak lateral rectus muscle.

The treatment is to eliminate the excessive accommodation by having the child wear the full hyperopic correction, as determined by a cycloplegic refraction. Amblyopia should be treated by patching the preferred eye, usually 1 week for each year of the child's age. The interval between examinations therefore depends on the child's age. If amblyopia persists, it should be treated with continued patching. If the vision is equal but esotropia remains with the glasses on, another cycloplegic refraction test should be performed and the glasses increased in strength if more hyperopia is found. If, after the vision is equal and the child has worn the strongest possible glasses that do not blur the vision (i.e., full plus), the condition continues, surgery should be considered for any remaining esotropia of more than 10 prism diopters.

If the glasses align the eyes initially, most children's eyes remain aligned with the proper glasses. The strength or degree of hyperopia tends to increase until about 6 years of age. It then gradually decreases until the child stops growing.

The other type of accommodative esotropia is the convergence excess or high AC/A type (Fig. 11.7). In this condition, the normal accommodation to fix on a near target results in excessive convergence. The child then looks at the near object with one eye and turns in the other eye. This is often first noticed by the parents at meal time. The child may be sitting across from the parents, probably holding the head up and looking at food in a spoon or on a fork, and the parents can see both eyes clearly. This condition is intermittent. It occurs only during near viewing. It may be present

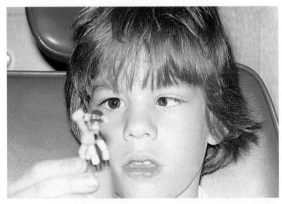
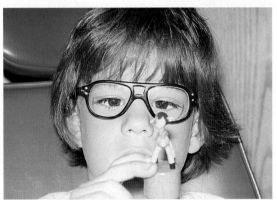

FIGURE 11.7. Accommodative esotropia of the high accommodative convergence–to–accommodation ratio type. **A:** The esotropia at near viewing is eliminated **(B)** with the use of bifocals.

only when viewing small near objects. It may be present only when the child is tired or sick. Amblyopia is less common than in the refractive type of accommodative esotropia and is usually of low degree. Unlike refractive accommodative esotropia, this type in its pure form is not associated with high hyperopia. The average refractive error is about 2 diopters of hyperopia.

The treatment of this condition is controversial but there are a number of management options for the variations that occur in this type of accommodative esotropia. If the esotropia at near focus is of low frequency and occurs only while viewing very small objects, observation is a good option. If the child is hyperopic to a moderate degree (e.g., +2.50 diopters), single vision glasses may reduce the accommodative requirements at near range sufficiently that there is no longer any esotropia at near viewing. If, despite the full plus glasses, the eyes remain straight at distant viewing and esotropic at near viewing, bifocals can be used so accommodation is not needed when looking at near objects. The bifocals should be the weakest strength possible that eliminates the near esotropia. Surgery may be an option in certain situations. If, despite all plus glasses, there remains an esotropia at distant viewing and a larger esotropia at near viewing, surgery can be performed for the angle of the deviation at near viewing. For many children, this restores binocular function.

Lateral Rectus Palsy

Children may develop a lateral rectus palsy, and this should be kept in mind when dealing with children with esotropia. Esotropia is so common and lateral rectus palsy in children is so uncommon that it is possible to overlook a lateral rectus palsy in managing children with esotropia. The angle of the deviation in the typical childhood onset of esotropia should be about the same in primary, left, and right gaze. Otherwise healthy children are rarely born with a lateral rectus palsy that persists. Newborns may rarely get a transient lateral rectus weakness. If there is a persistent congenital deficit of abduction, it almost certainly is a Duane's syndrome. However, children of any age can acquire a lateral rectus palsy (Fig. 11.8). It may occur after severe head trauma, after infections of the central nervous system, as the first sign of an intracranial mass, or after a presumed viral illness. The latter is called benign sixth nerve palsy of childhood.

Benign sixth nerve palsy typically occurs 1 or 2 weeks after a mild febrile illness. Its onset is typically sudden, within a day or overnight. The child usually has diplopia and may close or cover one eye to avoid the second image. The child may also adopt a face turn to the side of the weakened lateral rectus muscle. The ocular and neurologic examinations are otherwise normal. Neuroimaging of the brain is indicated to exclude a more serious cause. The lateral rectus

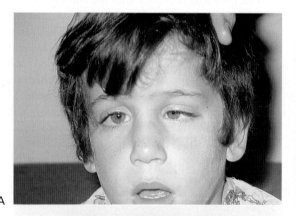
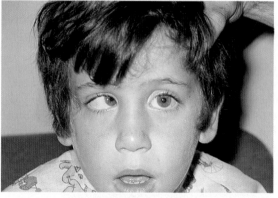
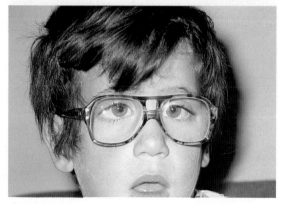

FIGURE 11.8. A: Acquired lateral rectus palsy. **B:** The esotropia increases in left gaze, with no abduction of the left eye past the midline. **C:** Glasses for the hyperopia reduced the esotropia enough that turning the face to the left restored single vision.

weakness typically goes away in several months. In some patients, the lateral rectus weakness may be recurrent. Until it resolves, steps should be taken to avoid the suppression scotoma that children typically develop in response to the diplopia from strabismus. If the child can see singly with a face turn, he or she should be allowed and encouraged to do so. If the esotropia is so large that a face turn cannot achieve single vision, diplopia should be avoided by alternately occluding each eye. Sometimes, the esotropia is increased by hyperopia that was causing no symptoms before the onset of the lateral rectus palsy. In that instance, full plus glasses may reduce the esotropia enough that a face turn can restore single vision.

Exotropia

There are three types of reasonably comitant exotropia: *childhood onset exotropia* (i.e., typical divergence excess), *sensory exotropia,* and *convergence insufficiency.*

Childhood-Onset Exotropia

Childhood-onset exotropia is an awkward name for what is the most common type of exotropia. Many children develop an exotropia that typically begins intermittently. The average age at onset is about 2.5 years (range, 6 months to 6 years), about the same time of onset as for accommodative esotropia. The cause is unknown. It may be weakly hereditary, because few children with this condition have parents or siblings with the same condition. It is useful to think of this entity as passing through several phases or stages.

The first phase of this condition is exophoria only. It is rarely seen because it is rarely symptomatic. If a child happened to be examined at this time in the evolution of this condition, the examiner would find only an exophoria. Testing would reveal a latent deviation, detected only by the cover test.

Several months later, the child may progress into the second phase: intermittent exotropia. With fatigue, illness, or inattention and when looking at a distance of several meters or more, one of the eyes turns out for several seconds. The child then becomes aware of diplopia and makes some unconscious effort to restore the alignment of the eyes. When the child looks at a distant object, an intermittent exotropia is revealed by the cover test. The covered eye turns out and, after the cover is removed, may remain turned out for several seconds or until the next blink, at which time the eyes would be straight. Examination using a near target would probably be normal at this stage. The fusional convergence mechanism at this stage is adequate most of the time to control the tendency for one eye to turn out.

Weeks or months later, the condition may evolve into a third phase, the phase when the fusional convergence mechanism is no longer adequate to control the tendency for exodeviation at distant looking (Fig. 11.9). The child is forced to deal with the exodeviation and the resultant diplopia in some manner. One common way is to close the deviating eye. This is frequently seen in brightly illuminated environments, such as outside. Alternately, a suppression scotoma may develop. If that occurs, the child is no longer bothered by the exodeviation. One eye remains in an exotropic position as long as the child continues to look at some distant object. Regardless of the mechanism employed to deal with the symptom of diplopia at distant fixation, at near fixation the alignment is likely to be orthophoric, exophoric, or intermittent exotropic. It is at this stage, when it is apparent that the child cannot control the progressive tendency for exodeviation, that surgery is indicated. Because there is still normal binocular function at near viewing, normal binocular function probably can be restored.

The fourth phase, constant exotropia at far and near viewing, develops months to years later. A suppression scotoma is well established to avoid all symptoms of diplopia. Except for the cosmetic problem, the patient is asymptomatic. Surgery at this point is primarily cosmetic, with a smaller chance of regaining binocularity.

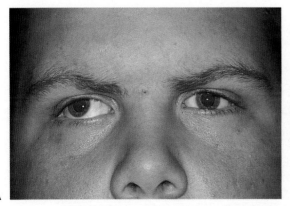 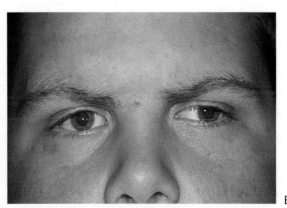

A   B

FIGURE 11.9. Childhood-onset exotropia. **A:** The left eye is fixating electively. **B:** The right eye is fixating electively. This alternate fixation almost certainly indicates equal vision in each eye.

Sensory Exotropia

This is another common type of exotropia, especially in adults. The name suggests that the primary etiologic factor is not a motor abnormality but some defect in the afferent or sensory system. If two eyes do not have good binocular function, it is likely that the poorer or nondominant eye will gradually turn out or become exotropic (Fig. 11.10). However, if the dominant or fixing eye is hyperopic and not optically corrected, the resultant accommodative convergence will often lead to a turning in of the poorer or nondominant eye. This may be called a sensory esotropia, although it is often an accommodative esotropia. However, assuming no excessive accommodation in the fixing eye, the poorer seeing eye will gradually turn outward. This process may take years before the exotropia is large enough to be a cosmetically significant problem for the patient.

Surgery is warranted on the poorer eye when the patient feels the size of the deviation has reached that point. Surgery usually involves recession of the lateral rectus muscle and, if the deviation is large enough, resection of the medial rectus muscle. The extent of surgery is usually based on the distant deviation, because the deviation at near viewing is usually smaller.

Convergence Insufficiency

A third type of exotropia is an apparent weakness of convergence, called convergence insufficiency (Fig. 11.11). The entity frequently affects young adults and is a major cause of asthenopia, or tired eyes, while doing near work in this age group. In this condition, the eyes are straight at distant fixation and without symptoms. However, at near viewing there is an exodeviation, sometimes an exophoria or sometimes an intermittent exotropia with transient diplopia. The deviation at near viewing is relatively small, never larger than 18 prism diopters, as determined by alternate cover testing. However, even a much smaller deviation can produce asthenopic symptoms.

There is often a remote near point of convergence. As a small target is brought closer to the patient in the primary position, the patient cannot continue to converge on the target as it approaches. Several inches or more away one eye deviates outward. Treatment is usually nonsurgical, consisting primarily of near point exercises. The patient is instructed to hold a small target at arm's length and bring it closer to the nose, until convergence is no longer possible and diplopia is appreciated. The patient is asked to do this exercise often, for short periods throughout the day. The goal is to improve the convergence mechanism, as measured by the near point of convergence. If that fails, reading glasses with base-in prisms can be used. Rarely is surgery needed, but a resection of each medial rectus muscle can be considered in selected cases.

Vertical Deviations

Vertical misalignment of the eyes involves an abnormality of one or more of the four vertically acting muscles in each eye: the superior rectus, the inferior rectus, the superior oblique, and the inferior oblique. Because each of these muscles also has a secondary cyclo- or torsional action that controls the position of the eye around the anteroposterior axis, the vertical deviations are sometimes called cyclovertical deviations.

If one eye is higher than the other, one eye is also lower than the other. If, for example, the right eye is higher than the left, the condition may be called a right hypertropia or a left hypotropia. It is usually easier to understand and to communicate if the nonfixing eye is labeled. If the higher right eye is the fixing eye and the left eye is low, it is probably easier to communicate if that condition is called a left hypotropia. However, in applying the three-step test to aid in the diagnosis of a cyclovertical palsy, it is traditional to speak of and think about hypertropia in the various positions of gaze.

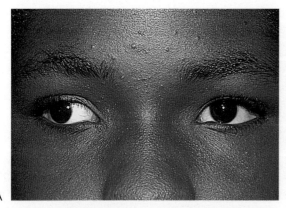
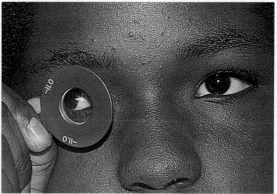

A   B

FIGURE 11.10. Sensory exotropia. **A:** There is a large right exotropia associated with poor sight in that eye. **B:** The cause of poor sight is amblyopia associated with high myopia.

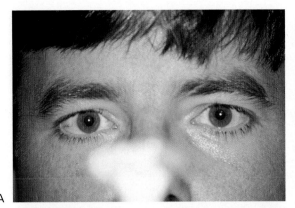

A

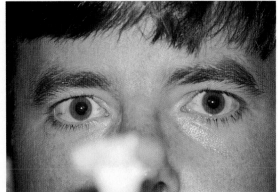

B

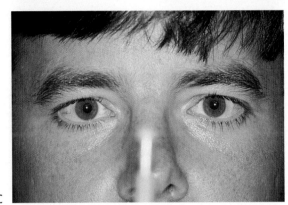

C

FIGURE 11.11. Convergence insufficiency. **A:** The patient is fixing on a near target with both eyes and single vision. **B:** When the target is moved a bit closer (too close for the patient to converge on the target), one eye drifts, with resultant diplopia. The patient has a remote near point of convergence. **C:** The patient is practicing near-point exercises, repeatedly moving a near target closer to improve the convergence ability.

Superior Oblique Palsy

The superior oblique muscle is innervated by the fourth cranial nerve, the trochlear nerve. Weakness of that muscle is commonly called superior oblique muscle palsy, trochlear nerve palsy, or fourth nerve palsy. Among cyclovertical palsies, it is by far the most common. It may be congenital or acquired. The acquired form frequently follows blunt head trauma. It may also occur in older adults as a result of presumed microvascular disease.

All unilateral superior oblique palsies have one eye higher than the other. That determination is the first step of the diagnostic three-step test. In both types, the vertical separation of the eyes is greater in lateral gaze to the side of the lower eye. Determining whether the vertical separation is greater in left or right gaze is the second step of the three-step test. In all unilateral superior oblique palsies, the vertical separation is larger than the deviation in primary position when the head is tilted to the side of the higher eye. Determining whether the vertical separation is greater on left or right head tilt is the third step of the three-step test. If the right eye is the higher eye in primary gaze, the deviation is greater on left gaze and right head tilt. If the left eye is higher in primary gaze in a patient with a superior oblique palsy, the deviation is larger on right gaze and left head tilt.

In addition to being a depressor, the superior oblique muscle is also an intorter. Usually, there is extorsion of the involved eye, which can be seen with indirect ophthalmoscopy, because the field of view is large enough to see the macula and the disc. Normally, the macula occupies a position directly horizontal to the lower third of the optic disc. If the eye is extorted, the disc is higher than the macula, or the macula is below the bottom of the disc. That view could be seen in a photograph. In the inverted view of the indirect ophthalmoscope, the normal position of the macula is horizontal to the upper third of the disc. If there is extorsion of the eye, the macula appears to be above the disc. In older children or adults, the examiner can measure the extorsion with a Maddox rod placed such that the perceived line is about horizontal. The patient then is asked to rotate the Maddox rod until the perceived line is exactly level or horizontal. The extorsion can be measured in degrees.

Congenital superior oblique palsy occurs in otherwise healthy children for no apparent reason. It is not familial, although it is common enough that a parent and a child may both have this condition. Typically, children present with a head tilt (Fig. 11.12). The head tilt may be apparent as soon as the child is old enough to sit. The head is tilted to the side opposite the high eye, where the vertical deviation is least. There may also be a face turn-away from the field of action of the weak superior oblique muscle, and there may be a chin-down position. A child with a congenital right superior oblique palsy tilts the head to the left, turns the face to the left to look right, and puts the chin down to look up slightly.

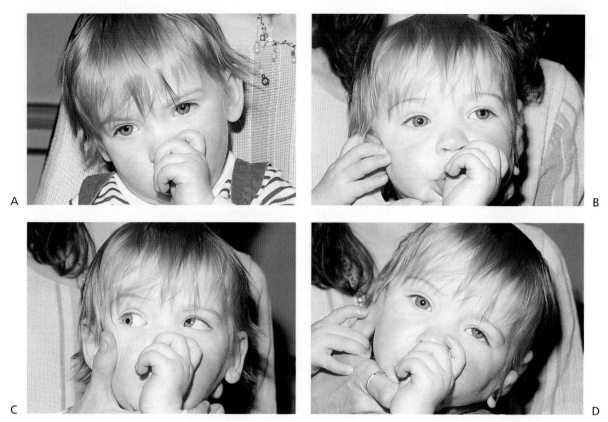

FIGURE 11.12. Congenital superior oblique palsy of the left eye. **A:** A typical abnormal head position is shown. The head is tilted away from the side of the palsied muscle. The chin is tilted downward slightly. **B:** There is a small left hypertropia in primary gaze when the head is nearly straightened. **C:** A large left hypertropia is present in right gaze. **D:** A large left hypertropia is seen on forced (by the mother's hand) left head tilt.

In this position, the child functions well and has binocular vision. Amblyopia is uncommon. If untreated, the condition continues, and the head tilt and the face turn become larger.

Adults frequently present because the compensatory head position is no longer adequate, and they begin to experience intermittent diplopia. They may close one eye to avoid the diplopia. In older children and adults, it is possible to measure the vertical fusional vergence. Patients with congenital superior oblique palsies have large vertical fusional vergences. A normal person can tolerate up to about 2 prism diopters placed vertically before one eye until he or she sees double. In patients with congenital superior oblique palsies, the vertical fusional range may be very large—as much as 25 or 30 prism diopters. A simple way to measure this is to ask the patient to place the head in a position where there is single vision. As the head is moved toward the normal position, the patient experiences diplopia. The vertical deviation measured at that head position is the vertical fusional amplitude. Patients with an acquired superior oblique palsy have the normal, small vertical fusional amplitude. The measurement of the vertical fusional amplitudes is probably the best way to differentiate congenital from acquired superior oblique palsies.

There are other differences. An acquired palsy usually has the greatest vertical deviation in the field of action of the palsied superior oblique muscle (Fig. 11.13). A congenital palsy frequently has a large overaction of the antagonist of the superior oblique muscle, the inferior oblique muscle. The greatest vertical deviation often is in that field of gaze. The complaints and measurements of tilting or torsion are generally less in congenital palsies, despite large vertical deviations. However, the vertical deviation in an acquired palsy is typically smaller, 10 prism diopters or less, but the awareness of and the measured size of the torsion are larger in relation to the size of the vertical deviation.

The treatment may be optical or surgical. Because acquired palsies are often relatively small, the patient can find relief with the appropriate prisms in glasses, especially if he or she is already wearing glasses and if the deviation is relatively comitant (i.e., about the same size in primary and downgaze and, to a lesser extent, in left and right gaze). If there is doubt about the efficacy of prisms, it is prudent to try them before surgery.

When surgery is indicated, it is best to perform that surgery on muscles whose field of action is in the field of gaze where there is the greatest vertical deviation. In the case of a right superior oblique palsy, if the greatest vertical devi-

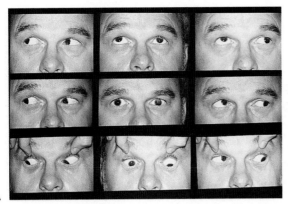 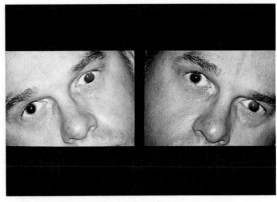

A   B

FIGURE 11.13. Right superior oblique palsy in an adult. **A:** The composite pictures show all of the typical features of a superior oblique palsy. There is right hypertropia that is greater in straight left gaze and **(B)** greater on right head tilt. When gazing up and to the patient's left, there is overaction of the right inferior oblique muscle. When gazing down and to the patient's left, there is underaction of the right superior oblique muscle. In straight upgaze, there is a small exotropia or V pattern from the secondary abducting action of the overacting inferior oblique. In gazing down and to the patient's right, the left eye is slightly lower, reflecting the slight overaction of the normal left superior oblique muscle. This may be caused by a contracted or tight right superior rectus muscle from the chronic, longstanding higher right eye. The overaction of the opposite superior oblique is a common finding in these patients.

ation is in gaze down and to the left, the reasonable surgical options are to strengthen the palsied right superior oblique by a tuck of the tendon or to weaken by a recession the yoke of the palsied muscle, the left inferior rectus muscle. This recession is often done by an adjustable suture technique to improve the precision of the surgical adjustment because of the accuracy needed with the typical small fusional vergence. Because this is the typical finding in an acquired superior oblique palsy, one of these procedures usually is performed. In patients with right congenital superior oblique palsy, the greatest vertical deviation is often in the field of the antagonist, the right inferior oblique muscle, in gaze up and to the left. A weakening procedure on that muscle would be the appropriate surgery. If the deviation is very large, surgery may be performed on two muscles. However, a patient with a congenital right superior oblique palsy would have large vertical fusional vergences for a right hyperdeviation, but very small or normal fusional vergences for a right hypotropia or left hypertropia. Surgery for these patients should approach but not overcorrect the vertical deviation. Correcting a large portion of the vertical deviation eliminates the symptoms.

Despite the rather common occurrence of unilateral congenital superior oblique palsies, congenital *bilateral superior oblique palsies* are rare. Severe blunt head trauma is the most common cause. All of the findings of two unilateral superior oblique palsies are typically present, but because the right hypertropia and the left hypertropia tend to cancel each other, all of the vertical deviations are relatively small. A subjective test of some sort, such as a Maddox rod, a red lens, or a Lancaster or Hess screen, is needed to detect the vertical deviations. There are vertical, horizontal, and torsional misalignments that vary in each position of gaze, and the pa-

tient often does not give a well-defined history of diplopia. The symptoms may sound like asthenopia.

In the primary position, there is a small or no hypertropia. In left gaze, there is a small right hypertropia and a small left hypertropia in right gaze. With the head tilted left, there is a left hypertropia and a right hypertropia with right head tilt. Typically, there is esotropia on downgaze and exotropia on upgaze (Fig. 11.14). Sometimes, these are the only deviations large enough to be seen by the examiner on cover testing. These findings strongly suggest bilateral fourth nerve palsy and should prompt a more thorough test for vertical and torsional defects, using some subjective methods as described previously. The hallmark of bilateral fourth nerve palsy is a

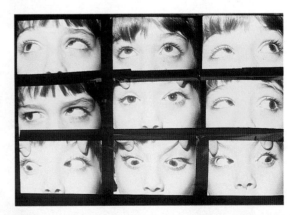

FIGURE 11.14. Bilateral superior oblique palsy. In the primary position the eyes are aligned, but in downgaze esotropia occurs, and in upgaze exotropia with a V pattern occurs. There is a right hypertropia in left gaze and a left hypertropia in right gaze. There is underaction of each superior oblique and overaction of each inferior oblique muscle.

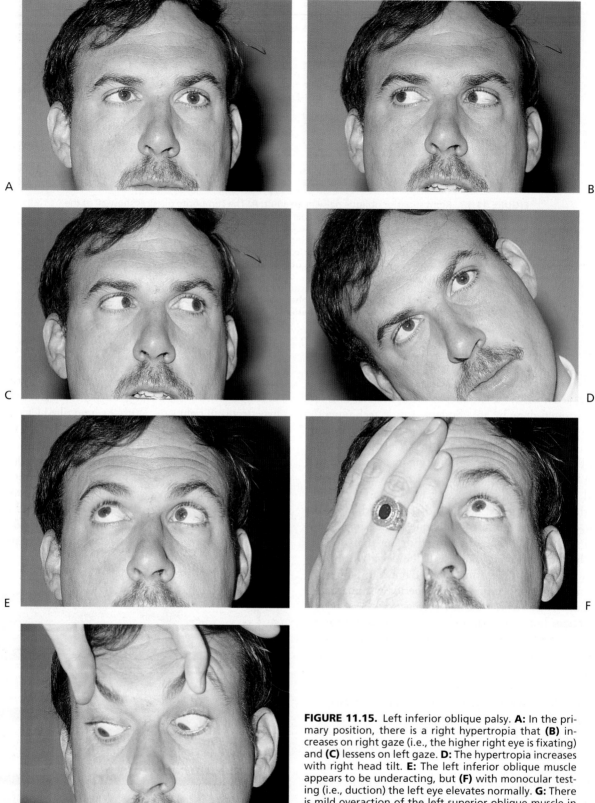

FIGURE 11.15. Left inferior oblique palsy. **A:** In the primary position, there is a right hypertropia that **(B)** increases on right gaze (i.e., the higher right eye is fixating) and **(C)** lessens on left gaze. **D:** The hypertropia increases with right head tilt. **E:** The left inferior oblique muscle appears to be underacting, but **(F)** with monocular testing (i.e., duction) the left eye elevates normally. **G:** There is mild overaction of the left superior oblique muscle in down and right gaze.

large amount of extorsion in primary gaze, usually greater than 10 degrees, which increases in downgaze.

The treatment is usually surgical. The anterior one half of each superior oblique tendon should be moved posterior to the superior pole of the lateral rectus muscle (i.e., Harato Ito procedure). This approach should correct the torsional defect and the esotropia in downgaze. If there is a large vertical deviation in primary gaze, appropriate surgery should be performed, based on the field of action where that vertical deviation is greatest.

Inferior Oblique Palsy

Although much less common than superior oblique palsies, inferior oblique palsies do exist. It is difficult to postulate where or what the lesion may be that creates such an isolated muscle weakness without any involvement of the pupil, because the two nerves share a common pathway after leaving the oculomotor nerve. These palsies appear to be congenital and idiopathic. They are not associated with trauma.

An inferior oblique palsy is diagnosed by the three-step test. There is a hypertropia in primary gaze that increases in gaze to the side of the hyperdeviation and increases with head tilt to that same side. If, for example, there is a right hyperdeviation in primary, it will be larger on right gaze and right head tilt (Fig. 11.15). That is characteristic of a left inferior oblique palsy. There is usually underaction of the left inferior oblique on testing versions with both eyes open, and it is possible to confuse that finding with Brown's syndrome. However, with monocular or duction testing, the eye in question moves up and in normally. There may be overaction of the ipsilateral superior oblique muscle with divergence in downgaze, an A pattern.

Treatment, if symptomatic, depends on where the deviation is greater: in the field of the palsied inferior oblique or its antagonist, the superior oblique. If the former, a recession of the yoke, the opposite superior rectus muscle, would be indicated; if the latter, a weakening procedure of the overacting superior oblique muscle.

Inferior Rectus Palsy

An inferior rectus palsy is usually a sequela of blunt trauma to the eye that produced a blow-out fracture of the orbital floor. There may be limitation of upgaze because of the trapped muscle in the orbital floor fracture. This condition is forced duction positive. There may also be limitation of downgaze, which is forced duction negative. The limitation is likely to be from an injury to the inferior rectus muscle. It may persist after the floor fracture is repaired. Occasionally, such trauma produces only the inferior rectus weakness without any fracture, as if the muscle were contused by the trauma. Occasionally, sharp, pointed objects can enter under the eyeball through the conjunctiva and injure the inferior rectus muscle.

Typically, the hypertropia in primary gaze increases to the side of the hypertropia and increases in downgaze, but it does not increase on head tilt to the opposite side, as the three-step test suggests that it would (Fig. 11.16).

Treatment should be conservative initially, especially after blunt trauma, because the weakness sometimes improves with time. When no further improvement is occurring, an inferior rectus resection of the palsied muscle or an inferior rectus recession of the opposite eye should be performed. If there is still bothersome diplopia in downgaze, a posterior fixation suture (i.e., Faden) can be employed on the opposite inferior rectus muscle to limit the extreme excursion of that muscle.

Dissociated Vertical Deviation

The vertical deviations that have been discussed have, to a large extent, followed Hering's law, which states that there is equal innervation (and therefore muscle function) to yoke muscles in any gaze. From a practical or clinical standpoint, as the deviation is being measured and neutralized with prisms in the alternate cover test, the movement ceases in each eye as the appropriate prism is placed before one or the other eye. Dissociated vertical deviation (DVD) is not associated with Hering's law. This accounts for part of its name. Most of these deviations have a large vertical component, accounting for the other part of the name.

DVD is most commonly seen with or especially after congenital esotropia. However, it may be seen in other types of horizontal strabismus or even without any form of horizontal strabismus. It is characterized by one eye rising spontaneously (i.e., manifest DVD) or only when the involved eye is covered or blurred (i.e., latent DVD) while the other eye is fixing (Fig. 11.17). If the fixing eye is covered, the high eye, the one with the DVD, lowers to take up fixation, but as this involved eye depresses to fixate, the other eye does not lower or depress. The other eye does not obey Hering's

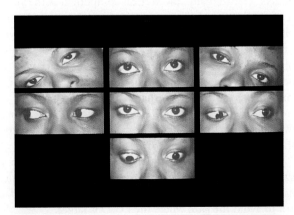

FIGURE 11.16. Right inferior rectus palsy. There is a right hypertropia in primary gaze, increasing on downgaze and right gaze. This patient is unusual in that the hypertropia increases with left head tilt, fulfilling the diagnostic criteria of the three-step test.

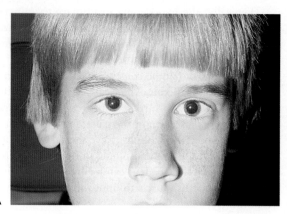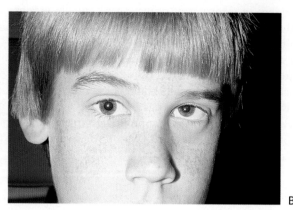

FIGURE 11.17. Dissociated vertical deviation. **A:** The right eye has risen spontaneously. **B:** The left eye has risen. In most patients with dissociated vertical deviation, one eye may rise easily. Usually, the other eye rises only when covered.

law, and it is this feature that is unique. Usually, both eyes have DVD. One eye may be the preferred or dominant eye, and it maintains fixation on the object of interest. The other eye may spontaneously rise intermittently, returning to level with a blink or remaining elevated. If the dominant or fixing eye is covered, the high eye assumes fixation, and the dominant eye rises behind the cover. It usually rises to a smaller degree than the nondominant eye. Occasionally, either eye may spontaneously be used for fixation; at first, one eye rises, and a moment later, it fixates, while the other eye rises.

The involved or rising eye usually extorts and abducts to some degree while it rises. When it lowers to be aligned with the other eye or when it takes up fixation, it intorts and adducts to return to its original position. The vertical movement usually is much larger than the horizontal or torsional movement. If a cover or occlude is alternately placed before each eye, the eye behind the cover exhibits the DVD phenomenon: elevation predominantly, along with extorsion and abduction. As the cover is removed to be placed before the other eye, the newly uncovered eye lowers, intorts, and adducts. Occasionally, the vertical component is the smallest of the three, and alternate cover produces only extorsion behind the cover and intorsion when the cover is removed. If the horizontal component is the major portion, the involved eye abducts spontaneously or under cover with no abduction of the other eye when the first eye takes up fixation. In this situation, alternate cover would produce exotropia when one eye is covered, but not the other. Hering's law is not obeyed. This entity is called dissociated horizontal deviation.

Usually, DVD is roughly of the same magnitude in all gazes, but less frequently there may be a substantial difference between lateral gazes. The difference can lead to a face turn to avoid the gaze where the DVD is larger.

To measure the magnitude of the vertical deviation, increasing strengths of base-down prisms are placed before the eye being measured while the eye is covered. The cover is

then moved to cover the fixing eye. When the movement of the eye being measured is neutralized with the appropriate-sized prism, that prism represents the size of the vertical deviation of that eye. As the movement of the eye is neutralized with the prism, the other or original fixing eye rises in a typical DVD movement. In this condition, it is impossible to eliminate all movement on alternate cover with prisms.

If the deviation, vertical or horizontal, is frequent enough that it is a cosmetic problem, is causing symptoms of a face turn, or is producing diplopia, therapy is indicated. Patching the fixing eye, as if treating amblyopia, can reduce the frequency of the deviation. If that fails, surgery is indicated.

This entity began to be recognized several decades ago. The originally proposed and performed treatment was to resect the inferior rectus muscle. It gradually became apparent that this was not totally effective. Later, larger recessions of the superior rectus muscle became popular. Most advocated surgery on only the habitually rising eye, but others advocated very large recessions of both superior rectus muscles. Some have advocated what is called an anteriorization of the inferior oblique muscle, a recession of that muscle but attaching it just lateral or anterior to the lateral border of the inferior rectus muscle. In this position, it limits the elevation of the treated eye. For dissociated horizontal deviation—which is, in effect, a monocular exotropia—a recession of the lateral rectus is indicated.

Oblique Muscle Dysfunction and A and V Syndromes

Overaction and Underaction of the Superior and Inferior Oblique Muscles

The primary action of the superior oblique muscle is to direct the eye down and in. For the right eye, that is gaze down and to the left. The primary action of the inferior oblique muscle is to direct the eye up and in. For the right eye, that is gaze up and to the left. Each of the oblique muscles has a secondary action of divergence. That secondary action increases as the direction of the eye moves away from the primary field of action of the muscle, in adduction, and up or down, toward the abducted position.

Either of the oblique muscles may overact. The overaction is usually bilateral and relatively symmetric between the two eyes, but occasionally it is not. Some patients have secondary overactions of the oblique muscles if the antagonists are palsied or weakened, which is common in superior oblique and inferior oblique palsies. In most patients with overaction of the oblique muscles, the mechanism is idiopathic, a primary overaction.

Overaction is revealed in the field of action of the muscle by a greater vertical action (Fig. 11.18). In the case of the right inferior oblique muscle, the patient's gaze is directed up and to the left. If the right eye is higher than the left eye, there is relative overaction of the right oblique muscle. The vertical disparity is best observed in the relative heights of the 6-o'clock position of each limbus. To detect overaction of the right superior oblique muscle, the patient's gaze is directed down and to the left (Fig. 11.19). For superior oblique overaction, the vertical disparity between the two

eyes is documented by comparing the relative heights of the 12-o'clock limbus position of each eye. If there is a weakness of elevation, it appears that the opposite inferior oblique muscle is overacting and elevating excessively; this could be called pseudooveraction of the inferior oblique muscle. The same holds true for a limitation of depression, such as an inferior rectus muscle weakness. This would look as if the superior oblique of the opposite eye were overacting.

Generally, if one set of oblique muscles is overacting, the pair of antagonists are underacting, although usually to a lesser degree. For instance, if both inferior oblique muscles are overacting, the superior oblique muscles usually are underacting to some degree. In patients with large angle exotropia, all four oblique muscles may overact. Correcting the exotropia surgically usually eliminates the overactions.

Overaction and underaction are usually graded on a scale of 1 to 4, with grade 1 being only slight overaction or underaction and grade 4 being marked overaction or underaction. One way to provide some uniformity among observers is to label a 1-mm vertical difference between the appropriate limbus of each eye as grade 1 and a 4-mm difference as grade 4.

Overaction of the inferior oblique muscles is commonly seen with or after the surgical correction of congenital

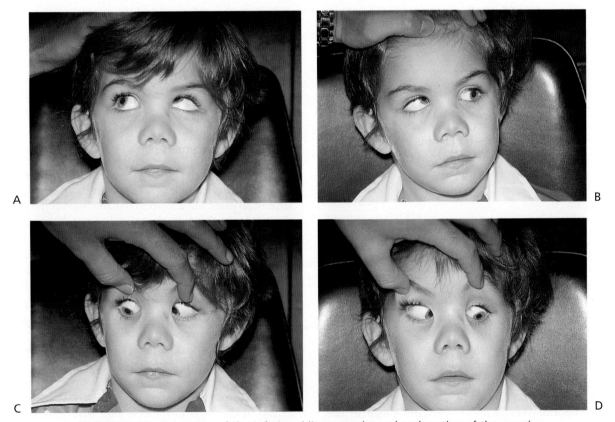

FIGURE 11.18. Overaction of the inferior oblique muscles and underaction of the superior oblique muscles. **A, B:** The overaction of the inferior oblique muscles could be graded as +4. **C, D:** Typically, the degree of underaction of the antagonist pair, the superior oblique muscles, is +2 or +3.

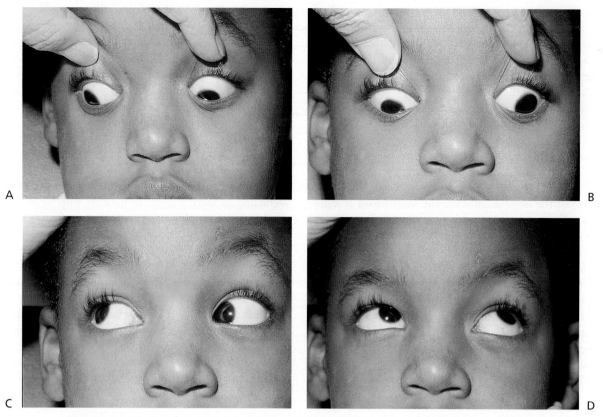

FIGURE 11.19. Overaction of the superior oblique muscles and underaction of the inferior oblique muscles. **A, B:** The overaction of the superior oblique muscles could be graded +3, and **(C, D)** the underaction of the inferior oblique muscles could be graded +2 for the left eye and +1 for the right eye.

esotropia. Although congenital esotropia typically starts at several months of age, the overaction of the inferior oblique muscles is usually noticed after 1 year of age. Overaction of the superior oblique muscles occurs much less frequently with or after the correction of congenital esotropia. Overaction of the oblique muscles is less frequently seen with exotropia. It may occur in patients with no horizontal strabismus.

The treatment for overaction and underaction of the oblique muscles is surgical. If the overaction or underaction is relatively equal, there is no vertical deviation in the primary position. The degree of overaction, especially of the inferior oblique muscles, may be large enough in side gaze that surgical treatment is indicated for cosmetic reasons. In patients who are binocular, the vertical misalignment in side gaze causes diplopia. To expand the field of single vision, surgery is indicated. In patients who are binocular and in whom the overaction or underaction is unequal between the two eyes, there may be vertical deviation in the primary gaze position that the patients avoid by a face turn to the side of the more abnormal oblique muscle, permitting them to look in the gaze of the less abnormal oblique muscle. Surgical correction of the oblique abnormality should eliminate the face turn. However, the most common reason for surgery on

a pair of oblique muscles is correction of an A or V syndrome.

A and V Syndromes

Horizontal strabismus in childhood is usually comitant; the angle of the deviation in cases of esotropia or exotropia is the same in all gazes while fixation is maintained at the same distance. The angle of the deviation commonly is different at different fixation distances, especially in exotropia (i.e., less at near viewing) and less commonly in esotropia (i.e., more at near viewing). Some patients may exhibit a difference in the angle of the deviation between primary or straight-ahead gaze and the angle of the deviation in straight upgaze and straight downgaze. Those types of strabismus are called A and V syndromes or patterns.

Regardless of the deviation in primary gaze, whether esotropia or exotropia, if the angle of the deviation diverges more or converges less in upgaze and diverges less or converges more in downgaze, it is called a V pattern (Fig. 11.20). If the angle of the deviation were graphed, the resulting line would resemble the letter V. Conversely, if the eyes diverge more in downgaze and converge more in upgaze relative to the primary position deviation, the condi-

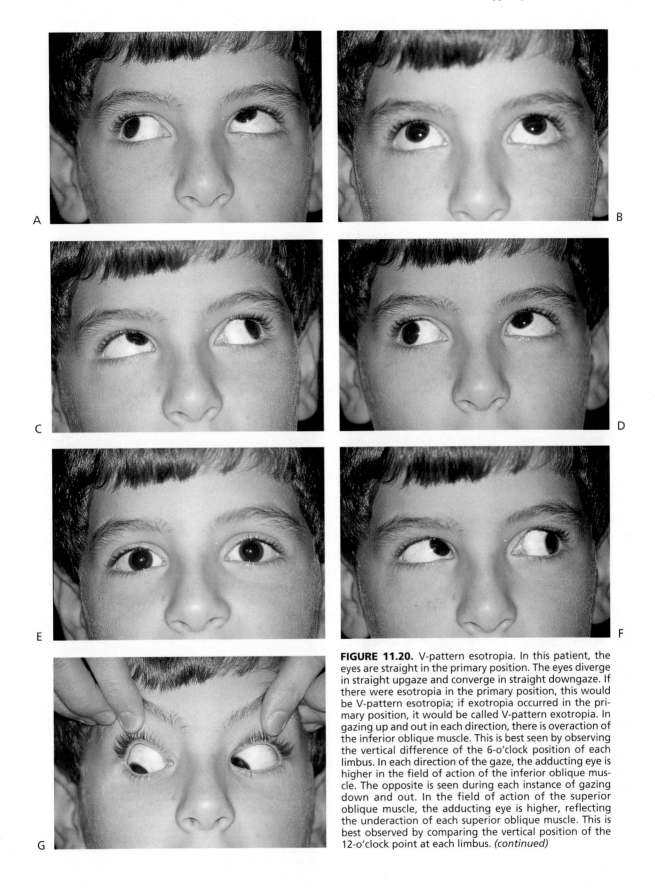

FIGURE 11.20. V-pattern esotropia. In this patient, the eyes are straight in the primary position. The eyes diverge in straight upgaze and converge in straight downgaze. If there were esotropia in the primary position, this would be V-pattern esotropia; if exotropia occurred in the primary position, it would be called V-pattern exotropia. In gazing up and out in each direction, there is overaction of the inferior oblique muscle. This is best seen by observing the vertical difference of the 6-o'clock position of each limbus. In each direction of the gaze, the adducting eye is higher in the field of action of the inferior oblique muscle. The opposite is seen during each instance of gazing down and out. In the field of action of the superior oblique muscle, the adducting eye is higher, reflecting the underaction of each superior oblique muscle. This is best observed by comparing the vertical position of the 12-o'clock point at each limbus. *(continued)*

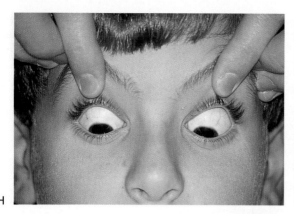
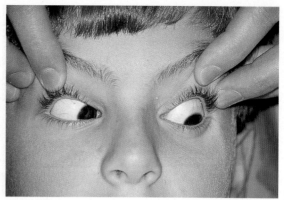

FIGURE 11.20. *Continued.*

tion is called an A pattern (Fig. 11.21). Some examples are provided in Table 11.1.

The secondary action of the superior and the inferior oblique muscles is divergence. If either muscle is overactive, there is secondary divergence or less convergence. Overaction of the superior oblique muscles produces more divergence in downgaze, an A pattern. Overaction of the inferior oblique muscles produces more divergence in upgaze, a V pattern.

For most A or V syndromes, there is corresponding overaction of the oblique muscles. To treat the A or V syndrome, the appropriate overacting oblique muscle is weakened surgically along with the appropriate surgery for the horizontal deviation in the primary position. In some patients with A or V syndrome, there is no overaction of the oblique muscles to account for the differences in the size of the deviation between primary gaze and upgaze and downgaze. If the deviation in the primary position warrants correction, surgery is performed on the appropriate horizontal rectus muscles.

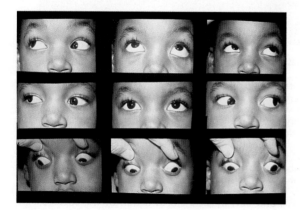

FIGURE 11.21. A-pattern exotropia. The small exotropia increases markedly during downgaze and is associated with overaction of each superior oblique muscle. The overaction is best observed by gazing down and out in each direction. The 12-o'clock position on the limbus is lower in the adducting eye than the corresponding point in the adducting eye. Because the lower adducting eye is in the field of action of the superior oblique muscle, it is called overaction of that muscle.

The A or V pattern is treated by offsetting or moving up or down by one-half tendon width the insertion of the horizontal muscle undergoing surgery. The new insertion is moved in the direction in which less effect is desired. For example, if there is excessive divergence in upgaze, the new insertion of the lateral rectus muscle should be moved up one-half tendon width, regardless of whether a recession or resection is performed. If the medial rectus is undergoing surgery, its new insertion should be moved down one-half tendon width. By similar reasoning through each of the four types of patterns possible with each horizontal muscle, the medial rectus muscle is always moved toward the apex of the A or V, and the lateral rectus muscle is moved toward the open end of the A or V, whether one or both eyes are undergoing surgery.

Divergence in Upgaze Not Associated With Inferior Oblique Muscle Overaction

One disorder can mimic a V-pattern exotropia. In affected patients, the eyes are usually straight in primary gaze and downgaze. However, on upgaze, there is a very large divergence or exotropia of the nonfixing eye (Fig. 11.22). This disorder is sometimes associated with some retraction of the eye away from the lower lid. This entity differs from the typical V pattern in that there is no overaction of the inferior oblique muscle on lateral gaze. The disorder probably represents co-firing or co-contraction of the lateral rectus muscle when the superior rectus muscle is innervated on upgaze.

TABLE 11.1. TYPICAL A AND V PATTERNS (DEVIATION IN PRISM DIOPTERS)

Direction of Gaze	A-Pattern ET	A-Pattern XT	V-Pattern ET	V-Pattern XT
Upgaze	40	5	10	50
Primary Gaze	ET = 20	XT = 20	ET = 30	XT = 30
Downgaze	10	50	40	10

ET, esotropia; XT, exotropia.

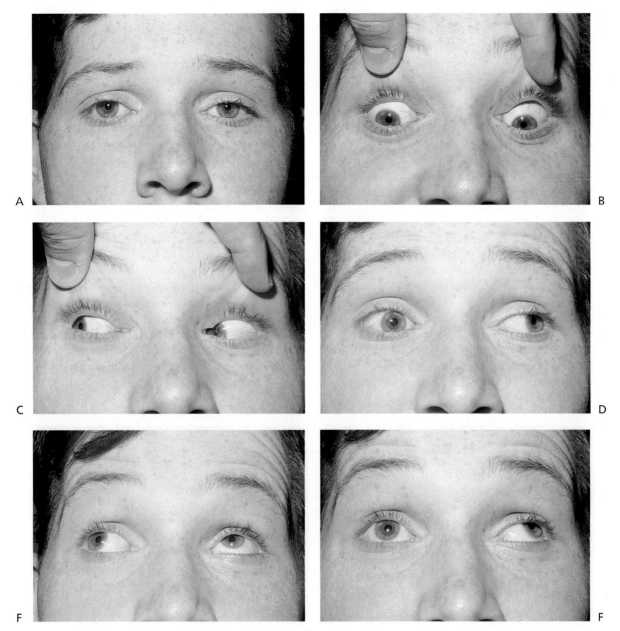

FIGURE 11.22. Divergence in upgaze. In primary gaze **(A)** and downgaze **(B)**, the eyes are aligned. **C, D:** In right and left gaze, there is no overaction of the inferior oblique muscle and no elevation of the adducting eye. **E, F:** In straight upgaze, with either eye fixing, there is a large exotropia of the nonfixing eye.

Most of the patients are relatively asymptomatic. This condition is not altered by weakening the inferior oblique muscle.

Strabismus Syndromes

Some types of strabismus do not fit into the well-defined categories of esotropia, exotropia, and hypertropia. These syndromes, palsies, and other disorders are frequently encountered in the practice of pediatric ophthalmology and must be recognized for proper management.

Brown's Syndrome

Brown's syndrome is a condition in which the affected eye cannot look up and in normally in the position of gaze that is the primary field of the inferior oblique muscle. It was first described in 1950 by Harold W. Brown. It was thought that the sheath of the superior oblique tendon was inelastic and therefore restricted the affected eye from moving into this position; the condition was originally called the superior oblique tendon sheath syndrome. Gradually, it became apparent that the superior oblique had no sheath and that the restriction was in the superior oblique muscle or its tendon.

A patient with this condition in one eye appears to have a weakness of the inferior oblique muscle (Fig. 11.23). The affected eye gives the appearance of underaction of that muscle. However, the inability to look up and in is forced duction positive. After the eye is anesthetized, the eye cannot passively be moved into that field with forceps, because there is a mechanical or physical restriction to the movement. As with other conditions, the degree of involvement varies. A normal eye can look about 45 degrees to 50 degrees from primary position in any direction. In an eye with Brown's syndrome, it is as if there is a wedge or sector in which the involved eye cannot look. The center or broad part of that wedge is always up and in, and the apex of the wedge is close to or at the primary position.

In mild cases, the wedge is narrow, and the limitation is noticed only when the eye looks up and in. In severe cases, the wedge of restricted gaze is 90 degrees to 120 degrees. The severely affected eye cannot adduct in straight lateral gaze and must depress under the restricted area for lateral gaze, a condition called down-shoot on lateral gaze. The severely involved eye cannot look straight up, and it can elevate fully only in a slightly abducted position, just lateral to the wedge of restriction. Because the normal eye is looking straight up, the abducted eye is divergent, constituting a pseudo–V pattern.

Brown's syndrome usually is congenital and unilateral. Occasionally, it is bilateral, and it is rarely intermittent. A patient with the intermittent form may hear or feel a click in the area of the trochlea as the eye returns to normal movement. Brown's syndrome may occur after trauma to the area of the trochlea, or it may be acquired without any trauma to the area. Mild tenderness may or may not be experienced in the area of the trochlea.

There is debate about whether Brown's syndrome resolves after periods of years to decades. In the typical strabismus practice, the condition is much more commonly seen in children than in adults.

Treatment is indicated when the restriction causes a vertical deviation in the primary position and a compensatory face turn. The patient usually assumes a face turn to gaze in abduction, away from the restriction in adduction. Surgical treatment weakens the tight superior oblique muscle. Because only the tendon can be approached surgically, the tendon is weakened by a tenotomy, tenectomy, disinsertion, or tendon-lengthening procedure. Some surgeons weaken the antagonist inferior oblique muscle at the same time to

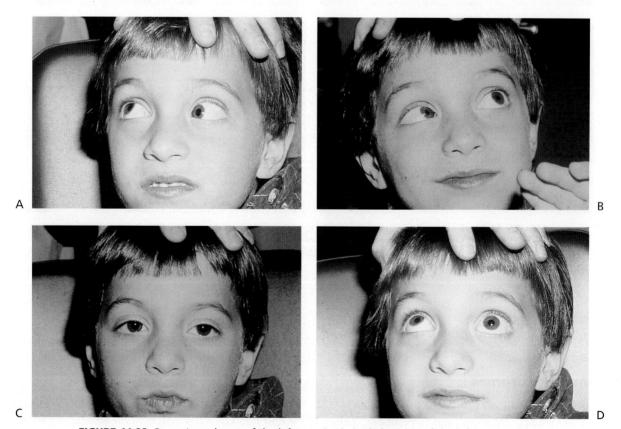

FIGURE 11.23. Brown's syndrome of the left eye. **A:** Limited elevation of the left eye in adduction with **(B)** normal elevation in abduction. **C:** Because the eyes are straight in the primary position, there is no compensatory face turn. **D:** In straight upgaze, there is divergence of the eyes, a V pattern, as the left eye "looks around" the restricted area.

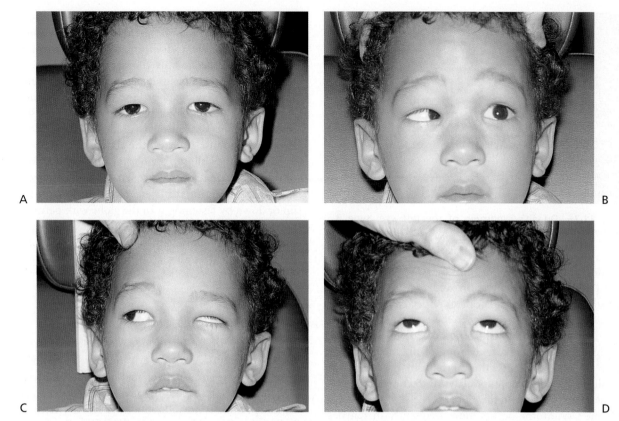

FIGURE 11.24. Duane's syndrome of the left eye, type 1. **A:** Eyes are straight in primary position. **B:** Notice the limitation of abduction and **(C)** the very large up-shoot effect on attempted adduction. **D:** Upgaze is normal.

reduce the likelihood of a superior oblique palsy, a frequent sequela in the surgical treatment of Brown's syndrome.

Duane's Syndrome

At the beginning of the 20th century, Alexander Duane described a series of patients with the following characteristics (Fig. 11.24):

Congenital onset of the disorder
Inability to abduct the involved eye
Slight limitation of adduction of the involved eye as manifested by
> Small exotropia in the field of adduction
> Remote near point of convergence
Narrowing of the fissure in the involved eye with adduction
Retraction of the globe of the involved eye with adduction

By studying the affected patients with electromyographic techniques in which a thin needle electrode is inserted into the ocular muscles under topical anesthesia to record the muscles' electrical activity, it became apparent that Duane's syndrome is a congenital defect of innervation. The lateral rectus muscle does not fire or recruit on lateral gaze to that side. With adduction of the involved eye, the lateral and the medial rectus muscles fire or contract, causing limitation of adduction and narrowing of the fissure as the globe is pulled posterior by the simultaneous firing of both horizontal rectus muscles. However, not all patients have exactly these characteristics.

Using electromyographic techniques and clinical observations, Huber divided Duane's syndrome into three types. Type 1 was previously described. Type 2 is the reverse of type 1, with a large deficit of adduction and normal abduction (Fig. 11.25). Patients with type 3 have severely limited

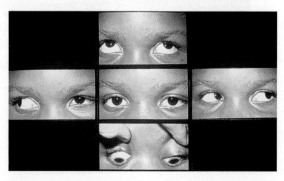

FIGURE 11.25. Duane's syndrome of the left eye, type 2. There is limited adduction, with apparently normal abduction.

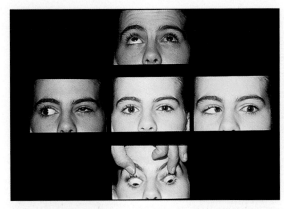

FIGURE 11.26. Duane's syndrome of the left eye, type 3. Adduction and abduction of the involved left eye are limited.

adduction and abduction (Fig. 11.26). Any type may have marked elevation or depression with adduction or attempted adduction, which is called, respectively, up-shoot and down-shoot. In some patients, these actions are caused by simultaneous firing or contraction of the superior or inferior rectus muscle along with firing of the medial rectus muscle. In other patients, the mechanism is thought to cause slippage of the inappropriately contracting lateral rectus muscle up or down on the globe.

Duane's syndrome occurs more frequently in females and in left eyes, although it may also be bilateral. Rarely is it inherited as an autosomal-dominant trait.

Patients with Duane's syndrome function quite well. They spontaneously learn to turn their necks to look to the involved side and maintain binocularity. On causal questioning, such patients deny diplopia in gaze to the involved side, but with a red lens before either eye, many admit to seeing double.

About half of the patients with Duane's syndrome of any type have their eyes aligned in straight-ahead gaze. These patients have no compensatory face turn. The other patients have their eyes aligned in some gaze other than straight ahead, and they turn their faces to maintain alignment. If

and when the face turn becomes a cosmetic and functional handicap, surgery may be performed to align the eyes in straight-ahead gaze and eliminate the face turn. Surgery should be a recession of the appropriate muscle, even though it appears to be underacting. Resection of an underacting muscle may aggravate the narrowing of the fissure and globe retraction. Some ophthalmologists have suggested transposing the vertical rectus muscles to the underacting lateral rectus muscle to treat the abduction deficit.

Treatment of the up-shoot and down-shoot patterns is difficult and therefore controversial. Some surgeons have suggested preventing the lateral rectus muscle from slipping up or down by fastening it to the globe with permanent sutures. Others have suggested splitting the insertional end of the lateral rectus muscle to create a Y shape and attaching the ends of the split muscle above and below the normal insertion point.

Möbius' Syndrome

Möbius' syndrome is a congenital defect of the cranial nerves to the muscles of the eye and face. Typically, there is paralysis of the abducens (cranial nerve VI) and facial (cranial nerve VII) nerves, usually bilaterally (Fig. 11.27). Although there is no abduction, the eyes are often straight, indicating bilateral horizontal gaze palsies. The facial palsies often are symmetric and may spare the lower part of the face. The hypoglossal nerve (cranial nerve XII) is often involved, with atrophy and furrowing of half or all of the tongue. Patients may have partial oculomotor (cranial nerve III) palsy, corneal anesthesia, abnormalities of the hands or feet, and pectoralis muscle defects. The flat, emotionless face gives the illusion of retardation, but few of these patients have below-normal intelligence. The role of the ophthalmologist is to treat amblyopia, align the eyes if esotropia is present, and to follow the patient for drying of the cornea. In most cases, elevation of the eyes on attempted lid closure prevents corneal desiccation.

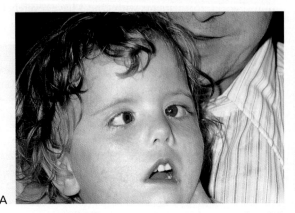
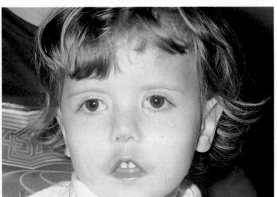

FIGURE 11.27. Möbius' syndrome. Before **(A)** and after **(B)** surgery to align eyes. Notice the bilateral facial palsies characteristic of this syndrome.

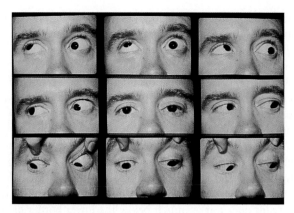

FIGURE 11.28. Double elevator palsy of the left eye. Notice the small left hypotropia and slight pseudoptosis. This patient preferred a small chin elevation.

Double Elevator Palsy

Double elevator palsy is a congenital defect, usually isolated, in which one eye can elevate (Fig. 11.28). The position of the affected eye may be level with the normal eye in straight-ahead gaze, in which case the head position is normal for viewing objects straight ahead. The affected eye may be lower than the normal eye, in which case the patient assumes a chin-up position to look at objects directly in front.

If the affected eye is lower than the normal eye in straight-ahead gaze, the lid is also lower, but this is most often a pseudoptosis. After the eye is surgically elevated, the lid assumes a more normal position in relation to the other normal lid. In a few patients, the affected eye rises normally with forced closure, indicating that the defect is supranuclear. In some patients, the elevation is restricted to passive movement, a positive forced duction, and the primary defect therefore must be an inferior rectus fibrosis.

Surgical treatment is indicated if there is a compensatory chin elevation, indicating that the affected eye is low relative to the normal eye. If there is resistance to passive elevation, the inferior rectus must be recessed. If the affected eye is about 30 prism diopters too low, the medial and lateral rectus muscles can be transposed adjacent to the superior rectus muscle (i.e., Knapp procedure). For smaller deviations, recession of the inferior rectus and resection of the superior rectus muscle can be performed.

Congenital Fibrosis Syndrome

A patient with congenital fibrosis syndrome has defects of elevation of both eyes and both lids (Fig. 11.29). Most patients present with a compensatory chin-up position. The eyes and the lids are lower than normal, but the lids are in a

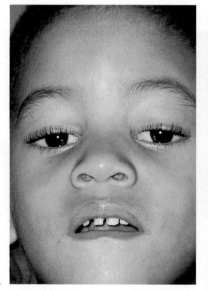

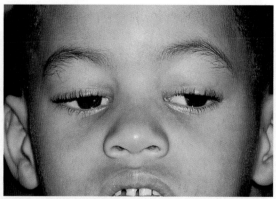

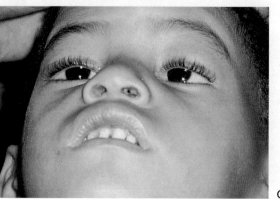

FIGURE 11.29. Congenital fibrosis syndrome. **A:** The typical chin-up position is illustrated. In some patients, the chin is elevated even more. **B:** Attempted downgaze causes a divergence of the eyes. **C:** Attempted upgaze causes some convergence.

relatively normal position on the depressed eyes. Although this can be an isolated defect in one family member, it is typically an autosomal-dominant trait. On attempted upgaze, there may be convergent movements of both eyes. On attempted downgaze, there may be divergence of the eyes, a pseudo–A pattern. Horizontal movements are usually limited. In a few patients, one of the lids may open normally with sucking or chewing, a condition called the Marcus-Gunn jaw-winking phenomenon. Under topical or general anesthesia, passive movement of the eyes is restricted in all directions. If the eyes alone are surgically elevated, the limitation of elevation of the lids becomes apparent as a ptosis.

Most patients warrant surgical treatment, consisting of very large recessions or disinsertion of the tight inferior rectus muscles. The ptosis may be repaired at the same time or later. The levator function deficiency mandates a frontalis suspension procedure on each lid. The goal is to allow the head to be in a more nearly normal position for viewing. A normal or level head position is difficult to achieve.

CONGENITAL PTOSIS

Otherwise healthy children may be born with one or both upper eyelids that are abnormally low, a condition called congenital ptosis. The history may indicate that the involved lid was swollen at birth and opened later than the normal one. By several months of age, the drooping lid becomes obvious to the parents.

Congenital ptosis is an autosomal-dominant trait, and either parent may have mild or severe ptosis of one or both eyelids. In congenital ptosis, some of the normal levator muscle is replaced by fibrous tissue, roughly in proportion to the degree of ptosis, and the upper lid does not relax normally during downgaze. As a result, there may be lid lag in downgaze, even though there is ptosis in primary gaze (Fig. 11.30). Even in severe congenital ptosis, the margin of the upper lid does not go much below the lower border of the pupil. If the upper lid is lower than that, the physician should consider a neurogenic cause. Infants with ptosis of one or both lids elevate the brows with the frontalis muscle in an attempt to raise the ptotic lid or lids even farther. Because the frontalis muscle tires easily, the lid position may be lower when the child is sick or tired. This is normal in congenital ptosis and should not be confused with myasthenia gravis.

If one or both ptotic lids cover the upper portion of the pupils, the infant or child must maintain a chin-up position to look at something straight ahead. This problem becomes apparent as soon as the infant has good head control, usu-

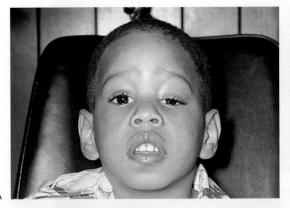
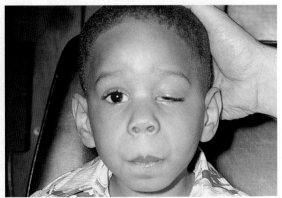
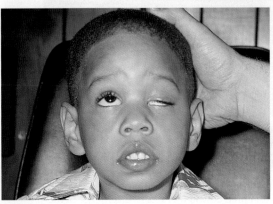

FIGURE 11.30. Congenital ptosis of the left upper lid. **A:** The chin-up position. The arched brows show that maximum frontalis muscle contraction is being used in an attempt to raise the lid. **B:** The head is level, and the left upper lid is below the pupil. **C:** Upgaze elevated the left lid very little, indicating very poor levator function.

ally by 4 or 5 months of age. However, the chin-up position indicates that each eye is seeing reasonably well and unaffected by amblyopia.

Treatment is indicated to restore the upper eyelids to a normal position. If severe ptosis mandates a compensatory chin-up position to look at something straight ahead, the surgery should be performed in the first year of life, even as early as 6 or 7 months of age. In severe ptosis, the levator function usually is so poor that a frontalis suspension procedure is required. If the ptosis is moderate and no compensatory chin-up position is used, the surgery may be delayed for several years.

CONGENITAL DACRYOCELE

Infants will frequently have a nasolacrimal duct at birth with an impatent valve of Hasner. Less commonly, a ball valve effect will occur where the canaliculus enters the lacrimal sac,

allowing fluid to enter the sac but not exit distally or proximally. The lacrimal sac enlarges, appearing as a firm, often blue, mass nasally on the lower lid (Fig. 11.31). It displaces the medial canthal tendon causing an upward slant to the lid fissure nasally. In nearly all cases, the membrane obstructing the valve of Hasner will distend, causing a cystic lesion within the nose. The majority of dacryoceles will resolve with massage of the swollen lacrimal sac within a few days. Dacryoceles that do not resolve can be probed. Probing may not be successful due to the failure of the probe to break through the wall of the associated intranasal cyst. Therefore, most authors recommend that the intranasal cyst be marsupialized at the time of surgery. Dacryoceles are at risk for infection, capable of producing dacryocystitis and preseptal cellulitis in the neonate. If infection does occur, prompt antibiotic therapy in the appropriate setting is necessary. In addition, neonates with bilateral dacryoceles are reported to be at risk for respiratory distress secondary to the intranasal cyst.

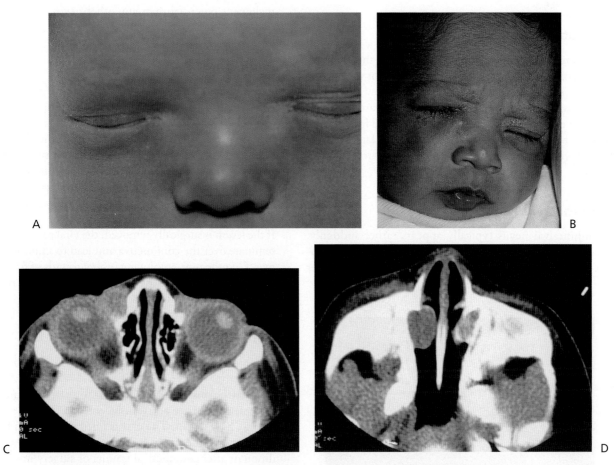

FIGURE 11.31. Congenital dacryocele. **A:** Bilateral dacryocele. The bluish swelling is most evident on the left. **B:** Right dacryocele. Note the upward slant to the lid fissure nasally in the right eye. **C:** Computed tomography (CT) of right dacryocele, demonstrating enlargement of lacrimal sac. **D:** CT scan showing associated intranasal cyst on right.

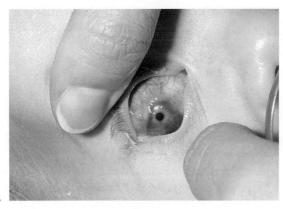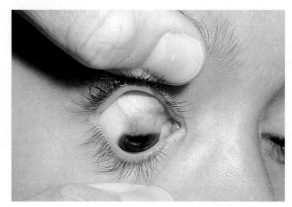

A   B

FIGURE 11.32. Choristomatous malformations of the conjunctiva.

CONJUNCTIVAL ABNORMALITIES

Some abnormalities of the conjunctiva that are common in infants and children are discussed in this section. Other abnormalities are found in the sections on the conjunctiva and cornea.

Choristomatous Malformations

Choristomas are congenital malformations of the conjunctiva or epibulbar region, usually in the superior part of the eye, that are present at birth but do not grow thereafter. These lesions typically appear raised and vascular (Fig. 11.32). Treatment is excision, largely performed for cosmetic reasons. Histologically, these lesions contain fatty and ectopic lacrimal tissue, as well as epidermal structures (Fig. 11.33).

Conjunctival Nevus

A conjunctival nevus typically appears rather suddenly, within several weeks, usually near the limbus on the temporal conjunctiva of adolescents (Fig. 11.34). Usually, it is not

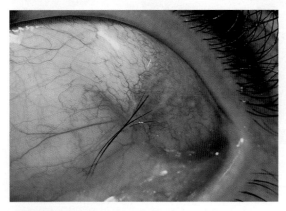

FIGURE 11.33. Dermolipoma with an associated hair.

pigmented, and it appears as a slightly raised, granular or microcytic, red mass that is several millimeters in diameter. There is typically a prominent conjunctival vessel feeding the lesion. After formation, the size of the nevus tends to remain constant. Treatment is excision if it is a cosmetic blemish or its presence causes concern. However, it has no more malignant potential than any other nevus. If incompletely excised, it may recur.

Papilloma

A papilloma of the conjunctiva presents as a raised, sometimes pedunculated lesion on the conjunctiva, lids, or caruncle (Fig. 11.35). Typically, it is fleshy and pink, but it may be paler. With the magnification of the slit lamp, the examiner can see through the translucent surface tissue to the red "dots" that represent the vascular core. Because they are of viral origin, papillomas may be multiple or affect several members of the same family. They may resolve spontaneously, and conservative treatment may be the best choice. If the lesion is surgically removed, the viral particles may disseminate over the conjunctiva and lead to multiple papillomas. Cryotherapy, employing several rounds of freezing and thawing, may destroy the papilloma and reduce the likelihood of spreading the virus.

Conjunctival Inclusion Cyst

If conjunctival tissue becomes located under the normal conjunctiva, it will grow to form a cyst (Fig. 11.36). This cyst may be only a few millimeters to several centimeters in diameter. It is raised and translucent, and the contents of the cyst are gray or tan. The cyst is filled with mucus from the goblet cells of the cyst wall. It may occur as a congenital condition or after conjunctival trauma or surgery involving the conjunctiva. If and when it becomes a cosmetic defect, it may be excised. The cyst is covered by normal conjunctiva that separates from the cyst easily. However, the cyst is very thin walled and ruptures easily. Rupture is less likely if a cry-

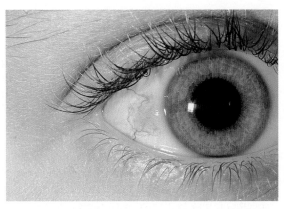 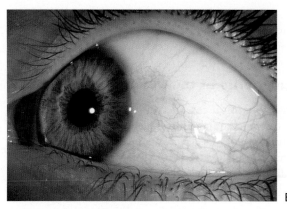

A　　　　　　　　　　　　　　　　　　　　　　　　　　B

FIGURE 11.34. The nonpigmented conjunctival nevus is typical in appearance and location.

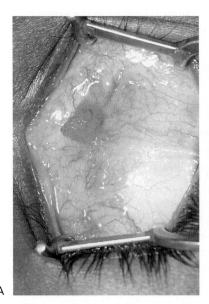 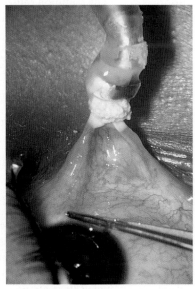

A　　　　　　　　　　　　　　　　　　　　　　　　　　B

FIGURE 11.35. Papilloma of the conjunctiva. **A:** The papilloma is in the medial conjunctiva. **B:** The papilloma is being treated with cryotherapy.

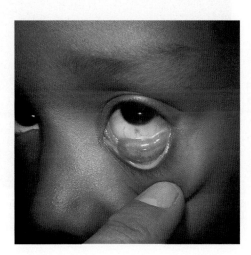

FIGURE 11.36. Conjunctival inclusion cyst.

oprobe is applied to the cyst to aid in traction and the blunt dissection after the normal overlying conjunctiva is reflected.

Conjunctivitis of the Newborn

Although gonorrheal conjunctivitis of the newborn is a vision-threatening conjunctival infection, it is rarely seen in the ophthalmologist's office. Its incubation period is so short that it usually is recognized in the newborn nursery and is diagnosed and treated by the pediatrician. However, an ophthalmologist may be called into the nursery to see the patient.

Gonorrheal conjunctivitis usually is seen within the first several days of life (Fig. 11.37A). It is characterized by marked purulent discharge and swollen lids. The purulent material may be trapped behind the swollen lids and spurt out on the examiner as the lids are forcibly opened. If an infection by *Neisseria gonorrhoeae* is suspected, appropriate smears and cultures should be taken. If the infection is caused by *N. gonorrhoeae,* gram-negative intracellular diplococci are seen.

Systemic treatment has traditionally employed penicillin, but as more penicillin-resistant strains are found, third-generation cephalosporins are being used instead. The patient should be isolated. Local treatment consists of irrigating or wiping away the purulent material.

Much more often seen by the ophthalmologist is inclusion or chlamydial conjunctivitis in the newborn (Fig. 11.37B). The disease generally manifests in children 1 to 2 weeks of age with marked swelling of the lids, especially the lower; copious mucoid discharge; marked hyperemia of the conjunctiva of the lower lid; and minimal injection of the bulbar conjunctiva. The condition has often been treated previously with topical antibiotic drops with minimal effect. The diagnosis can be confirmed by one of the commercially available rapid tests for *Chlamydia* infections. Less reliable is detection by Giemsa staining of the characteristic cytoplas-

mic inclusion bodies in the epithelial cells obtained by scraping the conjunctiva. The treatment is 2 weeks of oral erythromycin (50 mg/kg/day in four divided doses). Topical erythromycin also may be used. The treatment with oral erythromycin greatly reduces the likelihood of subsequent pneumonitis and otitis that may follow topical treatment only. The mother, father, and sexual contacts should be treated.

Newborns may also develop a nonspecific conjunctivitis, usually from infection with *Haemophilus, Staphylococcus,* or *Streptococcus* organisms. Gonorrhea should be excluded by the appropriate smear and culture. If the infection is nonspecific, it may be treated with topical antibiotics or lid hygiene alone.

CORNEAL CLOUDINESS

The common causes of corneal clouding in the neonate can be remembered with the following mnemonic:

Sclerocornea
Tears in Descemet's
Ulcer
Metabolic
Peter's anomaly
Endothelial dystrophy (CHED)
Dermoid

Infantile glaucoma can cause corneal cloudiness as well.

Sclerocornea

Opaque scleral tissue extends onto the cornea (Fig. 11.38). This usually involves the peripheral cornea but can extend centrally and in severe cases involve the entire cornea. It is almost always bilateral but asymmetric. The cornea is flattened. It is often associated with other ocular and systemic abnormalities. Most cases are sporadic, but it can be inher-

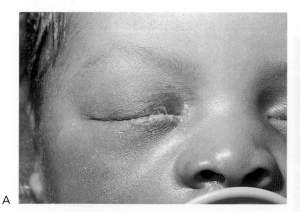 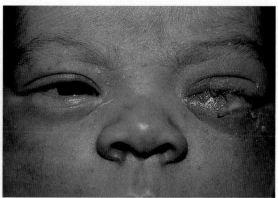

A   B

FIGURE 11.37. Neonatal conjunctivitis. **A:** Gonococcus infection of the newborn is responsible for the purulent material at the lid margins. Smears and cultures would be necessary for a certain diagnosis. **B:** Twelve-day-old with 5-day history of progressive lid swelling and discharge typical of chlamydial conjunctivitis.

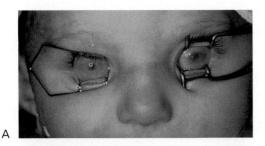

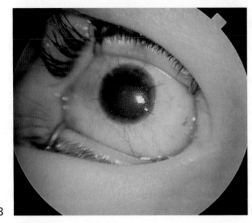

FIGURE 11.38. Four-month-old with sclerocornea. **A:** Both corneas appear opaque with an undetectable limbus. **B:** Right eye 2 weeks after penetrating keratoplasty. Pupil was pharmacologically dilated.

ited in an autosomal-dominant or -recessive form. If the central portion of the cornea is involved, keratoplasty can be performed.

Tears in Descemet's Membrane

Blunt trauma to the cornea during the birth process can result in a rupture of Descemet's membrane. Initially, the cornea will appear cloudy (Fig. 11.39). Usually, the cornea will clear after several days, revealing the Descemet's breaks. This is associated with corneal astigmatism, which can be as great as 10 diopters. The refractive error and resulting amblyopia need to be addressed to obtain a good visual outcome. In rare cases, the corneal cloudiness remains and penetrating keratoplasty is needed to obtain a clear visual axis.

The Descemet's breaks or Haab's striae from birth trauma tend to be vertical, while the Descemet's tears associated with congenital glaucoma tend to be horizontal or curvilinear.

Peter's Anomaly

Peter's anomaly involves a central corneal opacification associated with an underlying defect of Descemet's membrane and endothelium (Fig. 11.40). Iris adhesions and a cataract may be present. Over time, the corneal opacification may decrease. The peripheral cornea is typically clear. Enlarging

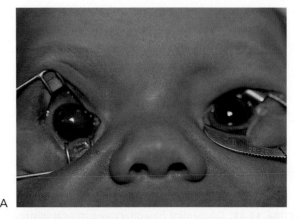

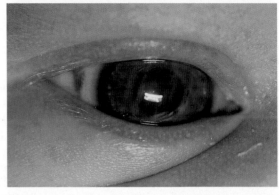

FIGURE 11.39. Descemet's tears secondary to birth trauma. **A:** Cloudy right cornea secondary to tears in Descemet's tears in a 2-day-old. The cornea cleared in a few days. **B:** Descemet's tears are oriented vertically. The same eye had a small hyphema. Blood can be seen at the edge of the Descemet's tears. The eye was left with 8 diopters of astigmatism.

the pupil pharmacologically or surgically may give the child an opportunity to see around the corneal opacification. Penetrating keratoplasty is performed when the opacification is large. There is an associated glaucoma in at least 50% of the affected eyes.

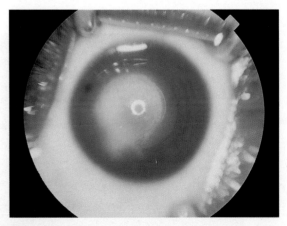

FIGURE 11.40. Peter's anomaly. Atropine was used to allow the child an opportunity to see around the central opacity. Over time, the opacification faded.

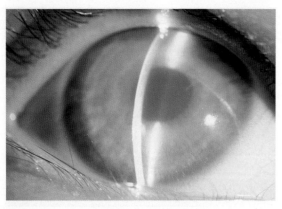

FIGURE 11.41. Congenital hereditary endothelial dystrophy. Notice the diffuse edema and the thickened cornea.

Congenital Hereditary Endothelial Dystrophy

Congenital hereditary endothelial dystrophy is an autosomal-recessive condition that is noticed at birth. Both corneas are hazy with diffuse epithelial edema (Fig. 11.41). There is no increase in the corneal diameter. Slit lamp examination reveals that the cornea is thicker than normal. The intraocular pressure is normal. These three findings differentiate this condition from congenital glaucoma. The condition remains unchanged, and vision is usually in the range of 20/50 to 20/100.

Dermoid

A corneal dermoid presents as a dense white congenital corneal opacification. The dermoid can be centrally located or involve the limbus (Fig. 11.42). It typically extends into the deeper stroma. A large dermoid can cause profound visual loss by blocking the visual axis. Peripheral dermoids can be associated with high astigmatism and amblyopia. If warranted, the dermoid can be excised by lamellar keratoplasty or shaving away the elevated portion of the lesion. Limbal

dermoids can be seen in association with other systemic abnormalities such as Goldenhar's syndrome.

CORNEAL ABNORMALITIES

Certain abnormalities of the cornea are more or less unique to children or are seen more often in children.

Congenital or Infantile Glaucoma

Corneal changes are the earliest findings in congenital glaucoma. Glaucoma that starts before age 2 years causes enlargement of the cornea and corneal edema (Fig. 11.43). The red reflex from a direct ophthalmoscope or a retinoscope is dulled by mild corneal edema. The dot-like light reflex on the cornea from a pen light is less well defined by corneal edema. Any apparent difference in the diameter of the cornea is congenital glaucoma until proven otherwise. Breaks in Descemet's membrane (i.e., Haab's striae) may be seen at the initial presentation, but their presence is not necessary for the diagnosis.

Megalocornea

Megalocornea is typically a sex-linked condition, manifested at birth by large corneas that are equally large in each eye (Fig. 11.44). There is no corneal edema, and the other signs of infantile glaucoma are not present. Vision and the refractive error are typically normal. The corneas are thinner than normal and perhaps more likely to rupture with blunt trauma. Protective glasses are a reasonable measure.

Cystinosis

Cystinosis occurs in three forms, all of which have the characteristic corneal crystals (Fig. 11.45). The infantile form is associated with growth retardation, renal failure, decreased

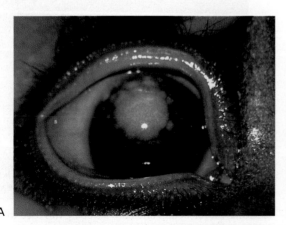
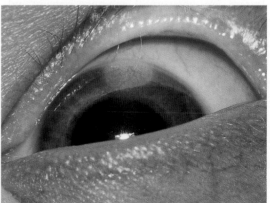

A

B

FIGURE 11.42. Corneal dermoid. **A:** Large central dermoid that was subsequently excised with 8.0 mm lamellar corneal transplant. **B:** Limbal dermoid that produced 2.25 diopters of astigmatism. Patient required treatment for anisometropic amblyopia.

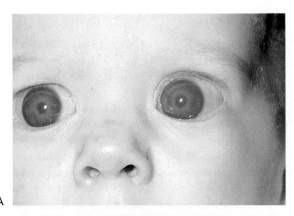

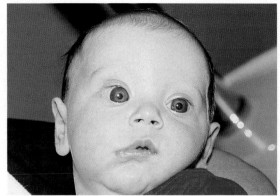

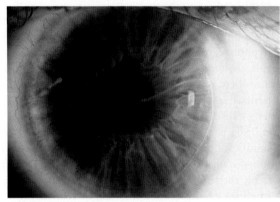

FIGURE 11.43. Congenital glaucoma. **A:** Both corneas are enlarged. The dot reflex from the flash of the camera is not sharp. **B:** The right cornea is larger than the left, probably because of glaucoma in the right eye. **C:** There is a transverse break in Desçemet's membrane crossing the pupil.

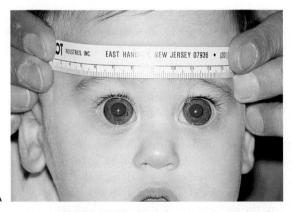

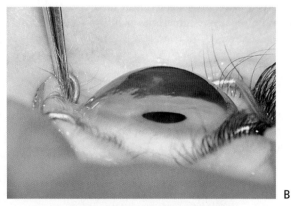

FIGURE 11.44. Megalocornea. **A:** Notice the corneal clarity as revealed by the red reflex. The ruler on the forehead allows the corneal diameter to be measured without an examination under anesthesia. **B:** The peripheral cornea is so steep that the angle can be viewed directly.

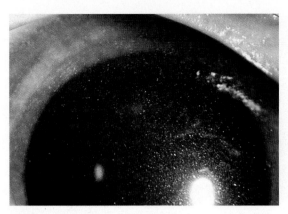

FIGURE 11.45. Cystinosis. The small crystals are easily seen with a slit lamp.

pigmentation, and early death. The adult form has no systemic manifestations. The adolescent form has only the renal complications. The crystals in the cornea are mainly in the anterior stroma.

Kayser-Fleischer Ring

Although a Kayser-Fleischer ring is not a disease, it is a corneal finding that is usually pathognomonic of Wilson's disease or hepatolenticular degeneration, an autosomal-recessive disorder of copper metabolism that affects the basal ganglia of the central nervous system, the liver, and the kidneys. Copper deposits in the periphery of Descemet's membrane impart a brown-green stain to that tissue (Fig. 11.46). The stain is usually most marked near the upper and lower limbus. Gonioscopy is sometimes helpful in determining mild or early cases.

IRIS ANOMALIES

Many pediatric patients present with congenital anomalies of the iris. Some of the most common are discussed in the following sections.

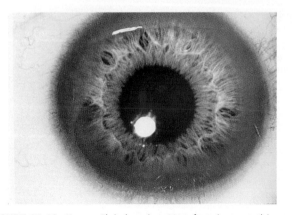

FIGURE 11.46. Kayser-Fleischer ring. Very few rings are this pronounced.

Aniridia

The name aniridia suggests that the iris is absent, but in this disorder, the iris is always present but hypoplastic, often hidden behind the sclera on direct view, and visible only by gonioscopy (Fig. 11.47). The condition is congenital, always bilateral, and often familial, transmitted in an autosomal-dominant fashion. A patient with the sporadic form of aniridia has a greatly increased chance of developing Wilms' tumor of the kidney. The risk is increased further if the patient has genitourinary anomalies or mental retardation. All patients with sporadic aniridia should have periodic ultrasound examinations of the kidney to detect such tumors early.

Patients with aniridia commonly have a nonvascularized and nonprogressive pannus of the cornea. Typically, there is hypoplasia of the fovea with no well-defined umbo. As a result, the typical vision is about 20/200, although some may have better vision, and nystagmus is common. These patients frequently have prominent deposits of the anterior lens capsule and cortical dot-like opacities. In a sense, aniridia is a progressive disease. Cataracts that are visually significant may develop, and the lens may partially dislocate. A major problem is the development of glaucoma that is difficult to treat. In about the second decade of life, the epithelium of the cornea may begin to become loose and slough away.

Coloboma

A coloboma of the iris is the external sign of a defect in the closure of the fetal fissure of the eye (Fig. 11.48). It may be unilateral or bilateral. It may be sporadic or an autosomal-dominant trait. It may be an isolated ocular defect or associated with cardiac, hearing, anal, choanal, central nervous system, and probably other defects. If it is an isolated iris defect, it is compatible with normal or near-normal vision. If there is a coloboma of the choroid (i.e., coloboma of the retina) that involves the optic nerve or macular area, vision may be greatly reduced. If the coloboma involves the ciliary body, the zonules in that area may be defective, causing a flattening or indentation of the lens equator in that area, which is erroneously called a lens coloboma. Typically, an eye with a coloboma is smaller than normal, a condition called colobomatous microphthalmos.

Persistent Pupillary Membranes

Persistent pupillary membranes are remnants of the anterior portion of the tunica vasculosa lentis, the vascular structure that surrounds the lens in utero (Fig. 11.49). One or several isolated persistent strands are common. The peripheral portion of the persistent pupillary membrane is always attached to the collarette of the iris. The central portion may attach

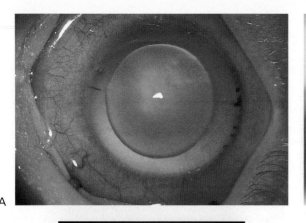

A

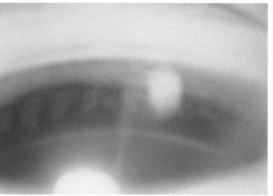

B

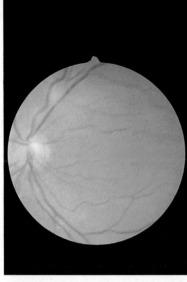

C

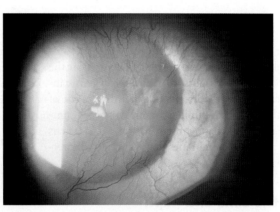

D

FIGURE 11.47. Aniridia. **A:** Typical external view of aniridia. The lens equator is visible against the red reflex. Ciliary processes are visible in the left side of the very large pupil. **B:** A gonioscopic view shows the hypoplastic iris stump with the easily visible ciliary processes. **C:** There is no foveal reflex. **D:** The dislocation of the lens is common. Against the red reflex, the roughened surface of the cornea is visible. This has stimulated some vascular pannus above and below.

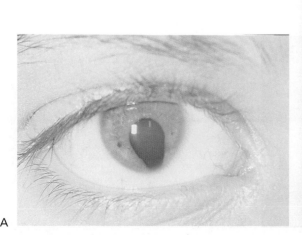

A

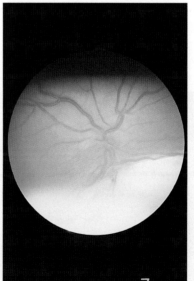

B

FIGURE 11.48. Coloboma. **A:** The right eye with the coloboma is in the typical location, down. **B:** The choroidal coloboma extends just inferior to the disc.

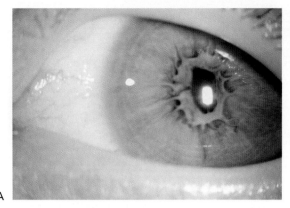

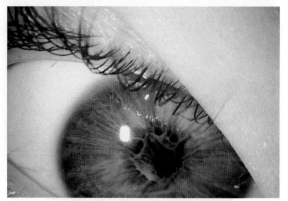

FIGURE 11.49. Persistent pupillary membranes. The membranes in these eyes are compatible with normal vision.

to the anterior lens capsule or break free from the lens attachment such that the central portion floats free in the anterior chamber. Pigment spots on the anterior lens capsule, called epicapsular stars, often mark the prior point of attachment. If the persistent pupillary membrane is circumferential, there may be no attachment to the anterior lens capsule. Rarely are these membranes dense enough to interfere with vision.

Ectopia of the Lens and Pupil

Ectopia of the lens and pupil (i.e., ectopia lentis et pupillae) is an autosomal-recessive condition in which the pupil becomes displaced in one direction, usually nasally, and the lens is displaced in the other, usually temporally (Fig. 11.50). The lenticular myopia of the dislocated lens is associated with axial myopia. A dislocation of the lens can be caused by trauma or a metabolic disorder, but it is not associated with displacement of the pupil. The affected child's vision often can be refracted as an aphake around the edge of the dislocated lens, with a good visual outcome.

Pupillary Nodules

Pupillary nodules or flocculi are an uncommon iris or pupil variant of no visual significance. These are very small cysts of the pigment epithelium at the edge of the pupil (Fig. 11.51). They may be isolated or scattered or occur around the entire pupil border. Typically, they become smaller with time. They are easily seen in the red reflex from the pupil as semicircular protrusions in the normally round reflection from the fundus. Except by the patient's history, they are indistinguishable from the pupillary cysts after prolonged use of long-acting anticholinesterase.

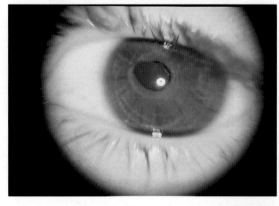

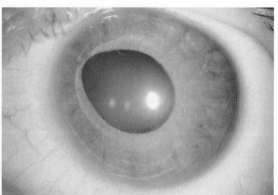

FIGURE 11.50. Ectopia lentis et pupillae. **A:** Before dilation. **B:** After dilation, the lens equator is faintly visible. There is ample space nasal to the lens for an "aphakic" refraction.

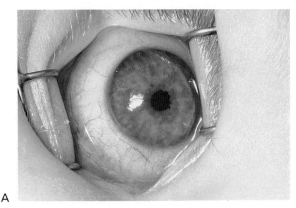
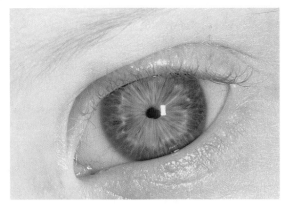

FIGURE 11.51. Pupillary nodules. **A:** The nodules are congenital and bilateral. **B:** The nodules indicate the chronic use of a long-acting anticholinesterase.

CATARACTS

Certain types of lens opacities are common in pediatric ophthalmology and unique to infants and children.

Anterior Polar Cataract

An opacity on the anterior pole of the lens is an anterior polar cataract (Fig. 11.52). It is always congenital, sometimes bilateral, and occasionally inherited in an autosomal-dominant fashion, although it is usually sporadic. There may be one or more persistent pupillary membranes attached to the front surface of the cataract. It is typically white and easily seen by the parents. The size ranges from a dot too small to measure to 1 or 2 mm in diameter. It is rarely large enough to cause a visual handicap. It often protrudes into the anterior chamber like a small cone. Normally, the lens cortex posterior to this type of cataract is clear for the first several years of life. With time, as new lens fibers grow behind the cataract, there is often visible an opacity in the cortex posterior to the cataract on the anterior pole but with a clear zone

of normal lens between. This condition could be called a reduplication cataract. Most anterior polar cataracts do not progress, but some do, especially with opacities in the cortex just posterior to the polar cataracts. Unilateral anterior polar cataracts may be associated with anisometropia with 20% to 30% of these patients developing amblyopia.

Zonular Cataracts

Most acquired cataracts in infants and children are zonular or lamellar. They begin in a zone or lamella of the cortex that is concentric to the surface of the lens. Initially, only the border or limit of the cataract is opaque. Gradually, the lens within the zone becomes less transparent (Fig. 11.53). At this stage, there may be "riders" peripheral to the opacified central zone, arcing over the periphery of the opacified zone in an anteroposterior direction. With time, the cortex peripheral to the zone becomes opacified to create a totally opacified lens.

The zonular cataract may manifest unilaterally or unequally, but it tends to be a bilateral process. They may be

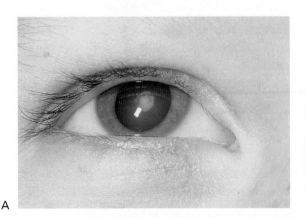
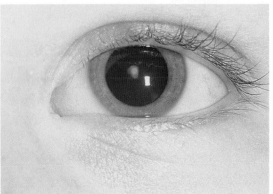

FIGURE 11.52. Anterior polar cataracts. Right eye **(A)** and left eye **(B)** of the same patient.

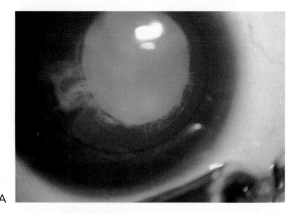
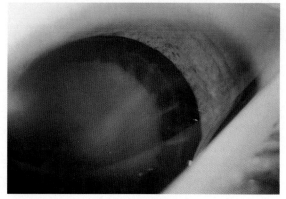

FIGURE 11.53. Zonular cataracts. **A, B:** The clear peripheral cortex is easily seen. The "riders" are visible in **B**.

sporadic or inherited in an autosomal-dominant fashion. They may start anytime during the first several years of life. A normal examination at birth in the child of a parent with zonular cataracts does not indicate that the child will not develop cataracts later. The appearance of the cataract does not suggest any specific cause. In otherwise healthy children, a search for a cause is usually fruitless.

Posterior Lenticonus

The most common type of acquired, unilateral, nontraumatic cataract in children is posterior lenticonus. Because the posterior protrusion is not a cone, some prefer to call the condition posterior lentiglobus. It may start at any age up to the midteens, although it is rarely detected at birth. It seems to start as a clear protrusion in the posterior lens capsule, usually in the central part of the lens or just nasal to the central part (Fig. 11.54). The protrusion is usually round and well circumscribed. Even though the protrusion is clear at this point, the red reflex through it is distorted, but the reflex around it is not. The next stage is an opacification in the protrusion. At this point, the vision may be reduced by only several lines, because the optics around this opacity are not distorted. The opacification then slowly moves anterior to involve the rest of the cortex. Posterior lenticonus sometimes is not recognized until surgery has removed the total cataract anterior to the posterior capsule, allowing the defect in the posterior capsule to be seen.

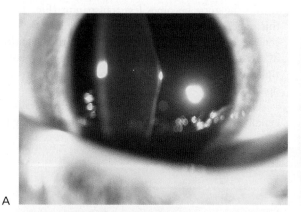
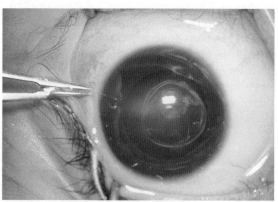

FIGURE 11.54. Posterior lenticonus. **A:** Only a small posterior protrusion is visible. **B:** There is a larger than typical, relatively clear protrusion. **C:** Characteristic opacification within the protrusion.

Many posterior protrusions do not progress. The evolutionary process just described may remain stationary for years or decades. If this condition starts within the first several years of life, amblyopia may be the major reason for the poor vision at presentation to the ophthalmologist later in childhood.

PERSISTENT HYPERPLASTIC PRIMARY VITREOUS

Persistent hyperplastic primary vitreous (PHPV) is the most common cause of a unilateral cataract in a newborn or infant. In utero, the posterior segment of the eye is filled with branches of the hyaloid artery emanating from the optic nerve. Embryologists call this blood-filled cavity the primary vitreous. In the normal process of embryogenesis, these blood vessels disappear, and the resulting space is filled by the secondary vitreous, creating the transparent and avascular vitreous cavity of the living human. If some blood vessels persist—typically, the hyaloid artery that runs from the disc to the posterior surface of the lens—the primary vitreous also persists. Associated with the hyaloid artery is glial tissue that becomes hyperplastic and grows along the posterior surface of the lens, a retrolental membrane that extends circumferentially to the ciliary processes. This membrane elongates the ciliary processes, pulling them into view in the pupil. It also acts as a diaphragm, pushing the lens and the iris forward.

An eye with PHPV usually is smaller than the normal fellow eye (Fig. 11.55). In mild PHPV, the only abnormality may be a persistent hyaloid artery, with or without a small

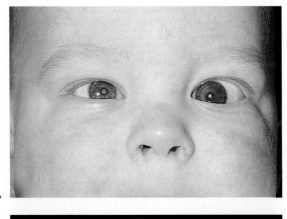
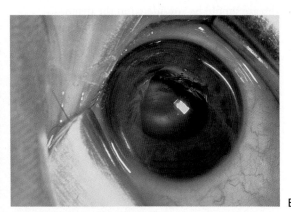
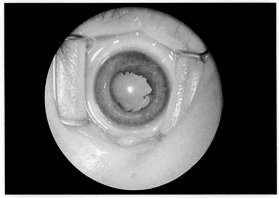
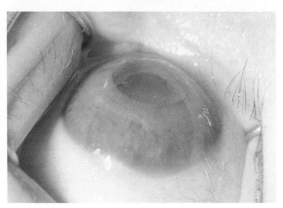
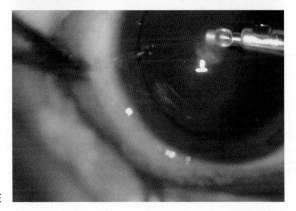

FIGURE 11.55. Persistent hyperplastic primary vitreous (PHPV). **A:** A typical presentation of esotropia, leukokoria, and microphthalmia. **B:** The plaque or membrane is on the posterior surface, and the overlying cataract is in the typical location. **C:** There is evidence of inflammation with posterior synechiae, a typical tan-colored cataract that is more dense posteriorly, and some blood vessels on the posterior lens surface. **D:** Very advanced PHPV with a flat anterior chamber. **E:** Completion of surgery for removal of a total cataract with a plaque on the posterior lens surface and the hyaloid artery posterior to the plaque.

opacity on the posterior surface of the lens. The opacity is usually just nasal to the center of the pupil. If the plaque is several millimeters in size, there may be blood vessels in it. In a more advanced stage, an opacity is detected in the posterior portion of the lens cortex. If the pupil dilates well, elongated ciliary processes may be seen. At this stage, the lens-iris plane is pushed forward, and the anterior chamber is more shallow than normal. The more advanced stage is characterized by a total cataract and a flat anterior chamber. The iris vessels may be prominent, and the pupil may be bound by posterior synechiae and may not dilate well. Vessels may be seen within the lens itself. If left untreated, secondary glaucoma usually develops, leading to a blind and painful eye.

This condition is usually unilateral. It is not inherited, and it is not associated with any systemic condition or disease. In the extremely unusual event that PHPV is bilateral, Norrie's disease should be considered in the diagnosis.

PHPV in the moderate or advanced stage is treated by removing the lens and the retrolental membrane. The visual outcome is usually poor because of the amblyopia characteristic of a unilateral cataract and the foveal hypoplasia that typically accompanies PHPV.

BIBLIOGRAPHY

Birch E, Stager D, Wright K, et al. The natural history of infantile esotropia during the first six months of life. *J AAPOS* 1998;2:325-328.

Jaafar MS, Robb RM. Congenital anterior polar cataract: a review of 63 cases. *Ophthalmology* 1984;91:249-254.

Kim T, Cohen EJ, Schnall BM. Ultrasound biomicroscopy and histopathology of sclerocornea. *Cornea* 1998;17:443-445.

Nelson LB. Harley's pediatric ophthalmology. 4th ed. Philadelphia: WB Saunders; 1998.

Paysee EA, Coats DK, Bernstein JM, et al. Management and complications of congenital dacryocele with concurrent intranasal mucocele. *J AAPOS* 2000;4:46-53.

Schnall BM, Christian CJ. Conservative treatment of congenital dacryocele. *J Pediatr Ophthalmol Strabismus* 1996;33:219-221.

Von Noordeen GK. Binocular vision and ocular motility. 5th ed. St. Louis: Mosby; 1996.

SUBJECT INDEX

References followed by *f* indicate figures; those followed by "t" denote tables